BRAIN ONCOLOGY

DEVELOPMENTS IN ONCOLOGY

Recent volumes

M.P. Hacker, E.B. Double and I. Krakoff, eds., Platinum Coordination Complexes in Cancer Chemotherapy. ISBN 0-89838-619-5
M.J. van Zwieten, The Rat as Animal Model in Breast Cancer Research: A Histopathological Study of Radiation- and Hormone-Induced Rat Mammary Tumors. ISBN 0-89838-624-1
B. Löwenberg and A. Hagenbeek, eds., Minimal Residual Disease in Acute Leukemia. ISBN 0-89838-630-6
I. van der Waal and G.B. Snow, eds., Oral Oncology. ISBN 0-89838-631-4
B.W. Hancock and A.H. Ward, eds., Immunological Aspects of Cancer. ISBN 0-89838-664-0
K.V. Honn and B.F. Sloane, Hemostatic Mechanisms and Metastasis. ISBN 0-89838-667-5
K.R. Harrap, W. Davis and A.H. Calvert, eds., Cancer Chemotherapy and Selective Drug Development. ISBN 0-89838-673-X
C.J.H. van de Velde and P.H. Sugarbaker, eds., Liver Metastasis. ISBN 0-89838-648-5
D.J. Ruiter, K. Welvaart and S. Ferrone, eds., Cutaneous Melanoma and Precursor Lesions. ISBN 0-89838-689-6
S.B. Howell, ed., Intra-arterial and Intracavitary Cancer Chemotherapy. ISBN 0-89838-691-8
D.L. Kisner and J.F. Smyth, eds., Interferon Alpha-2: Pre-Clinical and Clinical Evaluation. ISBN 0-89838-701-9
P. Furmanski, J.C. Hager and M.A. Rich, eds., RNA Tumor Viruses, Oncogenes, Human Cancer and Aids: On the Frontiers of Understanding. ISBN 0-89838-703-5
J. Talmadge, I.J. Fidler and R.K. Oldham, Screening for Biological Response Modifiers: Methods and Rationale. ISBN 0-89838-712-4
J.C. Bottino, R.W. Opfell and F.M. Muggia, eds., Liver Cancer. ISBN 0-89838-713-2
P.K. Pattengale, R.J. Lukes and C.R. Taylor, Lymphoproliferative Diseases: Pathogenesis, Diagnosis, Therapy. ISBN 0-89838-725-6
F. Cavalli, G. Bonadonna and M. Rozencweig, eds., Malignant Lymphomas and Hodgkin's Disease: Experimental and Therapeutic Advances. ISBN 0-89838-727-2
L. Baker, F. Valeriote and V. Ratanatharathorn, eds., Biology and Therapy of Acute Leukemia. ISBN 0-89838-728-0
J. Russo, ed., Immunocytochemistry in Tumor Diagnosis. ISBN 0-89838-737-X
R.L. Ceriani, ed., Monoclonal Antibodies and Breast Cancer. ISBN 0-89838-739-6
D.E. Peterson, G.E. Elias and S.T. Sonis, eds., Head and Neck Management of the Cancer Patient. ISBN 0-89838-747-7
D.M. Green, Diagnosis and Management of Malignant Solid Tumors in Infants and Children. ISBN 0-89838-750-7
K.A. Foon and A.C. Morgan, Jr., eds., Monoclonal Antibody Therapy of Human Cancer. ISBN 0-89838-754-X
J.G. McVie, W. Bakker, Sj.Sc. Wagenaar and D. Carney, eds., Clinical and Experimental Pathology of Lung Cancer. ISBN 0-89838-764-7
K.V. Honn, W.E. Powers and B.F. Sloane, eds., Mechanisms of Cancer Metastasis. ISBN 0-89838-765-5
K. Lapis, L.A. Liotta and A.S. Rabson, eds., Biochemistry and Molecular Genetics of Cancer Metastasis. ISBN 0-89838-785-X
A.J. Mastromarino, ed., Biology and Treatment of Colorectal Cancer Metastasis. ISBN 0-89838-786-8
M.A. Rich, J.C. Hager and J. Taylor-Papadimitriou, eds., Breast Cancer: Origins, Detection and Treatment. ISBN 0-89838-792-2
D.G. Poplack, L. Massimo and P. Cornaglia-Ferraris, eds., The Role of Pharmacology in Pediatric Oncology. ISBN 0-89838-795-7
A. Hagenbeek and B. Löwenberg, eds., Minimal Residual Disease in Acute Leukemia 1986. ISBN 0-89838-799-X
F.M. Muggia and M. Rozencweig, eds., Clinical Evaluations of Anti-Tumor Therapy. ISBN 0-89838-803-1
F.A. Valeriote and L. Baker, eds., Biochemical Modulation of Anticancer Agents: Experimental and Clinical Approaches. ISBN 0-89838-827-9
B.A. Stoll, ed., Pointers to Cancer Prognosis. ISBN 0-89838-841-4
K.H. Hollmann and J.M. Verley, eds., New Frontiers in Mammary Pathology 1986. ISBN 0-89838-852-X
D.J. Ruiter, G.J. Fleuren and S.O. Warnaar, eds., Application of Monoclonal Antibodies in Tumor Pathology. ISBN 0-89838-853-8
M. Chatel, F. Darcel and J. Pecker, eds., Brain Oncology. ISBN 0-89838-954-2

Brain Oncology

Biology, diagnosis and therapy

An international meeting on brain oncology, Rennes, France, September 4–5, 1986, held under the auspices of the Ministry of National Education, the University of Rennes and the Regional Hospital Rennes

edited by

M. Chatel
Department of Neurology,
University of Rennes, France

F. Darcel
Department of Neuropathology,
University of Rennes, France

J. Pecker
Department of Neurosurgery,
University of Rennes, France

With the collaboration of: Y. Adam, M. Carsin, J. Faivre, Y. Guegan, G. Guy, M. Jan, A. Javalet and J.M. Scarabin

1987 **MARTINUS NIJHOFF PUBLISHERS**
a member of the KLUWER ACADEMIC PUBLISHERS GROUP
DORDRECHT / BOSTON / LANCASTER

We wish to thank the PREUSS FOUNDATION for BRAIN TUMOR RESEARCH of SAN DIEGO, California, for their generous financial support in publishing this book.

Distributors

for the United States and Canada: Kluwer Academic Publishers, P.O. Box 358, Accord Station, Hingham, MA 02018-0358, USA
for the UK and Ireland: Kluwer Academic Publishers, MTP Press Limited, Falcon House, Queen Square, Lancaster LA1 1RN, UK
for all other countries: Kluwer Academic Publishers Group, Distribution Center, P.O. Box 322, 3300 AH Dordrecht, The Netherlands

Library of Congress Cataloging in Publication Data

International Meeting on Brain Oncology (1986 : Rennes, France)
Brain oncology.

(Developments in oncology)
Includes index.
1. Brain--Cancer--Congresses. I. Chatel, M. (Marcel)
II. Darcel, F. (Françoise) III. Pecker, J. (Jean)
IV. France. Ministère de l'éducation nationale.
V. Université de Rennes. VI. Centre hospitalier régional de Rennes. VII. Title. VIII. Series. [DNLM: 1. Brain Neoplasms--congresses. W1 DE998 / WL 358 I583 1986]
RC280.B7I544 1986 616.99'481 87-14154

ISBN-13: 978-94-010-8003-3 e-ISBN: 978-94-009-3347-7
DOI: 10.1007/978-94-009-3347-7

Copyright

PREFACE

The International Meeting on Brain Oncology in Rennes was organised in honor of Jean Pecker, to pay tribute to his contribution to the development of neurological sciences and to take stock of the current state of knowledge on brain tumors, a domain in which the role of neurosurgery has been and will continue to be primordial.

During the two-day conference, the major themes of brain oncology studies, both fundamental and clinical, were examined : oncogenesis, tumoral markers and immunology, metabolic and diagnosis imaging, prognostic factors and therapeutic strategies.

The large number and high quality of participations resulted in a genuinely synthetic view of current advances in research, of which this book presents the essentials.

We have attempted both to preserve the richness of scientific exchanges which occurred and to publish a great many oral and poster communications. The book respects the organization of conference sessions, and thus reflects the importance accorded to glial tumor studies.

This may seem disproportionate given their frequency of occurrence in proportion to total numbers of intracranial tumor processes, but their gravity and quasi-total resistance to current therapeutic methods are ample justification. Moreover, this is the domain in which hopes of progress are beginning to appear, and it is becoming possible to envisage treatment based on recently established fundamental knowledge.

Obviously these are only hopes as yet, since control of oncogene expression and immunity processes of gliomas are still not really feasible ; neither have therapies using monoclonal antibodies, the « suicidal enzymes » of polyamine metabolism or hormone receptor modulators yet given the results which experimental data seem to warrant ; nonetheless the continuation of new attempts based on ever-growing knowledge of tumor biology represents the sole available route to progress. The conference was planned as a landmark along this route ; this book is intended simply to prolong and widen its impact.

We should like to express our thanks to all those, authors, researchers and scientific personalities, who honored us by replying to our invitation, participating in the conference, presenting their work and contributing to the publication of this book.

M. CHATEL

EDITORIAL

In presenting the work of the International Meeting on Brain Oncology held in Rennes, I wonder what could be the underlying philosophy to this preface. In other words, what can we expect from it? Should the author justify the holding of the meeting and the choice of the topics; should he try to synthesize the views expressed. Should he pinpoint the importance of the achievements or on the contrary, should he point out the grey areas still existing and which could become future subjects for other studies, for other meetings ? And last but not least, should he leave aside his role as rapporteur and show his concern through his daily work on each case?

The answer to these questions becomes more difficult when researchers from different fields take part in the meeting. The table of contents might seem confusing for the reader. Undoubtedly he will find the usual chapters together with pathology, biology, medical imaging, therapy. Nonetheless it is odd to talk at the same time of such different lesions such as benign or malign gliomas, meningiomas, lymphomas.

It so happens that neuro-oncology must by its own essence, deal exhaustively with the different varieties of brain tumors. The complexity of the problems justifies this kind of encounter meeting ground for experts from different fields. The goal is not to verify the birth of a new speciality neuro-oncology; less still to give it an official stamp, but rather to show that in order to cure the brain tumors pooling of the knowledge is essential.

Presently, two main approaches can be identified:
— that of fundamental studies carried out in laboratories, anatomical, pathological, biological, immunological, genetical, physical etc. The notions of oncogenesis, resistance of the subject to the tumor, chemical sensitivity or chemical resistance and so on are related to the studies on general carcinology.
— that of studies on patients and for physicians, neurologists, neurosurgeons, neuroradiologists, the problem being the very nature of the brain which requires a very precise diagnosis concerning the localization. The search for a tissue diagnosis before any therapeutic decision is taken and the need to take into account the functional integrity of the brain.

It could be argued that there is nothing new or at least nothing revolutionary in this approach. Nevertheless it is true that the ever increasing knowledge and possibilities in different fields might lead to harmful attitudes. Laboratory searchers could be tempted by a too wide comprehension of the phenomena; on the other hand the physician is compelled to judge case by case. One of the lessons which could be drawn from the Rennes meeting is the need to set up **at the level of each hospital concerned with the treatment of brain tumors an interdisciplinary working group** interested both in the follow up of research in different fields and in the study, case by case, of the decisions concerning each patient.

The experience gained in Rennes allows us to draw some conclusions:

— the gap between the diagnostic and therapeutic methods has widened during the last twenty years: the medical imaging methods, the present wide use of stereotaxic biopsies, a better knowledge of tumoral markers, the possibilities offered by monoclonal antibodies permit us to avoid a biased pathological classification and to choose the best possible treatment taking into account the need for the functional integrity of the brain. On the contrary the range of treatments does not evolve but slowly: surgery thanks to the pre and intra-operatory explorations, less and less dangerous for a healthy brain and backed up by more efficacious reanimation techniques open new vistas but simultaneously realizes its limitations every time that the oncological problem prevails. Radiotherapy tries also to limit itself to the lesion sparing the necrosis of the healthy tissue, aiming after the relative failure of the interstitial irradiation, at the multibeam irradiation under stereotaxic conditions. New administration methods as well as the utilization of radiosensitizers attempt to reduce the pain and the length of the treatment but do not improve the results. Chemotherapy tries new drugs every day, thanks not only to a follow up of clinical results but also to in vitro trials in cell cultures and to tolerance and effectiveness tests on induced tumors in animals.

For man, the problems are heightened by the blood brain barrier; preparatory infusions of antiedematous or more and more focalised intra arterial administration could help to solve the problems. Here again there is hope that monoclonal antibodies behave as guided vehicles towards the tumor.

It is easy to verify that the therapeutical pattern of brain tumors has lately grealty advanced and therefore it will do so in the future. Tumors can no longer be divided into two groups: amenable to surgery or not.

Indeed the majority of extra-parenchymatous tumors fall almost exclusively in the realm of surgery. But a better knowledge of their induction and growth factors will give perhaps a role to some pharmacological agents such as the progesterone inhibitors. On the contrary few tumors which seemingly would have been excluded from any surgical possibility can nevertheless be removed today; for instance some MRI identified brain stem tumors.

For most of the intra parenchymatous tumors, surgery, radiotherapy, and chemotherapy are jointly utilised; not surprisingly several participants have coined the neologism of « multimodal therapies ». But one day we may well be witnesses to other choices than the three fold « surgery - radiotherapy -chemotherapy », thanks to further knowledge of the tumor induction factors and the relationship between the tumor and the host.

The lasting pessimism — unfortunately justified — of the physicians at facing therapeutical results in certain varieties of tumors, specially high grade gliomas, is nowadays tempered by the researchers: They open the door for the future: hope calms the medical and surgical team spirits and reflects itself on the quality of the management of the patient.

J. PECKER

CONTRIBUTORS

M. BAMBERG, Westdeutsches Tumor Zentrum Universitat
55 Hufelandstr. 4300 ESSEN, R.F.A.

David BATEMAN, Wessex Neurological Center, General Hospital
Shirley 777222, SOUHTAMPTON, U.K.

Julianne BEHNKE
Von Bar Strasse 8
D 3400 GOTTINGEN, R.F.A.

Mohammed BEN HASSEL, Centre Eugène Marquis, C.H.R.
Rue H. Le-Guilloux 35033 RENNES, FRANCE.

Alim Louis BENABID
Departement de Biophysique, C.H.U.
La Tronche 38700, GRENOBLE, FRANCE.

Sandra H. BIGNER
Laboratory of Neuropathology, Duke University Med. Center
B.O. Box 3156, DURHAM, North Carolina, U.S.A.

Ulrich BOGDAHN, Department of Neuroradiologie, University Wurzburg
11 Joseph Schneider Str., 8700 WURZBURG, R.F.A.

Jurgen BOHL, Abt. Neuropathologie, Institut J. Gutenberg
1 Lengenbeckstrasse, 6500 MAYENCE, R.F.A.

Robert BRADFORD Department of Neurological Surgery, Institute of Neurology
Gough Cooper Queen Square, WC1B 3BG, LONDRES, U.K.

Philippe BRET, Hopital Neurologique
B.P., Lyon Montchat, 69394 LYON CEDEX 3, FRANCE.

Giovanni BROGGI, Istituto Neurologico C. Besta
11 Via Celoria, 20133 MILANO, ITALY.

Jacques BROTCHI, Service de Neurochirurgie, Hopital Erasme
808 Rte de Lennik, B 1070 BRUXELLES, BELGIUM.

Jean-Marie BRUCHER, Unité de Neuropathologie
Université de Louvain, 52 av. Émile Mounier, B 1200 BRUXELLES, BELGIUM.

Volker BUDACH, Sreahlenklinik Westdeutsches Tumor Zentrum Universitat
55 Hufelandstr., 4300 ESSEN, R.F.A.

Roberto BUONAGUIDI, Institute of Neurosurgery, University of Pisa
57 Spedali S. Chiara, 56600 PISA, ITALIA.

Marcel CHATEL, Service de Neurologie, C.H.U.
Hôpital de Ponchaillou, 35000 RENNES, FRANCE.

Kyung CHO, Brain Tumor Research Center, University of California
94143 SAN FRANCISCO, California, U.S.A.

Hughes B. COAKHAM, Neurosurgery, Bristol Medical Center
BS16 1LE, BRISTOL, U.K.

E.V. COLAPINTO, Department of Pathology Duke, University Medal Center
P.O. Box 3156 27710 DURHAM, North Carolina, U.S.A.

Jean-Paul CONSTANS, Service de Neurochirurgie, Centre Hospitalier Sainte-Anne
1 rue Cabanis, 75674 PARIS, FRANCE.

Françoise DARCEL, Laboratoire de Neuropathologie, C.H.U.
Hôpital de Ponchaillou, 35000 RENNES, FRANCE.

John DARLING, Department of Neurological Surgery,
Institute of Neurology, Queen Square, WC 1N 3BG, LONDRES, U.K.

Stephen J. De ARMOND, Laboratory of Neuropathology
U.C.S.F. Parnassus, 94143 SAN FRANCISCO, California, U.S.A.

Jean-Michel DERLON, Service de Neurochirurgie
Centre Hospitalier Côte-de-Nacre, 14033 CAEN, FRANCE.

François DUBOIS, Service de Neurologie
Hôpital B, 59037 LILLE, FRANCE.

Vittorio Aldo FASANO, Institute of Neurosurgery
University of Turin, 15 Via Cherasco, 10126 TURINO, ITALY.

Kazuhisa FUJISAWA, Department of Neurosurgery
Fujita Gakuen Health University School of Medicine, 470 11 TOYOAKE AICHI JAPAN.

Daniel GEDOUIN, Centre Régional de Lutte contre le Cancer
Rue Henri-Le-Guilloux, 35000 RENNES, FRANCE.

Yvon GUEGAN, Service de Neurochirurgie, C.H.U.
Rue H.-Le-Guilloux, 35033 RENNES, FRANCE.

Jorge HILDEBRAND, Service de Neurologie
Hôpital Erasme, 808 Route de Lennik, 1070 BRUXELLES, BELGIUM.

Alfred HORACZEK, Klinik Neurochirurgie
18-20 Wahringer Gurtel, A 1090 VIENNE, AUSTRIA.

José IGLESIAS ROZAS, Abt fur Neurochirurgie
Rudolf Virchows-Krankenhaus, 1 Augustenburger Platz, 1000 BERLIN 65, R.F.A.

Bernard IRTHUM, Service de Neurochirurgie,
Hôpital Fontmaure, 63400 CHAMALIÈRES, FRANCE.

Roberto KNERICH, Department of Surgery, Neurosurgical section
Policlinico S. Matteo, 27100 PAVIA, ITALY.

Ivan KRIVOSIC, Laboratoire de Neuropathologie
Hôpital B LILLE, 59037 LILLE, FRANCE.

F. LABROUSSE, Laboratoire d'Anatomo-Cytologie
Hôpital Sainte-Anne, 1, rue Cabanis, 75014 PARIS, FRANCE.

Bernard LECHEVALIER, Laboratoire de Neuropathologie
Hôpital Côte-de-Nacre, 14040 CAEN, FRANCE.

Laurence LE MOYEC, Laboratoire de Biophysique
Faculté de Médecine, Av du Pr. Léon-Bernard, 35000 RENNES, FRANCE.

Édouard LEGALL, Service de Pédiatrie
C.H.U., Pontchaillou, 35033 RENNES, FRANCE.

G. LUCCARELLI, Istituto di Patologia
Universita Degli Studi, 31 Via Mangiagalli, 20133 MILANO, ITALY.

Jean-Philippe MAIRE, Service de Neurochirurgie
Hôpital St-André, 1, rue Jean-Burguet, 33075 BORDEAUX, FRANCE.

Thomas-Marc MARKWALDER, Service Neurochirurgie
Hôpital de l'Ile, 61 Seidenberggasschen, 3010 MURI/BERNE SWITZERLAND.

Sylvia MIESCHER, Laboratoire d'Oncologie
Institut Ludwig C.H.U.V., 1011 LAUSANNE, SWITZERLAND.

François MIKOL, Fondation Rotchshild
25 Rue Manin, 75019 PARIS, FRANCE.

Jacqueline MIKOL, Laboratoire d'Anatomie Pathologique
Hôpital Lariboisière, 2 Rue Ambroise-Paré, 75475 PARIS, FRANCE.

Richard MOSER, Anderson Hospital and Tumor Institute
6723 Bertner Avenue, 77030 HOUSTON, Texas, U.S.A.

Mikael MOSSKIN, Department of Neuroradiology
Karolinska Hospital, S 104 01 STOCKHOLM, SWEDEN.

Jacques-Philippe MOULINOUX, Laboratoire d'Histologie
Faculté de Médecine, 35033 RENNES, FRANCE.

H.F.V. NEWMAN Clinical Oncology Medical Research Council Centre
Hill Road, CB2 20H, CAMBRIDGE, U.K.

Maria PAMUCKA, Department of Radiotherapy
Hospital Opole, 66a Katowicka, 45060 OPOLE, POLOGNE.

Jean PECKER, Service de Neurochirurgie
C.H.U. Ponchaillou, 35033 RENNES, FRANCE.

Serge PRIER, Service de Neurologie
Hôpital Beaujon, 100 Avenue du Général-Leclerc, 92110 CLICHY, FRANCE.

Véronique QUEMENER, Laboratoire d'Histologie
Faculté de Médecine, 35033 RENNES, FRANCE.

Burckhard RAMA, Neurochirurgie Klinik der Universitat
40 Rob. Koch Str., D 3400 GOTTINGEN, R.F.A.

C. REMY, Département de Biophysique
C.H.U. La Tronche, 38700 GRENOBLE, FRANCE.

Norbert ROOSEN, Neurochirurgische Univ. Klinik
5 Moorenstrasse, 4000 DUSSELDORF 1, R.F.A.

Alain ROUGIER, Service de Neurochirurgie
C.H.U. Pellegrin Tripode, Place Améli-Raba-Léonie, 33076 BORDEAUX, FRANCE.

Lucien J. RUBINSTEIN, Laboratory of Neuropathology
University of Virginia, 22908 CHARLOTTESVILLE, Virginia, U.S.A.

Keiji SHIMIZU, Department of Neurosurgery
Osaka University Medical School, 1-1-50 Fukushima, Fukushima-ku 553 OSAKA, JAPAN.

Paolo SIMI, Department of Pediatrics
University of Pisa, 57 Via Roma, 56100 PISA, ITALY.

Umberto SIMI, Service of Istology
Spedali Santa Chiara, 57 Via Roma, 56100 PISA, ITALIA.

David J. STEWART, Ontario Cancer Treatment Center
Ottawa General Hospital, 501 Smyth Rd, KIN 8L6 OTTAWA, Ontario, CANADA.

Martienne TARDY, Unité 282 INSERM
Hôpital Henri-Mondor, 69 Avenue Gabriel-Péri, 94010 PARIS, FRANCE.

Jacques THERON, Neuroradiologie
C.H.U. Côte-de-Nacre, 14040 CAEN, FRANCE.

David G.T. THOMAS, Neurological Surgery
Institute of Neurology, Queen Square, WC 1N 3BG, LONDRES U.K.

Cornelis TIJSSEN, Department of Neurology
St. Elisabeth Hospital B.O., 90151, 5000 LC TILBURG, NETHERLANDS.

Jonathan VAFIDIS, Department of Neurosurgery
Manchester Royal Infirmary, M13 OWL, MANCHESTER, U.K.

Jan VERLOOY, Universitair Ziekenhuis Antwerpen
10 Wilrukstraat, B 2520 EDEGEM, BELGIQUE.

Louis VILLETTE, Neurochirurgie B
C.H.U., Place de Verdun, 59037 LILLE, FRANCE.

A.J. VOETS, Institute of Neurology, Catholic University
St Radboudziekenhuis, NIJMEGEN, NETHERLANDS.

Thomas WALLENFANG, Service de Neurochirurgie
Mainz University, 1 Langenbeckstrasse, 6500 MAINZ-WEISENAU, R.F.A.

Gerhardt WALTER, Institut Neuropathologie
Medizinische Hochschule, 8 Konstanty Gutschow Str., 3000 HANNOVER, R.F.A.

Wolfgang WECHSLER, Neuropathologische Inst.
5 Moorenstrasse, 4000 DUSSELDORF, R.F.A.

Roy WELLER, Neuropathology,
Southampton General Hospital, Tremona Road, SO9 4XY SOUTHAMPTON, U.K.

Bengt WESTERMARK, Department of Clinical Pathology
University Hospital, S- 751 85 UPPSALA, SWEDEN.

John WILDEN, Department of Neurosurgery
Southampton Hospital, 111222 SOUTHAMPTON, U.K.

Paolo ZAMPIERI, Divisione of Neurochirurgia
Ospedale Civile, Via Giustimiani, 35100 PADOVA, ITALY.

Patrick ZUBER, Service de Neurochirurgie
C.H.U.V., 1011 LAUSANNE, SWITZERLAND.

CONTENTS

PART I: ONCOGENESIS

PART II: NEUROPATHOLOGY

PART III: TUMORAL IMMUNOBIOLOGY AND ONCOBIOLOGY

PART IV: BIOLOGICAL AND DIAGNOSTIC IMAGING

PART V:
CLINICO-PATHOLOGICAL STUDIES

PART VI:
NEUROSURGICAL PROCEDURES AND RADIOTHERAPY TRENDS

PART VII:
CHEMOTHERAPY AND IMMUNOTHERAPY

PART I: ONCOGENESIS

Genetics of Neuroepithelial Brain Tumours

C.C. TIJSSEN

INTRODUCTION

Various etiologies, such as chemical carcinogens and oncogenic viruses, have been postulated to be important in the development of neuroepithelial brain tumours. However, their exact pathogenesis remains unknown and the influence of genetic factors is uncertain. A possible relationship between genetic factors and cerebral tumour development has been under discussion since as early as 1896 when Besold reported two sisters suffering from brain tumours (1). Koch in 1954 thought two factors at least necessary for the formation of a "glioma": 1. a local hereditary influence: neuroglial dysplasia in the region of the ventricular germinal centres with a tendency to tumour degeneration; he suggested a mutation in a pleiotropic gene to be responsible for this local disturbance. 2. a second or several factors, exogenous or endogenous, that initiate oncogenesis in these predisposed areas (2). This corresponds with the two-hit hypothesis later put forward by Knudson which supposes that cancer results from at least two events one of which could be transmitted genetically (3). In the hereditary forms of cancer, the first mutation occurs in a germinal cell and somatic mutations later occur at the same site, converting proto-oncogenes to oncogenes.

In this presentation, I will discuss the relevant data presently available concerning this subject, in order to evaluate if there is any indication for a relationship between genetic factors and the development of neuroepithelial brain tumours.

CASE REPORTS

To study this subject we are for a great part dependent on the cumulative case histories of familial occurrences that have been reported. These reports have been assembled until 1982 in a commented register (4). From then, an International Register of Familial Brain Tumours (IRFBT) has been established (5). The number of reported and registered cases are given in table 1, divided into the occurrence in twins, siblings and more generations. In the majority of reports (siblings and more generations) it concerned two affected relatives (79 reports), in 16 reports three affected relatives and four, six, seven and ten relatives were affected in 1 report. Many of these case reports, especially the older ones, are of limited value as several important data such as type of zigosity, associated physical conditions, the precise histological nature of the tumour, investigations of the family and other epidemiological factors are often not clearly indicated. Nevertheless, after analyzing these case reports, some remarks can be made:

TABLE 1

Familial occurences of neuroepithelial brain tumours (excluding neuronal tumours)

Type of Tumour	Twins	Siblings	More Generations
Astrocytic	2	11	9
Oligodendroglial	1	1	4
Ependymal and choroid plexus	1	5	3
Pineal cell	—	4	1
Glioblastoma	—	27	17
Medulloblastoma	2	9	—
Unspecified glioma	1	7	2

1. All affected twins were monozygotic and no reports about human dizygotic twins with concordant neuroepithelial brain tumours are available. The histological type of tumour and age at manifestation are strikingly similar in the majority of the separate twin pairs.

Department of Neurology, St. Elisabeth and Maria Hospitals, P.O. Box 90151, 5000 LC TILBURG, The Netherlands.

M. Chatel, F. Darcel and J. Pecker (eds.), Brain Oncology. ISBN-13: 978-94-010-8003-3

2. The majority of the case reports of neuroepithelial brain tumours deals with siblings. They often show a similarity in gender, age at onset, location and histological nature of the tumour in the separate families. Males are more affected than females and in a large number of cases the affected siblings are born consecutively. The mean age at symptom occurrence in siblings is approximately the same as in isolated cases.
3. In more generations mother-child(ren) and father-child(ren) occurrence of neuroepithelial brain tumours are approximately equal in number. The age at occurrence in children (second generation) is considerably lower than in the parent group, on average 20 years earlier. The mean age in the children group is also lower than that found in isolated cases.
4. The most frequently encountered histological types of neuro-epithelial brain tumours in familial occurrences are glioblastomas and medulloblastomas, which are classified among the poorly differentiated and embryonal tumours in the WHO classification of brain tumours, and the astrocytomas, predominantly of a higher degree of malignancy.
5. Some reports showed associated conditions in the patients or the family members indicating the presence of an hereditary disease complex such as neurofibromatosis, polyposis-colon syndrome and SBLA syndrome (see associated hereditary diseases). Other incidental associated conditions were also found such as hepatic focal nodular hyperplasia, hemophilia, congenital anomalies, presacral lipoma, head injury, alcoholism, multiple sclerosis and immunological disorders, but there was no consistency in these findings to characterize the population at high risk for familial occurrence. Cancer of the stomach was the most frequent malignancy noted among members of the reported families and there was a rather high number of deaths of unknown cause occurring at an early age among the close relatives.

In contrast with the several reports of familial occurrences of neuroepithelial brain tumours the appearance of such tumours in otherwise unrelated married people is very rare; only two reports on such conjugal cases are available concerning glioblastomas and astrocytomas in a husband and wife occurring within a two year period (6,7).

Congenital examples of neuroepithelial brain tumours also have been reported, some cases being found in still-births, so external factors could have had only a limited influence. The most common types were astrocytomas, glioblastomas, medulloblastomas and ependymal brain tumours.

ASSOCIATION WITH HEREDITARY DISEASES

Neuroepithelial brain tumours can appear more or less frequently in a number of hereditary diseases (table 2). The reported percentages of CNS tumours occurring in neurofibromatosis have a wide range varying from 4 to 45 percent, mainly due to a lack of uniform distinction between the different forms of the disease. In tuberous sclerosis, CNS tumours have been noted in to 5 percent of cases; in one report astrocytomas were diagnosed in two neonates soon after birth (10). The SBLA or Li-Fraumeni cancer syndrome is a rare familial cancer syndrome characterized by the aggregation of **S**: sarcoma, **B**: breastcancer and brain tumours, **L**: leukemia, laryngeal carcinoma and lungcancer and **A**: adrenal cortical carcinoma. Genetic analysis of the families, together with morphological findings of the tumours suggests that a dominantly inherited cancer-prone factor interacts with environmental factors. The brain tumours occurring in this syndrome (glioblastomas, medulloblastomas, astrocytomas) as well as in

TABLE 2

Hereditary diseases in which neuroepithelial brain tumours frequently occur

Autosomal dominant diseases	Type of tumour
Neurofibromatosis	astrocytoma, ependymoma, spongioblastoma, glioblastoma
Tuberous sclerosis or Bourneville's disease	astrocytoma, ependymoma, glioblastoma
SBLA or Li-Fraumeni cancer syndrome	glioblastoma, medullo-blastoma, astrocytoma
NBCC or multiple nevoid basal cell carcinoma or Gorlin syndrome	medulloblastoma
Glioma-polyposis or Turcot syndrome*	glioblastoma, medullo-blastoma
Autosomal recessive diseases	
Glioma-polyposis or Turcot syndrome*	glioblastoma, medullo-blastoma

* Mode of inheritance in discussion.

the NBCC syndrome (medulloblastomas) usually appear at an early age. Glioblastomas and medulloblastomas have also been described in association with polyposis of the colon (Turcot syndrome). Although an autosomal-dominant pattern has been established for familial polyposis coli, the mode of genetic transmission of this syndrome remains unclear (autosomal recessive or autosomal dominant with variable expression) (4).

TWIN AND FAMILY STUDIES

A number of twin studies and, controlled and uncontrolled, family studies for neuroepithelial brain tumour occurrence have been performed, which show rather divergent results. In general, studies on twin populations indicate that genetic factors are not of major importance in the etiology of these tumours. Studies of siblings and studies of relatives of "glioma" patients on the other hand have yielded conflicting results. Some investigators found no significant increased number of familial occurrences and concluded that there was no evidence for genetic factors in the etiology of these tumours. In most instances however, the number of familial occurrences was increased and more frequent than would be expected on a chance basis, especially for the group of astrocytomas, glioblastomas, medulloblastomas and unspecified gliomas (4). Also an association of central nervous system tumours, especially glioblastomas and medulloblastomas, with other malignancies such as leukemia and cancer of the bone and muscle has been found which was higher than expected (8, 9). In these studies no environmental or any other exogenous factor has been clearly demonstrated. The association with cancer of bone and muscle is of special interest as identical chromosomal abnormalities have been found in these tumour cells.

CYTOGENETIC STUDIES

Cytogenetic studies of neuroepithelial brain tumours show that a diversity of chromosomal abnormalities can be found, also related to the histological nature of the tumour. Especially high-grade tumours demonstrate extensive hetero geneity. In general, the majority of human glioma cells contains a most common number of chromosomes in the near-diploid region. The most frequent deviations in number are a gain of chromosome no. 7 and loss of chromosomes no. 10, 22 and the sex chromosomes. Abnormal (marker) chromosomes may be present in various degrees and numbers, the most prevalent structural abnormalities are double minutes and changes involving chromosome no. 9 (4, 11, 12). A major problem lies in the interpretation of these chromosomal abnormalities as to the genesis of these tumours. At present a single structural rearrangement has not been identified suggesting that it is a secundary event in the evolution of the neuroepithelial brain tumours. The specific chromosomal abnormalities observed in these tumours however may provide clues as to the genes important in glial transformation. Several investigations support the hypothesis that the mechanism by which abnormalities of chromosomes 7 ans 22 relate to glial malignancies may reside in the proto-oncogenes mapped to these chromosomes: c-erb-B to chromosome 7 and c-cis to chromosome 22 (12).

Chromosome studies on peripheral blood samples of familial occurrences of neuroepithelial brain tumours have been performed in some cases and demonstrated no abnormalities of karyotypes (13, 14, 15). Studies of the tumour cells in such cases were not available.

CONCLUSION

Summarizing the present data, no definite conclusions are permitted. There is only a strong suggestion that genetic factors play a role in the development of certain neuroepithelial brain tumours, especially the group of glioblastomas and medulloblastomas, in certain families. The characteristics of this subgroup with a familial predisposition for neuroepithelial brain tumours are not yet identified. Therefore in the future a further collection of case material is needed with careful evaluation of all associated conditions, possible environmental circumstances and extensive family investigations. Immunological and biochemical studies of these families should also be performed. For this reason, an International Register of Familial Brain Tumours (IRFBT) has been established (5). Case control studies of series of brain tumour patients with thorough relative investigations and long-term follow up also are of great importance. Another approach lies in comprehensive cytogenetic studies, including the determination of genetic markers and the modern linkage analysis techniques, of patients with brain tumours, especially the familial cases. This should be done both on blood samples and tumour cells. Furthermore investigations of the characteristics of the familial brain tumours through tissue culture techniques seem interesting.

KEY WORDS

Brain Tumours, Neuroepithelial tissue, Genetics, Familial occurrence.

REFERENCES

1. BESOLD (G.): Ueber zwei Fälle von Gehirntumor bei zwei Geschwistern. Dtsch Z Nervenheilk 8: 49-74 (1986).
2. KOCH (G.): Beitrag zur Erblichkeit der Hirngeschwülste. Acta Genet Med Gemellol 3: 170-191 (1954).
3. KNUDSON (A.G.), STRONG (L.C.), ANDERSON (D.E.): Heredity and cancer in man. Prog Med Genet 9: 113-158 (1973).
4. TIJSSEN (C.C.), HALPRIN (M.R.), ENDTZ (L.J.): Familial Brain Tumours (Martinus Nijhoff, 1982).
5. International Register of Familial Brain Tumours (IRFBT): Comprehensive Cancer Centre, Opaalstraat 5, 2332 TA Leyden, The Netherlands.
6. TUPCHONG (L.), LEVISON (D.A.), JONES (A.E.): Concomitant Conjugal Gliomas with Similar Histologic Features. Cancer 55: 864-869 (1985).
7. GRIFFIN (T.W.), SMITH (T.W.), LEVY (B.S.), RECHT (L.D.): Synchronous occurrence of glioblastoma multiforme in a husband and wife. J. Neuro-Onc 4: 75-78 (1986).
8. DRAPER (G.J.), HEAF (M.M.), KINNIER WILSON (L.M.): Occurrence of childhood cancers among sibs and estimation of familial risks. J. Med Gen 14: 81-90 (1977).
9. FARWELL (J.), FLANNERY (J.T.): Cancer in relatives of children with central-nervous-system neoplasms. N. Engl J Med 311: 749-753 (1984).
10. PAINTER (M.J.), PANG (D.), AHDAB-BARMADA (M.), BERGMAN (J.): Connatal brain tumors in patients with tuberous sclerosis. Neurosurgery 14: 570-573 (1984).
11. BIGNER (S.H.), BJVERKVIG (R.), LAERUM (O.D.): DNA content and chromosal composition of malignant human gliomas. Neuro Clin 3: 769-784 (1985).
12. SHAPIRO (J.R.): Biology of gliomas: heterogeneity, oncogenes, growth factors. Semin Oncol 13: 4-15 (1986).
13. CHADDUCK (W.N.), NETSKY (M.G.): Familial gliomas: report of four families, with chromosome studies. Neurosurgery 10: 445-449 (1982).
14. CHALLA (V.R.), GOODMAN (H.O.), DAVIS (C.H.): Familial Brain Tumors: Studies of Two Families and Review of Recent Literature. Neurosurgery 12: 18-23 (1983).
15. LEBLANC (R.), LOZANO (A.), ROBITAILLE (Y.): Familial mixed oligodendrocytic-astrocytic gliomas. Neurosurgery 18: 480-482 (1986).

Oncogenes, Growth Factors and the Pathogenesis of Human Glioma:
The 1986 Engelhardt Lecture (°)

B. WESTERMARK, M. NISTÉR, C.H. HELDIN.

Cancer is generally believed to evolve through a multihit mechanism involving several genetic lesions. Those genes, whose expression convert cells to a neoplastic phenotype, are collectively called oncogenes. In recent years, it has become evident that the oncogenes do not constitute a novel genetic material in the transformed cell but represent altered versions of normal cellular genes (proto-oncogenes). The latter can be activated to transforming oncogenes through specific genetic mechanisms, summarized in fig. 1.

Oncogenes were first identified as parts of the genome of acutely transforming retroviruses (v-onc); these viruses evolve through recombinatory events by which a mutated version of a proto-oncogene is integrated into a usually partially deleted retroviral genome (Bishop 1983). This converts the virus from a principally innocent particle to a highly oncogenic variant.

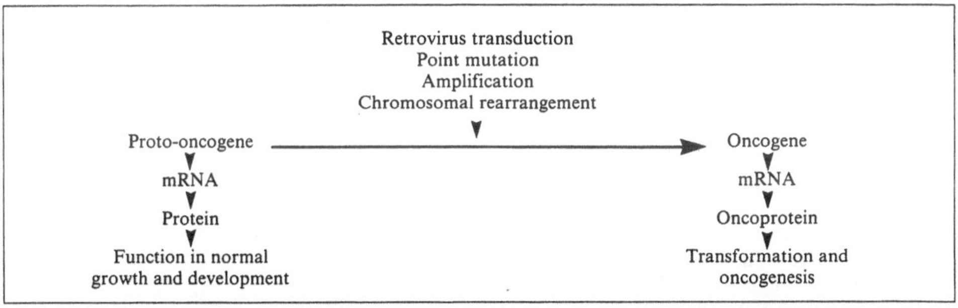

FIGURE 1. Evolution of oncogenes. Proto-oncogenes are normal cellular genes that encode proteins with key functions in normal growth and development. A proto-oncogene can be converted into a transforming oncogene by genetic mechanisms that affect its mode of expression and/or structure of the coding sequences. Adapted from Westermark et al., 1985.

There is no evidence that acutely transforming retroviruses have a role in the pathogenesis of human cancer. However, other genetic mechanisms than transduction by retroviruses, such as rearrangement, point mutation or amplification, seem to operate in the activation of oncogenes in human malignant neoplasms (fig. 1). These changes lead to the expression of qualitatively or quantitatively aberrant proteins.

Recent studies on oncogenes and their products (« oncoproteins ») in relation to growth factors and their mechanism of action have yielded a unifying concept of neoplastic transformation and normal mitogenesis. Specifically, a number of proto-oncogenes have been found to encode proteins with defined roles along growth factor-dependent pathways (Heldin and Westermark, 1984). A striking example is provided by the finding that the oncogene v-sis of simian sarcoma virus (SSV) is homologous to the cellular gene encoding the B chain of platelet-derived growth factor (Waterfield et al., 1983; Doolittle et al., 1983). Another example is v-erb B which represents a mutated form of the gene encoding the receptor for epidermal growth factor (Downward et al., 1984a). The current view is that proto-oncogene products fulfill a role in normal, regulated mitogenesis, whereas the corresponding oncoproteins subvert the growth stimulation (fig. 2). This concept is briefly reviewed

(°) Dr. Peter Engelhardt, a member of the EORTC BRAIN TUMOUR GROUP, died accidentally in 1982. Since then, an annual memorial lecture has been given during one of the Group meetings. We wish to thank the members of the Group for permitting the 1986 lecture to be presented to a wider audience.

M. Chatel, F. Darcel and J. Pecker (eds.), Brain Oncology. ISBN-13: 978-94-010-8003-3

and related to the pathogenesis of human glioma in the present communication (see also Westermark et al., 1985).

Oncogenes related to growth factors

The finding of a structural homology between the transforming gene product of SSV and the B chain of PDGF infers that SSV has acquired the B chain gene. Molecular cloning of the c-sis gene, i.e. the cellular counterpart of v-sis, proved the case (Josephs et al., 1984; Johnsson et al., 1984). This finding strongly suggests that SSV-transformation is mediated by a PDGF-like growth factor. Evidence in favor of this model has been provided by experiments showing that the transformed phenotype of SSV-transformed cells in culture is reverted by specific and nonspecific antagonists of PDGF activity. Thus, addition of PDGF antibodies, known to recognize and neutralize the v-sis gene product, normalizes the morphology of the transformed cells and retards their growth in serum-free medium (Johnsson et al., 1985). An even stronger reverting effect is obtained by the polycyclic compound suramin, which has been shown to displace receptor-bound PDGF (Williams et al., 1984). Suramin was found to revert the SSV-transformed phenotype totally, but reversibly (Betsholtz et al., 1986). Johnsson et al. recently addressed the question whether the phenotypic properties of SSV-transformed cells in all respects are identical to those of normal cells exposed to PDGF (Johnsson et al., 1986). It was found that SSV is not an immortalizing virus and that it does not induce anchorage independence beyond the effect of exogenously added PDGF. In conclusion, we would argue that the mechanism of SSV-transformation in culture is nearly clarified: SSV encodes a PDGF-like growth factor that is externalized and transforms cells by generating an autocrine mitogenic signal.

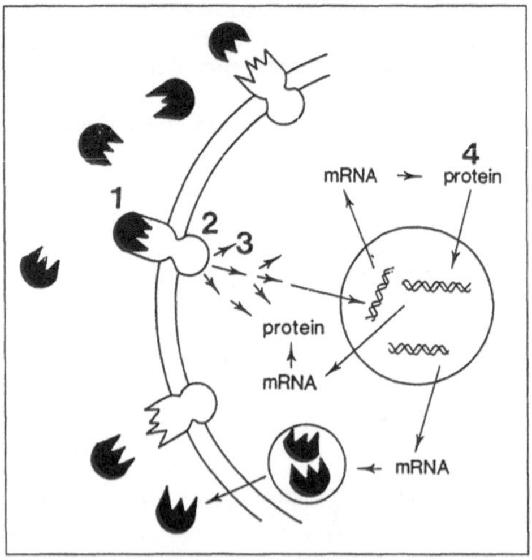

FIGURE 2. The molecular mechanism of normal mitogenesis in relation to transformation. The growth factor (1) binds to a specific cell surface receptor (2) which is thereby activated and triggers the post-receptor pathway (3). Specific genes are expressed, their products are synthesized (4) and then participate in the regulation of later events in the cell cycle. Oncogenes encode proteins that subvert the mitogenic pathway: v-sis encodes a PDGF-like growth factor that is externalized and activates the PDGF receptor (1). v-erb B encodes a truncated EGF receptor that mimicks an activated receptor. Other oncogenes, such as ras may encode proteins that subvert the postreceptor pathway (3) and fos and myc encode nuclear proteins which operate at level 4. Adapted from Westermark et al., 1985.

An important question that remains to be answered concerns the tumorigenic effect of SSV. Deinhardt and collaborators have shown that SSV induces malignant tumors when injected into newborn marmosets (Deinhardt, 1980). Intracerebral injection leads to the generation of tumors which have all the hallmarks of glioblastoma multiforme, including pleomorfism and proliferation of the vascular endothelium. Since the genotypic and phenotypic characteristics of SSV-induced tumors have not been subjected to a detailed analysis, the discussion on the relationship between transformation in culture and tumorigenicity in vivo has to be speculative. We consider it unlikely that an autocrine signal alone is sufficient to induce and maintain a fully malignant phenotype. Rather, we propose a model by which SSV elicits an autocrine response in a polyclonal population, in analogy with SSV-transformation in culture, and that this is only the first step in a multihit process that is complemented by subsequent changes in the host cell genome. These changes then lead to the emergence of a fully malignant subpopulation. As SSV-mediated tumorigenicity may constitute an interesting model for the role of autocrine growth stimulation in the genesis of malignant glioma, further studies on the molecular and biological properties of SSV-induced tumors are warranted.

The v-sis gene is an example of an oncogene that directly encodes a growth factor. Studies on certain virus-transformed cells have provided evidence that the expression of a v-onc may indirectly lead to the activation of a host cell growth factor gene. One such growth factor is transforming growth factor-α (TGF-α) which is structurally related to epidermal growth factor (Marquardt et al., 1983) and exerts its cellular activity by binding to the EGF receptor. The oncogenic potential of TGF-α has recently been demonstrated. Introduction of TGF-α coding sequences in the established Rat-1 fibroblast cell line results in autocrine growth stimulation in culture and tumorigenesis in animals (Rosenthal et al., 1986).

Oncogenes related to growth factor receptors

Growth factor receptors are usually transmembrane proteins with an external binding domain and an internal effector domain. The internal domains of a number of growth factor receptors are endowed with protein tyrosine kinase activities which become activated by growth factor binding (reviewed by Hunter and Cooper, 1985). The oncogenic potential of growth factor receptors became evident by the observation that avian erythroblastosis virus (AEV) has acquired cellular EGF receptor sequences (Downward et al., 1984a). The viral oncogene, v-erb B, encodes a truncated receptor that lacks the binding domain and part of the intracellular domain (Downward et al., 1984b). Owing to the loss of these sequences, the v-erb B product seems to mimic the activated EGF receptor and fires in a uncontrolled fashion.

Oncogenes related to factors along the postreceptor signal pathway

The finding that several growth factor receptors display tyrosine kinase activity has led to the assumption that tyrosine phosphorylated proteins have a key role in the transmission of the mitogenic signal from the activated receptor to the nucleus. Such a substrate has, however, not yet been identified. In other systems, transmembrane transduction of an extracellular signal is mediated by GTP- binding proteins (G proteins). Interestingly, the members of the ras oncogene family encode 21 kDa GTP-binding proteins which are localized to the cell membrane and which share amino acid sequences with the G proteins. The c-ras genes are converted to transforming oncogenes by point mutations, which in general lead to a decrease in the GTP-hydrolyzing activity of the $p21^{ras}$ product. It has been inferred from these observations that the ras proteins in the normal cell function as coupling factors in the transduction of the mitogenic signal and that the point mutations lead to a constitutive, i.e. growth factor independent, activity (reviewed by Heldin et al., 1987).

Oncogenes encoding nuclear proteins

A change in the expression of specific, cell cycle-related genes is an early response of growth factors. A particularly intriguing finding is that growth factors induce an increase in the mRNA levels of certain proto-oncogenes, e.g. c-fos (Greenberg and Ziff, 1984) and c-myc (Kelly et al., 1983). The involvement of the myc gene in transformation and oncogenesis has been the object of intense studies during recent years. The consensus is that deregulation of c-myc, as induced by retrovirus transduction, chromosomal translocation or gene amplification, is a contributory factor in the pathogenesis of a number of neoplasms, particularly in the lymphoid system. Most likely, both c-fos and c-myc encode proteins that have a function in rate limiting steps at the level of gene expression in normal mitogenesis. Constitutive expression of these genes therefore leads to growth factor independence and uncontrolled growth.

Oncogene expression in human glioma

Because of the remarkable oncogenic effect of SSV in the central nervous system it is relevant to ask the question whether the cellular homolog of v-sis (i.e. c-sis or the PDGF B chain gene) is involved in the pathogenesis of human glioma. This problem relates to studies performed in our laboratories over the last years, in which we have analysed a panel of human glioblastoma cell lines with regard to the production of PDGF-like growth factors and expression of corresponding genes. By a Northern blotting hybridization analysis, Nistér et al. studied the expression of the PDGF A and B chain genes in a number of glioblastoma cell lines (Nistér et al., in preparation). A remarkable observation was that glioblastoma cell lines express these genes at a remarkably high frequency and that the two genes are independently expressed. A few examples are given in fig. 3. Note for instance that the widely used U-251 MG sp cell line expresses a relatively high amount of c-sis transcripts and considerably less A chain mRNA.

Because of the variable expression of PDGF A and B chain mRNA among individual cell lines, one might ask the question whether there is also a clonal variation in expression within a single glioma cell line. A detailed study on the clonal variation of the production of a PDGF-like growth factor has been performed on sublines of the U-343 MG line, derived from a glioblastoma of a 64-year old man (Westermark et al., 1973). From this tumor, two cell lines with different phenotypic characteristics were derived. One of these, U-343 MG, does not contain the glial fibrillary acidic protein (GFAP) and produces an abundance of fibronectin, which becomes deposited in a pericellular matrix (Westermark et al., 1982). The other subline, designated U-343 MGa, has the inverse phenotype, i.e. produces no fibronectin and is homogeneously GFAP positive. It was initially observed that a clonal derivative (Cl 2) of the U-343 MGa subline produces relatively large amounts of PDGF-like growth factor activity (Nister et al. 1984). A similar analysis of a large number of clonal derivatives of the U-343 MGa line, obtained from low as well as from high passage cultures, has demonstrated a considerable clonal variation in growth factor production and PDGF A and B chain mRNA expression (Nister et al., 1986, 1987). A significant finding was that high passage cultures yielded growth factor producing clones at a considerably higher frequency than low passage cultures, indicating that the production of a PDGF like growth factor may confer a selective growth advantage. Analysis of the U-343 MG line, has shown only low levels od PDGF A chain expression and no consistent growth factor production. However, since only the parental cell line has been investigated, the existence of subclones with high expression of the PDGF and/or B chain gene cannot be excluded even in this line.

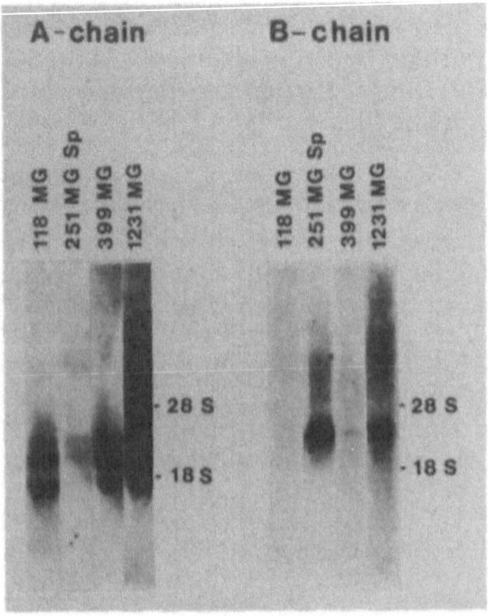

FIGURE 3. Northern blot hybridization analysis of PDGF A and B chain (c-sis) mRNA in human glioma cell lines. RNA was extracted from the cell lines using the Lice/urea method. Poly $(A)^+$ RNA was selected on oligo (dT) cellulose, electrophoresed in agarose gels and blotted onto nitrocellulose filters by standard techniques. The blots were probed with ^{32}P-labeled nick-translated cDNA probes.

Analysis of ^{125}I-PDGF binding and expression of PDGF receptor mRNA has provided evidence for the biosynthesis and expression of PDGF receptors in a number of glioma cell lines that concomitantly produce a PDGF-like growth factor. Although there is thus circumstantial evidence for an autocrine PDGF receptor activation in such cell lines, direct evidence for such a mechanism is lacking; thus no inhibitory activity of PDGF antibodies has been recorded. This may mean that an autocrine PDGF receptor mechanism is not implicated in the pathogenesis of human glioma. An alternative interpretation is that an autocrine growth stimulation is an early event in a multihit process that ultimately leads to the emergence of a fully malignant population and that the progressional changes during this development lead to a state of absolute growth factor independence, including endogenously synthesized factors. Hopefully, studies on the involvement of PDGF in experimentally induced gliomas will shed light on this problem. One should also regard the possibility that the expression of PDGF A and B chain genes in glioma cells may reflect an activity of the progenitor cell which simply persists in the malignant cell. Critical analyses of PDGF expression in normal brain at various stages of development are thus warranted.

Karyotypical analyses of human glioma have revealed a high frequency of tumors containing double minute chromosomes (Bigner et al., 1984). Such elements are known to harbor amplified

genes (Schimke, 1984). In experimental systems, gene amplification and formation of double minutes may be induced by applying a selective pressure on cell cultures, the classical example being an amplification of the dehydrofolate reductase gene in cells exposed to increasing concentrations of methotrexate (Schimke, 1984). In several instances have double minutes in human tumor cells been associated with an amplification of an oncogene, such as N-ras in neuroblastoma (Schwab et al., 1983). By applying Southern blot analysis using human c-erb B cDNA probes, Libermann et al. (1985) could demonstrate a high frequency of EGF receptor gene amplification in a material of primary human glioblastoma tissue. It is therefore likely that the double minute chromosomes in glioblastoma often harbor amplified EGF receptor gene sequences, although this has not yet been formally proven by in situ hybridization. How might an amplified EGF receptor in glioma cells confer a selective growth advantage? Firstly, the EGF receptor may be structurally changed and be constitutively active, i.e. « fire » without ligand binding and thus be functionally similar to the v-erb B product. The occurrence of new restriction fragments in the erb B gene in glioma may be indicative of a rearrangement in some instances (Libermann et al., 1985). Whether these changes give rise to a product with altered functional properties, however, is at present only a matter of speculation. Secondly, EGF (or TGF-α) may be present at low concentration in glioma. Cells with an overexpressed receptor will then at a given time contain a larger number of occupied (i.e. activated) receptors than a cell with a normal receptor number. Thirdly, glioma cells may produce their own ligand. This notion has recently been supported by the finding that a number of human glioma cell lines express TGF-α mRNA (Nistér et al., in preparation). Lastly, as even an unstimulated EGF receptor kinase may have a low, constitutive activity, this may in a cell with an amplified receptor reach the threshold level at which stimulation of growth occurs.
Evidence for an amplified c-myc gene in human glioblastoma was recently obtained by Trent et al. (1986). By selecting a tumor that contained double minute chromosomes for a Southern blot analysis using a number of oncogene probes, these investigators found a manyfold amplification of c-myc whereas other genes probed, including c-erb B, were present at normal copy numbers.

Growth factors as effectors in tumor growth

A malignant tumor, such as the glioma, not only consists of neoplastic cells but also contains normal, reactive cells that form a supportive stroma. An essential component of the stroma is the endothelial cells that invade the tumor and form a microvascular network in the tumor tissue. Folkman has pointed out that neovascularization is an absolute requirement for the progressive growth of a tumor and suggested that tumor-derived angiogenesis factors are effectors in this process (Folkman, 1986). Interestingly, a number of human glioma cell lines have recently been shown to produce acidic fibroblast growth factor and express corresponding mRNA (Libermann et al., 1987). As this factor is a potent endothelial cell growth factor, it may in the intact tumor be an important mediator of neovascularization. The surrounding reactive gliosis and the reactive glia cells found within the glioma tissue may be taken as other examples of normal cells that respond to growth factors produced by the tumor cells. Fig. 4 summarizes our current view on the role of locally produced growth factors in tumor growth. We would like to suggest that tumor cells may produce growth factors that function in an autocrine fashion, provided that the tumor cell concomitantly synthesises the corresponding receptor. Growth factors, produced both by tumor cells and normal stroma cells may function as paracrine stimulators. The coordinated growth of the

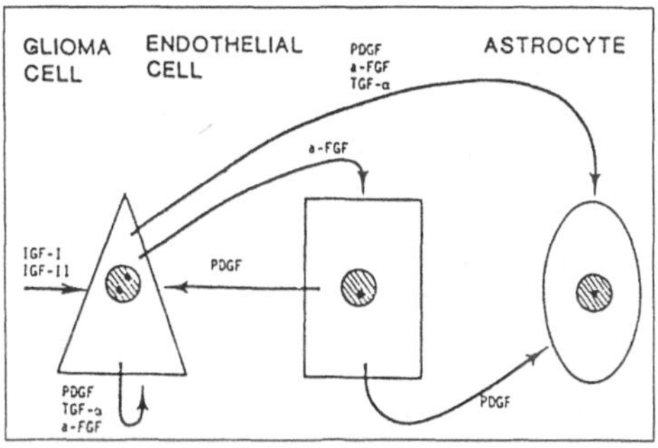

FIGURE 4. Cell-derived growth factors form a regulatory network in the growing glioma. The glioma cell may carry receptors for insulin-like growth factors (IGF-I and IGF-II) (Gammeltoft et al., 1987), PDGF, TGF-α and EGF (see text for references). Tumor cell-derived factors may stimulate the glioma cell by an autocrine loop and also stimulate infiltrating stroma cells by paracrine mechanisms. In conjunction with growth factors produced by the normal cells, these growth factors form a network by which a coordinated growth of all cellular compartments of the tumor is maintained. Adapted from Westermark et al., 1985.

whole tumor mass, including its normal constituents, is then the result of the concerted action of these factors.

Final remarks

The few reports on oncogenes in human glioma reviewed above form only the beginning of a new research anvenue, which will undoubtly lead to a better understanding of the molecular biology of glioma. As traditional investigators in brain tumor research become more aware of modern molecular genetics and its potentials, and as molecular geneticists become aware of glioma as a challenging tumor, we can foresee an interesting and fruitful future. It may also be anticipated that an insight into the molecular mechanisms involved in tumor growth may lead to the development of improved therapeutic modalites, that are more specific in their action than those that are available to-day.

ACKNOWLEDGMENTS

B. Westermark is supported by grants from the Swedish Cancer Society.

KEY WORDS

Oncogenes, Growth factors, Glioma.

REFERENCES

1. BETSHOLTZ (C.), JOHNSSON (A.), HELDIN (C.H.) and WESTERMARK (B.): Efficient reversion of simian sarcoma virus-transformation and inhibition of growth factor induced mitogenesis by suramin. Proc. Natl. Acad. Sci. USA **83**: 6440-6444 (1986).
2. BIGNER (S.H.), MARK (J.), MAHALEY (S.) and BIGNER (D.D.): Patterns of the early, gross chromosomal changes in human glioma. Hereditas 101: 103-113 (1984).
3. BISHOP (J.M.): Cellular oncogenes and retroviruses. Ann. Rev. Biochem. **52**: 301-354 (1983).
4. DEINHARDT (F.): The biology of primate retroviruses. *In* Viral Oncology, G. Klein. ed. Raven Press New York, pp. 359-398 (1980).
5. DOOLITTLE (R.F.), HUNKAPILLER (M.W.), HOOD (L.E.), DEVARE (S.G.), ROBBINS (K.C.), AARONSON (S.A.) and ANTONIADES (H.N.): Simian sarcoma virus onc gene, v-sis, is derived from the gene (or genes) encoding a platelet-derived growth factor. Science **221**: 275-277 (1983).
6. DOWNWARD (J.), YARDEN (Y.), MAYES (E.), SCRACE (G.), TOTTY (N.), STOCKWELL (P.), ULLRICH (A.), SCHLESSINGER (J.) and WATERFIELD (M.D.): Close similarity of epidermal growth factor receptor and v-erb B protein sequences. Nature **307**: 521-527 (1984a).
7. DOWNWARD (J.), PARKER (P.) and WATERFIELD (M.D.): Autophosphorylation sites on the epidermal growth factor receptor. Nature **311**: 483-485 (1984b).
8. FOLKMAN (J.): How is blood vessel growth regulated in normal and neoplastic tissue? Clowes memorial award lecture. Cancer Res. **46**: 467-473 (1986).
9. GREENBERG (M.E.) and ZIFF (E.B.): Stimulation of 3T3 cells induces transcription of the c-fos gene. Nature **312**: 433-438 (1984).
10. HELDIN (C.H.) and WESTERMARK (B.): Growth factors: mechanism of action and relation to oncogenes. Cell **37**: 9-20 (1984).
11. HELDIN (C.H.), BETSHOLTZ (C.), CLAESSON-WELSH (L.) and WESTERMARK (B.): Subversion of growth regulatory pathways in malignant transformation. Biochem. Biophys. Acta. in press.
12. HUNTER (T.) and COOPER (J.A.): Protein-tyrosine kinases. Annu. Rev. Biochem. **54**: 897-930 (1985).
13. JOHNSSON (A.), HELDIN (C.H.) WASTESON (A.), WESTERMARK (B.), DEUEL (T.F.), HUANG (J.S.) SEEBURG (P.H.) GRAY (E.), ULLRICH (A.), SCRACE (G.), STROOBANT (P.) and WATERFIELD (M.D.): The c-sis gene encodes a precursor of the B chain of platelet-derived growth factor. EMBO J. **3**: 921-928 (1984).
14. JOHNSSON (A.), BETSHOLTZ (C.), HELDIN (C.H.) and WESTERMARK (B.): Antibodies against platelet-derived growth factor inhibit acute transformation by simian sarcoma virus. Nature **317**: 438-440 (1985).
15. JOHNSSON (A.), BETSHOLTZ (C.), HELDIN (C.H.) and WESTERMARK (B.): The phenotypic characteristics of simian sarcoma virus-transformed human fibroblasts suggest that the v-sis gene product acts solely as a PDGF receptor agonist in cell transformation. EMBO J. **5**: 1535-1541 (1986).
16. JOSEPHS (S.F.), GUO (C.), RATNER (L.) and WONG-STAAL (F.): Human protooncogene nucleotide sequences corresponding to the transforming region of simian sarcoma virus. Science **223**: 487-490 (1984).
17. KELLY (K.), COCHRAN (B.H.), STILES (C.D.) and LEDER (P.): Cell-specific regulation of the c-myc gene by lymphocyte mitogens and platelet-derived growth factor. Cell **35**: 603-610 (1983).

18. LIBERMANN (T.A.), NUSBAUM (H.R.), RAZON (N.), KRIS (R.), LAX (I.), SOREQ (H.), WHITTLE (N.), WATERFIELD (M.D.), ULLRICH (A.) and SCHLESSINGER (J.): Amplification, enhanced expression and possible rearrangement of EGF receptor gene in primary human brain tumors of glial origin. Nature **313**: 144-147 (1985).

19. LIBERMANN (T.A.), FIESEL (R.), JAYE (M.), LYALL (R.M.), WESTERMARK (B.), DROHAN (W.), SCHMIDT (A.), MACIAG (T.) and SCHLESSINGER (J.): An angiogenetic factor is expressed in human glioma cells. Submitted (1987).

20. MARQUARDT (H.), HUNKAPILLER (M.W.), HOOD (L.E.), TWARDZIK (D.R.), DE LARCO (J.E.), STEPHENSON (J.R.) and TODARO (G.J.): Transforming growth factors produced by retrovirus-transformed rodent fibroblasts and human melanoma cells: amino acid sequence homology with epidermal growth factor. Proc. Natl. Acad. Sci. USA **80**: 4684-4688 (1983).

21. NISTÉR (M.), HELDIN (C.H.), WASTESON (A). and WESTERMARK (B.): A glioma-derived analog to platelet-derived growth factor: demonstration of receptor-competing activity and immunological crossreactivity. Proc. Natl. Acad. Sci. USA **81**: 926-930 (1984).

22. NISTÉR (M.), HELDIN (C.H.) and WESTERMARK (B.): Clonal variation in the production of a platelet-derived growth factor-like protein and expression of corresponding receptors in a human malignant glioma. Cancer Res. **46**: 332-340 (1986).

23. NISTÉR (M.), WEDELL (B.), BETSHOLTZ (C.), HELDIN (C.H.), WESTERMARK (B.) and MARK (J.): Evidence for progressional changes in the human malignant glioma line U-343 MGa: Analysis of karyotype and expression of the genes encoding the subunit chains of platelet-derived growth factor. Cancer Res. in press (1987).

24. ROSENTHAL (A.), LINDQUIST (P.B.), BRINGMAN (T.S.), GOEDDEL (D.V.) and DERYNCK (R.): Expression in rat fibroblasts of a human transforming growth factor-α cDNA results in transformation. Cell **46**: 301-309 (1986).

25. SCHIMKE (R.T.): Gene amplification in cultured animal cells. Cell **37**: 705-713 (1984).

26. SCHWAB (M.), ALITALO (K.), KLEMPNAUER (K.H.), VARMUS (H.E.), BISHOP (J.M.), GILBERT (F.), GOLDSTEIN (M.) and TRENT (J.): Amplified DNA with limited homology to myc cellular sequences is shared by human neuroblastoma cell lines and a neuroblastoma tumor. Nature **305**: 345-348 (1983).

27. SHERR (C.J.), RETTENMIER (C.W.), SACCA (R.), ROUSSEL (M.F.), LOOK (A.T.) and STANLEY (E.R.): The c-fms proto-oncogene product is related to the receptor for the mononuclear phagocyte growth factor, CSF-1. Cell **41**: 665-676 (1985).

28. TRENT (J.), MELTZER (P.), ROSENBLUM (M.), HARSH (G.), KINZLER (K.), MASHAL (R.), FEINBERG (A.) and VOGELSTEIN (B.): Evidence for rearrangement, amplification, and expression of c-myc in a human glioblastoma. Proc. Natl. Acad. Sci. USA **83**: 470-473 (1986).

29. WATERFIELD (M.D.), SCRACE (G.T.), WHITTLE (N.), STROOBANT (P.), JOHNSSON (A.), WASTESON (A.), WESTERMARK (B.), HELDIN (C.H.), HUANG (J.S.) and DEUEL (T.F.): Platelet-derived growth factor is structurally related to the putative transforming protein $p28^{sis}$ of simian sarcoma virus. Nature **304**: 35-39 (1983).

30. WESTERMARK (B.), PONTEN (J.) and HUGOSSON (R.): Determinants for the estabhishment for permanent tissue culture lines from human gliomas. Acta Path. Microbiol. Scand. section A. **81**: 791-805 (1973).

31. WESTERMARK (B.), NISTÉR (M.) and HELDIN (C.H.): Growth factors and oncogenes in human malignant glioma. Neurologic clinics 3: 785-799 (1985).

32. WESTERMARK (B.), MAGNUSSON (A.) and HELDIN (C.H.): Effect of epidermal growth factor on membrane motility and cell locomotion in cultures of human clonal glioma cells. J. Neurosci. Res. **8**: 491-507 (1982).

33. WILLIAMS (L.T.), TREMBLE (P.M.), LAVIN (M.F.) and SUNDAY (M.E.): Platelet-derived growth factor receptors form a high affinity state in membrane preparations. J. Biol. Chem. **259**: 5287-5294 (1984).

Amplification and Expression of Viral Sequences and Oncogenes in Human Brain Tumors

A.L. BENABID, C. CHAUVIN, A.M. FOOTE (°),
M. SUH, M. DANIK (°°), M. LAINE, M. CHAFFANET (°),
C. MERCIER (°°) and N. ROST (°).

INTRODUCTION

Although the cause of cancers is still unknown, experimental data of the last ten years have led to the theory that the abnormal growth pattern typical of cancer is related to changes in the genome of cells (11, 16, 18). The changes can be due to mutations in the gene sequence either spontaneously occurring or due to oncogenic agents (X-rays, chemicals or viruses) (9-14). The altered genes have been demonstrated to be responsible for the induction of malignant transformation in cell cultures or in animals. Oncogenic sequences have been found in the genomic material of cell lines derived from tumors or in solid tumors (11, 16). The purpose of this study was to investigate by hybridization methods the presence of such transforming genes in the genome of brain tumors, either as introduced by viruses (Herpes simplex virus, Simian Virus 40, Adenovirus type 2) or as analog to oncogenes of retroviruses.

MATERIAL AND METHOD

Human brain tumors

A bank of 90 human brain tumors have been constituted following neurosurgical excisions. During the neurosurgical procedure, the tumor tissue which was removed was immediately placed in sterile containers, frozen in liquid nitrogen and stored at -80 °C until processing. Clinical and pathological records were collected for each tumor sample, allowing future correlation with the molecular biological data.

DNA extraction from brain tumor tissues

High molecular weight DNA was prepared from brain tumor samples following a procedure which allowed simultaneous isolation of DNAs and RNAs: tissue samples were homogeneized in RSB-NP40 buffer (Tris 10 mM pH 7.4, NaCl 10 mM, MgCl2 1.5 mM, Nonidet-P40 0,5 %). Nuclei were released in the solution and pelleted by centrifugation for further isolation of DNA, and the supernatants containing RNA were saved. Nuclei were then broken in TEN buffer (Tris 10 mM, EDTA 1 mM, NaCl 100 mM, pH 8) and DNA was deproteinized by 2 or 3 phenol extractions and one chloroform extraction. The DNA was digested with RNases (20 μg/ml RNase A, 100 U/ml RNase T1) for 2 hours and dialysed against Tris 10 mM, EDTA 1 mM pH 8 (T.E.). The DNA was then concentrated by ethanol precipitation and dissolved in sterile water or T.E. The extracted DNAs were checked to control that they were not degraded. This was done by agarose gel electrophoresis, which demonstrated that the samples were made of high molecular weight DNAs and by Southern blot hybridization which demonstrated the presence of the human beta-globine gene (data not shown).

RNA extraction

From the supernatant obtained during the initial part of the DNA extraction procedure, the RNAs (total and messenger) were obtained according to the following procedure: the supernatant, adjusted to 10 mM EDTA in the aqueous phase was precipitated by ethanol, dried, dissolved in water and stored at -70 °C.

(°) LMCEC, Department of Biophysics, Grenoble University Medical School, 38700 La Tronche, France, (°°) Institut du Cancer et Departement de Neurochiruigie, Hôpital Notre-Dame, 1560 East Sherbrooke, Montréal, Québec, H2L4M1, Canada.

M. Chatel, F. Darcel and J. Pecker (eds.), Brain Oncology. ISBN-13: 978-94-010-8003-3

Hybridization probes

Viral and oncogenic DNA probes were used in this study. Herpes Simplex Virus type 1 and 2 (HSV-1 and -2) DNAs were purified at the Montreal Cancer Institute (19), Simian Virus 40 (SV 40) and Adenovirus type 2 (Ad 2) DNAs were a gift from Dr. E. Frost (Montreal Cancer Institute). 10 viral Oncogene probes (Ha- and Ki-ras, mos, myc, myb, N-myc, abl, erb-A, fes, sis) were purchased from ONCOR, USA.

Nick translation of the DNA probes

DNA probes were labeled according to Rigby et al. (1977) (15) using a nick translation kit (Amersham) and alpha -32P-dCTP 400 Ci/mmol to specific activities of 10^9 cpm/μg DNA. Unincorporated nuleotides were removed by gel filtration through a Sephadex G-50 column. The labeled probes were further purified by ethanol precipitation and controlled by agarose gel electrophoresis.

Blotting

A) Southern blots

After complete digestion with the restriction enzymes EcoR1, HindIII or BamH1 (Boehringer), the DNA fragments were separated in 0.7 % or 1.4 % agarose gels (1.5 V/cm overnight). Following exposure to 0.25 M HCl for 30 minutes, they were denatured in NaOH 0.3 M/NaCl 0.6 M (1 hour, 20 °C) and then neutralised in TRIS 1 M/NaCl 0.6 M. Transfer to nitrocellulose filters was made in 10xSSC according to Southern (1975) (17).

B) Northern blots

The RNAs denatured at 65 °C for 15 min in MOPS buffer 50 % formamide 6 % formaldehyde, were separated on denaturing 1 % agarose gels and transfered to nitrocellulose filters in 20 XSSC (12).

C) Dot blots

Parallel to the blotting of gels, DNAs and RNAs were also examined using direct application of the nucleic acids on nitrocellulose filters with a Biorad dot-blot apparatus.

Hybridization

Prehybridization was performed overnight at 42 °C in 50 % formamide, 5 x SSC, 5 x Denhardt, 50 mM Na phosphate pH 6.5, 1 % glycine, 200 μg/ml denatured Calf thymus DNA. DNA hybridization was carried out for 62 hours in 50 % formamide, 5 x SSC, 5 x Denhardt, 20 mM Na phosphate pH 6.5, 10 % Na Dextran sulfate 500, 100 μg/ml denatured Calf thymus DNA plus the hybridization probe. The hybridization were performed with 2×10^6 cpm/cm^2 of filter. The filters, were rinced, dried, and autoradiographed for periods of few hours to 30 days against XAR5 Kodak films. The intensity of the hybridization was estimated versus controls by densitometry.

RESULTS

Hybridization with HSV, SV40 and Ad2

28 human brain tumors (20 gliomas, 6 metastases, 1 gliosarcoma and 1 medulloblastoma), 4 chemically induced tumors of the nervous system of rats, 3 normal rat brains and 3 cell lines (C6 rat glioma, C4II human cervix cancer and NIH3T3 mouse fibroblasts) were investigated by Southern blot hybridization. None of these materials showed the presence of the three viral probes in their genomes. Positive controls with the human beta-globine gene demonstrated that the DNAs were not degraded (Data not shown).

DNA-DNA hybridization of oncogenes

39 human brain tumors (29 gliomas — 4 grade 2, 11 grade 3, 14 grade 4 —, 8 metastases, 1 medulloblastoma and 1 meningioma) were investigated by dot-blot hybridization (and for most of them by parallel Southern blot) with the 10 oncogenes available for this study. The intensity of the hybridization was measured by densitometry, relative to the normal human brain taken as a control. The results are displayed in Table 1.

TABLE 1

Frequency (%) of amplification of oncogenes in gliomas and in metastases

Oncogenes	Gliomas		Metastases	
Ki-ras	0	(0/28)	100	(6/6)
mos	5.5	(1/18)	83.3	(5/6)
myc	54.5	(12/22)	16.7	(1/6)
myb	65.4	(17/26)	0	(0/6)
erbA	60.7	(17/28)	16.7	(1/6)
abl	38.5	(10/26)	0	(0/5)
N-myc	34.6	(9/26)	0	(0/7)
sis	62.5	(15/24)	66.6	(4/6)
Ha-ras	34.8	(8/23)	42.8	(3/7)
fes	27.3	(6/22)	16.7	(1/6)

The numbers between brackets represent the number of tumors in which the oncogenes were amplified out of the number of tumors tested by DNA-DNA hybridization.

DNA-RNA hybridization of oncogenes

10 human brain tumors (6 gliomas — 2 grade 2, 2 grade 3, 2 grade 4 —, 2 meningiomas, 1 acoustic neurinoma, 1 medulloblastoma), 1 normal human brain and 3 normal rat brains were investigated by dot blot hybridization with 2 oncogenes, Ha-ras and Ki-ras. The results (Table 2) show no increased hybridization in brain tumors as compared to the normal human brain values. In contrast, the normal rat brains yield a much stronger signal than the normal human brain.

TABLE 2

Expression of HA-ras and Ki-ras in human brain tumors as compared to normal human and rat tissues (RNA-DNA Dot blot).

Sample		Ha-ras	Ki-ras
Glioma grade 2	n° 3	+	+
	n° 46	+	+
Glioma grade 3	n° 49	+	+
	n° 5	+	+
Glioma grade 4	n° 20	+	+
	n° 38	+	+
Medulloblastoma	n° 12	+	+
Meningioma	n° 31	+	+
	n° 33	+	+
Neurinoma	n° 50	+	+
Normal human brain		+	+
Normal rat brain	n° 8	+++	+++
	n° 9	+++	+++
	n° 10	+++	+++

9 human brain tumors (5 gliomas — 1 grade 2, 1 grade 3, 3 grade 4 —, 4 metastases), 1 human bladder carcinoma cell line EJ and 1 normal human brain were investigated by Northern blot analysis with the oncogene v-myc. The preliminary results are shown in Table 3.

TABLE 3

Expression of v-myc in gliomas and metastases (Northern hybridization)

Sample			v-myc
Glioma	grade 2	n° 3	++++
Glioma	grade 4	n° 40	++
Metastases		n° 5	++
		n° 23	+++
		n° 28	+++
		n° 41	+++++
Normal human brain			+

The densitometric intensity of the hybridization is expressed as compared to the normal human brain.

DISCUSSION

Involvement of HSV, SV40 and Ad2 viruses in human brain tumors

This study suggests that the viruses HSV, SV40 and Ad2 are not implicated in human brain tumors. These results are in agrement with others (2,8) but contrast with the reports of those (5, 7, 10,13) who detected viral genomic sequences in tissue removed from subjects exhibiting different brain diseases (mental illness, multiple sclerosis, brain tumors) or in various tissues (1, 3, 4). These positive results have been criticized by Jones and Hyman (1983) (8) on the basis of methodological conditions of stringency which could have been responsible for these false positive results. The three viruses may have no responsability in neuroconcogenesis. However, one must keep in mind that the viral genome may be highly dispersed among the host genome and therefore not detectable during the latent phase of the infection. It may be also possible that viruses are oncogenic by a "hit-and-run" mechanism (6).

Amplification of oncogenes in human brain tumors

The results of DNA-DNA hybridization displayed in Table 1 show that the level of amplification of the oncogenes varies depending on the type of tumor and also from one oncogene to another. From these preliminary results, it is possible to distinguish a pattern of amplification of the oncogenes studied with tumor type. A first group of oncogenes (Ki-ras and mos) is almost always amplified in the metastases and almost never in the gliomas. A second group (myc, myb, erb-A, abl, N-myc) is preferentially amplified in the gliomas and never in the metastases. The third group (sis, fes, Ha-ras) is amplified in about 20 % to 60 % of both types of tumors.

Expression of oncogenes in human brain tumors

The results of DNA-RNA hybridization displayed in Tables 2 and 3 show that Ha-ras and Ki-ras are not overexpressed in the gliomas. As it appeared from DNA-DNA hybridization experiments that Ki-ras was also not amplified in gliomas, the involvement of the Ki-ras encoded protein in the determinism of the human brain tumors does not appear either on gene amplification or on an increased transcriptional activity. It remains possible that the Ki-ras product may be activated during post-translationnal steps. For instance, it might be only a point mutation, as demonstrated in the bladder carcinoma EJ, which could be responsible for the abnormal cellular phenotype although the amount of DNA, RNA and protein would stay normal. The Northern analysis shows that v-myc, which was not amplified in metastases, is overexpressed in this same type of brain tumor. This would suggest that, if v-myc is involved in the mechanism of induction of these tumors, it is at the level of RNA expression or stability that abnormal cell proliferation is triggered. These preliminary results must be verified before stating any definitive conclusion.

CONCLUSION

From this preliminary study of the presence, amplification and expression of certain viral genomic sequences and oncogenes, it appears that :

— Genomic components of HSV, SV40 and Ad2 are not detectable in human brain tumors of various types, including gliomas and metastases.

— Oncogenes are differentially amplified in gliomas and metastases and can be separated into three groups on this basis. The present data are too preliminary for allowing any correlation between the type of glioma and the pattern of amplification-expression of the oncogenes.

— Ki-ras, which is neither amplified nor overexpressed in gliomas, is either not involved in the process of malignant transformation of these tumors or is involved at the level of its translationnal protein product which could be deleterious due to a structural mutation.

SUMMARY

39 human brain tumors (29 gliomas: 4 grade 2, 11 grade 3, 14 grade 4. 8 metastases. 1 medulloblastoma and 1 meningioma), were sampled in sterile conditions during neurosurgical procedures and were used as a tumor bank material, stored at -80 °C. The purpose of the present work was to study in the genomes of these brain tumors the presence of genomic sequences which could be responsible for cancer induction. The first approach was to detect in the tumor genomic material DNA sequences belonging to viruses like Herpes Virus Simplex, Simian virus 40 and Adenovirus type 2. This was done by Southern blot hybridization of high molecular weight DNA of brain tumors with viral DNA probes nick-translated with 32P-labeled nucleotides. 28 human brain tumors (20 gliomas, 6 metastases, 1 gliosarcoma and 1 medulloblastoma), 4 chemically induced tumors of the nervous system in rats, 3 normal rat brains and 3 cell lines (C6 rat glioma, C4II human cervix cancer and NIH3T3 mouse fibroblasts) were investigated. None of these materials showed the presence of the 3 viral probes in their genomes. Positive controls with the human globine gene demonstrated that the tumor DNAs were not degraded.

The second approach was to look for the presence, amplification and expression of 10 oncogenes (Ha-and Ki-ras, mos, myc, myb, N-myc, abl, erb-A, fes, sis), using Southern, Northern and Dot Blots methods, in 28 gliomas and 8 metastases. As compared to the level of these oncogenes in the genoma of normal human brain, an amplification of Ki-ras and mos was observed in metastases, while myc, myb, erbA, abl and N-myc were amplified in gliomas. The other oncogenes (Ha-ras, sis and fes) had complex patterns of amplification in both types of tumors. Preliminary results (21 tumors tested) of Northern blots and RNA-DNA dot blots bring additionnal informations about the overexpression of Ha-ras, Ki-ras and myc in these human brain tumors.

KEY-WORDS

Brain tumors, Oncogenes, Herpes Simplex Virus, Simian Virus 40, Adenovirus type 2.

AKNOWLEDGEMENTS

Histological and pathological examinations of the human tumors were done by Pr. C. MOURIQUAND and Dr. B. PASQUIER. This work was supported by grants from FRANCE-QUEBEC Research Program, ESPOIR, FCLCC, LCC, the Scientific Council of the Grenoble University Medical School and by a post-doctoral fellowship from EMBO to Dr. A.M. FOOTE.

REFERENCES

1. ALONI (Y.), WINOCOUR (E.), SACHS (L.), TORTEN (J.): Hybridization between SV40 DNA and cellular DNA's. J. Mol. Biol., 44, 333-345 (1969).
2. AULAKH (G.S.), ALBRECHT (P.), TOURTELOTTE (W.W.): Search for cytomegalovirus and Herpes Simplex virus genetic information in multiple sclerosis. Neurology, 10, 530-532 (1980).
3. BARINGER (J.R.), SWOVELAND (P.): Recovery of HSV from human trigeminal ganglions. N. Engl. J. Med., 288, 648-650 (1973).
4. CONRAD (S.E.), BOTCHAN (M.R.): Isolation and characterization of human DNA fragments with nucleotide sequence homologies with the simian virus 40 regulatory region. Mol. Cell. Biol., 2, 949-965 (1982).
5. FRASER (N.W.), LAWRENCE (W.C.), WROBLEWSKA (A.), GILDEN (D.H.), KOPROWSKI (H.): Herpes simplex type 1 DNA in human brain tissue. Proc. Natl. Acad. Sci. USA, 78, 6461-6465 (1981).
6. GALLOWAY (D.A.), Mc DOUGALL (J.K.): The oncogenic potential of herpes simplex virus: evidence for a "hit-and-run" mechanism. Nature, 302, 21-24 (1983).
7. IBELGAUFTS (H.): DNA viruses and brain tumors. Trends in Neuro Sci., 5, 16-19 (1982).
8. JONES (T.R.) and HYMAN (R.W.): Specious hybridization between Herpes Simplex virus DNA and human cellular DNA. Virology, 131, 555-560 (1983).
9. KLEIN (G.): Advances in viral oncology: cell derived oncogene (Raven, New York) (1981).
10. KRIEG (P.), AMTMANN (E.), JONAS (D.), FISCHER (H.), ZANG (K.), SAUER (G.): Episomal simian virus 40 genomes in human brain tumors. Proc. Natl. Acad. Sci. USA, 78, 6446-6450 (1981).
11. KRONTIRIS (T.G.), COOPER (M.): Transforming activity of human tumor DNA's. Proc. Natl. Acad. Sci. USA, 78, 1181-1184 (1981).
12. MANIATIS (T.): Molecular cloning, Cold Spring Harbor Laboratory (1982).
13. MEINKE (W.), GOLDSTEIN (D.) and SMITH (R.): SV40 related DNA sequences in a human brain tumor. Neurology, 29, 1590-1594 (1979).
14. PORTOLANI (M.), BARBANTI-BRODANO (G.) and LA PLACA (M.): Malignant transformation of hamster kidney cells by BK virus. J. Virol., 15, 420-422 (1975).
15. RIGBY (P.W.), DIECKMANN (M.), RHODES (C.), BERG (P.): Labelling deoxyribonucleic acid to high specific activity in vitro by Nick translation with DNA polymerase I. J. Mol. Biol., 113, 237-251 (1977).
16. SLAMON (D.J.), de KERNION (J.B.), VERMA (I.M.), CLINE (M.J.): Expression of cellular oncogenes in human malignancies. Science, 224, 256-262 (1984).
17. SOUTHERN (E.M.): Detection of specific sequences among DNA fragments separated by gel electrophoresis. J. Mol. Biol., 98, 503-517 (1975).
18. STEHELIN (D.), VARMUS (H.E.), BISHOP (J.M.), VOGT (P.K.): DNA related to the transforming gene(s) of avian sarcoma virus is present in normal avian DNA. Nature, 260, 170-173 (1976).
19. SUH (M.), CHAUVIN (C.), FILION (M.), SHORE (G.), FROST (E.): Localization of the coding region for a 35 000 Dalton polypeptide on the genome of Herpes Simplex virus type 2. J. Gen. Virol., 64, 2079-2085 (1983).

Chromosomal Studies in Malignant Gliomas

S.H. BIGNER (°).

INTRODUCTION

Karyotypic evaluation of lymphomas, leukemias and solid tumors has demonstrated that specific chromosomal abnormalities characterize many of these processes (1). There are now several examples of tumor types in which the chromosomes involved in specific translocations have pointed the way to genes which are important in the evolution of these neoplasms. For example, the 9; 22 translocation of chronic granulocytic leukemia places c-abl in proximity to a breakpoint cluster region on 22q. (2). The protein coded by the rearranged sequence resembles the product of the transforming viral sequence, v-abl. (2). Similary, the 8; 14, 2; 8, and 8;22 translocations of Burkitt's lymphoma move the c-myc gene to location near the genes which code for the light and heavy immunoglobulin chains (3).

In 1971, Mark published the first large series of karyotypes of malignant human gliomas (MG). He established that the majority of these tumors had stemlines in the near-diploid region, that multiple sidelines were often present, and that double minute chromosomes (DMs) were often present in them. But since the studies were performed before chromosomal banding techniques were available, it was not possible to determine which individual chromosomes were involved in numerical or structural deviations. G-banded studies of established cultured cell lines derived from MG were carried out in the 1970's and common patterns of chromosomal deviations were described (5, 7). The karyotypes of these lines were so complex, however, that the primary abnormalities that had been present in the original tumors could not be distinguished from later evolutionary changes that had occured *in vitro.*

In 1981 we began to karyotype MG biopsies using g-banding in direct preparations and short-term cultures. We have, to date, presented karyotypic data on 54 MG (8, 10). The purpose of the present communication is to summarize these findings and to demonstrate how karyotypic abnormalities relate to amplification of the epidermal growth factor receptor (EGFR) gene in MG.

Chromosomal Analyses

We have karyotyped a total of 54 MGs using direct preparations and short term culture to determine their patterns of chromosomal deviations (8, 10). In 4 tumors, mitoses were too few and chromosomes were too poorly banded for complete evaluation. The remaining 50 cases could be divided into 3 groups. Group I tumors [(8 glioblastomas (GBM) and 4 anaplastic astrocytomas (AA)] had either normal stemlines or only lacked one sex chromosome. Group II tumors (6 GBM) had near-triploid or near-tetraploid stemlines. Four Group II tumors lacked 2 copies of chromosome No. 22. Group III tumors [1 mixed glioma, 25 GBM, 1 AA, 3 gliosarcomas, and 2 giant cell glioblastomas] had near-diploid stemlines. 26 of 32 Group III tumors had gains of normal or abnormal chromosome No. 7 and 19, had losses of chromosome No. 10. The most common structural abnormalities were the presence of DMs, and rearrangements involving 9p. DMs characterized 4 Group II and 17 Group III tumors, and 3 of the 4 tumors which were not completely characterized. Thirteen Group III tumors had deletions or translocations of chromosome 9 with breakpoints within the short arm or at the centromere. In three of these tumors, both copies of chromosome 9 were abnormal. Other chromosomes commonly involved in structural abnormalities were Nos. 1, 6, and 11.

(°) *Department of Pathology Duke University Medical Center Durham, North Carolina 27710, USA.*

M. Chatel, F. Darcel and J. Pecker (eds.), Brain Oncology. ISBN-13: 978-94-010-8003-3

Gene Amplification

Almost 50% of MG's have been shown to contain amplified genes, the most frequent of which is the EGFR gene (11, 12). The usual chromosomal manifestations of gene amplification are DMs, homogeneously staining regions (HSR) and structurally abnormal chromosomes with abnormal banding regions (ABR) (13). DMs are seen in approximately one half of MG biopsies, suggesting that these structures may be a chromosomal manifestation of gene amplification in MG. The EGFR gene is normally located on human chromosome No. 7 (14). The presence of polysomy 7 in a large proportion of MG raises the possibility that it may play a role in amplification and/or expression of the EGFR gene.

In a series of 64 MG's studied with Southern blot analysis and probes against EGFR, N-**myc**, c-**myc** and **gli**, Wong et al. demonstrated amplification of the EGFR in 25 cases, 2 examples of N-**myc** amplification, 1 case of **gli** amplification, and no examples of amplified c-**myc** (12). Since karyotypes were available on original biopsies from 32 of these tumors, we compared the distribution of gene amplification to the presence of DMs on one hand and polysomy 7 on the other to determine which of these chromosomal abnormalities was responsible for the amplified gene (15).

Sixteen of these 32 MG's contained amplified (more than 8 gene copies per cell) genes as determined by Southern blot analysis. The amplified gene was EGFR in 15 cases and n-myc in one case. Twelve of the 15 (80%) evaluable tumors with amplification contained DMs, while only 4 of the 16 (25%) MG's without amplification contained these structures. Polysomy 7, in contrast, characterized 7/12 (58%) evaluable MG with EGFR amplification and 9 of 17 (53%) evaluable MG without amplification of the gene, supporting the concept the EGFR amplification and polysomy 7 are unrelated in MG.

DISCUSSION

The most frequent chromosomal abnormalities of MG are gains of chromosome 7, losses of chromosome 10, structural abnormalities of chromosome 9 and the presence of DMs (10). We have shown that DMs are usually associated with gene amplification (15); the gene which is most commonly amplified codes for the EGFR. Polysomy 7, however, is not related to amplification of this gene. Although an association between polysomy 7 and EGFR expression has been suggested for cultured glioma lines (16, 17), such a relationship for MG biopsies remains to be demonstrated and the molecular mechanism for such an association has not been determined. The possibility remains that the molecular basis for the high incidence of polysomy 7 in MG may involve a gene other than the EGFR.

Although DMs have been identified in the majority of MG with EGFR amplification, 3 tumors did not contain these structures. It is possible that DMs were missed due to sampling or were simply too small to be detected in these tumors. Alternatively, EGFR amplification may be due to a structural abnormality of the p arm of chromosome 7 which was identified in one case. Further studies, including *in situ* hybridization will be necessary to resolve this question.

The molecular explanation for the specific chromosomal abnormalities seen in MG are only beginning to be elucidated. As those studies progress, genetic mechanisms controlling the proliferation and differentiation of MG will be defined and perhaps will lead to new approaches for stopping the growth of these tumors.

SUMMARY

The most frequent chromosomal abnormalities of malignant human gliomas (MG) are gains of chromosome No. 7, losses of chromosome No. 10, structural abnormalities of chromosome No. 9 and the presence of double minute chromosomes (DMs). Almost 50% of MG's contain gene amplification; the gene which is usually amplified codes for the epidermal growth factor receptor (EGFR). We have shown that gene amplification is associated with DMs in the majority of tumors, but that structural abnormalities of 7p may be responsible for EGFR amplification in a small proportion of these tumors. Polysomy 7, however, is probably unrelated to amplification of this gene.

KEY WORDS

Chromosomes, Karyotypes, Gliomas, Brain tumors.

ACKNOWLEDGEMENTS

Supported in part by PO1 NS0023 from the National Institute of Neurological and Communicative Diseases and Stroke and RO1 CA43722 from the National Cancer Institute.

REFERENCES

1. YUNIS (J.J.): The Chromosomal Basis of Human Neoplasia. Science **221**: 227-235 (1983).

2. BEN-NERIAH (Y.), DALEY (G.Q.), MES-MASSON (A.M.), WITTE (O.N.), BALTIMORE (D.): The Chronic Myelogenous Leukemia-Specific P210 Protein is the Product of the bcr/abl Hybrid Gene. Science **233**: 212-214 (1986).

3. CROCE (C.M.), TSUJMOTO (Y.), ERIKSON (J.), NOWELL (P.): Chromosome Translocation and B Cell Neoplasia. Lab Invest **51**: 258-267 (1984).

4. MARK (J.): Chromosomal Characteristics of Neurogenic Tumours in Adults. Hereditas **68**: 61-100 (1971).

5. MARK (J.), PONTÉN (J.) and WESTERMARK (B.): G-band Analyses of an Established Cell Line of Human Malignant Glioma. Humangenetik **22**: 323-326 (1974).

6. MARK (J.), PONTÉN (J.) and WESTERMARK (B.): Cytogenetical Studies with G-band Technique of Established Cell Lines of Human Malignant Gliomas. Hereditas **78**: 304-308 (1974).

7. MARK (J.), WESTERMARK (B.), PONTÉN (J.) and HUGOSON (R.): Banding Patterns in Human Glioma Cell Lines. Hereditas **87**: 243-260 (1977).

8. BIGNER (S.H.), MARK (J.), MAHALEY (M.S.) and BIGNER (D.D.): Patterns of the Early, Gross Chromosomal Changes in Malignant Human Gliomas. Hereditas **101**: 103-113 (1984).

9. BIGNER (S.H.), MARK (J.), BULLARD (D.E.), MAHALEY (M.S.), Jr., and BIGNER (D.D.): Chromosomal Evolution in Malignant Human Gliomas Starts With Specific and Usually Numerical Deviations. Cancer Genet Cytogenet **22**: 121-135 (1986).

10. BIGNER (S.H.), MARK (J.), MAHALEY (M.S.), Jr., BULLARD (D.E.), MULHBAIR (L.J.) and BIGNER (D.D.): Specific Chromosomal Abnormalities Characterize Malignant Human Gliomas. Submitted (1986).

11. LIBERMANN (T.A.), NUSBAUM (H.R.), RAZON (W.), KRIS (R.), LAX (I.), SOREQ (H.), WHITTLE (N.), WATERFIELD (M.D.), ULLRICH (A.) and SCHLESSINGER (J.): Amplification Enhanced Expression, and Possible Rearrangement of the EGF Receptor Gene in Primary Human Brain Tumours of Glial Origin. Nature **313**: 144-147 (1985).

12. WONG (A.J.), BIGNER (S.H.), BIGNER (D.D.), KENZLER (K.W.), HAMILTON (S.R.) and VOGELSTEIN (B.): Increased Expression of the EGF Receptor Gene in Malignant Gliomas is Invariably Associated With Gene Amplification. Submitted (1986).

13. COWEL (J.K.): Double Minutes and Homogeneously Staining Regions: Gene Amplification in Mammalian Cells, Am Rev. Genet **16**: 21-59 (1982).

14. YANG-FENG (T.L.), SCHECHTER (A.L.), WEINBERG (R.A.) and FRANKE (U.): Oncogene from rat neuro/glioblastomas (human gene symbol **NGL** is located on the proximal long arm of human chromosome 17 and **EGFR** is confirmed at 7p13-q11.2. Cytogenet Cell Genet **40**: 784 (1985).

15. BIGNER (S.H.), WONG (A.J.), MARK (J.), MUHLBAIER (L.H.), KINZLER (K.W.), VOGELSTEIN (B.) and BIGNER (D.D.): Relationship Between Gene Amplification and Chromosomal Deviations in Malignant Human Gliomas. Submitted (1986).

16. BELL (C.), HARSH (I.V.), (G.), ROSENBLUM (M.), MELTZER (P.) and TRENT (J.): Numeric and Structural Alterations of Chromosome 7 in Human Brain Tumors: Correlation With Expression of Epidermal Growth Factor Receptor (EGFR). Proc. AACR **27**: 37 (1986).

17. HENN (W.), BLIN (N.), ZANG (K.D.): Polysomy of Chromosome 7 is Correlated With Overexpression of the erbB Oncogene in Human Glioblastoma Cell Lines. Human Genet **74**: 104-106 (1986).

Karyotype Patterns in Forty Human Meningiomas

P. SIMI (°), E. TARANTINO (°), D. PARRINI (°),
M.-C. CAGNO (°°) and R. BUONAGUIDI (°°).

INTRODUCTION

It is well established that chromosome abnormalities are not random in human neoplasias (1).

Human solid brain tumors have been extensively studied with cytogenetic investigations. The chromosome 22 abnormalities, monosomy or more rarely deletion of its long arm, have been reported as a specific anomaly in meningiomas (2) (3) (4). Other chromosomes often involved were n. 1, n. 8 (most frequent), n. 9, n. 14 and n. 15 (5).

The loss of either the X or Y has been reported in a significant number of meningiomas accompanied by other chromosomal changes (5).

In the present study we report the results of the cytogenetic findings in 25 out of 40 utilized human meningiomas.

According to the literature, several tumors showed chromosome n. 22 abnormalities (monosomy and rearrangement), chromosome n. 8 monosomy and trisomy, chromosomes rearrangement n. 1, n. 7 and n. 9. In a small number of tumors the chromosomes X or Y were lost.

MATERIAL AND METHODS

The tumoral tissue was minced with fine scissors or scalpels to make a cell suspension. The fragments and disaggreagated cells were introduced into a culture flask (25 cm). Then 3 ml of Ham's F10 culture medium containing antiblastics supplemented with 15 % of fetal calf serum was added and incubated at 37 °C for different periods of time. The culture medium was regulary replaced every 3 days. They were harvested 8 to 16 days later after treatment with 0,2 ug Colcemid per ml medium for 2-3 hours. The cells were removed by trypsinization; hypotonic treatment and fixation were performed with a 0,075 M Kcl solution for 20-30 min. and methanol-acetic acid air method. Q-banding technique was used for chromosome identification (6).

Karyotypes were determined by microscopic analysis and by arranging photographed metaphases. The chromosome constitution of the tumor was expressed with the complete formula of clonal lines when the sufficient number of cells examined and the nature of the aberrations made it possible. The constitutional karyotype was determined in peripheral blood and found to be normal in all patients.

RESULTS

Cytogenetic studies were successful in 25 out of 40 cases of meningiomas. Clonal chromosome abnormalities were found in 13 of the 25 tumors studied.

The tumor karyotypes are given in table 1. Patients were 8 male and 17 female, the age range was 32 to 66 years.

Anatomical localization of the studied meningiomas was as follows: 11 were of the base of the skull, 13 at the convexity of the skull and 1 was a meningioma of the spinal cord. Chromosome analysis was performed after 8-16 days of culture and always on cells from primary cultures. Direct chromosome preparations, performed in seven cases, was successful only in case n. 24. Our cytogenetic findings can be summarized as follows:

(°) Department of Pediatrics University of Pisa, (°°) Department of Neurosurgery University of Pisa.

M. Chatel, F. Darcel and J. Pecker (eds.), Brain Oncology. ISBN-13: 978-94-010-8003-3

The cases n. 2, 4, 5, 6, 7, 8, 10, 12, 14, 17, 22 and 25 were karyotypically normal. Monosomy 22 was present in three cases: n. 11 in all cells, n. 16 in five cells and n. 20 in twenty cells, as the only abnormality; in four cases it was associated with trisomy n. 8 (case n. 1), with chromosome monosomy n. 8, n. 13, n. 16 and the loss of X (case 19); in case n. 21, eight cells showed loss of both chromosomes n. 22 associated with monosomy n. 8. At last in case 24, the 22 monosomy was associated with the loss of Y chromosome.

Other abnormalities were found in case n. 13 del (1) (p. 21 ?) (fig. 1) and in case n. 23 as 9q+ (fig. 2).

An interesting abnormal karyotype was present in cases 3 and 9 defined rispectively as der (7) (pter-q31:: ?), 9p+, der (22) (pter-q11:: ?) (fig. 3) and 46, XX, -22, +der (22) (pter- q11::q11- pter) (fig. 4 a-b).

DISCUSSION

The presence of chromosome abnormalities in meningiomas and in particular the specific involvement of chromosome n. 22 already noted by other investigators, is confirmed in the present study. In fact, out of 25 cases utilized for cytogenetic analysis 13 revealed an abnormal karyotype. The incidence of chromosome abnormalities in meningiomas was 96,3 % in Sweden (7), 56,6 % in Germany (7) and 71 % in Japan (8). We found 52 %. Monosomy 22 was present in about 95 % of abnormal karyotype in Germany, Sweden and Japan. Our data confirmed this specific involvement of chromosome n. 22 in meningiomas.

In fact, out of 13 abnormal cases, nine (69 %) revealed an involvement of n. 22 in monosomy or rearrangements. Other defined chromosome abnormalities present in our samples are monosomy 8, 13, 16, trisomy 8, and loss of one sex chromosome (X or Y). The deletion of the short arm of chromosome n. 1 has been previously reported in meningiomas (9) just as the 9 q+ has also been observed by Mark (10) and Katsuyama (11). A reilevant aspect of the present report are the cases without monosomy of chromosome n. 22 but with unusual rearrangement of the same chromosome. The marker der (22) (pter--q11::?) and der (22) (pter--q11::q11--pter) found in cases 3 and 9 are interesting because these two cases have rearrangements involving the region of the 22q11 band. These data support the non-random involvement of this break points q11 in meningiomas.

Finally, no correlation was found between particular karyotypic patterns of the tumors studied and then histopathological characteristic. However we can confirm that meningiomas with normal karyotypes were mostly found at the base of the skull (12). In fact, in our material only two of 11 meningiomas from the base had an abnormal karyotype, while these were 10 of 13 cases from the convexity.

SUMMARY

Cytogenetic studies using Q-Banding technique, involving 25 out of 40 human meningiomas utilized for this investigation, revealed clonal abnormality in 13 of them. Monosomy 22 was present in three cases as the only abnormality, in four it was associated with other anomalies. Rearrangement of chromosomes n. 1, n. 7, n. 9, monosomy and trisomy of chromosome n. 8 have also been observed.

These data support the hypotesis of the association of n. 22 chromosome abnormalities with meningiomas.

KEY-WORDS

Brain Tumors, Karyotypes, Genome.

AKNOWLEDGEMENTS

We wish to thank Doctors Rosario Casalone and Paola Granada (Institute of Medical Genetics, University of Pavia) for help in the preparation of this paper.

REFERENCES

1. MITELMAN (F.), LEVAN (G.): Clustering of aberrations to specific chromosomes in human neoplasmas. - IV a survey of 1 871 cases. Hereditas, **95**, 79-139, 1981.
2. MARK (T.): Chromosomal abnormalities and their specificity in human neoplasmas. An assessement of recent observation by banding techniques. Adv. Cancer Res., **24**, 165-222, 1977.
3. ZANKL (H.), ZANG (K.D.): Correlations between blinical and cytogenetical data in 180 meningiomas. Cancer Genet Cytogenet, 1, 351-356, 1980.
4. REY (J.A., BELLO (J.M.), DE CAMPO (J.M.), BENITEZ (T.), AYUSO (MC), VALCARCEL (E.): Chromosome studies in two human brain tumors. Cancer Genet Cytogenet **10**: 159-165, 1983.
5. SANDBEERG (E.A.): The Chromosomes in Human Cancer and Leukemia. Elsevier N.Y., 1980.
6. PARIS CONFÉRENCE 1971: Standardization in human Cytogenetics. Birth defects. Original article series IX, **9**: 1975. The National Foundation N.Y.
7. MITELMAN (F.), LEVAN (G.): Clustering of aberrations to specific chromosomes in human neoplasmas. Incidence and geographic distribution of chromosomes aberrations in 856 cases. Hereditas **89**: 207-232. 1978.
8. YAMADA (K.), KONDO (T.), YOSHIODA (M.), OAMI (H.): Cytogenetic studies in twenty human brain tumors: association of n. 22 chromosome abnormalities with tumors of the brain. Cancer Genet Cytogenet **2**: 293-307, 1980.
9. MITELMAN (F.): Catalogue of chromosome aberrations in cancer. Cancer Genet Cytogenet **36**: 1, 1983.
10. MARK (J.): Chromosomal abnormalities and their specificity in human neoplasms: an assessment of recent observations by banding techniques. Adv. Cancer Res. **24**: 165-222, 1976.
11. KATSUYAMA (J.), PAPENHAUSEN (P.R.), HERZ (F.), GAVIZODA (P.), HIRANO (A.), KOSS (L.G.): Chromosome abnormalities in meningiomas. Cancer Genet Cytogenet **2**: 63-68, 1986.
12. ZANKL (H.), ZANG (K.D.): Correlations between clinical and cytogenetical data in 180 meningiomas. Cancer Genet Cytogenet **1**: 351-356, 1980.

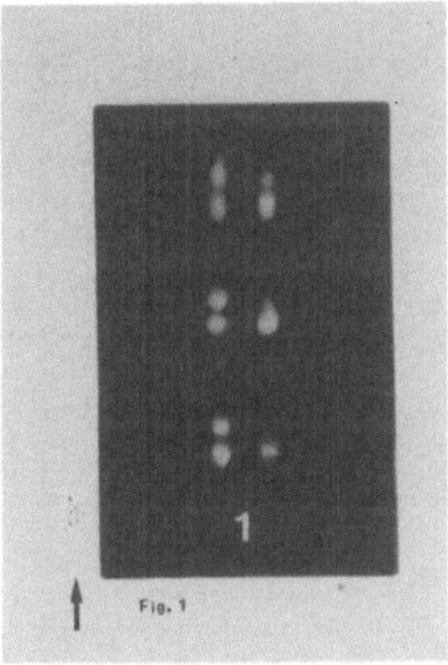

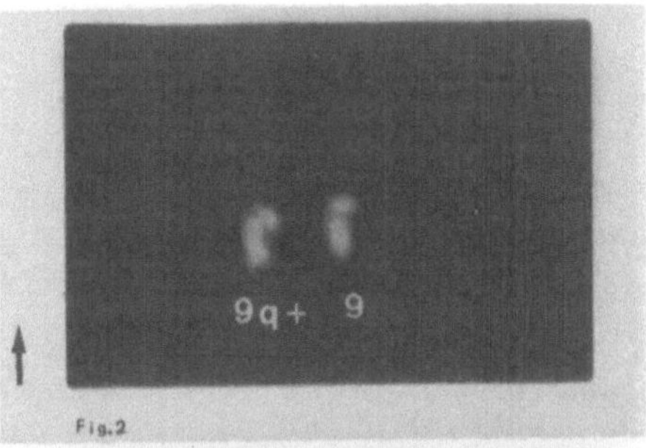

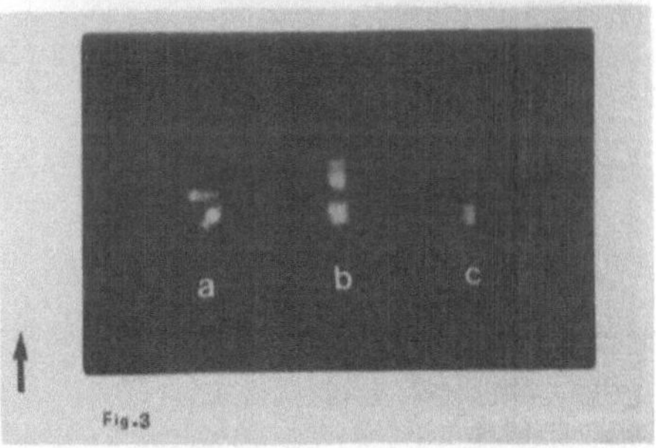

FIGURE 1. Chromosome n. 1 from different mitoses of case 13 showing the marker del (1) (p21 ?).

FIGURE 2. The chromosome 9q+ in case 23.

FIGURE 3. Relevant chromosomes n. 22 from different mitoses of case 3 showing the markers a) der (7)(pter--q31::?); b) 9p+ c) der (22)(pter--q11::?).

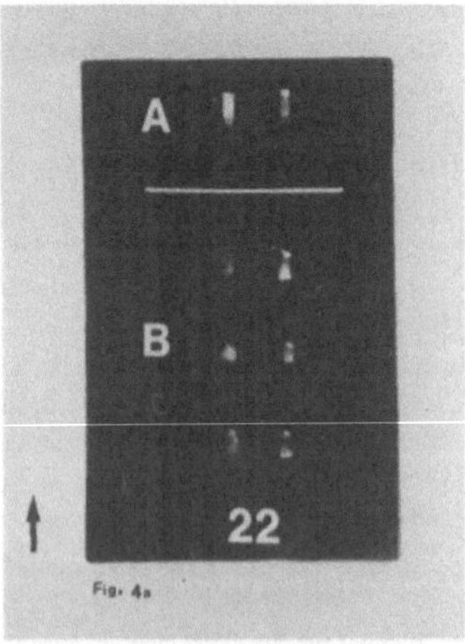

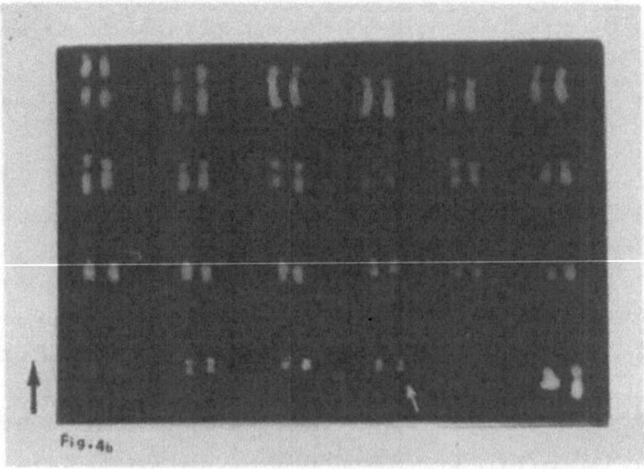

FIGURE 4. Chromosomes 22 from different mitoses of case 9 :
a) Cultured peripheral blood lymphocytes: at the right the n. 22 with brigthly fluorescent satellites.
b) Tumor cells: at the right the der (22) (pter--q11::q11--pter) with brightly fluorescent satellites at both ends).

PART II: NEUROPATHOLOGY

Immunohistochemistry in Neuro-Oncology: Markers or Signposts?

L.J. RUBINSTEIN (°).

The contributions of immunohistochemical techniques to the interpretation and further study of central nervous system (CNS) tumors are well known. Recent reviews have described the scope of these techniques in neurosurgical diagnosis and illustrated how proteins with diverse neural specificity are being employed today as markers of developing, normal adult, and pathological cells of the nervous system (1-3). These proteins may be structural (therefore related to the cytoskeleton or the cell membranes), or soluble (some having enzymatic activity); others may be concerned with neuroendocrine functions, and others again behave as neurotransmitters. While these markers are often highly sensitive, their cell-specificity varies. Consequently some of their immunomorphological reactions are currently raising a number of questions which necessitate a reappraisal of their role as indicators of cytogenesis. In reality the antigenic determinants revealed by these methods often prove to be not so much markers of histogenesis, as signposts — or signals — pointing towards one or more potential lines of neoplastic differentiation. We have discussed in greater detail elsewhere the implications that may be drawn from the various manifestations of this phenomenon (4). In this brief review, we propose to summarize some of these points.

Many reports, originating from centers world-wide, have established glial fibrillary acidic (GFA) protein as the most reliable and the most frequently used of the immunohistochemical markers employed to resolve diagnostic problems in CNS tumors (1). The characteristics of this protein, which is the major chemical subunit of the glial intermediate filaments of differentiated astrocytes, have been described repeatedly (5). The reasons for its importance in neurosurgical diagnosis are evident. First, gliomas numerically constitute the most important group of primary intracranial neoplasms and, by reason of their protean morphological manifestations, are also those which pose the greatest number of difficulties from the diagnostic viewpoint. Secondly, GFA protein has proved to be a marker which is at the same time highly specific and highly sensitive. It is also one which, as might have been expected, has raised several problems in regard to some of its immunopositive reactions.

GFA protein is the chief diagnostic antigenic determinant of normal, reactive and neoplastic astrocytes, but it is well-recognized that it may be found in neuroglial tumor cells that are not of astrocytic origin, such as in ependymomas and oligodendrogliomas. Ependymocytes have long been known to contain intracellular glial filaments, which become most prominent when these cells become reactive or neoplastic. Moreover it is apparent that normal ependymal cells will transiently express GFA protein in embryonal development (6). Thus its presence in reactive and neoplastic ependymocytes may reflect a normal transitory developmental phase of these cells, i.e. the protein, momentarily expressed in the fetal stage and then suppressed in the adult cell, reappears when the cell undergoes pathological change. The immunopositivity of neoplastic oligodendrocytes for GFA protein (7, 8) may perhaps be explained on the same lines. It should be stressed that positivity for GFA protein is to be found, in this context, not merely in the astrocytic component of composite oligoastrocytomas (7), but in cells which have the typical morphological features of oligodendroglioma. In our experience, some 40 percent of oligodendrogliomas contain GFA protein-positive oligodendroglial cells (8). We believe, with others (7, 9), that this feature may be related to the fact that, in the course of ontogeny, immature oligodendrocytes express GFA protein immediately before myelinogenesis. According to some workers, this is linked to the presumed origin of oligodendrocytes, which in common with mature astrocytes are derived from the GFA

(°) Division of Neuropathology, Department of Pathology, University of Virginia School of Medicine, Charlottesville, Virginia, USA.

M. Chatel, F. Darcel and J. Pecker (eds.), Brain Oncology. ISBN-13: 978-94-010-8003-3

protein-positive embryonal radial glia (9). Mixed oligodendrogliomas and astrocytomas are a very common occurrence in human neuro-oncology. Thus one could speculate that the cell which is the target in the initial step of neoplastic transformation might be a glial precursor cell that is still uncommitted to either astrocytic or oligodendroglial differentiation, but whose descendants may exhibit either phenotype.

A different interpretative problem is raised by the occasional presence of GFA protein in the stromal cells of capillary hemangioblastomas (10, 11). Some workers have suggested that these cells form a heterogeneous group which includes astrocytic as well as other cells, and that cell lipidization may be common to all (10). An alternative explanation is that GFA protein uptake by angiogenic cells may occur when intense gliosis is present in the vicinity (11). This hypothesis is supported by the electron microscopic demonstration of a considerable micropinocytotic activity on the part of the hemangioblastoma cells. However, experimental proof is still lacking that stromal cells are capable of taking up GFA protein released by neighboring astrocytes.

Choroid plexus papillomas may include a number of epithelial tumor cells which are positive for GFA protein (12, 13). This is perhaps evidence of ependymal differentiation, in the sense that the GFA protein-positive tumor cells, having retained the genetic information of· their primitive neuroepithelial precursors, may express glial phenotypic features that would normally have been present had the descendants of these precursor cells differentiated into ependymocytes. We have referred to this phenomenon as an instance of aberrant differentiation expressing an ontogenetic memory (4).

The five distinct biochemical and antigenic varieties of intermediate filament protein that have been identified in different cell types, either normal or neoplastic, have been extensively documented (14). There is increasing recognition, however, that the same tumor may express two or even three of these proteins and that in a number of instances more than one intermediate filament protein may be coexpressed within the same tumor cell. This is exemplified by the presence of neurofilament protein and of cytokeratin in a number of neuroendocrine tumors and in parathyroid adenomas (15). It is therefore not surprising that cytokeratin has been found to be expressed in the epithelial cells of choroid plexus papillomas (16) and in the cells of some meningiomas (17). A group of supratentorial desmoplastic neuroepithelial neoplasms of infancy, termed "desmoplastic infantile gangliogliomas", has been documented in which dual glial and neuronal differentiation has been confirmed by the presence of GFA protein on the one hand, and of the 200 Kd neurofilament protein triplet recognized by a monoclonal antibody on the other; the identification of this tumor is of clinical importance because of the favorable prognosis attached to this rare type of embryonal neoplasm (18). Certain glioblastomas and gliosarcomas which contain compact foci of small undifferentiated epithelial-like cells may demonstrate, in the same foci, immunopositivity for cytokeratin (19). In the same keratin-positive areas, clear-cut squamous differentiation may also be recognized in routine stains.

Neuron-specific enolase, a cytoplasmic enzyme of the glycolytic cycle, therefore a non-structural marker, provides another instance in which the protein may be expressed in neoplastic cells and not in their normal equivalents. In this case it is assumed that the enzyme is needed to augment the rate of glycolysis postulated to occur in neoplastic proliferation. The form of the enzyme, originally known as the 14-3-2 protein, is normally characteristic of, but not specific for, ganglion cells, endocrine cells, and cells of the amine precursor uptake and decarboxylation (APUD) system. It is, however, also demonstrable in CNS tumors of non-neuronal origin such as gliomas, meningiomas, choroid plexus papillomas, etc., as well as in a number of tumors outside the central nervous system which do not form part of the endocrine or neuroendocrine systems (20). The same reactive or neoplastic astrocytes may simultaneously express both GFA protein and neuron-specific enolase (21)

Neuron-specific enolase, occasionally the 68 Kd neurofilament protein, and GFA protein may variously be expressed in the subependymal giant cell astrocytoma, a unique neoplasm which may or may not be associated with tuberous sclerosis. The significance and possible cytogenetic implications of these immunohistochemical reactions in that remarkable type of glial tumor have been considered (22). The immunomorphological features indicate that the cellular composition of these neoplasms is more heterogeneous than is suggested by their uniform cytological appearance in routine stains. In this instance the difficulty lies in relating the tumor cells to a recognized normal mature or immature neuroepithelial cell type. The most plausible explanation is that the tumor originates from a dysplastic cell in which the potential for astrocytic and, to a much lesser extent, ganglionic differentiation, is aberrantly or incompletely expressed.

There is increasing awareness (see references in 5) that immunoreactivity to GFA protein may be found in several cell types outside the CNS. These include non-myelin-forming Schwanns cells in peripheral and enteric autonomic nerves, the satellite (or capsular) cells of sensory and sympathetic ganglia, the epithelial cells of the crystalline lens, the Kupffer cells of the liver, the folliculostellate cells of the normal and neoplastic anterior pituitary gland, the cells of Rathke's cleft, and a number of normal epithelial and neoplastic cells of human salivary glands. Some of those studies have shown that the antigen(s) recognized by the antiserum share properties with astrocytic GFA protein, namely similar molecular weight by immunoblooting, whereas others have suggested that the immunoreactivity may represent non-specific cross-reactivity with other filamentous proteins or non-immune binding. In any event, there is evidence that the neoplastic cells of human peripheral nerve shealth tumors may, like glial cells, demonstrate immunopositivity for GFA protein (23).

The immune system and the nervous system have been shown to possess common antigenic determinants, and cross-reactivity between lymphoid and neural cells has been reported in several instances. Of special interest from the diagnostic viewpoint of neural tumors is the cross-reactivity that has been defined with anti-Leu 7 (HNK1), a mouse monoclonal antibody obtained from a human lymphoblasttoma. This antibody, a marker of lymphoid cells with natural killer activity, has been shown to be capable of reacting, in the nervous system, with myelin sheath elements, including their cellular components. It has been studied in a number of nerve sheath tumors (24) and in CNS neoplasms (25), especially — but not exclusively — in oligodendrogliomas (8, 25). Although it may be of considerable ancillary help in the elucidation of specific differential diagnostic problems that cannot be resolved by traditional histological techniques, it is clear that the marker is not specific for any particular neural or non-neural cell type. Unlike the reaction obtained with intermediate filament proteins, the cells that are immunopositive for the Leu 7 antibody generally demonstrate the reaction along their cytoplasmic membranes only. It is of interest that the central neurocytoma (26), a tumor which by traditional light microscopy closely resembles the oligodendroglioma but differs from it by its electron microscopic features, reacts with the antibody in a manner identical with that of the oligodendroglioma, whereas the more primitive cerebral neuroblastomas are immunonegative. It has been suggested that the cell membranes recognized by the anti-Leu 7 antibody are, more often than, those of well-differentiated neuroepithelial tumors, since most of the embryonal CNS neoplasms are negative with this marker (25). Here again, therefore, the immunohistochemical reaction is likely to be related to cell differenciation rather than to tumor cytogenesis. However, further work is needed to test this hypothesis.

The examples quoted above illustrate the need of readjusting some of our thinking on the differentiating potential of CNS tumors. They also reinforce the importance of caution in the interpretation of unexpected immunomorphological reactions, not only in rare and difficult cases, but also in well-established entities.

KEY WORDS

Immunocytochemistry, Brain Tumours, Differentiation Markers, Histopathology.

REFERENCES

1. BONNIN (J.M.), RUBINSTEIN (L.J.) (1984): Immunohistochemistry of central nervous system tumors. Its contributions to neurosurgical diagnosis. Journal of Neurosurgery, 60, 1121-1133.
2. COAKHAM (H.B.), GARSON (J.A.), ALLAN (P.M.), HARPER (E.I.), BROWNELL (B.), KEMSHEAD (J.T.), LANE (E.B.) (1985): Immunohistological diagnosis of central nervous system tumors using a monoclonal antibody panel. Journal of Clinical Pathology, 38, 165-173.
3. RUBINSTEIN (L.J.) (1986): Contribution des méthodes immunohistochimiques à l'étude des tumeurs du système nerveux central. Annales de Pathologie, 6, 157-163.
4. RUBINSTEIN (L.J.) (1986): Immunohistochemical signposts — not markers — in neural tumour differentiation. Neuropathology and Applied Neurobiology in press.
5. ENGL (L.F.) (1985): Glial fibrillary acidic protein (GFAP): the major protein in glial intermediate filaments in differentiated astrocytes. Journal of Neuroimmunology 8, 203-214.

6. ROESSMANN (U.), VELASCO (M.E.), SINDELY (S.D.), GAMBETTI (P.) (1980): Glial fibrillary acidic protein (GFAP) in ependymal during development. An immunocytochemical study. Brain Research 200, 13-21.

7. HERPERS (M.J.H.M.), BUDKA (H.) (1984): Glial fibrillary acidic protein (GFAP) in oligodendroglial tumors. Gliofibrillary oligodendroglioma and transitional oligoastrocytoma as subtypes of oligodendroglioma. Acta Neuropathologica 64, 265-272.

8. NAKAGAWA (Y.), PERENTES (E.), RUBINSTEIN (L.J.) (1986): Immunohistochemical characterization of oligodendrogliomas. An analysis of multiple markers. Acta Neuropathologica 72, 15-22.

9. CHOI (B.H.), KIM (R.C.) (1984): Expression of glial fibrillary acidic protein in immature oligodendroglia. Science 223, 407-409.

10. KEPES (J.J.), RENGACHARY (S.S.), LEE (S.H.) (1979): Astrocytes in hemangioblastomas of the central nervous system and their relationship to stromal cells. Acta Neuropathologica 47, 99-104.

11. DECK (J.H.N.), RUBINSTEIN (L.J.) (1981): Glial fibrillary acidic protein in stromal cells of some capillary hemangioblastomas. Significance and possible implications of an immunoperoxidase study. Acta Neuropathologica 54, 173-181.

12. RUBINSTEIN (L.J.), BRUCHER (J.M.) (1981): Focal ependymal differentiation in choroid plexus papillomas. An immunoperoxidase study. Acta Neuropathologica 53, 29-33.

13. TARATUTO (A.L.), MOLINO (H.), MONGES (J.) (1983): Choroid plexus tumors in infancy and childhood. Focal ependymal differentiation. An immunoperoxidase study. Acta Neuropathologica 59, 304-308.

14. MIETTINEN (M.), LEHTO (V.P.), VIRTANEN (I.) (1984): Antibodies to intermediate filament proteins in the diagnosis and classification of human tumors. Ultrastructural Pathology 7, 83-107.

15. GOULD (V.E.) (1985): The coexpression of distinct classes of intermediate filaments in human neoplasms. Archives of Pathology and Laboratory Medicine 109, 984-985.

16. COFFIN (C.M.), WICK (M.R.), BRAUN (J.T.), DEHNER (L.P.) (1986): Choroid plexus neoplasms. Clinicopathologic and immunohistochemical studies. American Journal of Surgical Pathology 10, 394-404.

17. KEPES (J.J.) (1986): The histopathology of meningiomas. A reflection of origins and expected behavior? Journal of Neuropathology and Experimental Neurology 45, 95-107.

18. VANDENBERG (S.R.), MAY (E.E.), RUBINSTEIN (L.J.), HERMAN (M.M.), PERENTES (E.), VINORES (S.A.), COLLINS (V.P.), PARK (T.S.) (1987): Desmoplastic supratentorial neuroepithelial tumors of infancy with divergent differentiation potential ('desmoplastic infantile gangliogliomas'). A report on 11 cases of a distinctive embryonal tumor with favorable prognosis. Journal of Neurosurgery 66, 58-71.

19. RUBINSTEIN (L.J.), MÖRK (S.J.), KEPES (J.J.), UPHOFF (D.F.) (1986): Squamous differentiation of epithelial-like formations in glioblastoma and gliosarcoma. Journal of Neuropathology and Experimental Neurology 45, 327 (abstr.).

20. VINORES (S.A.), BONNIN (J.M.), RUBINSTEIN (L.J.), MARANGOS (P.J.) (1984): Immunohistochemical demonstration of neuron-specific enolase in neoplasms of the CNS and other tissues. Archives of Pathology and Laboratory Medicine 108, 536-540.

21. VINORES (S.A.), RUBINSTEIN (L.J.) (1985): Simultaneous expression of glial fibrillary acidic (GFA) protein and neuron-specific enolase (NSE) by the same reactive or neoplastic astrocytes. Neuropathology and Applied Neurobiology 11, 349-359.

22. BONNIN (J.M.), RUBINSTEIN (L.J.), PAPASOZOMENOS (S.Ch.), MARANGOS (P.J.) (1984): Subependymal giant cell astrocytoma. Significance and possible cytogenetic implications of an immunohistochemical study. Acta Neuropathologica 62, 185-193.

23. MEMOLI (V.A.), BROWN (E.F.), GOULD (V.E.) (1984): Glial fibrillary acidic protein (GFAP) immunoreactivity in peripheral nerve sheath tumors. Ultrastructural Pathology 7, 269-275.

24. PERENTES (E.), RUBINSTEIN (L.J.) (1985): Immunohistochemical recognition of human nerve sheath tumors by anti-Leu 7 (HNK-1) monoclonal antibody. Acta Neuropathologica 68, 319-324.

25. PERENTES (E.), RUBINSTEIN (L.J.) (1986): Immunohistochemical recognition of human neuroepithelial tumors by anti-Leu 7 (HNK-1) monoclonal antibody. Acta Neuropathologica 69, 227-233.

26. HASSOUN (J.), GAMBARELLI (D.), GRISOLI (F.), PELLET (W.), SALOMON (G.), PELLISSIER (J.F.), TOGA (M.) (1982): Central neurocytoma. An electron-microscopic study of two cases. Acta Neuropathologica 56, 151-156.

Immunocytochemistry and the Pathological Diagnosis of Cerebral Tumours

R. O. WELLER (°).

INTRODUCTION

Traditionally, the diagnosis of cerebral tumours has been based upon histological morphology and the resemblance of tumour cells to normal tissues (1). With the introduction of immunocytochemistry, it became possible to identifiy cellular elements in normal brain and other tissues by the presence of specific intracellular elements such as intermediate filaments, other cell proteins and cell products (Table 1) or by the expression of cell surface antigens (2). However, it also became clear that, as a reflection of changes in the DNA of tumour cells, normal cell components or surface antigens of the proposed cell of origin were not always appropriately expressed by the tumour cells (3). Some neoplastic cells **retain** appropriate marker proteins, whereas, in other tumours, the cells **lose** marker proteins or even **gain** markers that are inappropriate for the apparent cell of origin. The main use of immunocytochemistry in the diagnosis of cerebral tumours lies in 3 main areas:

a) Definition of the cell of origin of a tumour but taking into the account the loss or gain of marker proteins by tumour cells.

b) Identification of normal and reactive nervous tissue cells and their relationships to tumour cells. Immunocytochemistry has supplemented or even replaced the use of capricious silver stains and dye techniques for light microscopy and has reduced the need for electron microscopy in tumour diagnosis.

c) Detection of inflammatory cells and lymphocyte subsets within tumours and the use of similar techniques for the diagnosis and classification of lymphomas.

MATERIAL AND METHODS

Five-micron paraffin sections of formalin-fixed biopsy tumour tissue or cryostat sections of fresh tumour tissue were stained by the peroxidase-anti-perixodase (PAP) technique (4) or by immunofluorescence for the polyclonal and monoclonal antibodies listed in Table 1.

TABLE 1

Some immunocytochemical markers in the adult nervous system	
Neurons:	Neurofilament proteins (intermediate filaments) Neuron-specific enolase
Astrocytes:	Glial fibrillary acidic protein (GFAP) (intermediate filaments)
Oligodendrocytes:	Carbonic anhydrase C
Endothelial cells:	Factor VIII related antigen
Arachnoid and pia mater:	Vimentin (intermediate filaments) Desmosomal proteins
Choroid plexus:	Carbonic Anhydrase C
Schwann cells:	S100 protein (also glia)
Lymphocyte subsets:	Monoclonal antibodies (MCA) to cell surface components
Macrophages:	Alpha-1-antichymotrypsin and MCA

RESULTS

Glial fibrillary acidic protein (GFAP) is probably the single most valuable immunocytochemical marker for the diagnosis of **gliomas** (2). The combination of tumour cell staining and the demonstration of reactive astrocytes within the tissue invaded by the tumour produces a clearer picture of the tumour biology than can be obtained from most other stains. GFAP is not, however, a specific marker for any particular tumour.

(°) Department of Neuropathology, Southampton General Hospital, Southampton S09 4XY, England.

M. Chatel, F. Darcel and J. Pecker (eds.), Brain Oncology. ISBN-13: 978-94-010-8003-3

In well-differentiated and poorly-differentiated **astrocytomas** the tumour cells show varying degrees of nuclear pleomorphism but may still be difficult to distinguish from reactive astrocytes. Except for gemistocytic astrocytomas, neoplastic astrocytes, stained for GFAP, usually have fewer cell processes and less abundant paranuclear cytoplasm than reactive astrocytes. In **anaplastic astrocytomas** there is often variable staining for GFAP (fig. 1); some tumour cells may not express this marker although they may contain vimentin. Small rod-shaped anaplastic tumour cells typical of **glioblastoma multiforme** usually do not express GFAP. These cells resemble microglia which are also present in glioblastomas, but the tumour cells do not contain alpha-1-antichymotrypsin. Variable expression of GFAP is seen in the large bizarre giant cells in the centre of many glioblastomas; some of these cells do not express GFAP. Capillary endothelial proliferation in glioblastomas is well-demonstrated in reticulin stains but can also be characterised by staining the endothelial cells for Factor VIII related antigen. Such staining reveals the complex glomeruloid formation of capillaries and the absence of staining in pericytes and supporting cells.

In **gliosarcomas,** there is a mixture of glial elements and nonglial spindle cells. A reticulin stain may allow the unstained glial areas to be distinguished from the reticulin-rich spindle cell elements, but, in small biopsies, immunocytochemistry for GFAP may be very valuable for identifying with certainty the islands of glial tumour cells. The spindle cells in gliosarcomas may express alpha-1-antichymotrypsin but do not usually contain Factor VIII related antigen.

Oligodendroglioma cells do not usually contain the Carbonic Anhydrase C that is present in normal oligodendroglia, although frequently a proportion of the tumour cells show positive staining for GFAP in their cytoplasm. Conversely normal ependymal cells do not express GFAP except during fetal life and in certain areas of the brain, but **ependymomas** typically show a pattern of fine GFAP positive fibrillary processes forming pseudorosettes around blood vessels even in the poorly-differentiated tumours.

Some confusion may arise in the diagnosis of **choroid plexus papillomas** as, histologically, these tumours may resemble well-differentiated papillary adenocarcinomas or ependymomas. Using a panel of antibodies, immunocytochemistry supplements other histological stains in distinguishing between these tumours (5). In 10 choroid plexus papillomas studied, all were positive for Carbonic Anhydrase C (fig. 2a), even the poorly differentiated papillomas. All tumours contained areas of epithelium that were positive for S100 protein and, in all but one poorly-differentiated papilloma, there was patchy staining in the epithelium for GFAP (fig. 2b), despite the absence of this intermediate filament in normal choroid plexus epithelium. This pattern of staining distinguishes choroid plexus papillomas from ependymomas which do not contain Carbonic Anhydrase C and from metastatic carcinomas which are negative for all three markers.

Primitive neuroectodermal tumours (PNET) include medulloblastomas of the cerebellum and cerebral neuroblastomas (6); they occur mainly in children but are also seen in adults. Histologically, the tumour cell nuclei are moderately pleomorphic and have a diffuse hazy hyperchromasia. Small groups of cells expressing GFAP in the perinuclear cytoplasm and in fine short processes are present in a high proportion of PNET although the majority of cells may not express this marker (fig. 3). GFAP-positive reactive astrocytes are also present within most PNET and can be distinguished from the tumour cells by their multiple long processes and copious paranuclear cytoplasm. Ependymal elements may be seen within PNET and striated muscle fibres, identified by immunocytochemical staining for myoglobin (7), may also be present. Cerebral PNET may show areas of astrocyte or oligodendroglial differentiation particularly in adults. The combination of histology and immunocytochemical staining for GFAP in the primitive areas of the tumour are valuable in distinguishing the radiosensitive PNET from glioblastoma multiforme in older patients.

The neuronal elements in **ganglioneuroblastomas, ganglioneuromas** and **gangliogliomas** do not contain GFAP but they do stain for neuron-specific enolase; neurofilament proteins may also be detected in axonal processes and in some tumour cell bodies. Neuron-specific enolase is not a specific marker for neurons in cerebral tumours and many astrocytic tumours also contain this enzyme.

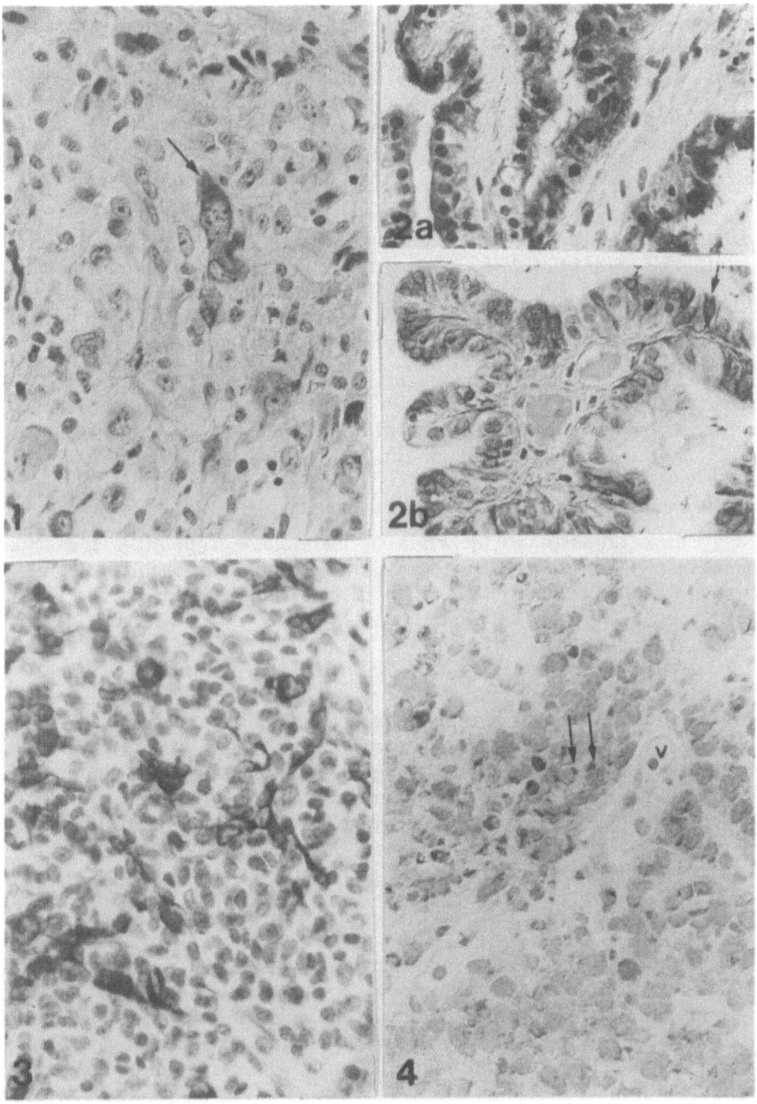

FIGURE 1. Anaplastic astrocytoma: a cell in the centre (arrow) contains GFAP but many others are not stained for this astrocyte marker.
Peroxidase-anti-peroxidase (PAP) for GFAP x400.

FIGURE 2. Choroid plexus papilloma showing positive staining in the epithelium for :
a) Carbonic Anhydrase C and
b) GFAP in the epithelial cells (e.g. arrow - top right).
PAP for Carbonic Anhydrase C x330.

FIGURE 3. Primitive neuroectodermal tumour (medulloblastoma) showing positive GFAP staining in a small number of cells.
PAP for GFAP x400

FIGURE 4. Primary cerebral lymphoma: punctate staining (arrows) for the B-cell monoclonal antibody marker RB411 is seen in lymphoma cells around a blood vessel (v).
Immunoperoxidase on cryostat section x330.

Most **meningiomas** are recognisable by their histological features. The majority have desmosomal junctions between the tumour cells which can be identified by electron microscopy or by immunocytochemistry for desmosomal proteins (8). Meningioma cells contain vimentin intermediate filaments. Occasionally, there may be difficulty in distinguishing meningiomas from Schwannomas, particularly when they arise in the cerebellopontine angle or within the spinal canal. In general, however, meningiomas lack an intimate reticulin network, except in the angioblastic type, whereas Schwannomas cells are rich in reticulin (7). Only occasionally do meningiomas contain S100 protein.

Schwannomas and **neurofibromas** contain Schwann cells which can be identified by immunocytochemical staining for S100 protein. Distinction between neurofibromas and Schwannomas often lies in the relationship of nerve fibres to the tumour. Immunocytochemistry for neurofilament protein is a valuable technique for detecting the axons that run through neurofibromas and the uninvolved nerve fascicles that are often attached to the side of Schwannomas. Although Schwannoma cells are positive for S100 protein, perineurial cells do not contain this marker.

Many **metastatic carcinomas** in the brain can be characterised immunocytochemically by the presence of cytokeratins stained by monoclonal antibodies such as CAM 5.2 (9) and by the absence of GFAP. However, not all carcinomas stain for CAM 5.2, nor do all gliomas contain GFAP. Furthermore GFAP positive reactive astrocytes may cause confusion as they are often incorporated into the stroma of metastatic tumours. **Malignant melanomas** usually stain for S100 protein.

Lymphomas may arise primarily in the brain or metastasize from other sites. Spinal cord compression may result from lymphoma in the extradural space and occasionally lymphomas arise primarily in this site. Monoclonal antibodies to cell surface components of lymphocyte subsets and monocyte-macrophages are used to characterise lymphomas. The primary diagnosis of lymphoma and its distinction from anaplastic carcinoma can be made by staining for a common leukocyte antigen and further characterised using panels of monoclonal antibodies (fig. 4) and the cytological features of the tumour cells. Most primary lymphomas of the central nervous system characterised in this way are B cell lymphomas (centroblastic/centrocytic) (10). The tumours were originally thought to be 'microgliomas' but the microglial cells in the tumours are reactive and the name 'microglioma' is now obsolete. A wide variety of lymphomas has been characterised in the extradural space of the spinal column. If a lymphoma is suspected clinically, it is most important to preserve fresh frozen tissue for cryostat sections and to make touch preparations of fresh tissue at the time of biopsy for cytological and immunocytochemical evaluation.

DISCUSSION

Immunocytochemistry has immeasurably enhanced the capacity of histopathologists to distinguish and define cerebral tumours, but its appropriate use depends upon the maintenance of well-controlled techniques and adequate correlation with clinical data and routine histological appearances. In some cases, the accuracy of diagnosis may be increased by using panels of polyclonal or monoclonal antibodies in tumour diagnosis. The use of immunocytochemistry has brought a change in attitude to the classification of cerebral tumours, and may play an increasingly important role in defining more appropriate treatment.

SUMMARY

Many of the different cellular components of the normal nervous system can be identified by immunocytochemistry using antibodies against cell components. However, expression of these cell markers is inconstant in cerebral tumours. Thus, immunocytochemistry is of most value in the diagnosis of cerebral tumours, when the detection of normal cell markers is used in combination with the evaluation of histological features of the tumour. Tissue reactions to the presence of tumour cells may also be evaluated using immunocytochemical techniques as general histological stains. To compensate for the lack of specificity of many tumour markers, panels of polyclonal or monoclonal antibodies have been employed for the diagnosis of cerebral tumours; examples of the use of immunocytochemistry in this way are discussed.

KEY WORDS

Immunocytochemistry; Brain-tumours; Diagnosis.

AKNOWLEDGEMENTS

I would like to thank the Staff of the Neuropathology Laboratory in Southampton for technical assistance and Margaret Harris for typing the manuscript. This study was supported by the Wessex Neurological Centre Brain Tumour Research Fund.

REFERENCES

1. ZULCH (K.J.) (ed.): Histological typing of tumours of the central nervous system (WHO, 1979).
2. BONIN (J.M.), RUBINSTEIN (L.J.): Immunohistochemistry of central nervous system tumours. Journal of Neurosurgery, **60**, 1121-1133 (1984).
3. GOULD (V.E.): Histogenesis and differentiation. A reevaluation of these concepts as criteria for the classification of tumors. Human Pathology, **17**, 212-215 (1986).
4. STERNBERGER (L.A.): Immunocytochemistry, 2nd Edition (Wiley, 1979).
5. WELLER (R.O.), STEART (P.V.), MOORE (I.E.): Carbonic Anhydrase C as a marker antigen in the diagnosis of choroid plexus papillomas and other tumours: an immunoperoxidase study. *In:* Biology of Brain Tumour. Eds Walker MD and Thomas DGT (Martinus Nijhoff and Dr W Junk 1986), p. 115-120.
6. RORKE (L.B.): The cerebellar medulloblastoma and its relationship to primitive neuroectodermal tumors. Journal of Neuropathology and Experimental Neurology, **42**, 1-15 (1983).
7. WELLER (R.O.): Color atlas of Neuropathology (Harvey Miller and Oxford University Press, 1984).
8. PARRISH (E.P.), GARROD (D.R.), MATTEY (D.L.), HAND (L.), STEART (P.V.), WELLER (R.O.): Mouse antisera specific for desmosomal adhesion molecules of suprabasal skin cells, meninges and meningioma. Proceedings of National Academy of Sciences, USA, **83**, 2657-2661 (1986).
9. MAKIN (C.A.), BORROW (L.G.), BODMER (W.F.): Monoclonal antibody to cytokeratin for use in routine histopathology. Journal of Clinical Pathology, **37**, 975-983 (1984).
10. GRANT (J.W.), GALLAGHER (P.J.), JONES (D.B.): Primary Cerebral Lymphoma. A histological and immunohistochemical study of 6 cases. Archives of Pathology and Laboratory medicine **110**, 897-901 (1986).

GFAP Immunoreactivity of Oligoastrocytomas
Study of 120 Cases

J.R. IGLESIAS, E. KAZNER (°), C. ARUFFO (°°).

INTRODUCTION

Glial fibrillary acidic protein (GFAP) is a distinct cytoskeletal protein (1) which represents the principal constituent of glial filaments (3). Because of its easy immunocytochemical detection it has been used as a specific glial marker in studies of glial cytology in CNS neoplasms (2-4). Very few reports exist in which the immune reactivity of oligoastrocytomas is described (6, 8). We wish to present our results in a large series of primary oligoastrocytomas.

MATERIALS AND METHODS

One hundred and twenty oligoastrocytomas were studied histologically. All tumours were biopsies from the Institute of Neuropathology of the Free University of Berlin. They were classified as oligoastrocytomas according to the WHO classification (11). The diagnosis was confirmed with the expert system "TUMOR" (see Iglesias *et al.* in this volume). The tumour specimens were fixed in 10% neutral formalin and embedded in paraffin. Routine stains were made for every tumour. For every tumoural sample at least two GFAP immunostainings (DAKO) were performed on 6μ thick sections. The peroxidase-antiperoxidase (PAP) technique of Sternberg (10) was used. All those cases in which the immunostaining presented artifacts or in which positivity was only seen in one of the preparations were eliminated. Thus only 99 cases were used for our final immunohistological evaluation.

RESULTS

With routine histopathology three different types of oligoastrocytomas could be identified. Those in which oligodendroglial and astroglial tumoural cells were intermingled (OAOA) (Fig. 1). These corresponded to 100 cases (83%). The second type in which two separate populations of tumoural cells existed, on the one hand oligodendroglial and on the other astroglial tumoural cells (OOAA) (Fig. 2), correspond to 14% (16 cases of our casuistic). Both tumoural cell types boarder with one another. The type of oligoastrocytoma less frequently observed (4 cases = 3%) was that in which intermediary cells (IC) predominated (Fig. 3). In HE and silver impregnations these cells have morphological characteristics which make them similar to both oligodendrocytes and astrocytes. They are small cells with a round nucleus and halo cytoplasm. However, they have small processes which resemble astrocytic processes. In most oligoastrocytomas more than one cellular pattern (OAOA; OOAA; IC) was seen in the same case. Thus, they were classified according to the pattern which predominated.

With GFAP it was seen that positive astrocytes predominated in all three types of oligoastrocytomas (Table I). Positive oligodendrocytes (Fig. 4) were seen in 30 to 50% of the cases. Positive intermediary cells were less frequently seen (Table I). Blasts were positive in 18% of all cases studied (Fig. 5). When positive they were very intensely positive. Negative oligodendrocytes and astrocytes were seen in 100% of the cases in a higher or lesser degree. With GFAP intermediary cells were positive. Although they could be considered as positive oligodendrocytes they were not classified as such because they were more or less isolated among astroglial cells and were not found constituting honey-comb formations.

(°) Neurosurgical Clinic, Rudolf Virchow Krankenhaus. Augustenburger Platz 1, 1000 Berlin 65. (°°) Institute of Neuropathology, Klinikum Steglitz der Freien Universität Berlin, Hidenburgdamm 30, 1000 Berlin 45, FRG. On leave from the IIBM-UNAM, Mexico with a DAAD fellowship.

M. Chatel, F. Darcel and J. Pecker (eds.), Brain Oncology. ISBN-13: 978-94-010-8003-3

Intracellular patterns of GFAP positivity varied greatly from cell to cell and from tumour type to tumour type (see Tables II-IV). In most cells GFAP positivity was diffusely distributed throughout the cytoplasma, whereas in others it was granularly positive or formed a ring around the nucleus. In approximately 50% of the positive cells the processes were likewise positive (Tables II-IV). Positivity was always diffuse and most frequently seen in astrocytes in all three types of oligoastrocytomas. In very few cases the processes were positive whereas the cell bodies were negative. Ring and granular positivity were practically only seen in the OAOA type of oligoastrocytomas and was localized in astrocytes. The positivity of the neuropile varied widely as can be seen in Table V.

TABLE I

GFAP positive immunoreactivity in the different cellular types seen in Oligoastrocytomas

	CELL TYPES			
Pattern	Oligo-dendrocytes	Astrocytes	Intermediary	Blasts
OAOA 82 cases	31 (38%)	79 (96%)	25 (29%)	15 (18%)
OOAA 14 cases	8 (57%)	13 (93%)	1 (7%)	1 (7%)
IC 3 cases	1 (33%)	2 (66%)	2 (66%)	2 (66%)

Table II

Patterns of intracellular GFAP positivity in OAOA Oligoastrocytomas

	PATTERN AND SITE			
CELL	Ring Cytoplasm	Granular Cytoplasm	Diffuse Cytoplasm	Diffuse Processes
Oligodendrocytes (+ in 31 cases)	—	1	31	1
Astrocytes (+ in 79 cases)	12	10	75	1
Intermediary (+ in 25 cases)	—	—	25	7
Total Nr. of cases = 82				

Table III

Patterns of intracellular GFAP positivity in OOAA Oligoastrocytomas

	PATTERN AND SITE			
CELL	Ring Cytoplasm	Granular Cytoplasm	Diffuse Cytoplasm	Diffuse Processes
Oligodendrocytes (+ in 8 cases)	—	—	7	1
Astrocytes (+ in 13 cases)	1	—	10	9
Intermediary (+ in 1 case)	—	—	1	1
Total Nr. of cases = 14				

Table IV

Patterns of intracellular GFAP positivity in IC Oligoastrocytomas

	PATTERN AND SITE			
CELL	Ring Cytoplasm	Granular Cytoplasm	Diffuse Cytoplasm	Diffuse Processes
Oligodendrocytes (+ in 1 case)	—	—	1	1
Astrocytes (+ in 2 cases)	—	1	1	1
Intermediary (+ in 2 cases)	—	—	1	1
Total Nr. of cases = 3				

TABLE V

Type of GFAP positive immunoreactivity of the intercellular matrix in the different types of Oligoastrocytomas

Type of tumour	OAOA	OOAA	IC
Fibrillary Neuropile	55	9	1
Granular Neuropile	23	1	1
Foot Plates	43	5	2

DISCUSSION

Herpes and Budka (8) have described oligoastrocytomas with GFAP. In 12% of their 16 cases they found GFAP positive oligodendroglial cells. This led them to classify these tumours as transitional oligoastrocytomas. Gullotta *et al.* (7) have also described the presence of positive oligodendrocytic components in some oligoastrocytomas. In 40% of the oligoastrocytomas studied by us numerous oligodendrocytes were clearly positive. These findings speak in favour of the fact that GFAP is not astrocyte specific, at least from a morphological stand point. Although up to now it has been thought that oligodendrocytes and astrocytes are totally independent types of cells, oligodendroglial GFAP positivity has led us to think that a certain immunological relationship exists between them. This fact is further supported by the presence of intermediary cells. These correspond to a new type of cells which do not differentiate into oligodendrocytes nor into astrocytes. The presence of morphologically blastic cells which are very positive and the fact that not all astroglial cells are GFAP positive although glial fibers were seen with polarization, speak for an asynchronic differentiation of tumour cells. In other words, glial cells which are morphologically blastic are GFAP positive indicating an immunological maturity. On the other hand, morphologically mature astroglial cells may be GFAP negative.

Granular and ring positivity could correspond to the granulations and ring formations described by Ravens and Calvo (9) in silver impregnations of senile brains. Such a pattern of GFAP positivity could also be an expression of secondary degenerative changes. This could account for the few cases in which this pattern of positivity was seen. This is further corroborated by the fact that only very few of the tumours studied by us had necrosis.

Oligoastrocytomas are oligodendroglial and astroglial cell containing tumours in which both tumoural cell types are seen forming an entity. This has been confirmed by our study in which we have seen that both types of cells are immunologicaly interrelated. The reason why some tumours grow forming a given pattern is not yet known. It might be related to the speed at which each tumoural cell type reproduces itself. However, it is interesting to notice that there is no definitive correlation between the histological and the immunohistological patterns of oligoastrocytomas. This is subject of further studies in our laboratory.

SUMMARY

All those tumours which contain both oligodendroglial and astroglial tumoural cells were classified as oligoastrocytomas or mixed gliomas. Histologically three types of oligoastrocytomas were seen. The classification depended on the distribution of the tumoural cells. The pattern most frequently seen was that in which oligodendroglial and astroglial tumoural cells were intermingled. These corresponded to 83% of all cases studied. Less frequently seen were the tumours in which a clear delimitation existed between the oligodendroglial and the astroglial tumoural components (14%). Very rare were those tumours in which intermediary cells predominated (3%). Under intermediary cells we have groupped those isolated cells which have a morphology between oligodendrocytes and astrocytes and react positively to GFAP. The intracellular localization of GFAP reactivity is described in all cellular populations.

KEY WORDS

Oligoastrocytomas, Mixed gliomas, GFAP, Histopathology, Immunocytochemistry.

REFERENCES

1. BIGNAMI (A.), ENG (L.F.), DAHL (D.), UYEDA (C.T.): Localization of the glial fibrillary acidic protein in astrocytes by immunofluorescence. Brain Res. **43:** 429-435, 1972.
2. ARMOND (S.L. de), ENG (L.F.), RUBINSTEIN (L.J.): The application of glial fibrillary acidic protein immunohistochemistry in neurooncology. Pathol. Res. Pract. **168**: 374-394, 1980.
3. ENG (L.F.), VANDERHAEGHEN (J.J.), BIGNIAMI (A.), GERSTL (B.): An acidic protein isolated from fibrous astrocytes. Brain Res. **28:** 351-354, 1971.
4. ENG (L.F.), RUBINSTEIN (L.J.): Contribution of immunohistochemistry to diagnostic problems of human cerebral tumours. J. Histochem. Cytochem. **26**: 513-522, 1978.
5. ENG (L.F.), ARMOND (S.L. de): Immunochemical studies of astrocytes in normal development and disease. Adv. Cell Neurobiol. **3**: 145-171, 1982.
6. FIGOLS (J.), IGLESIAS-ROZAS (J.R.), KAZNER (E.): Myelin basic protein (MBP) in human gliomas: A study of twenty five cases. Clinical Neuropath. **4:**116-120, 1985.
7. GULLOTTA (F.), SCHINDLER (F.), SCHMUTZLER (R.), WEEKS-SEIFERT (A.): GFAP in brain tumour diagnosis: Possibilities and limitations. Path. Res. Pract. **180**: 54-60, 1985.
8. HERPES (J.H.M.), BUDKA (H.): Glial fibrillary acidic protein (GFAP) in oligodendroglial tumours: Glial fibrillary oligodendroglioma and transitional oligoastrocytoma as subtypes of oligodendroglioma. Acta Neuropath. (Berl.), **64**: 265-272, 1984.
9. RAVENS (J.R.), CALVO (W.): Neuroglial changes in the senile brain. Proc. 5th Int. Congr. Neuropath. Zürich, 1965.
10. STERNBERG (L.A.): *Immunocytochemistry.* Wiley and Sons, New York, 1979.
11. ZÜLCH (K.J.): Historical development of the classification of brain tumours and the new proposal of the world health organization (WHO). Neurosurg. Rev. **4**: 123-127, 1981.

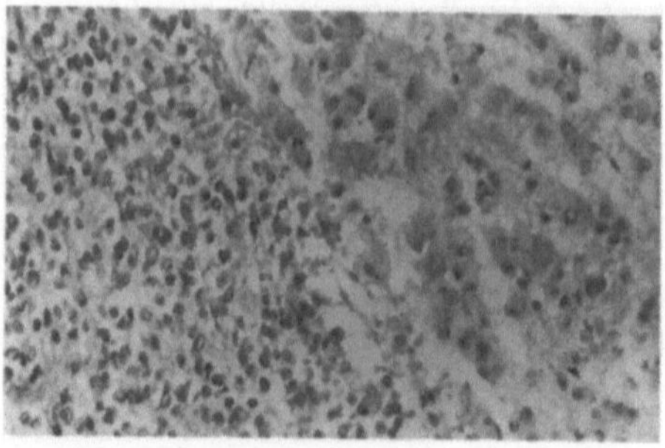

FIGURE 1. OAOA oligoastrocytoma. Oligodendrocytes and astrocytes are intermingled (HE x160).

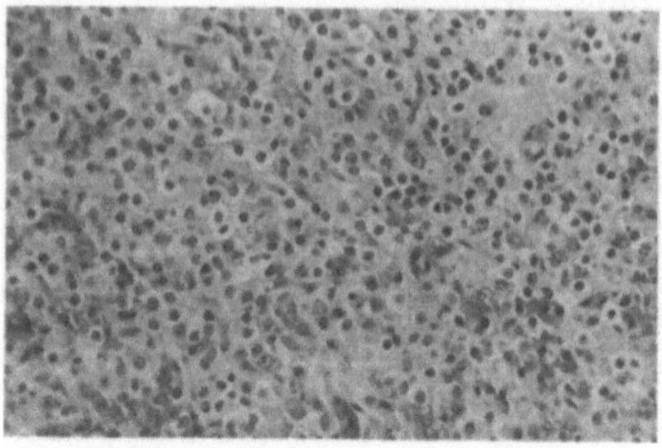

FIGURE 2. OOAA oligoastrocytoma. Oligodendrocytic area on the left, astrocytic on the right (HE x160).

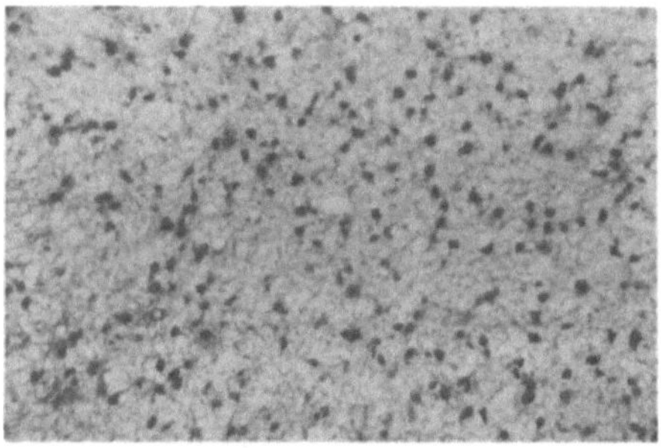

FIGURE 3. IC oligoastrocytoma. GFAP positive intermediary cells predominate (GFAP x160).

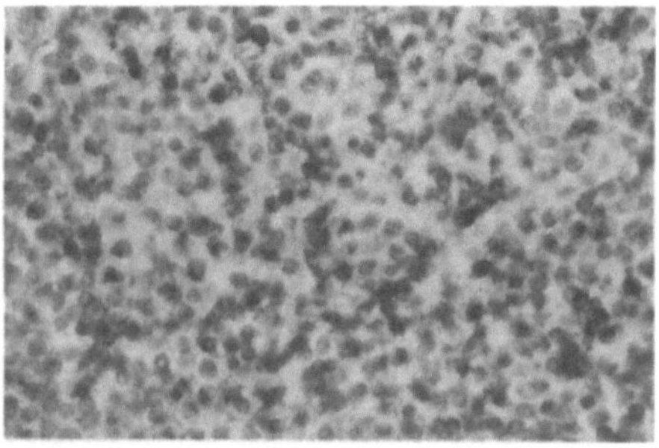

FIGURE 4. OAOA oligoastrocytoma with GFAP positive oligodendrocytes (GFAP x250).

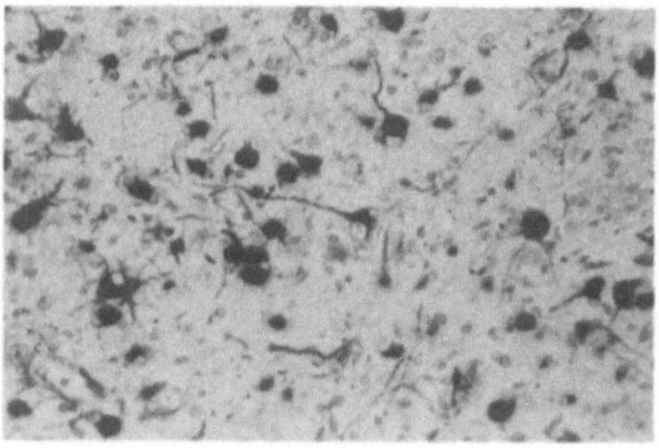

FIGURE 5. OAOA oligoastrocytoma with positive large blastic and small intermediary cells (GFAP x160).

GFA and S 100 Proteins in Low Grade Astrocytomas

B. LECHEVALIER (°), F. CHAPON (°), J.F. VIEL (°°), J.P. HOUTTEVILLE (°°°).

INTRODUCTION

Two glia specific proteins have been identified by biochimists and immunologists: the glial fibrillary acidic (GFA) protein (2, 3, 10) and the S 100 protein (13, 17, 18, 19).

Many authors have used these proteins as markers for glial tumors, specially for astrocytomas (1, 4-9, 11, 12, 16). These studies dealt with astrocytomas of all grades, from Kernohan's grade 1 to grade 4 (15) and with glioblastomas.

Some authors reported that the higher the protein content, the better differenciated the tumor was.

Whereas prognosis appears to be clearly different for low-grade versus high grade astrocytomas, it seems more difficult to anticipate the evolution of Kernohan's grade 1 and 2.

To our knowledge, a quantitative study comparing the content of GFA and S 100 proteins with the evolution of these low grade tumors has not been carried out so far. The present report studies the correlations between these immunochemistric findings and evolutive data on thirty cases of so called low grade astrocytomas.

MATERIALS AND METHODS

Selection of patients

Only patients with low grade supratentorial astrocytic tumors referred from 1973 to 1984 were selected.

Clinical and evolutive data are given in figure 1.

Methods

a - Neuropathology

Surgical specimens were fixed in 10% formalin and embedded in paraffin. Three micrometer thick sections were deparaffinized in toluene for 6 min. After rehydratation in a graded ethanol series and blockage of the endogenous peroxidase activity with hydrogen peroxide (3% in H_2O for 30 min.), immunochistochemical stainings were performed using the peroxidase antiperoxidase (PAP) method of Sternberger (20) with anti-GFAP antibody (DAKO, Santa Barbara, CA, USA) or anti-S 100 protein antibody (Courtesy of Dr C.M. Jacque, INSERM U 134, Hôpital de la Salpétrière, Paris, France). The reaction was revealed by amino ethyl carbazole.

Two criteria were chosen to quantify the GFA and S 100 protein cell content: the intensity of reaction and the percentage of stained cells. The intensity of staining was studied by grading tumors in four groups A, B, C, D. The percentage of stained cells was measured on at least three hundred cells in ten or more microscopic fields, using a X 40 objective and a X 10 ocular magnification. The fields were taken at random.

b - Statistical analysis

Kaplan-Meïer survival curves were drawn (± SD) for every group in order to relate the proportion of surviving patients to the trial time (this time was post operative survival time until death or last

(°) Laboratoire de neuropathologie; (°°) Laboratoire d'informatique médicale et d'épidémiologie; (°°°) Service de neurochirurgie, C.H.U. Côte de Nacre, 14040 Caen (France).

M. Chatel, F. Darcel and J. Pecker (eds.), Brain Oncology. ISBN-13: 978-94-010-8003-3

Case	Sex	Age	Localization	Trial Time (months)	Follow-up Status Dead (D) / Alive (A)
1	M	70	Occipital	1	D
2	M	60	Temporal	1	D
3	F	25	Temporal	6	D
4	M	57	Frontal	8	D
5	M	39	Frontal	13	D
6	F	46	Frontal-Parietal	18	A
7	M	31	Frontal	20	D
8	F	16	V3	24	A
9	F	28	Frontal	27	A
10	M	49	Parietal-Temporal	29	D
11	M	51	Frontal	30	D
12	M	25	Frontal	34	D
13	M	29	Frontal	36	D
14	F	23	Frontal	40	D
15	M	35	Parietal	41	D
16	M	40	V3	41	D
17	F	37	Frontal	43	A
18	M	45	Frontal	44	A
19	M	34	Frontal	48	A
20	F	32	Frontal	50	A
21	M	36	Frontal	57	A
22	F	23	Frontal	60	A
23	M	50	Parietal-Occipital	64	D
24	F	24	Temporal	66	D
25	F	18	Fornix	72	A
26	F	34	Temporal	72	A
27	M	26	Temporal	72	A
28	F	26	Frontal	73	A
29	F	45	Temporal	8	A
30	M	31	Frontal	96	A

FIGURE 1. Clinical and evolutive data

news). Statistical significance was assessed by a logrank test. For statistical analysis the cases were distributed into 4 groups according to the percentage of stained cells. The limits of each group were chosen in order to obtain an homogeneous distribution of cases (figure 2).

	Group	Number of cases	Percentage of stained cells
GFA	PG1	6	> 60
	PG2	8	30 to 60
	PG3	9	15 to 30
	PG4	7	< 15
S 100	Ps1	7	> 50
	Ps2	7	40 to 50
	Ps3	9	25 to 40
	Ps4	7	< 25

FIGURE 2. Percentage of stained cells. Definition of groups.

In addition we used non parametric tests :

— A Spearman test was applied to dead patients only in search of a correlation between post operative survival time and percentages of stained cells;

— a Wilcoxon test compared the percentages of stained cells between the following 2 groups: 1) patients dead within 5 years post operatively; 2) patients with 5 years or more survival time whether alive or dead;

— the intensity of staining, both for S 100 and GFAP, was compared within the same groups by means of a Yate rectified chi-square test.

RESULTS

All the data are given in figure 3.

— Survival curves obtained for each of the previously described parameters are drawn on figure 4.

The logrank test demonstrated a positive correlation between intensity of S 100 staining and survival time: X^2 3DF = 9.02, $p < 0.05$.

The comparison of groups two by two yielded significant results for:

A/D: X^2 1DF = 1.94, $p < 0.05$
A/C: X^2 1DF = 5.78, $p < 0.02$
B/C: X^2 1DF = 7.08, $p < 0.01$

No significant correlation was found between any of the three remaining parameters and survival time.

Howewer when considering the percentage of S 100 stained cells, survival time was found to be longer in groups P_S1 - P_S2 taken as a whole than in groups P_S3 - P_S4 (λ^2 1DF = 3.97, $p < 0.05$, logrank test).

Non parametric tests

— A positive correlation was found between survival length and percentage of GFA and S 100 stained cells ($p < 0.01$, Spearman test, dead patients only);

— A survival time of 5 years or more was associated with a higher percentage of S 100 stained cells ($p < 0.01$, Wilcoxon test);

— Intensity of GFA staining was positively correlated with survival time when comparing group A to the remaining cases ($2\,p < 0.05$, Yates'rectified X^2 test).

Case	GFA		S 100	
	Percentage	Intensity	Percentage	Intensity
1	12,25	B	33,90	A
2	15,65	C	21	A
3	26,60	B	32,75	B
4	16,60	D	23,40	C
5	15,40	C	19,40	D
6	16,40	C	40,80	B
7	28,90	C	32,30	B
8	13	B	62	B
9	17	B	40,50	B
10	5,50	B	41,10	A
11	66,25	B	23,90	C
12	17,55	C	23,40	C
13	11,80	C	49,35	A
14	56,30	A	50,50	A
15	71,20	C	34	D
16	3	D	27,70	D
17	17,30	C	28,80	B
18	15,40	A	46,70	A
19	41,70	A	24,10	A
20	14,60	B	21,50	B
21	37,30	C	39,60	B
22	54,60	A	45,80	B
23	52,40	B	68,50	B
24	19,70	A	32,40	A
25	64,90	B	89	A
26	3	D	53,70	B
27	72	A	33,40	A
28	74,90	A	81,60	A
29	28,30	A	41	A
30	61,60	B	65,90	B

FIGURE 3. Neuropathological data for each case.

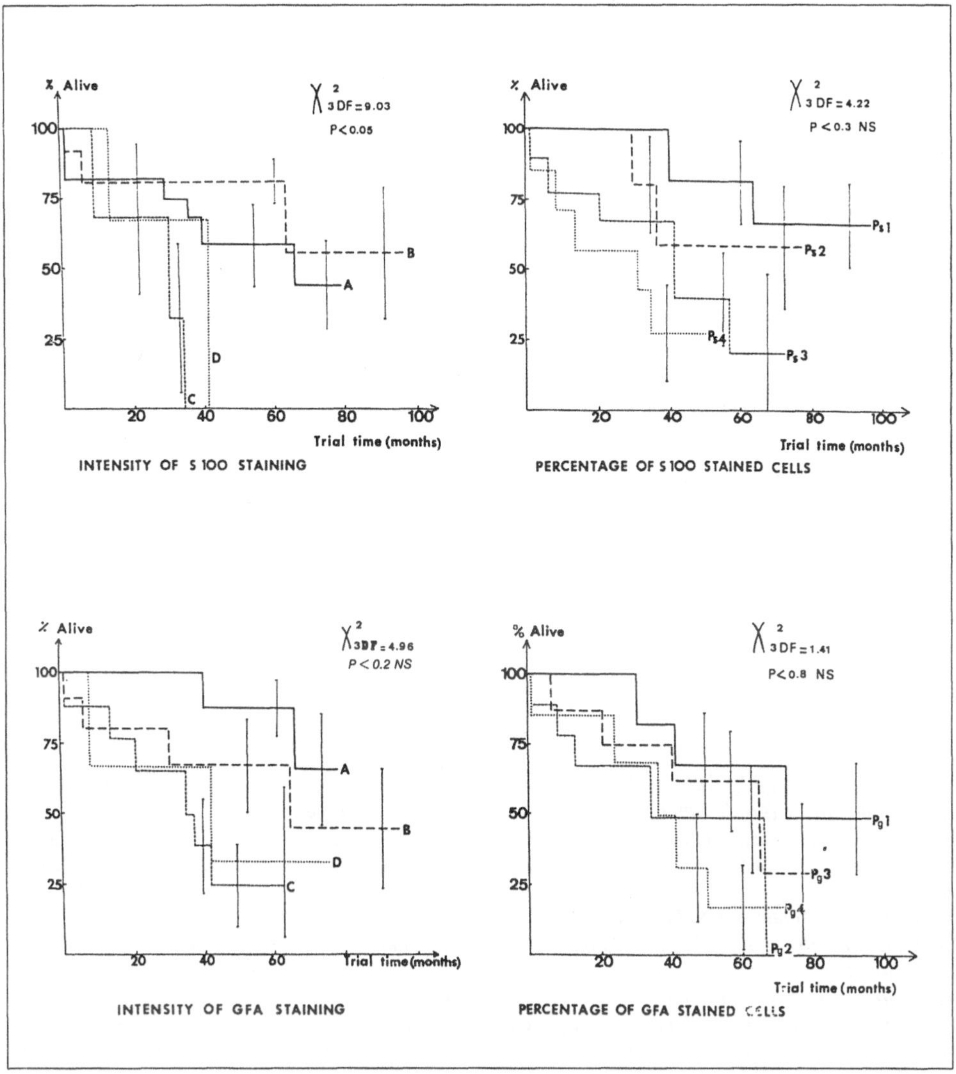

FIGURE 4. Survival curves for each parameter

DISCUSSION

Our study showed several positive correlations between GFA or S 100 proteins staining and survival times in low grade astrocytomas.

However a few points have to be discussed:

— Our material is heterogeneous for age, localization (superficial or deep seated), complete or incomplete surgical removal and for postoperative treatment (radiotherapy, and chimotherapy).

— Throughout our study, the quality of protein staining has not depended on the time of sampling, showing that these antigens were not altered by long duration paraffin embedding. Retrospective studies are thus reliable.

Futhermore, we have been counting the stained cells rather than using a colorimetric method which might have over estimated the cellular protein content by inclusion of perivascular and background staining in the measurements.

— Concerning the Kaplan Meïer survival curves, the only statistically significant result is a positive correlation between the length of survival and the intensity of S 100 protein staining. These results might be partly explained by the small size and heterogeneity of the sample, and, for some cases, by the shortness of the survey period. These drow-backs have been overcome by means of non-parametric tests.

— The results reported by others about the content of GFA and S 100 proteins concerned astrocytomas of all grades. Delpech et al. (7), Eng and Rubinstein (11) concluded there is no evident relation between the importance of the GFA protein staining and the degree of neoplasia. On the contrary, Jacque et al. (14) showed that the lower the GFAP content, the more malignant the tumor was, but they found no correlation for the S 100 protein. However Haglid et al. (12) reported that rates of soluble S 100 Protein in 12 astroglial tumors decreased with shorter post operative survival time. Dohan et al. (8) found only a very weak positive correlation for S 100 protein on their 14 cases of astrocytomas and glioblastomas. These authors explained these results by the greater heterogeneity of their material (10 glioblastomas and only 4 astrocytomas) with a median survival time of 6,5 months (24 months for the patients of Haglid et al.). Morever, in glioblastomas, data may be biased by microscopic areas of necrosis or hemorrhage even if macroscopic necrotic or hemorrhagic portions were cut away before analysis. For this reason we chose to work on histologic slides and to directly count stained cells instead of using colorimetric method.

CONCLUSION

This preliminary work has demonstrated positive correlations between GFA or S 100 protein staining and survival times in low grade astrocytomas.

These methods seem to allow a more accurate evaluation of prognosis and need further investigations.

SUMMARY

The content of GFA and S 100 proteins was determined in thirty cases of supratentorial so-called low grade astrocytomas (grade I and II according to Kernohan's classification).

For this purpose, we used an immunoperoxidasic method suitable for "routinely processed" tissue on paraffin sections. Both the staining intensity and the number of stained astrocytes were analysed for various fields.

The data were compared with both the histological type and the clinical evolution.

Preliminary results indicated often strong GFA protein staining without correlation with the evolution and histological types.

On the other hand, we found a positive relationship between the S 100 protein staining and the length of evolution: cases with a more than five year post operative survey showed the most important staining. The lowest staining was observed in cases with a lower than forty month post operative survey. The intensity of S 100 staining seems to provide a valuable indication for the prognosis of low grade astrocytomas.

KEY WORDS

Immunocytochemistry, Histopathology Markers, Differentiation, Grading.

REFERENCES

1. BENDA (P.) (1968): Protéine S-100 et tumeurs humaines. Rev. Neurol. 118, 368-372.
2. BIGNAMI (A.), ENG (L.F.), DAHL (D.), UYEDA (C.T.) (1973): Localization of the glial fibrillary acidic protein in astrocytes by immunofluorescence. Brain Res. 43, 429-435.
3. BIGNAMI (A.), DAHL (D.) (1977): Specificity of the glial fibrillary acidic protein for astroglia. J. Histochem. Cytochem. 25, 466-469.
4. CONLEY (F.K.) (1979): The immunocytochemical localization of GFA Protein in Experimental Murine CNS Tumors. Acta Neuropathol. (Berl.), 45, 9-16.

5. DECK (J.H.), ENG (L.F.), BIGBEE (J.) (1976): A preliminary study of glioma morphology using the peroxidase-antiperoxidase immunohistological method for glial fibrillary acidic protein. J. Neuropath. Exp. Neurol., 35, 362.

6. DECK (J.H.), ENG (L.F.), BIGBEE (J.), WOODCOCK (S.M.) (1978): The role of glial fibrillary acidic protein in the diagnosis of central nervous system tumors. Acta Neuropathologica (Berl.), 42, 183-190.

7. DELPECH (B.), DELPECH (A.), VIDARD (M.N.), GIRARD (N.), TAYOT (J.), CLEMENT (J.C.), CREISSARD (P.) (1978): Glial fibrillary acidic protein in tumors of the nervous system. Br. J. Cancer 37, 33-40.

8. DOHAN (F.C.), KORNBLITH (P.L.), WELLUM (G.R.), PFEIFFER (S.E.), LEVINE (L.) (1977): S-100 Protein and 2', 3' -Cyclic Nucleotide 3'-Phosphohydrolase in Human Brain Tumors. Acta Neuropathol. (Berl.) 40, 123-128.

9. DUFFY (P.E.), GRAF (L.), RAPPORT (M.M.) (1977): Identification of glial fibrillary acidic protein by the immunoperoxidase method in human brain tumors. J. Neuropath. Exp. Neurol. 36, 645-652.

10. ENG (L.F.), VANDERHAEGHEN (J.J.), BIGNAMI (A.), GERSTL (B.) (1971): An acidic protein isolated from fibrous astrocytes. Brain Res. 28, 351-354.

11. ENG (L.F.), RUBINSTEIN (L.) (1978): Contribution of immunohistochemistry to diagnostic problems of human cerebral tumors. J. Histochem. Cytochem. 26, 513-523.

12. HAGLID (K.G.), STRAVROU (D.), RONNBACK (L.), CARLISSON (C.A.), WEIDENBACH (W.) (1973): The S-100 protein in water-soluble and pentanol-extractable forms in normal human brain and tumors of the human nervous system: A quantitative study. J. Neurol. Sci. 20, 103-111.

13. HYDEN (H.), MCEWEN (N.) (1966): A glial protein specific for the nervous system. Proc. Nat. Acad. Sci. 55, 354-358.

14. JACQUE (C.M.), KUJAS (M.), POREAU (A.), RAOUL (M.), COLLIER (P.), RACADOT (J.), BAUMANN (N.) (1979): GFA and S-100 Protein levels as an index for malignancy in human gliomas and neurinomas. J. Natl. Cancer Inst. 62, 479-483.

15. KERNOHAN (J.W.), SAYRE (G.P.) (1952): Tumors of the central nervous system. Fascicule 35, Atlas of Tumor Pathology Washington: Armed Forces Institutes of Pathology (AFIP).

16. MAUNOURY (R.), DELPECH (A.), DELPECH (B.), VIDARD (M.N.), VEDRENNE (C.), CONSTANS (J.P.), HILLEREAU (J.) (1977): Localisation de la protéine gliofibrillaire (GFAP) par immunocytochimie dans les tumeurs cérébrales humaines. Neuro-Chirurgie 23, 173-185.

17. MOORE (B.W.) (1965): A soluble protein characteristic of the nervous system. Biochemical and biophysical research communications 19, 739-744.

18. MOORE (B.W.) (1972): Chemistry and biology of two proteins S-100 and 14-3-2, specific to the nervous system. International review of Neurobiology 15, 215-225.

19. PFEIFFER (S.E.), HERSCHMAN (H.R.), LIGHTBODY (J.) and SATO (G.V.) (1970): Synthesis by a clonal line of rat glial cell of a protein unique to the nervous system. J. Cell. Physiol. 75, 329-339.

20. STERNBERGER (L.A.) and CUCULIS (J.J.) (1969): Method for enzymatic intensification of the immuno cytochemical reaction without use of labelled antibodies. J. Histochem. Cytochem. 17, 190.

Intermediate Filaments in Fresh Frozen Tissue in Neuro-Oncology - About a Series of 1000 Peroperative Biopsies -

Y. KRIVOSIC (1), M. JOMIN (2), J.L. CHRISTIAENS (3), P. DHELLEMMES (4), G. COMBELLES (3), F. LESOIN (2), G. LOZES (2), L. VILETTE (2), J.P. LEJEUNE (3), T. DUPARD (3), S. BLOND (3), A. AUTRIQUE (2), H. REYFORD (5), A. DUPONT (1).

Intermediate filaments represent a class of identical ultra-structure (intracellular filaments 70-100 Angström in diameter), yet biologically different according to their cell of origin, thus allowing the production of specific sera and monoclonal antibodies for their identification by histoimmunological technique (LAZARIDES E. 1980).

Previous studies have established the specificity of intermediate antifilament sera and monoclonal antibody for different types of tumours. Specific sera and monoclonal antibody: keratin for epithelial tumours; vimentin for mesenchymatous tumours; desmin for muscle tumours; GFAP for astrocytic tumours and neurofilaments for neuronal tumours.

ALTMANNSBERGER M., OSBORN M., SCHUER A. (1981); CORSON J.M., PINKUS G.S. (1982); DAHL D. (1982); DECK J.H.N. (1978); DENK H. (1983); DUFFY Ph. E., GRAF L., RAPPORT M.M. (1977); DUFFY Ph. E. (1979); ESPINOZA C.G., AZAR H.A. (1982); GABIANI G. (1981); LEHTO V.P. (1983); PASQUIER B. (1983); VAN DER MEULEN J.D.M., HOUTHOFF H.J., EBELS E.J. (1978); VELASCO M.E. (1980).

On the other hand, the results of histoimmunological studies can be verified by confrontation with studies under the electron microscope as far as quality and type of distribution of intermediate filament is concerned. We have combined histoimmunological studies of serum and monoclonal antibodies specific to intermediate filaments (prokeratin; GFAP; vimentin; protein originating from neurofilament 70 K, 160 K, 210 K, desmin) on fresh frozen tissue section and cytology of fresh crushed tissue as well as classical histopathology and electron microscopy.

The latter have been completed in typical and special cases by a histoimmunological study of serial semi-thin section in order to correlate between amount, mode of distribution of filaments under electron microscope with the intensity and nature of histoimmunological reactions.

The histoimmunological reactions have been performed in series of a dozen cases together with controls for serum and monoclonal antibody as well as for variety of cells. The tests were performed in parallel with positive and negative controls and included a study of the aspect and intensity of the histoimmunological reaction. The characteristics of the histoimmunological reactions on the cells concerns on one hand the surface of the cells which were positive (whole surface or part of the surface being positive) and on the other hand the aspects of this reaction. We have identified a homogenous dense reaction (example: GFAP on certain bodies and astrocytic projections); a cotton wool appareance; motted or reticular (example: vimentin on a meningioma). The intensity of the reaction is expressed with respect to controls: 4+ intensity corresponds to a maximal reaction obtained and realised on controls whose cytoplasm was completly filled with intermediate filaments; 3+ intensity corresponds to 3/4 (75 %) of the maximal intensity; 2+ corresponds to 1/2 (50 %) of the maxima intensity; 1+ corresponds to a histoimmunological reaction less than 2+ but always clearcut.

Doubtful reactions are quantified 0.1+ to 0.9+; our subjective quantification was controlled by photometry. The quantification and the aspect of the reaction give an idea, histoimmunologically, of the ultrastructural distribution of intermediate filaments.

(1) Laboratoire de Neuropathologie (Chef de Service : Prof. A. DUPONT). (2) Service de Neurochirurgie B (Chef de Service : Prof. M. JOMIN). (3) Service de Neurochirurgie A (Chef de Service : Prof. J.-L. CHRISTIAENS. (4) Service de Neurochirurgie C (Chef de Service : Prof. P. DHELLEMMES. (5) Service d'Anesthésie A (Chef de Service : Prof. R. KRIVOSIC-HORBER), Hôpital B, C.H.U. Lille.

M. Chatel, F. Darcel and J. Pecker (eds.), Brain Oncology. ISBN-13: 978-94-010-8003-3

Using this technique, we have been able to identify:

1. **Cells or part of typical cells rich in intermediate filaments, with selective histoimmunological reactions** (normal fibrillar astrocytes, reactionnal and neoplasic astrocytes, axons, certains dystrophic neurons, fibrocytes, metastasis of malpighian epithelioma differenciated rhabdosarcoma cells). All the histoimmunological techniques allowed the identification of the type of intermediate filaments by reaction to specific sera and monoclonal antibody (anti-keratin, anti-vimentin, anti-GFAP, anti-neurofilament, anti-desmine). Certains specific anti-GFAP sera give rise to a weaker reaction on frozen tissue than an formalin fixed and paraffin embeded tissue. This technique allows a good visualisation of the cells by identification, of cells body and extensions. The shape of cells body together with the existence of irregulary intricated projections were suggestive of the degree of malignancy (very malignant cells had more irregular projections which were more hapfazardly intricated). In others circumstances, the shape of the cells allowed the identification of cells due to a reactionnal gliosis characterised by cells with fine and regular projections (example: identification of reactional gliosis in a malignant lymphoma facilitates its differenciation with a malignant glial tumour in which the neoplastic cells had more irregularly intricated projections). Cells rich in intermediate filaments were identified even if necrotic.
2. **Typical cells rich in intermediate filaments identified by complex histoimmunological reactions combined a positive reaction to two or more sera** (meningiomas, schwannomas, certain fibrillar astrocytes, certain astrocytomas, certain neuronal cells, certain epithelial cells and certain mesenchymatous cells). This combined reaction sems to correspond to varied conditions:

   a. The most frequent association being a positive reaction to anti-vimentin serum combined with another intermediate anti-filament sera (GFAP, neurofilaments, keratine, desmine). The positive histoimmunological reaction to anti-vimentine sera is observed in all varieties of tumours. Sometimes it is stronger than the reaction to specific filament sera of the cells concerned (example: certain astrocytomas were more strongly positive on the frozen sample to anti-vimentine specific sera than to anti GFAP serum). In certain cases the positive reaction to anti-vimentine specific sera did not arise in the same part of the cells or the same neoplastic cells than that of the intermediate filament specific of this type of cells. In other cases a positive reaction existed in the same cells with however a different aspect. If a positive reaction to anti-vimentine specific sera does not permit to eliminate a particular type of cell, its absence in cells rich in intermediate filaments permits the elimination of a mesenchymatous origin.

   b. Association in a metaplastic tendendy. Several glioblastomas give rise to change of a malpighian type positive to anti-keratin specific sera.

   c. Association in cells ontogenetically related. Example: schwannomas and meningiomas cells were often positive to serum specific for glial cells (GFAP) and to anti-vimentine specific sera. Certains gliomas showed to crossed reactions with anti-neurofilaments specific sera (filaments specific of nervous cells). These reactions were often of weak intensity and existed only on fresh frozen tissue.

   d. Crossed reactions in cells ontogenetically different. Example: cells of chondromas, chordomas, mixed parotid tumours, giant cells tumours of bone were often positive to anti-vimentine specific sera as well as anti-neurofilaments and anti-gliofilaments specific sera. These cells were rich in intermediate filaments and we could raise the biochemical question as to whether this positivity did not correspond to common biochemical sequences of different intermediate filaments. The other interpretation concerns the possibility of existence of several types of filaments in the same type of cells. The reactions make one wonder whether the increase in the number of immunised animals and monoclonal antibodies could allow the production of more specific sera. In case of university research the cost of production does not allow the possibility of multiplication. In practice, these features implies that the verification of sera does not only entail immuno-absorption test and their typing on immunoblot but also on specific controls. Before using the serum produced by us, we have tested it on samples of every organ of the human body as well.
3. **Atypical cells without a hint as to their origin, on histopathological examination, but rich in intermediate filaments at electron microscopy and positive to several specific sera** and intermediate antifilaments monoclonal antibody.

Some of the reactions to sera and monoclonal antibodies were present only with fresh frozen tissue whereas those fixed and paraffin embedded tissue did not react with the same specific sera and monoclonal antibodies. The interpretation of this situation is delicate for it may concern on one hand sera and antibodies highly specific to a site strongly characteristic of an intermediate filament only accessible on frozen tissues, and on the other hand of a positive reaction on frozen tissue in relation to a non specific site on a given intermediate filament. This latter situation is therefore delicate as it may entail altered cellular structures, reduced to a mass of filamentous structures to which the antibody can link. Sometimes the absence of certain reactions on paraffin fixed tissue allows an easier identification of the type of cell. For example, certain undifferenciated astrocytomas had cell bodies and projections highly positive to anti-vimentin sera on fresh frozen tissue whereas this reaction was weakly positive on fixed tissue, but nevertherless gave a clearcut positive reaction to characteristic antifilament serum to gliofilament (antiGFAP). An electron microscopic examination is required in such cases. It is the combination of results obtained by different techniques which permits the diagnosis to be established.

4. **Atypical cells poor in intermediate filaments.**
It concerns cells whose identification is not possible by classical histopathological examination (certain undifferenciated small cells astrocytomas, undifferenciated oligodendrogliomas, undifferenciated ependymomas, metastases with undifferenciated small cells, certain neuroblastomas). Histoimmunological reaction to anti-protein specific sera to intermediate filaments are positive only on fresh unfixed tissue which is rapidly frozen (delay between sampling and freezing less than 30 mn). These reactions are often weak (0.1+ to 0.5+) and of delicate interpretation specially as far as artefacts are concerned. They are however useful and indicate an origin. Electron microscopic examination were performed in these cases. The combination of features obtained by histoimmunological study and electron microscopy allowed a more rational interpretation rather than a simple classic histo-pathological examination.

5. **Atypical cells devoid of intermediate filaments on ultrastructural examination, negative to reaction with serum of intermediate filament proteins.**
These cases represent the limitation of this technique. Ultrastructural examination concerning the search for a type of organite or group of organites permits sometimes in similar cases a more realistic approach of the diagnosis.

6. **False positive**
   a) Intracellular false positive
   Intracellular false positive concerns cytoplasmic structures which adhere or absorp specific antibodies on normal and altered structures. The adhesion to intracellular normal structures concerns nucleus and cytoplasmic fibrillar proteins Altered intracellular filamentous structures are of varied composition and origin.
   They include:
   — denatured intermediate filaments clumped together,
   — filamentous material originating from degraded nucleus,
   — filamentous material originating from degraded mitochondrias,
   — filamentous material originating from degraded endoplasmic reticulum.

Compared to the absorption in irregular lumps on necrosed cells, the absorption on degraded filamentous structures can present as regular shapes difficult to distinghuish from a true reaction. Comparative study under electron microscopy allowed in such cases to verify structures responsible for the positive reactions.

   b) Extracellular false positive
   The adhesion of polyvalent sera antibodies and certain monoclonal antibodies were observed in two types of circumstances on differents types of non altered collagen fibres and in relation with altered collagen fibers including sometimes cellular debris.
   — non altered collagen fibers.
   Collagen fibers absorbing sera or (and) giving to crossed reactions were more often fine protocollagen fibers observed in meningiomas, schwannomas, myxomas, chordomas, chondromas, bony tumours, mixed parotid tumours. One can wonder whether part of this

adherence of specific sera antibody does not correspond to true crossed histoimmunological reactions with sites common to the interstitial filamentous proteines of collagen and intermediate intracellular filaments.

— altered collagen fibers.

Another situation concerns adhesion to dissociating collagenous fibers which becomes larger than normal and separated in elemantary units. In this circumstance, the denatured collagen is often associated with fragments of cell debris which represent a mechanical absorption substratum identified by its irregular spoted aspect.

7. **Histometry**

Instantaneous freezing does not alter, contrary to fixation and embedding, cerebral and tumoral tissue sampling, and permits the realisation of comparative histometric studies concerning cells, projections of cells and vessels. Histoimmunological reaction allowed precise histometric studies particulary, comparative studies between normal brain tissue, non tumoral pathological brain tissue, cerebral tissue starting to be invaded by tumors and different stages of neoplastic invasion. The extent of invasion is expressed as a percentage of surface occupied by tumoral cells. In all stages of invasion we can study quantitatively and qualitatively the normal cerebral tissue and its remnants more clearly identified by histochemical than classical histopathological techniques.

GENERAL CONCLUSION

We have combined the histoimmunological studies of serum and monoclonal antibodies specific of intermediate filaments (prokeratin, GFAP, Vimentin, proteins of neurofilaments 70 K, 160 K, 210 K, Desmine) on fresh frozen tissue sections and cytology of fresh smeared tissue with the electron microscopic study and histoimmunological study on semi-thin serial sections which permitted a correlation between quantity, aspect of distribution of filaments under electron microscopy, with the intensity and aspects of histoimmunological reactions.

Using this technique, we have been able to identify:

1. Cells or parts of typical cells rich in intermediate filaments, with selective histoimmunological reactions.
2. Typical cells rich in intermediate filaments characterized by complex histoimmunological reactions combining positivity to 2 or more sera.
3. Atypical cells with a hint of their origin at histopathological examination, but rich in intermediate filaments under electron microscope and positive to several specific sera and intermediate antifilaments monoclonal antibodies.
4. Atypical cells poor in intermediate filaments.
5. Atypical cells deprived of intermediate filaments at ultrastructural examination, negative to reactions with sera of proteins of intermediate filaments.

Histoimmunological study of proteins of the cytoskeleton associated with other histochemical techiques has modified the analysis of lesions in neuro-oncology. These features have however not transformed histopathological examination into chemical examination, but the features of the histochemical study has considerably widen the possibilities of histopathological interpretation of neuro-oncological lesions.

KEY WORDS

Histopathology, Immunocytochemistry Markers, Differentiation references.

REFERENCES

1. ALTMANNSBERGER (M.), OSBORN (M.), SCHUER (A.): Antibodies to different intermediate filament proteins: Cell type-specific markers on paraffin embedded human tissues. Lab. Invest. **41**: 427-434 (1981).

2. CORSON (J.M.), PINKUS (G.S.): Mesothelioma: Profile of Keratin proteins and Carcinoembryonic Antigen An Immunoperoxydase study of 20 cases and comparison with Pulmonary Adenocarcinomas. Am. J. Pathol. 1982, **108**: 80-88 (1982).

3. DAHL (D.), CHI (N.H.), MILES (L.E.), NGUYEN (B.T.) and BIGNAMI (A.): Glial Fibrillary Acidic (GFA) Protein in Schwann Cells: Fact or Artifact? The Journal of Histochemistry and Cytoch., **30**: 912-918 (1982).

4. DECK (J.H.N.) ENG (L.F.), BIGBEE and WOODCOCK (S.M.): The Role of Glial Fibrillary Acidic Protein in the Diagnosis of Central Nervous System Tumors. Acta Neuropath. **42**: 183-190 (1978).

5. DENK (H.), KREPLER (R.), ARTLIEB (V.), GABIANI (G.), RUNGGER-BRANDLE (E.), LEONCINI (P.), G. FRANK (W.): Proteins of Intermediate Filaments. An Immunohistochemical and Biochemical Approach to the Classification of Soft tissue tumors. American Journ. Path.: **110**: 193-208 (1983).

6. DUFFY (Ph. E.), GRAF (L.), RAPPORT (M.M.): Identification of glial fibrillary acidic protein by the immunoperoxydase method in human brain tumors. Journal Neuropath & Exp. Neurol. **36**: 645-662 (1977).

7. DUFFY (Ph. E.), GRAF (L.), HUANG (Y.) Y and RAPPORT (M.M.): Glial fibrillary acidic protein in ependymomas and other brain tumors. Journal of Neurological Sciences, **40**: 133-146 (1979).

8. ESPINOZA (C.G.), AZAR (H.A.): Immunohistochemical localisation of Keratin-Type Proteins in Epithelial Neoplasms. Am. J. Clin. Path. **78**: 500-506 (1982).

9. GABIANI (G.), KAPANCI (Y.), BARAZZON (Ph.), FRANK (W.). Immunochemical Identification of Intermediate Sized Filaments in Human Neoplastic cells. A Diagnostic Aid for the Surgical Pathologist. Am. J. Pathol. **104**: 206-216 (1981).

10. LAZARIDES (E.): Intermediate filaments as mechanical integrators of cellular space. Nature **283**: 249-256 (1980).

11. LEHTO (V.P.), VIRTANEN (I.), MIETTINEN (M.), DAHL (D.), KAHRI (A.): Neurofilaments in Adrenal and Extra-adrenal Pheochromocytoma Arch Pathol. Lab. Med. **107**: 492-494 (1983).

12. PASQUIER (B.), LACHARD (A.), PASQUIER (D.), COUDERC (P.), DELPECH (B.), COUREL (M.N.): Proteine gliofibrillaire acide (GFA) et tumeurs nerveuses centrales. Etude immunohistochimique d'une série de 207 cas. Ann. Pathol. **3**: 127-135 (1983).

13. VAN DER MEULEN (J.D.M.), HOUTHOFF (H.J) and EBELS (E.J.): Glial Fibrillary Acidic Protein in human gliomas Neuropath. & Applied Neurob. **4**: 177-190 (1978).

14. VELASCO (M.E.), DAHL (D.), ROESSMANN (U.), GAMBETTI (P.): Immunohistochemical Localisation of Glial Fibrillary Acidic Protein in Human Glial Neoplasms. Cancer **45**: 484-494 (1980).

FIGURE 1

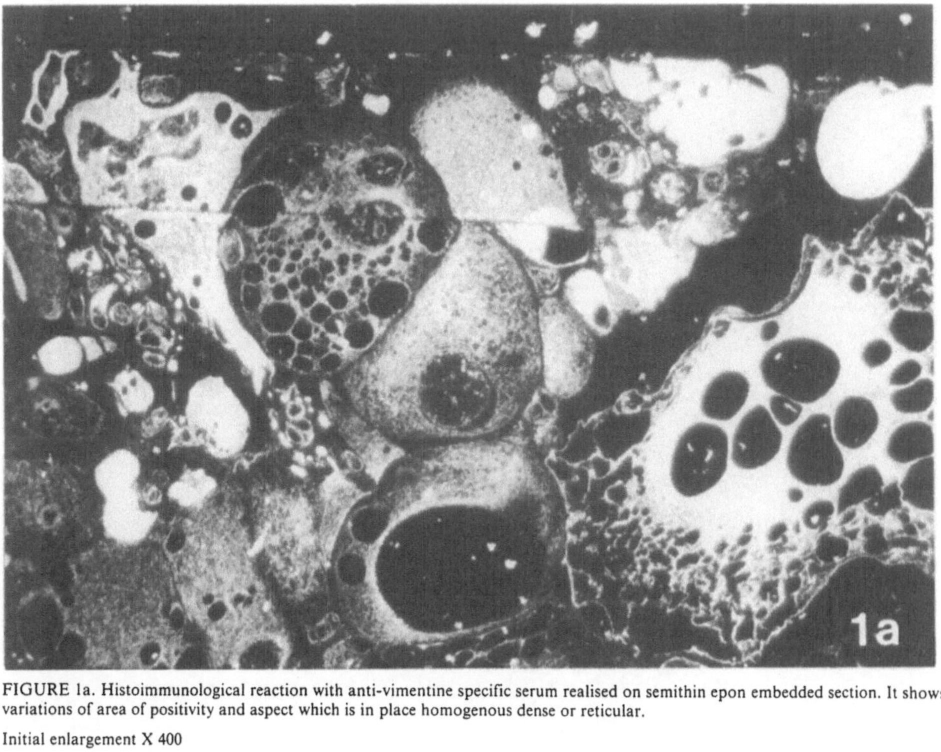

FIGURE 1a. Histoimmunological reaction with anti-vimentine specific serum realised on semithin epon embedded section. It shows variations of area of positivity and aspect which is in place homogenous dense or reticular.

Initial enlargement X 400

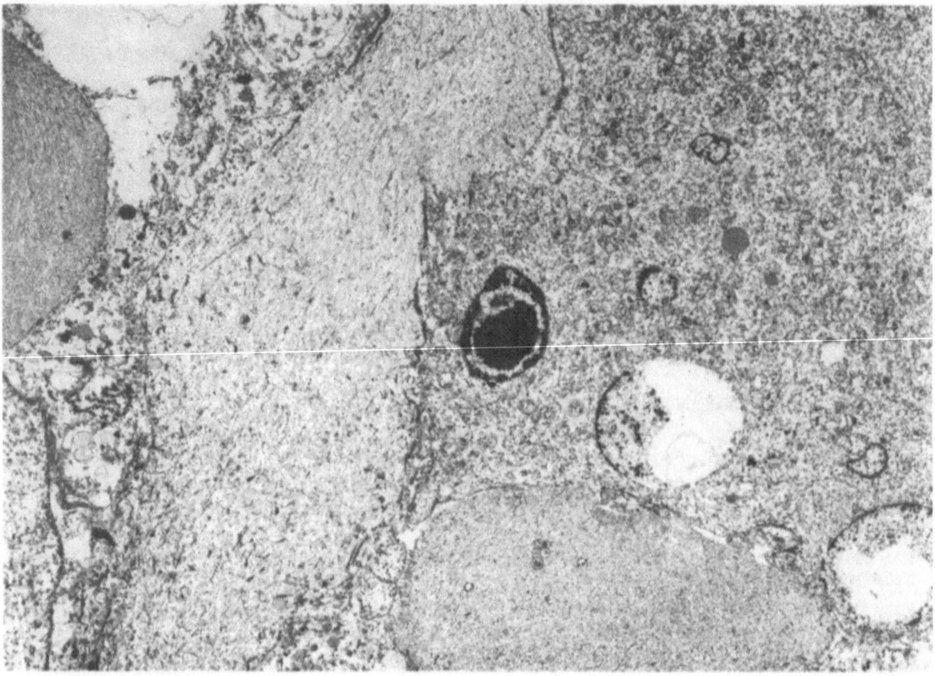

FIGURE 1b. Electron microscopical examination shows serial section of the same specimens as 1a. Some cells contain intermediate filaments densely packed while in others these filaments are rarefied.

Glutamine Synthetase, a Marker of an Astroglial Subpopulation in Mouse Brain

M. TARDY (°), C. FAGES (°), M. KHELI (°), B. ROLLAND (°).

The elucidation of the molecular mechanism of brain detoxification is an important neurochemical problem. Ammonia neutralization in brain is performed by astrocytes through the effect of an enzyme directly implicated in glutamate metabolism: glutamine synthetase (GS) (L-glutamate-ammonia ligase, ADP-forming, EC 6.3.1.2.). Glutamine is formed from glutamate and is a diffusible molecule that can be released directly by astrocytes. GS is subject to a variety of control mechanisms in bacterial (1). In mammalian cells, hormonal regulation of GS has been shown in liver cells (2, 3), in chick retina (4), and, more recently, in astrocytes (5-7). GS activity in brain was immunochemically restricted to astrocytes (8, 9), but in astrocytic primary cultures the assay of GS-specific activity did not reflect preferential localization. Two possibilities may exist:

1. The astrocytic population considered is not evenly implicated in glutamine formation from glutamate.
2. Other factors are implicated in GS reactivity which are absent in cell cultures.

To elucidate this problem, we studied the development of GS activity and immunolabelling in primary astroglial cultures from four mouse brain areas: Cerebral Hemispheres (CH), Cerebellum (Ce), Medulla Oblongata (MO) and Olfactory bulbs (OB).

MATERIALS AND METHODS

Primary cultures highly enriched in astrocytes were obtained as previously described (10) by mechanical dissociation of newborn mouse brain areas. For the study of the action of hormonal and other effectors, cells were switched 48 h before cell harvesting to standard growth medium supplemented with the given concentration of each effector. Cell homogenates were obtained after cell harvesting with a rubber policeman and sonication (2 × 15 s) at 4 °C.

Brain homogenates were prepared from freshly sacrificed mice as previously described (5). Enzyme assay was performed according to the very sensitive and specific method developed by Pishak and Phillips (12), with slight modifications as mentioned in a previous report (5).

For immunofluorescence staining, cells were fixed directly on Corning plastic dishes with cold methanol (-20 °C) for 10 min., washed twice with 10 ml phosphate-buffered saline (PBS) for 5 min., and incubated in a humidified chamber (30 min., room temperature) successively with 50 μl GS antiserum (1:50 with PBS) or rabbit preimmune serum as control (1:50) and fluorescein-labeled goat antirabbit IgG (1:50 dilution). After each incubation step, the cells were washed twice in PBS (10 min., room temperature). Finally, they were washed with deionized water air-dried, and round pieces of plastic plates were mounted on microscopic slides. After sealing, the preparations were viewed in a Leitz fluorescence microscope (oil-immersed, phase contrast objective, final magnification X 800).

RESULTS

Characterization of Astroglial Primary Cultures

Astroglial cells obtained in our laboratory have been biochemically well characterized (10, 14, 15). They are highly enriched in protoplasmic-like astrocytes as well as in fibrous-like cells according to classical morphological criteria. They still contain darker bipolar cells which appear later in development (12th day *in vitro*) and myelin basic protein (MBP), an oligodendrocytic marker present in myelin. About 85% of the cells are glial fibrillary acidic protein (GFAP)-positive (an astrocyte marker) (Fig. 1A) in the four areas cultures.

(°) INSERM U 282, Hôpital Henri-Mondor, 94010 Créteil - France.

M. Chatel, F. Darcel and J. Pecker (eds.), Brain Oncology. ISBN-13: 978-94-010-8003-3

Glutamine synthetase activity

GS activity in the four area homogenates show some heterogeneity. The highest specific activity was found in the OB area during the whole postnatal developmental period and the lowest in the MO.

Considering astroglial cell extracts from the corresponding brain areas, CH cells present the highest activity whereas OB cells seemed to need different additional factors to reach its homogenate equivalent.

GS activity increased all over postnatal development in both, brain homogenates and cell cultures, but at various degrees depending the area considered.

Effect of hydrocortisone on GS activity

In the presence of lμM hydrocortisone for 48h, GS activity was increased in astroglial cultures. This increase could be due either to the activation of enzyme or to synthesis of more enzyme protein. Exposure to cycloheximide (lμM) an inhibitor of the protein synthesis, decreased both the protein content and the GS activity in all areas astrocytes. These results showed that the GS activity increase, requires de novo protein synthesis. GS induction was heterogenous and varied with the area considered and with the stage of development of the cells (Table I). In presence of the hormone, GS specific activity reached and overpassed the corresponding activity of the brain area homogenate in CH, Ce and MO but not in OB.

TABLE I

Glutamine synthetase (GS) specific activity during postnatal development

	7 days			18 days			30 days		
BRAIN AREA	H	C_c	C_I	H	C_c	C_I	H	C_c	C_I
Cerebral hemispheres	6±1	6±0.8	12±1.3	12±2	12±2	15±2	12±1	12±1	20±2
Cerebellum	3±0.5	3±0.8	3±1	8±0.5	8±1	10±1.3	9±1	10±1	20±3
Modulla oblongata	6±1	2±0.1	6±1	10±1	5±0.5	18±1	11±2	8±1	15±2
Olfactory bulbs	12±2	4±1	4±1	18±1	6±1	15±2	20±3	8±2.2	12±1

H = brain homogenates; C_c = astroglial (from control) cultures extracts; C_I = astroglial (from lμM hydrocortisone induced) cultures extracts. Results are expressed as nmoles/min/mgP. Mean ±SEM (n = 4-6).

GS immunohistochemical analysis

GS labeling has been performed using a polyclonal antibody raised in rabbit from pig brain purified GS. This antiserum was monospecific and cross-reacted with the mouse antigen.

GS positivity of the cells appeared as soon as 7 days *in vitro*. At that period large clusters of protoplasmic-like (type I) astroblasts were labeled. Labeling was diffuse and dispersed in the cell cytoplasm however showing a denser intensity in the perinuclear area of the cell. During *in vitro* development, the number of GS positive cells increased and the intensity of these labeled cells reached an optimum between 20 and 30 days *in vitro*. At that period, we observed a net heterogeneity in the number of GS labeled cells compared with the number of GFA labeled cells. While about 85%-90% of the astroglial cultures appeared GFA-positive only 50 to 60% of the cells were GS-positive and here too, an heterogeneity was observed depending the considered area.

Double labeling experiments using a goat polyclonal GFA antibody and the rabbit GS antiserum showed that, at maturation, there exist at least two types of "protoplasmic-like" astrocytes in culture, one which express both GFA and GS and another which do not express GS (Fig. 1_B).

DISCUSSION

Brain areas primary cultures were developped from postnatal mouse Cerebral Hemispheres (CH), Cerebellum (Ce), Olfactory Bulbs (OB) and Medulla (MO). The cultures were highly enriched in astroglial cells since about 85-90% of these cells express GFA, an astroglial marker. These cells reach a morphological apparent maturation between 21 and 30 days *in vitro*. This model has been used to study GS activity development and inductibility by hydrocortisone in the four brain astrocyte cultures.

The regulation of GS has been studied in various tissues, such as retina, fibroblasts, hepatomas, and astroglial cells. In all these mammalian cells, GS is a strategic target for hormonal regulation of nitrogen metabolism. Glucocorticoids induced de novo synthesis of GS in all cells studied, but the hormonal induction was modulated by various factors. In retina, induction is totally dependent on the histotypic cell association (4). In adipocytes, cyclic nucleotides and insulin modulate this induction. In astrocytes obtained in primary cultures from different brain areas, GS induction was dependent on the age of the cells and on the area investigated.

GS labeling showed an heterogeneity between the various areas and in a given area, between the astroglial population.

Distinct subpopulations of astrocytes with characteristic biochemical properties have been described (16). In the present study, we found that astrocytes, even within the same brain region differ so that some of them are capable to express both the glial fibrillary acidic protein and the glutamine synthetase protein and some of them only express GFA.

Finally, GS appeared as a protein marker of a subpopulation of astrocytes. Immunohistochemical observations confirmed the rather protoplasmic nature of the GS-labeled cells. This family of cells could have the capacity either of ammoniac detoxication and/or of aminoacid transmitter metabolism and could be correlated to subareas enriched in GABA ergic or Glutamatergic terminals in situ.

SUMMARY

Glutamine synthetase (GS) catalyzes the synthesis of glutamine from glutamate and ammonium ions. GS was found to be localized in the glial cells in the brain. This work involves determination of GS activity and of GS immunolabeling in primary cultures from 4 specific mouse brain areas: cerebral hemispheres (CH), cerebellum (Ce), olfactory bulbs (OB) and medulla oblongata (MO). The purpose was to evaluate whether astroglial cells were able to express differences concerning this functional parameter and whether such differences were affected by the time in culture, by the genetic program of the cells or by the cellular interactions.

Highly enriched astroglial primary cultures present a GS activity which appears early in the four considered areas. CH showed the highest specific activity at 7DIV whereas the MO appeared as the area where GS activity was the lowest at that stage of development. Glucocorticoids were abble to induce GS activity particularly in CH and MO. GS activity reached its optimum values between 18DIV and 30DIV and the glucocorticoid stimulation was effective all over the culture period, but at various degrees depending on the considered areas.

Indirect single or double labeling with GS or GFA antisera showed:

1) *that most GS-labeled cells were type I (protoplasmic-like) astrocytes with two major aspects. One flat epithelioid-like cell and a more elongated, denser, smaller, process bearing cell type,*
2) *that in all the four area cultures the number of GFA-labeled cells was higher than the GS-stained cells,*
3) *that it exists at least two populations of astroglial type I astrocytes* in vitro. *One which expresses both GS and GFA and another type which only expresses GFA.*

GS has been localized in astroglial cells during postnatal development. The GS activity has been suggested to reflect a maturation of the neuron-astrocytic interaction in the metabolism of Aa neurotransmitter. When GABA or Glutamate are released from the nerve terminals, they are taken up into astroglial cells where they can be converted into glutamine by GS. Differences in GS activity and in the number of GS-stained cells between the brain areas might strengthen the idea of an astroglial heterogeneity which can be determined either by the genetic program of the cells, or/and by cellular contacts, and/or humoral factors.

KEY WORDS

Glutamine synthetase, Astroglia, Markers, Glia.

REFERENCES

1. GINSBURG (A.), STADTMAN (E.R.): Regulation of glutamine synthetase in E. Coli. In: Prusiner (S.), Stadtman (E.R.), eds. The enzymes of glutamine metabolism. New York: Academic Press, 1973, 9-43.
2. KULKA (R.G.), COHEN (H.): Regulation of glutamine synthetase activity of hepatoma tissue culture cells by glutamine and dexamethasone. J. Biol. Chem. 1973, 248-6738-48.
3. CROOK (R.B.), LONIE (M.), DENEL (T.F.), TOMKINS (G.M.): Regulation of glutamine synthetase by dexamethasone in hepatoma tissue culture cells. J. Biol. Chem. 1978, 253: 6125-31.
4. MOSCONA (M.), FRANKEL (N.), MOSCONA (A.A.): Regulatory mechanisms in the induction of glutamine synthetase in the embryonic retina: immunochemical studies. Dev. Biol. 1972, 8: 229-41.
5. GALDANI (M.), ROLLAND (B.), FAGES (C.), TARDY (M.): Glutamine synthetase activity during mouse brain development. Experientia 1982; 38: 1199-1202.
6. HALLENMAYER (K.), HARMENING (C.), HAMPRECHT (B.): Cellular localization and regulation of glutamine synthetase in primary cultures of brain cells from newborn mice. J. Neurochem. 1981, 37: 43-52.
7. HERTZ (L.), SCHOUSBOE (A.), BOECKLER (N.), MERKERJI (S.), FEDOROFF (S.): Kinetic characteristics of the glutamate uptake to normal astrocytes in cultures. Neurochem. Res. 1978; 3: 10-4.
8. NOREMBERG (M.D.), MARTINEZ-HERNANDEZ (A.): Fine structural localization of glutamine synthetase in astrocytes of rat brain. Brain Res. 1979, 161: 303-10.
9. PATEL (A.J.), HUNT (A.), TAHOURNIN (C.S.M.): Regional development of glutamine synthetase activity in the rat brain and its association with the differentiation of astrocytes. Dev. Brain Res., 1983, 8: 31-7.
10. BARDAKDJIAN (J.), TARDY (M.), PIMOULE (C.), GONNARD (P.): GABA metabolism in cultured glial cells. Neurochem. Res. 1979: 4: 519-29.
11. PETTMANN (B.), DELAUNOY (J.P.), COURANGEOT (J.), DEVILLIERS (G.), SENSENBRENNER (M.): Rat brain glial cells in culture. Effect of brain extracts on the development of oligodendroglia-like cells. Dev. Biol. 1980, 75: 278.
12. PISHAK (M.R.), PHILLIPS (A.T.): Glucocorticoid stimulation of glutamine synthetase production in cultured rat glioma cells. J. Neurochem. 1980, 34: 866-72.
13. CAMPAGNONI (A.T.), CAREY (G.D.), YIE-TEH (Y.): In vitro synthesis of the myelin basic proteins: subcellular site of synthesis. J. Neurochem. 1980, 34: 677-86.
14. TARDY (M.), FAGES (C.), GONNARD (P.): cGMP in primary cultures in glial cells. J. Neurochem. 1980, 35: 612-5.
15. TARDY (M.), FAGES (C.), ROLLAND (B.), BARDAKDJIAN (J.), GONNARD (P.): Effect of prostaglandins and dBc AMP on the morphology of cells in primary astroglial cultures and on metabolic enzymes of GABA and glutamate metabolism. Experientia 1981, 37: 19-20.
16. RAFF (M.), MILLER (M.) and NOBLE (M.): A glial progenitor cell that develops in vitro into an astrocyte or an oligodendrocyte depending on culture medium. Nature 1983, 303: 390.

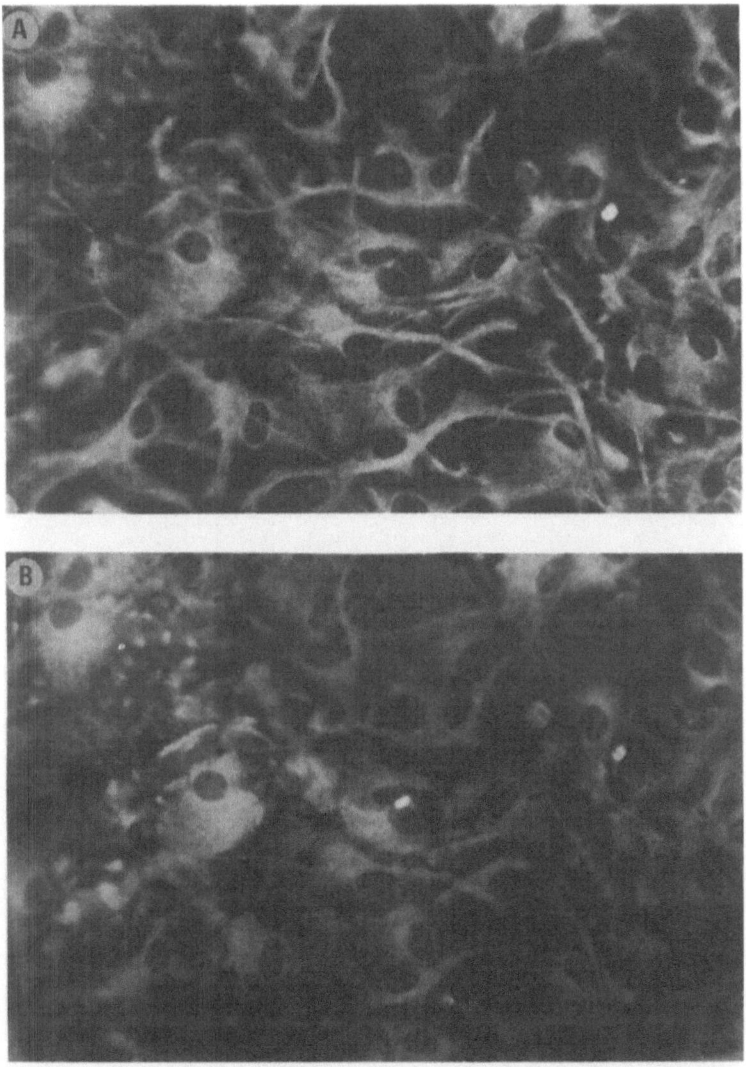

FIGURE 1. Primary astroglial cells from mouse cerebral hemispheres after 21 DIV.

Immunofluorescence double staining with (A) goat anti GFA serum and (B) rabbit anti GS serum (x400).

GFA is present in 85-90% of the cells whereas GS is expressed only in some of them.

Correlation of in situ cell Kinetics and Degree of Anaplasia in Human Brain Tumors: Identification of S-phase cells with anti-BUdR Antibodies

S.J. De ARMOND (°), T. NAGASHIMA (°°), K.G. CHO (°°), J.A. MUROVIC (°°), R.L. DAVIS (°°), and T. HOSHINO (°°).

INTRODUCTION AND BACKGROUND

The goal of the neuropathological examination of a cerebral neoplasm is to obtain an accurate measure of its proliferative potential. The underlying assumption made by those who must treat patients is that there is a direct correlation between the histological characteristics of a brain tumor and its prognosis and its response to treatment. However, experience has shown that there is often a considerable variation in the clinical behavior and rate of proliferation of neoplasms with the same histological characteristics.

Dr Takao Hoshino at the University of California, San Francisco (UCSF) has been studying cell kinetics in human brain neoplasms for over 10 years. Initially, ^{3}H-thymidine was used for these studies in human subjects (Hoshino, et al., 1972; Johnson, et al., 1980). However, H^3-thymidine was not practical as an adjunct to neurooncological treatment of patients because it took 1 to 2 months to obtain results by autoradiography and because the radioactive thymidine was potentially hazardous to the patient. In 1982, a methodological breakthrough occurred which made it practical and safe to directly assess the proliferative potential of human neoplasms in situ. This breakthrough was the development by Gratzner (1982) of a monoclonal antibody (MAb) to bromodeoxyuridine (BUdR). BUdR is a thymidine analogue which becomes incorporated into chromosomal DNA during the DNA synthesis phase (the S-phase) of the cell cycle. With the advent of anti-BUdR Mab's, it has become possible to identify cells which have incorporated BUdR into their DNA using standard immunohistochemical techniques such as immunofluorescence or peroxidase immunohistochemistry. The ratio of the number of cells labeled to the total number of cells is known as the "labeling index". For tissues sections, we prefer indirect peroxidase immunohistochemistry because the diaminobenzidine reaction product which is specifically deposited in BUdR containing nuclei is permanent and because non-labeled nuclei can be counterstained with a nuclear stain such as hematoxylin (Nagashima et al., 1985). Fluorescein isothiocyanate-conjugated anti-BUdR MAb's for fluorescence immunocytochemistry remains important for flow cytometric analysis of single cell suspensions (Hoshino, et al., 1986a; Nagashima and Hoshino, 1985). Single-cell suspensions can be made from solid tumors removed at surgery by treating them with an enzyme cocktail (0.02% collagenase II, 139 units/mg; 0.02% DNAse I, 7×10^4 DNAse units/mg; and 0.05% pronase, 45 proteolytic units Kalken/ml, B-grade; at 37°C for 30 min.) followed by filtration through a 37 micron Nitex mesh in 70% ethanol for 30 mins. The labeling index of brain tumor cell suspensions determined by flow cytometry has been found to be identical to that determined by counting immunoperoxidase labeled nuclei in tissue sections. For instance, the flow cytometric measurements of six glioblastoma multiforme neoplasms were $9.6 \pm 2.0\%$ and those from tissue sections were $9.8 \pm 1.6\%$ (Hoshino et al., 1986a). Furthermore, the values for labeling index obtained by BUdR immunohistochemistry are identical to those previously obtained with ^{3}H-thymidine (Hoshino, et al., 1986a).

Prior to trials with human subjects, approximate doses of BUdR were determined in rats bearing 9L brain tumor cells (Nagashima and Hoshino, 1985). In those studies, labeling index of a solid tumor grown in rats was calculated from flow cytometric analysis of single-cell suspensions stained with

(°) The Department of Pathology (Neuropathology Unit) and (°°) The Department of Neurological Surgery, Brain Tumor Research Center, School of Medicine, University of California, San Francisco, 94/43.

M. Chatel, F. Darcel and J. Pecker (eds.), Brain Oncology. ISBN-13: 978-94-010-8003-3

fluorescein-labeled anti-BUdR MAb and was compared to the number of S-phase cells calculated independently from DNA histograms of the same cells. It was found that the labeling index was not dependent on the dose of BUdR administered since doses from 1 to 40 mg/kg administered intraperitoneally resulted in average values which were similar to the values calculated from DNA histograms (16% vs 17% respectively) and to the values from previously published tritiated thymidine studies (12.8% to 19%) (Barker, et al., 1983; Hoshino and Wilson, 1979). The intensity of nuclear fluorescence was found to increase proportionally with the dose of BUdR administered. It was very encouraging that BUdR labeled cells were detected even when the rats were given doses as low as 1 mg/kg (7 mg/m^2) of BUdR. BUdR is rapidly degraded by the liver with more than 90% of a single bolus metabolized within 20 mins (Kris and Revesz, 1962). Pharmacokinetics studies have shown that the mean serum level of BUdR following a 1 hour intravenous infusion of 200 mg/m^2 is 2.48 μg/ml (8 μM) (Hoshino et al., 1985). Flow cytometric methods were able to detect fluorescence antibody labeling of BUdR treated cells at doses as low as 0.6 μM in 9L cells grown in vitro (Nagashima and Hoshino, 1985). Russo et al. (1984) found that an infusion rate of 108 mg/m^2/hr produced a serum level of 3.9 μM.

These in vitro and in vivo studies indicated that a serum BUdR level of 5 μM for one hour is sufficient to label S-phase cells and that a 1-hour BUdR infusion of 150-250 mg/m^2 in human subjects would be adequate to achieve the required serum levels. This is a relatively low dose since, when BUdR is used as a radiosensitizing agent for treatment of brain tumors, doses of 500-1000 mg/m^2/day are given for 4-5 weeks without serious side effects (Bagshaw et al., 1967; Hoshino and Sano, 1969; Kinsella et al., 1984; Mitchell et al., 1983; Russo et al., 1984; Sano et al., 1968). Kinsella, et al., (1984) found that myelo-suppression occurred at doses above 700 mg/m^2/day.

BUdR is known to have toxic and mutagenic effects on cultured cells at high concentrations and after long exposures (Goz, 1978). In addition, there is considerable evidence that incorporation of BUdR into DNA sensitizes the cell to ionizing radiation (Szybalski, 1974). Therefore, it became very important to know the lowest BUdR concentration which causes minimal cytotoxic or mutagenic effects. Answers to these questions have been of deep concern to clinicians who intend to administer BUdR to human subjects for diagnostic purposes. To answer these questions Zhang et al. (submitted) developed an in vitro assay using rat 9L gliosarcoma cells to test the effects of various concentrations of BUdR on colony-forming efficiency (CFE) and sister chromatid exchange (SCE). The SCE assay is considered to be a rapid and sensitive method for measuring the effects of agents that modulate DNA (Perry and Wolff, 1974). BUdR is known to induce exchanges (cross-overs) between sister chromatids which are detectable after two rounds of cell replication (Davidson et al., 1980; Heartlein et al., 1982; Perry and Wolff, 1974). Cell cultures of 9L cells were treated for 1 or 2 hours with varying concentrations of BUdR. SCE's were only increased at a concentration of 100 μM for 1 hour or 20 μM for 2 hours. For comparison, a 1 hour intravenous infusion of 200 mg/m^2 of BUdR in human subjects is equivalent to about 8 μM/ml in tissue culture. Furthermore, the highest dose (1000 μM BUdR) produced very little cell kill (5%) with a 1 hour exposure. This in vitro study, therefore, has provided further evidence that the BUdR dose proposed for human subjects for in situ cell kinetic studies is safe.

METHODS

Over the past two years at UCSF about 200 patients have been given BUdR at the time of surgery and the number of S-phase cells in their neoplasms determined. The methods are as follows. Immediately after induction of anesthesia, patients are given a 30 min. to 1 hour intravenous infusion of 150-200 mg/m^2 of BUdR. Following biopsy of the neoplasm, one portion is sent to pathology for diagnosis and another is immediately immersed in chilled 70% ethanol for a minimum of 12 hours. Occasionally, a portion of the biopsy specimen is treated with the enzyme cocktail described above to produce a single-cell suspension to be reacted with fluorescein labeled anti-BUdR MAb for flow cytometric measurement of labeling index. The ethanol fixed tissue is embedded in paraffin and 6 micron thick sections are cut. A modified immunoperoxidase procedure is then performed. After deparaffinization, the tissue is incubated for 1 hour with 2N HCl. It is then neutralized with 0.1 M borax and rinsed with phosphate buffered saline (PBS). A 1:30 dilution of anti-BUdR MAb (Becton-Dickinson, Mountain View, CA) is placed on the tissue for 45 mins. After a rinse with PBS, the tissue is reacted with a 1:50 dilution of peroxidase-conjugated anti-mouse IgG (Zymed, S. San Francisco, CA) for 45 mins. Following a final PBS rinse, the tissue is incubated for 15 min. with diaminobenzidine tetrahydrochloride (DAB) reaction product (0.0125% DAB in 50 mM Tris-HCl buffer, pH 7.6, with 0.0025% H_2O_2, freshly made). A brown precipitate indicates positive reaction. To identify unlabeled nuclei, the tissue is conterstained lightly with hematoxylin. For neoplasms in which vascular endothelial proliferation is prominent, the tissue is counterstained with periodic acid Schiff (PAS) to help delineate vascular structures. In the example provided (Figure 1), BUdR immunostained nuclei in a mature teratoma of the thoracic spine are easily distinguishable from BUdR-negative nuclei counterstained with hematoxylin (Murovic, et al., 1986).

Although the best immunostaining for BUdR is obtained with ethanol-fixed sections, specific staining can also be achieved on formalin-fixed paraffin-embedded specimens. The technique is modified as follows. After deparaffinization, the sections are incubated with 0.3% pepsin in 0.01N HCl for 30 min. at 37°C. The sections are rinsed with PBS and placed in methanol with 3% H_2O_2 for 30 min. to block endogenous peroxidase activity. After another PBS rinse, the rest of the procedure is identical to that used for ethanol-fixed tissues.

RESULTS

Glial neoplasms

The classification scheme for astrocytic neoplasms used at UCSF is based on a simple additive system of cellular and architectural abnormalities (Liu et al., submitted). Infiltrating cerebral astrocytomas have been divided into five subgroups. The histological criteria used for each subgroup are presented in Table I. We have found that this classification scheme accurately predicts the behavior of each subtype in context of the treatment protocols used at UCSF. The median survival for each subgroup is presented in Table II. None of the patients in that study had mildly anaplastic astrocytoma. The differences in survival between highly anaplastic astrocytoma and glioblastoma multiforme and between moderately anaplastic astrocytoma and glioblastoma multiforme are statistically significant after adjustment for age and Karnoski performance score. It should be noted that necrosis is not a criterion for classification. In addition, the diagnosis of glioblastoma multiforme is made even when the criteria are fulfilled only focally.

BUdR labeling indices of 127 neuroectodermal neoplasms is presented in Table III (Hoshino et al., 1986b). The highest labeling index occurred in medulloblastomas (12%) which is comparable

TABLE I

UCSF criteria for classification of supratentorial malignant tumors

Glioblastoma Multiforme
- A glial neoplasm that is at least focally highly cellular
- Nuclear pleomorphism
- Cytoplasmic pleomorphism
- Vascular endothelial proliferation

Gemistocytic Astrocytoma
- Not a glioblastoma multiforme
- An astrocytoma composed of at least 60% gemistocytes

Highly Anaplastic Astrocytoma (Infiltrating)
- Not a glioblastoma multiforme
- At least focally moderately to highly cellular
- Two of the following characteristics:
  - High nuclear: cytoplasmic ratio
  - Coarse nuclear chromatin
  - Much mitotic activity
  - Nuclear pleomorphism
  - Cytoplasmic pleomorphism

Moderately Anaplastic Astrocytoma (Infiltrating)
- Not a highly anaplastic astrocytoma
- Mildly to moderately increased cellularity
- Enlarged nuclei
- Relatively uniform cytoplasm

Mildy Anaplastic Astrocytoma (Infiltrating)
- Not a moderately anaplastic astrocytoma
- Mildly increased cellularity
- Enlarged but regular nuclei
- Uniform cytoplasm

TABLE II

Median survival times of 258 patients with gliomas at UCSF

	N*	Survival (weeks)
Glioblastoma multiforme	134	63
Gemistocytic astrocytoma	24	104
Highly anaplastic astrocytoma	60	123
Moderately anaplastic astrocytoma	40	192

N*: Number of patients

TABLE III

BUdR labeling indices of nervous system neoplasms

Tumor Type	No of Cases	LABELING INDEX (%)		No. OF CASES OF LI		
		Median	Ranges	< 1%	1-5	> 5%
Medulloblastoma	8	12.0	4.0-28.6	0	1	7
Glioblastoma Multiforme	38	7.3	1.3-26.1	0	2	21
Highly anaplastic astrocytoma	19	4.2	< 1.0-38.1	4	7	8
Moderately anaplastic astrocytoma	36	< 1.0	< 1.0-9.3	23	11	2
Ependymoma	9	< 1.0	< 1.0-18.9	5	3	1
Juvenile pilocytic astrocytoma	8	1.7	< 1.0-3.1	4	4	0
Mixed glioma*	5	4.4	< 1.0-8.1	1	2	2
Ganglioglioma	4	< 1.0	< 1.0-2.4	3	2	0
Meningioma	47	< 1.0	< 1.0-5.4	30	4	3
Pituitary adenoma	29	< 1.0	< 1.0-1.5	26	3	0
Metastatic neoplasms	9	14.9	5.9-28.6	0	0	9

* Mixed oligodendroglioma-astrocytoma

to metastatic neoplasms (14%). Glioblastoma multiforme had the next highest labeling index (7.3%) followed by highly anaplastic astrocytoma (4.2%) and mixed malignant oligodendroglioma-astrocytoma (4.4%). While the median labeling indices correlate very well with the median survival time, the range of labeling indices varies considerably even among relatively slower growing neoplasms. For instance, two patients with moderately anaplastic astrocytomas had labeling indices greater than 5% which is close to the average for glioblastoma multiforme. Sufficient time has not yet elapsed in this study to determine whether the labeling index can predict patient survival within a subclass of astrocytomas. It may explain why some patients with moderately anaplastic astrocytomas have short survivals and why some patients with glioblastoma multiforme are still alive in our series more than 2 years after diagnosis. Our goal in the coming years will be to determine what weight the labeling index has as compared with other factors known to influence prognosis such as patient age and location and size of the neoplasm.

Meningioma

The most precise correlation between the rate of neoplastic growth and the labeling index has been found for neoplasms of the meninges (Cho et al., 1986). Forty-five neoplasms originating from leptomeningeal cells proper (meningiomas) and two angioglastic meningiomas of the hemangiopericytic type have been examined with BUdR labeling. The great majority of meningiomas are generally accepted to be benign neoplasms and it is generally accepted that the most significant factor determining rate of recurrence is the extent of surgical removal (Skullerud and Loken, 1974). Among the various histological and cytological criteria used to estimate recurrence, only the degree of cellularity has been found to be significant (Skullerud and Loken, 1974) although increased mitotic activity, focal necrosis, and infiltration of the brain substance have also been found to be important (Crompton and Gautier-Smith, 1970). However, the behavior of meningiomas remains very difficult to predict from classical histological features alone and the definitions of atypical and malignant meningiomas are still ambiguous.

Eight recurrent meningiomas, including two non-malignant meningotheliomatous meningiomas, four malignant meningiomas (classification based on increased cellularity, increased number of mitoses, and frank invasion of the central nervous system) and two angioblastic meningiomas of the hemangiopericytic type have been subjected to in situ BUdR labeling (Figure 2). The logarithm of the doubling time, estimated from serial computed tomography scans, was found to be directly proportional to the labeling index (Figure 3). BUdR labeling index measurements in each of the eight cases was performed at the time of recurrence. Six of the measurements were made at the time of the first recurrence and two at the time of the third recurrence. In four of the cases (marked with a star in Figure 1), doubling time was calculated from the preoperative growth since no further postoperative growth has been detected in these patients. In the other four, doubling time was calculated from postoperative growth estimated by computerized tomography scans. These preliminary data indicate that BUdR labeling indices of meningiomas will be an important adjunct to histological classification for predicting clinical behavior.

Pituitary Adenoma

Twenty-nine pituitary adenomas have been examined to date (Nagashima, et al., 1986). The great majority, 26 out of 29, had labeling indices of less than 1% and, of these, almost 50% had labeling indices less than 0.1%. Two patients had labeling indices greater than 1% (1.46 and 1.26%) and both of these suffered from Nelson's syndrome. In Nelson's syndrome, an ACTH-secreting pituitary adenoma becomes manifest after bilateral adrenalectomy for pre-existing Cushing's disease. Surgical removal of the adrenal glands eliminates the suppressing effects of cortical steroids on the rate of cellular proliferation in the pre-existing microadenoma.

CONCLUSIONS

The thymidine analogue, BUdR becomes incorporated into DNA during the DNA synthesis phase of the cell cycle. Monoclonal antibodies specific for BUdR are commercially available which makes it possible to identify cell nuclei which contain BUdR in their chromosomal DNA and, therefore, to identify cells which have gone through the S-phase of the cell cycle. The proportion of cells which immunostain for BUdR is termed the labeling index and is directly related to the proliferation rate of a neoplasm. Although the labeling index is related to the rate at which daughter cells are made, it is not the only factor which determines the doubling time of a neoplasm. Doubling time is also directly related to the rates of cell death and loss and, at present, there is no way to assess these in situ. For meningiomas and hemangiopericytomas occuring in the meninges, the labeling index appears to be sufficient to predict tumor doubling time suggesting that the rate of cell loss is constant and the same in these two categories of meningeal neoplasms. It is not yet known whether or not a similar relationship exists for glial neoplasms. As a general rule, the number of mitotic figures does not correlate with the labeling index. With regard to patient safety, the combined results of clinical, pharmacokinetic and in vitro studies indicate that the doses of BUdR required to obtain strong specific immunostaining of S-phase cells are far below levels which are hazardous. It is not yet known whether all cells within CNS tumors have equal access to intravenously infused BUdR; however, our initial results are comparable to those obtained previously with ^{3}H-Thymidine. Because it is possible to determine the labeling index within three days of a brain tumor biopsy by immunohistochemistry, it has the potential to be useful for designing individualized treatment schedules for patients. Of equal importance, because the labeling index of a large number of neoplasms will be studied and their clinical course accurately documented, we hope to gain a clearer understanding of the pathobiology of neoplasia.

KEY WORDS

Cell Kinetics, Grading, BUdR Antilodies.

ACKNOWLEDGEMENTS

This work was supported by Grand PD159 from the American Cancer Society and Grant CA13525 from the National Cancer Institute.

REFERENCES

1. BAGSHAW (M.A.), DOGGETT (R.L.S.), SMITH (K.C.), KAPLAN (H.S.) and NELSON (T.S.) (1967): Intra-arterial 5-bromodeoxyuridine and X-ray therapy. Amer. J. Radiol. 99, 886-894.
2. BARKER (M.), HOSHINO (T.), GURCAY (O.), WILSON (C.B.), NIELSEN (S.L.), DOWNIE (R.) and ELIASON (J.) (1973): Development of an animal brain tumor model and its response to therapy with 1,3-bis(2-chloroethyl)-1-nitrosourea. Cancer Res. 33, 971-986.
3. CHO (K.G.), HOSHINO (T.), NAGASHIMA (T.), MUROVIC (J.A.) and WILSON (C.B.) (1986): The prediction of tumor doubling time in recurrent meningiomas: Cell kinetics studies with bromodeoxyuridine labeling. J. Neurosurg. 65, 790-794.
4. CROMPTON (M.R.) and GAUTIER-SMITH (P.C.) (1970): The prediction of recurrence in meningiomas. J. Neurol. Psychiat. 33, 80-87.
5. DAVIDSON (R.L.), KAUFMAN (E.R.), DOUGHERTY (C.P.), OUELLETTE (A.M.), DIFOLCO (C.M.) and LATT (S.A.) (1980): Induction of sister chromatid exchanges by BUdR is largely independent of the BUdR content of DNA. Nature, 284, 74-76.
6. GOZ (B.) (1978): The effects of incorporation of 5-halogenated deoxyuridines into the DNA of eukaryotic cells. Pharmacol. Rev. 29, 249-272.
7. GRATZNER (H.G.) (1982): Monoclonal antibody to 5-bromo- and 5-iododeoxyuridine: a new reagent for detection of DNA replication. Science 218, 474-475.
8. HEARTLEIN (M.W.), O'NEILL (J.P.), PAL (B.C.) and PRESTON (R.J.) (1982): The induction of specific-locus mutations and sister-chromatid exchanges by 5-bromo- and 5-chloro-deoxyuridine. Mutation Research 92, 411-416.
9. HOSHINO (T.) and SANO (K.) (1969): Radiosensitization of malignant brain tumors with bromouridine (thymidine analogue). Acta Radiol. Ther. Phys. Biol. 8, 15-21.
10. HOSHINO (T.) and WILSON (C.B.) (1979): Cell kinetic analysis of human malignant brain tumors (gliomas). Cancer 44, 956-962.
11. HOSHINO (T.), BAKER (M.), WILSON (C.B.), BOLDREY (E.B.) and FEWER (D.) (1972): Cell kinetics of human gliomas. J. Neurosurg. 37, 15-26.
12. HOSHINO (T.), NAGASHIMA (T.), MUROVIC (J.), LEVIN (E.M.), LEVIN (V.A.) and RUPP (S.M.) (1985): Cell kinetic studies of in situ human brain tumors with bromo-deoxyuridine. Cytometry 6, 627-732.
13. HOSHINO (T.), NAGASHIMA (T.), MUROVIC (J.A.), WILSON (C.B.), EDWARDS (M.S.B.), GUTIN (P.), DAVIS (R.L.) and DE ARMOND (S.J.) (1986a): In situ cell kinetics studies on human neuroectodermal tumors with bromodeoxyuridine labeling. J. Neurosurg. 64, 453-459.
14. HOSHINO (T.), NAGASHIMA (T.), CHO (K.G.), MUROVIC (J.A.), HODES (J.E.), WILSON (C.B.), EDWARDS (M.S.B.) and PITTS (L.H.) (1986b): S-phase fraction of human brain tumors in situ measured by uptake of bromodeoxyuridine. Int. J. Cancer 38, 369-374.
15. JOHNSON (H.A.), HAYMAKER (W.E.), RUBINI (J.R.), FLIEDNER (T.M.), BOND (V.P.), CRONKITE (E.P.) and HUGHES (W.L.) (1960): A radioautographic study of a human brain and glioblastoma multiforme after the in vivo uptake of tritiated thymidine. Cancer 13, 636-642.
16. KINSELLA (T.J.), RUSSO (A.), MITCHELL (J.B.), ROWLAND (J.), JENKINS (J.), SCHWADE (J.), MYERS (C.E.), COLLINS (J.M.), SPEYER (J.), KORNBLITH (P.), SMITH (B.), KUFTA (C.) and GLATSTEIN (E.A.) (1984): A phase I study of intermittent intravenous bromodeoxyuridine (BUdR) with conventional fractionated irradiation. Int. J. Rad. Oncol. Biol. Phys. 10, 69-76.
17. KRISS (J.P.) and REVESZ (L.) (1962): The distribution and fate of bromodeoxyuridine in the mouse and rat. Cancer Res. 22, 254-265.
18. LIU (H.C.), DAVIS (R.L.), HANNIGAN (J.), SILVER (P.) and LEVIN (V.A.) (submitted): Diagnosis of supratentorial malignant gliomas: histologic criteria and correlation with survival.
19. MITCHELL (J.B.), KINSELLA (T.J.), RUSSO (A.), MCPHERSON (S.), ROWLAND (J.), KORNBLITH (P.), and GLATSTEIN (E.A.) (1983): Radiosensitization of hematopoietic precursor cells (CFUc) in glioblastoma patients receiving intermittent intravenous infusions of bromodeoxyuridine (BUdR). Int. J. Radiat. Oncol. Biol. Phys. 9, 457-463.
20. MUROVIC (J.A.), DE ARMOND (S.), NAGASHIMA (T.), EDWARDS (M.S.B.) and HOSHINO (T.) (1986): Cell kinetics analysis in a case of teratoma of the thoracic spine. J. Neurosurg. 65, 331-334.
21. NAGASHIMA (T.) and HOSHINO (T.) (1985): Rapid detection of S-phase cells by anti-bromodeoxyuridine monoclonal antibody in 9L brain tumor cells in vitro and in situ. Acta Neuropathol. (Berl) 66, 12-17.

22. NAGASHIMA (T.), DE ARMOND (S.J.), MUROVIC (J.) and HOSHINO (T.) (1985): Immunocytochemical demonstration of S-phase cells by anti-bromodeoxyuridine monoclonal antibody in human brain tumor tissues. Acta Neuropathol. (Berl) 67, 155-159.

23. NAGASHIMA (T.), MUROVIC (J.A.), HOSHINO (T.), WILSON (C.B.), and DE ARMOND (S.J.) (1986): The proliferative potential of human pituitary tumors in situ. J. Neurosurg. 64, 588-593.

24. PERRY (P.) and WOLFF (S.) (1974): New Giemsa method for the differential staining of sister chromatids. Nature 251, 156-158.

25. RUSSO (A.), GIANNI (L.), KINSELLA (T.J.), KLECKER (R.W.), JENKINS (J.), ROWLAND (J.), GLATSTEIN (E.A.), MITCHELL (J.B.), COLLINS (J.), and MYERS (C.): Pharmacological evaluation of intravenous delivery of 5-bromodeoxyuridine to patients with brain tumors. Cancer Res. 44, 1702-1705.

26. SANO (K.), HOSHINO (T.) and NAGAI (M.) (1968): Radiosensitization of brain tumor cells with a thymidine analogue (bromouridine). J. Neurosurg. 28, 530-538.

27. SKULLERUD (K.) and LOKEN (A.C.) (1974): The prognosis in meningiomas. Acta Neuropath. (Berl) 29, 337-344.

28. SZYBALSKI (W.) (1974): X-ray sensitization by halopyrimidines. Cancer Chemother. 58, 539-557.

29. ZHANG (R.X.), NAGASHIMA (T.) and HOSHINO (T.) (submitted): Effect of brief exposure to bromodeoxyuridine on exponentially growing rat 9L gliosarcoma cells.

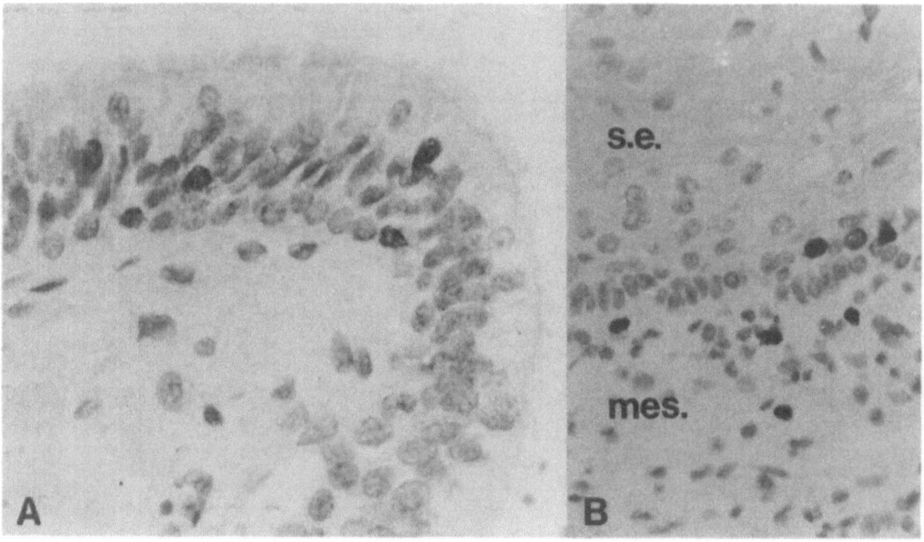

FIGURE 1. Immunohistochemical localization of BUdR in a mature teratoma. The immunopositive BUdR containing nuclei can be distinguished from hematoxylin stained nuclei which do not contain BUdR.

A. Ciliated, pseudotratified columnar epithelium (respiratory epithelium) has five BUdR containing nuclei in this field.

B. Stratified squamous epithelium (s.e.) has two BUdR containing nuclei in its basal layer and the subepithelial loose mesenchyme (mes.) contains four positive nuclei.

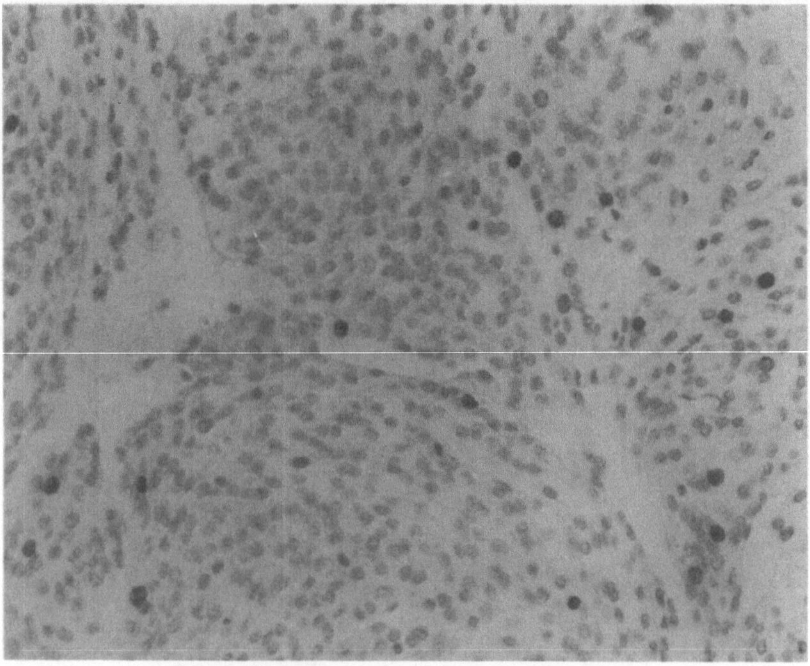

FIGURE 2. BUdR localization in a malignant meningioma. Immunopositive nuclei are scattered throughout the neoplasm giving a labeling index of 3.8%. Peroxidase immunohistochemistry with hematoxylin counterstain.

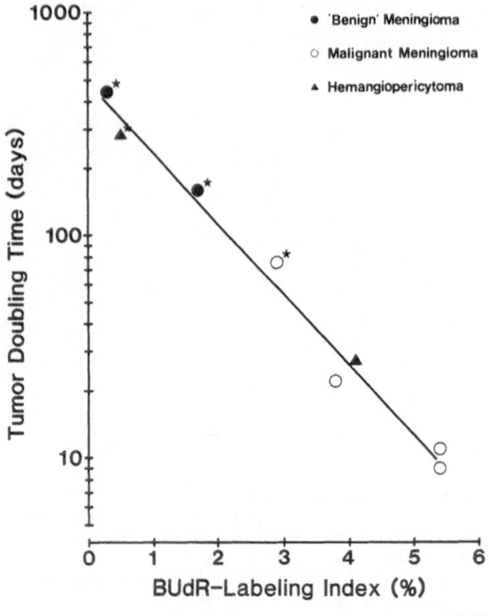

FIGURE 3. The relationship of tumor doubling time to BUdR labeling index among 8 recurrent meningeal neoplasms. See text for further details. The figure was adapted from Cho et al. (1986).

Prognostic Value of Labeling Index in Stereotactic Biopsies of Glial Tumours

G. BROGGI (°), A. FRANZINI (°), S. FERRARESI (°), C. GIORGI (°), A. ALLEGRANZA (°°).

INTRODUCTION

Prognostic data from stereotactic serial biopsies of glial tumours are usually derived following the histological grading of the WHO Committee (11) and/or the spatial classification proposed by French Authors (3). Nevertheless the histological grading based only on morphological and cytological features may not be considered strictly prognostic.

In mature astrocytomas i.e. the histological diagnosis provides data regarding the tumor as it appears at the time of biopsy but no data are given about its possible evolution or about the lasting of the slow-growing resting phase.

The tumor growth may be estimated on the basis of the proliferative activity by different methods: Thomas et al. (10) recently proposed the cell culture from biopsic specimens; Kleihues et al. (7) developped monoclonal antibodies for immunohistochemical detection of proliferating cells; Hoshino since 1975 utilized the 3H-Thymidine method for in vivo labeling of cells in the S phase of the mitotic cycle (5, 6).

The last method has been modified for in vitro application according to Silvestrini et al. (9) and finally adapted to serial stereotactic biopsies (2, 4).

Preliminary results obtained by this technique are reported and discussed in view of their value to optimize the choice of treatments in glial tumours.

PATIENTS AND METHODS

This study has been performed in a randomized series including 23 consecutive patients which underwent stereotactic biopsy for glial tumours between July and December 1983 (12 were males, and the age ranged from 11 to 62 years).

In each patient the stereotactic biopsy was performed following the mathematical reconstruction of CT and NMR images; the intraoperative neurophysiological monitoring and smear examination confirmed the neuroradiological targets (1).

The fragments of tissue have been obtained by the original Sedan instrument and each sample has been longitudinally divided for two separate double-blind examinations: the first consisted in conventional staining (H.E. Masson GFAP) and the second has been processed for labeling cells in S phase of the mitotic cycle.

H3-Thymidine and autoradiographic technique has been utilized according to the method described by Hoshino (5) and modified for in vitro application according to Silvestrini et al. (9) and Livingston et al. (8). Finally the number of H3-Thymidine labeled cells has been expressed as Labeling Index (LI) which means the ratio between the cells in S phase (x 100) and the total number of cells within the specimen.

The count of cells was made by optical microscopy and manual technique: an average value of at least 1000 units has been counted for each specimen.

The full methodology has been previously described in details (4).

(°) Dept. of Neurosurgery, Istituto Neurologico "C. Besta", Milano, Italy. (°°) Consultant Neuropathologist.

M. Chatel, F. Darcel and J. Pecker (eds.), Brain Oncology. ISBN-13: 978-94-010-8003-3

Since the stereotactic procedure provides 3-5 specimens from different targets, the highest value of LI detected along the trajectory has been considered representative of the tumor proliferating activity; in previous feasibility-studies the LI considered representative of each single case was assumed as the average of the all LI values detected along the stereotactic trajectory (2, 4). In the present study the need to compare the LI with the histological diagnosis and with the prognosis suggested to consider only the intratumoral target where the maximum LI is detected.

This series of patients has been carefully reviewed at serial follow-up times every three months (C.T. examinations) for at least three years. The LI, the definitive histological grading and the clinical history have been matched and the relationships between these different parameters have been investigated.

RESULTS AND DISCUSSION

The whole series of patients has been divided into three groups according to the follow-up: the first group includes 12 patients still alive at least three years after biopsy (no patient of these series died within the third year after the biopsy); the second group includes 5 patients died during the second year after biopsy; the third group includes 6 patients who died during the six months after stereotactic biopsy.

These groups have been correlated to the LI independently of the histological grading. In other words the groups were homogeneous concerning the survival time and dishomogeneous as far as the histological diagnosis is concerned. The LI value representative of each single group has been considered as the average of the highest LI values detected along the stereotactic trajectory in each single patient belonging to the group.

The average value of LI resulted 1.6% in the first group (alive at three years follow-up), 7.8% in the group of patients died 6-24 months after biopsy and 15.2% in the group with the worst clinical history (Fig. 1).

These results have been also retrospectively matched to the histological grading: astrocytomas considered mature were present also in the second and third groups with poor prognosis; these data suggest the existence of "active gliomas" even without anaplasic features at conventional morphological examinations.

Moreover the mature astrocytoma series have been analysed in view to study the intratumoral variability of LI along the trajectory of serial sampling.

Preliminary results suggest that major variability is present in patients having the worst prognosis.

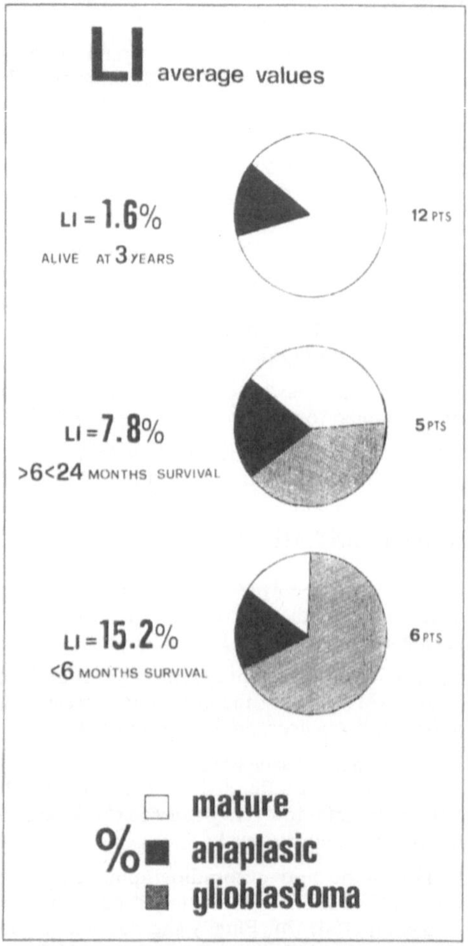

FIGURE 1. The LI average value of patients still alive at 3 years follow-up resulted 1.6%. The group includes 12 patients and the percentage of the different histological conventional classes is graphically represented. The LI average value of patients died between 6 and 24 months after the stereotactic biopsy resulted 7.8% and the presence of the three glioma classes is graphically represented. The last group includes patients died within the first six months after biopsy and the highest LI average value has been found in these series. The prevalence of glioblastoma in this group is clearly shown. The LI value considered representative of each single group has been considered as the average of the highest LI values detected along the stereotactic trajectory in each single patient belonging to the group.

On the contrary the LI showed homogeneous values in the different targets in patients being still alive at two years follow-up (Fig. 2).

In conclusion the preliminary data suggest the following remarks:

A) A clearcut relationship between LI and life expectancy has been demonstrated in the whole series.

B) In mature astrocytomas LI resulted more predictive than histological grading and the presence of a high LI intratumoral variability suggests the existence of potentially active tumours.

These encouraging data stress the values of LI study in the strategy of glial tumour treatment: the indications to invasive or conservative treatments in mature astrocytomas may be reviewed at the light of LI values with particular regard to the existence of latent fast-growing "active" lesions.

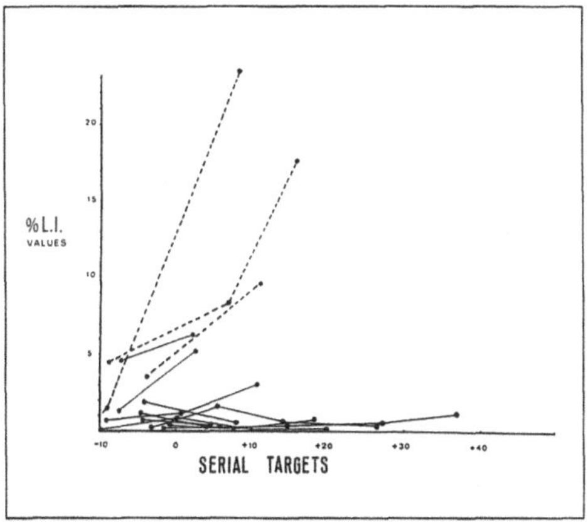

FIGURE 2. This figure concerns only mature astrocytomas. On the abscissa the serial targets along the stereotactic transtumoral trajectories are represented. The estimated outer boundary of the tumor have been assumed as 0, while intratumoral samples were +10, +20, +30, etc. On the ordinates the LI values are indicated. Each sample is marked by a black dot. Scattered lines indicate patients died within three years after the stereotactic biopsy: they display an high intratumoral LI variability. The filled line refers to the patients still alive at three years follow-up.

SUMMARY

Between July and December 1983, 23 consecutive patients affected from glial tumours underwent serial stereotactic biopsy and labeling index (LI) in vitro determination by H3-Thymidine method. The clinical history at 3 years follow-up, the conventional histological grading and the LI have been matched each other to study retrospectively the prognostic values of kinetic investigations during stereotactic biopsy. Our results suggest more accuracy of LI to predict the life expectancy versus conventional histological examinations.

ACKNOWLEDGEMENTS

Supported in part by grant n 84.00474.44 of the Consiglio Nazionale delle Ricerche, Rome, Italy.

KEY WORDS

Stereotactic Biopsy, Glial Tumours, Cell Kinetics, Labeling Index, Gliomas.

REFERENCES

1. BROGGI (G.), FRANZINI (A.): Value of serial stereotactic biopsies and impedance monitoring in the treatment of deep brain tumours. J. Neurol. Neurosurg. Psychiatry. 44: 397-401 (1981).
2. BROGGI (G.), FRANZINI (A.), COSTA (A.), MELCARNE (A.), ALLEGRANZA (A.): Cell kinetics of neuroepithelial tumors in serial stereotactic biopsies. A new combined approach. Appl. Neurophysiol. 48: 472-476 (1985).
3. DAUMAS-DUPORT (C.), MONSAINGEON (V.), SZENTHE (L.), SZIKLA (G.): Serial stereotactic biopsies: a double histological code of gliomas according to malignancy and 3D configuration. as an aid to therapeutic decision and assessment of results. Appl. Neurophysiol. 45: 431-437 (1982).
4. FRANZINI (A.), BROGGI (G.), ALLEGRANZA (A.), VENTURA (L.), COSTA (A.): Cell kinetics of gliomas by serial stereotactic biopsy. Basic Appl. Histochem. 30: 203-207 (1986).
5. HOSHINO (T.): A commentary on the biology and growth kinetics of low-grade and high-grade gliomas. J. Neurosurg. 61: 895-900 (1984).
6. HOSHINO (T.), BARKER (M.), WILSON (C.B.), BOLDREY (E.B.), FEWER (D.): Cell kinetics of human gliomas. J. Neurosurg. 37: 15-26 (1972).

7. KLEIHUES (P.), SHIBATA (T.), BURGER (P.C.): The use of monoclonal antibody Ki-67 in the identification of proliferating cells: application to surgical pathology. VI th Meeting of Swiss Neuropathologists with international participation. St. Moritz, March 15th-19th, 1986.

8. LIVINGSTON (R.B.), AMBUS (U.), GEORGE (S.L.), FREIREICH (E.J.), HART (J.S.): In vitro determination of thymidine 3H labeling index in human solid tumors. Cancer Res. 34: 1376-1380 (1974).

9. SILVESTRINI (R.), DAIDONE (M.G.), COSTA (A.), SANFILIPPO (O.): Cell kinetics and in vitro chemosensitivity as a tool for improved management of patients. Eur. J. Cancer Clin. Oncol. 21: 371-378 (1985).

10. THOMAS (D.G.T.), DARLING (J.L.), WATKINS (B.A.), HINE MARIA (C.): A simple method for the growth of cell cultures from small biopsies of brain tumors taken during C.T. directed stereotactic procedures. Acta Neurochir. 33 Suppl.: 243-245 (1984).

11. W.H.O.: Histological classification of tumours of the nervous system. Geneva, 1979.

Proliferative Potential of Malignant and Non-Malignant Meningiomas

K.G. CHO (°), T. HOSHINO (°), T. NAGASHIMA (°) and R.L. DAVIS (°°).

INTRODUCTION

Meningiomas are common neoplasms in the central nervous system. Although most of these tumors are encapsulated and grow very slowly, some meningiomas invade into adjacent brain tissue and skull, grow faster, and recur more frequently than classic meningiomas. These malignant meningiomas, however, are not well defined histopathologically, and their biological characteristics have never been well documented. We studied the cell kinetics of human meningiomas immunohistochemically using a monoclonal antibody against bromodeoxyuridine (BUdR) (2), a thymidine analogue that is incorporated into nuclear DNA during the synthesis phase of the cell cycle. BUdR-labeled S-phase cells can be identified by anti-BUdR monoclonal antibodies, which can then be detected by indirect immunoperoxiase methods (3, 6).

MATERIAL AND METHODS

Forty-five patients aged 8 to 80 years with various types of primary or recurrent meningiomas (33 non-malignant, 10 malignant, and 2 hemangiopericytic) were included in this study. Sixteen of the patients were males and 29 were females. Malignant meningiomas were more common in males by a ratio of 6:4. The pathological diagnosis of malignant meningioma was based on the presence of mitoses, cellularity, necrosis, and signs of anaplasia; all meningiomas that showed signs of invasiveness were also diagnosed as malignant.

All patients were given an intravenous infusion of BUdR (200 mg/m^2) at the time of surgery, but before biopsy of the tumor. The excised tumor specimens were fixed in chilled 70% ethanol for at least 12 hours and embedded in paraffin. After deparaffinization, the tissue sections were incubated for 30 minutes in methanol with 0.1% H_2O_2 to avoid endogenous peroxidase activity, and for 60 minutes in 2 N HCI to denature DNA. The sections were neutralized with 0.1 M Borax, covered with a 1:30 dilution of purified anti-BUdR monoclonal antibody in phosphate-buffered saline (PBS) solution containing 1% bovine serum albumin and 0.5% Tween 20, and left for 60 minutes at room temperature in a 100% humidified atmosphere. The slides were rinsed, covered with a 1:50 dilution of peroxidase-conjugated anti-mouse IgG antibody in PBS, and left for 60 minutes at room temperature in a 100% humidified atmosphere. The slides were reacted for 10 to 15 minutes with diaminobenzidine and H_2O_2 in Tris buffer, lightly counterstained by immersion in 10% Gill No. 1 hematoxylin solution, dehydrated, and mounted in routine fashion. BUdR-labeled cells were counted in six to 15 microscopic fields to determine the average BUdR labeling index (LI), which was expressed as a percentage of the total number of cells scored.

To determine whether the rate of tumor growth could be predicted from the BUdR LI, the tumor doubling time (Tds) was estimated from serial computed tomographic (CT) scans of eight patients with recurrent meningiomas (four malignant, two hemangiopericytic, and two non-malignant). One recurrent malignant meningioma was excluded from this analysis because the CT scans and clinical history could not be obtained. The area of tumor in each scan was determined by planimetry; tumor volume was calculated as the sum of the products of the area multiplied by the slice thickness. Td was calculated as $t \times \log 2/(\log V_B - \log V_A)$, where V_A is the initial volume of the tumor and V_B the volume of the tumor after t days (8).

(°) Brain Tumor Research Center, Department of Neurological Surgery. (°°) Department of Neuropathology, School of Medicine, University of California, San Francisco, San Francisco. California 94143.

M. Chatel, F. Darcel and J. Pecker (eds.), Brain Oncology. ISBN-13: 978-94-010-8003-3

RESULTS AND DISCUSSION

The average LI was less than 1% in 27 (82%) of 33 non-malignant meningiomas, whereas it was 3.6% in 10 histologically malignant meningiomas. All of the malignant meningiomas had an LI greater than 2.7%, except for one that was diagnosed solely on the basis of invasiveness (Table I). The two hemangiopericytomas had LIs of 0.5% and 4.1%, respectively. Five of the 10 malignant meningiomas and both hemangiopericytomas were recurrent tumors. Most of these tumors recurred within 2 years after surgery, with the exception of the hemangiopericytoma with an LI of 0.5%, which recurred after 8 years (Table II). Nine (56%) of 16 meningiomas with LIs greater than 1% were recurrent, whereas only three (10%) of 29 meningiomas with LIs less than 1% were recurrent (Table I). Thus, meningiomas with LIs greater than 1% appear to grow faster and recur more frequently than those with LIs less than 1%. These results agree with our previous observations (3-5,7).

TABLE I

BUdR labeling indices of 45 meningiomas

Type of tumor	No. of Cases	Age (yrs)	Sex (M/F)	BUdR LI $<1\%$	BUdR LI $>1\%$
Nonmalignant	33 (5)*	10 to 80	9/24	27 (2)	6 (3)
Malignant	10 (5)	8 to 69	6/4	1** (0)	9 (5)
Hemangiopericytoma	2 (2)	25 to 34	1/1	1 (1)	1 (1)
Total	45 (12)	8 to 80	16/25	29 (3)	16 (9)

* Numbers in parentheses indicate recurrent tumors.
** Diagnosed on the basis of invasiveness only.

TABLE II

Characteristics of patients with malignant meningioma and hemangiopericytoma

Case No.	Age (yrs)/Sex	Tumor Location	BUdR LI (%) (mean ± SD)	Recurrence (Interval/No. of Surgeries)
Malignant Meningioma				
1	41/M	L C-P angle	2.7 ± 0.3	No
2	69/M	L parietal	2.9 ± 0.3	Yes (2 years/2)
3	46/F	Tentorial	3.1 ± 0.8	No
4	58/M	Tentorial	3.5 ± 0.5	No
5	48/M	R parasagittal	3.8 ± 0.4	Yes (6 months/2)
6	58/M	R parasagittal	3.8 ± 0.6	No
7	69/M	R parietal	5.1 ± 1.1	Yes (4 years/2)
8	8/F	Falx	5.4 ± 0.6	Yes (4 years/4)
9	49/M	L parietal	5.4 ± 0.2	Yes (2 years/2)
10*	59/F	Orbital	<1.0	No
Hemangiopericytoma				
11	34/M	R temporal	0.53 ± 0.05	Yes (8 years/2)
12	25/F	R ventricle	4.1 ± 0.7	Yes (4 years/4)

* Diagnosed on the basis of invasiveness alone.
C-P = cerebellopontine.

Two of the eight patients in whom the rate of tumor growth was estimated from serial CT scans had low BUdR LIs (0.3% and 0.5%); the time to recurrence in these two cases was more than 5 years and the Tds were 440 days and 281 days, respectively. The remaining six patients, whose tumors had an LI greater than 1%, including one nonmalignant meningioma with an LI of 1.7%, had a recurrence of their tumor within 2 years. The Tds of these eight recurrent meningiomas were plotted in logarithmic scale against the BUdR LIs (1). A semilogarithmic linear regression analysis revealed a correlation coefficient of 0.99. Td may be calculated with the formula Td = 500 x Exp (- 0.73 x LI) (1). The results of this preliminary study suggest that by providing an estimate of both the proliferative potential and the growth rate of meningiomas, the BUdR LI may supplement the histopathological diagnosis and improve both the determination of prognosis and the design of treatment regiments for individual patients.

SUMMARY

Forty-five patients with meningiomas of various types were given an intravenous infusion of the thymidine analogue bromodeoxyuridine (BUdR, 200 mg/m^2) at the time of surgery, to label cells in the DNA synthesis phase. Labeled cells were detected immunohistochemically with anti BUdR monoclonal antibodies. The average labeling index (LI), or percentage of BUdR-labeled cells, was less than 1% in 27 (82%) of 33 non-malignant meningiomas, but was 3.6% in 10 histologically malignant meningiomas. Two hemangiopericytomas had LIs of 0.5% and 4.1%. Five of 10 malignant menginiomas and both hemangiopericytomas were recurrent tumors. All but one of these tumors recurred with 2 years after surgery; the hemangiopericytoma that had an LI of 0.5% recurred after 8 years. Nine (56%) of 16 meningiomas with LIs greater than 1% were recurrent tumors, whereas only 3 (10%) of 29 meningiomas with LIs less than 1% were recurrent tumors. The tumor doubling times (Tds) were estimated from serial computed tomographic scans of eight patients with recurrent meningiomas. Tds ranged from 8 to 440 days and showed a close inverse correlation with the BUdR LIs. A semilogarithmic linear regression analysis of these values yielded a correlation coefficient of 0.99.

Td may be estimated using the formula Td = 500 × Exp (-0.73 × LI). The LIs obtained by BUdR studies may increase the accuracy with which the proliferative potential of meningiomas can be predicted.

By supplementing the histological diagnosis, the BUdR LI may help to improve the determination of prognosis and the design of treatment for individual patients.

AKNOWLEDGMENTS

This study was supported in part by grants PDT-159 from the American Cancer Society and CA 13525 from the National Cancer Institute.

KEY WORDS

Meningiomas, Labeling Index, BUdR.

REFERENCES

1. CHO (K.G.), HOSHINO (T.), NAGASHIMA (T.) et al.: The prediction of tumor doubling time in recurrent meningiomas: Cell kinetics studies with bromodeoxyuridine. J. Neurosurg. **65**: 790-794, 1986.
2. GRATZNER (H.G.): Monoclonal antibody to 5-bromo- and 5-iododeoxyuridine: A new reagent for detection of DNA replication. Science 218: 474-476, 1982.
3. HOSHINO (T.), NAGASHIMA (T.), MUROVIC (J.) et al.: Cell kinetic studies of *in situ* human brain tumors with bromodeoxyuridine. Cytometry 6: 627-632, 1985.
4. HOSHINO (T.), NAGASHIMA (T.), MUROVIC (J.A.), et al.: Proliferative potential of human meningiomas of brain: A cell kinetic study with bromodeoxyuridine. Cancer **58**: 1466-1472, 1986.
5. HOSHINO (T.), NAGASHIMA (T.), MUROVIC (J.A.), et al.: *In situ* cell kinetics studies on human neuroectodermal tumors using bromodeoxyuridine. J. Neurosurg. 64: 453-459, 1986.
6. NAGASHIMA (T.), ARMOND (S.J. de), MUROVIC (J.) et al.: Immunocytochemical demonstration of S-phase cells by anti-bromodeoxyuridine monoclonal antibody in human brain tumor tissues. Acta Neuropathol 67: 155-159, 1985.
7. NAGASHIMA (T.), MUROVIC (J.A.), HOSHINO (T.) et al.: The proliferative potential of human pituitary tumors *in situ*. J. Neurosurg. 64: 588-593, 1986.
8. JAASKELAININ (J.), HALTIA (M.), LAASONEN (E.), et al.: The growth rate of intracranial meningiomas and its relation to histology. Surg. Neurol. 24: 165-271, 1985.

Histological Patterns in Germ Cell Tumors

J. VERLOOY (°), P. CRAS (°°), P. SELOSSE (°),
J.J. MARTIN (°°).

INTRODUCTION

Two patients, who had a recurrence of a germ cell tumor are presented. In both cases, the first diagnosis was a benign teratoma; however, the second neuropathological diagnosis was: germinoma. This changing histological pattern of germ cell tumors is considered as a pitfall in the diagnosis and a difficulty in planning the treatment.

Case 1 :

A 17 year old man presented with vertical gaze paralysis, disturbed convergence and diffuse headaches. Neuroradiological investigations demonstrated a calcified pineal tumor. A right, supratentorial, suboccipital approach was used. A heterogenous, firm lesion, 2,5 cm in diameter, containing numerous cysts was macroscopically fully resected.

The tumor contained ecto-, meso-, and endodermal elements. Cysts, lined by mucus secreting or ciliated, pseudostratified columnar epithelia were surrounded by loose connective tissue and found next to stratified squamous epithelium. Interspersed were numerous islets of hyaline cartilage. However, some regions contained a high cell density of fusiform cells with pale, isomorphic nuclei, little cytoplasm and numerous mitoses. A diagnosis of **teratoma** was made. After the initial resection, the patient was not irradiated and was without complaints. Following a 2 - months interval, he complained of diplopia on upward gaze, dysarthria and disturbed gait. Clinical examination showed a right cerebellar syndrome in addition to a Parinaud syndrome and signs of intracranial hypertension. A large, contrast enhancing mass in the pineal region was found on CT scan. The lesion invaded the right lateral ventricle and the posterior fossa. Serum concentrations of AFPand HCG were elevated about 5- foldly. After performing a ventriculo-peritoneal shunt operation, the general condition of the patient continued to deteriorate and the pineal region was reexposed. The biopsied tissue was gray-red and consisted of large polygonal cells with large nuclei and numerous mitoses. The stroma was infiltrated by lymphocytes. A few multinucleated giant cells were present. All sections examined were characteristic of **germinoma** (Fig. 1). Teratomatous areas were no longer present.

The patient died in the immediate postoperative period. Autopsy could not demonstrate other tumoral localisations. Cerebral autopsy confirmed a large interoccipital mass with interoccipito-cerebellar extension to the right. The mesencephalon and cerebellar white matter were invaded by gray-red, necrotic tumor tissue. The histological pattern was analogous to the second biopsy.

Case 2 :

A 9 year old boy presented with signs of intracranial hypertension due to an obstructive hydrocephalus. CT scan revealed a third ventricle tumor, which was completely resected macroscopically.

The neuropathological examination showed a benign **teratoma** with epidermal cells, dermal tissue, blood vessels, mesenchymal cells and hair follicles of different age (Fig. 2).

A few zones of cylindrical ciliated epithelium are found, as well as zones with numerous psammoma bodies.

At the age of 13, the patient started complaining again of headaches, fatigue and difficulties in learning. A CT scan revealed a recurrence of the tumor, which had a suprasellar and a pineal localization.

The suprasellar part was macroscopically completely resected; the neuropathological diagnosis was: **germinoma.**

Different zones were present in the tumor: typical germinomatous zones were found with great, pale cells and small lymphocyte-like cells. Channels, lined by ciliated epithelium were present in association with cylindrical epithelial cells, papillary structures and uni- and multinucleated giant cells.

Multiple mitoses were present.

Postoperatively, radiotherapy was given and after 6 weeks, the tumor had disappeared on control CT scan and NMR.

(°) Department of Neurosurgery, University Hospital Antwerp, Belgium. (°°) Born-Bunge Foundation, University of Antwerp, Antwerp, Belgium.

M. Chatel, F. Darcel and J. Pecker (eds.), Brain Oncology. ISBN-13: 978-94-010-8003-3

CONCLUSION

We conclude that germ cell tumors are not only able to present with mixed histological patterns, but that the predominating picture is liable to change in the course of time.

The influence of abstinence of radiation therapy in the proliferation of a germinomatous component has to be considered.

SUMMARY

Some of our patients with germ cell tumors are presented.

Emphasis is placed on the mixed histological patterns, on the change of the predominating histological pattern in the course of time and on the recurrence of these tumors.

The influence of abstinence of radiation therapy in the proliferation of a germinatous component has to be considered.

KEY WORDS

Germinoma, Teratoma.

REFERENCES

1. ABAY (E.) et al.: J. Neurosurg. 55: 889-895, 1981.
2. JENNINGS (M.) et al.: J. Neurosurg. 63: 155-167, 1985.
3. SANO (K.): Clin. Neurosurg., 30: 59-91, 1982.

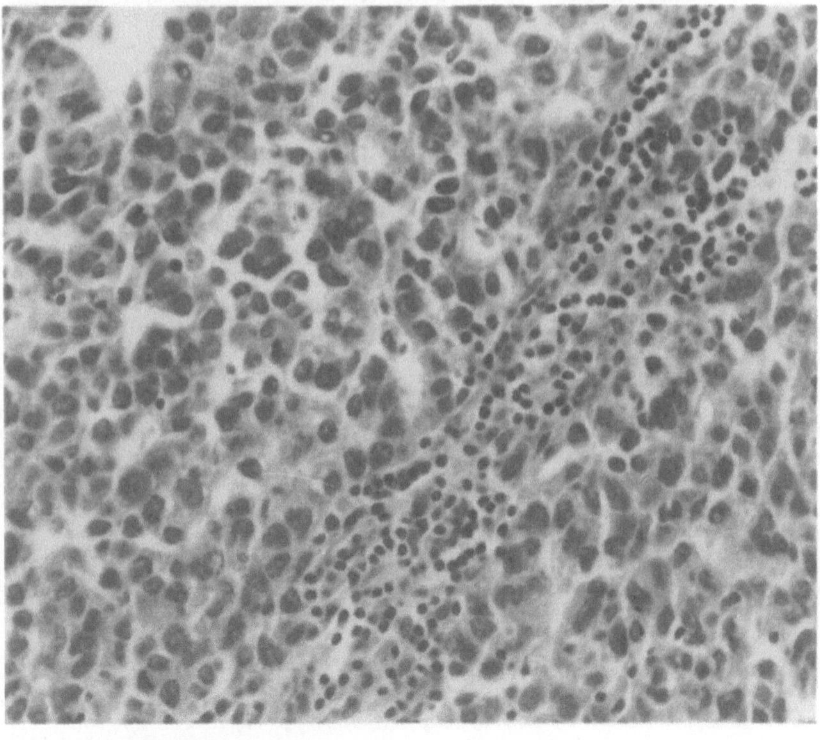

FIGURE 1:
Germinoma: Large polygonal cells and lymphocytic infiltrates.

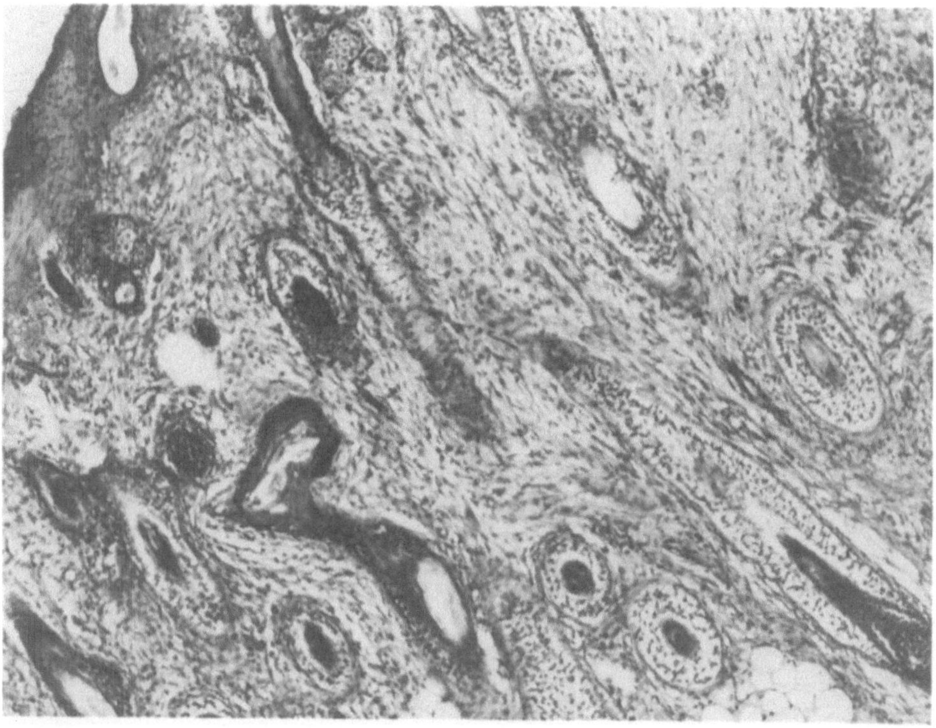

FIGURE 2:
Teratoma: Skin and appendages.

Dysontogenetic Brain Tumours. Morphological Variability and Problems of Classification

G.F. WALTER (°).

INTRODUCTION

The international classification of central nervous system tumours by WHO (9) does not give an extensive classification of germ cell tumours and other malformative tumours and tumour-like lesions. The neuropathologist usually has to fall back on the classification of germ cell tumours of the testis by WHO (7). But in that classification the peculiarities of dysontogenetic brain tumours are not taken into account. The best description of dysontogenetic brain tumours in the AFIP-series (8) is not accompanied by a clear conception of classification.

In this study, examples of transitional cases of dysontogenetic brain tumours are given and a more detailed classification is suggested.

CASE REPORTS AND NEUROPATHOLOGICAL FINDINGS

Case 1 :

A 66 years old man suffered from bitemporal hemianopsia since one year before death. 10 days before death, part of a suprasellar tumour has been removed. He died of a massive bronchopneumonia. In autopsy, the brain weighed 1290 g. The main finding consisted of a walnut-size suprasellar pearly tumour with the macroscopic aspect of an epidermoid cyst. Histologically, the wall of the cyst contained bone and undifferentiated glands next to the typical epidermal layer lining the cyst with keratin lamellae as content (Fig. 1).

Case 2 :

A 67 years old man has been operated in the age of 12 (thus 55 years ago) from a "brain tumour". There are no more exact informations on the histological type available. Since then he suffered from epileptic seizures of grand mal-type. Six months before death a spastic hemiparesis of the right side occurred. In computerized tomography, a very large calcified tumour of the left parietal lobe was seen. The neurosurgeon considered it to be inoperable. The seizures occurred more and more frequent. He died with signs of increased intracranial pressure. In autopsy, the brain weighed 1350 g. The left parietal and occipital lobes were extremely displaced by a 12:8:7 cm large, well demarcated cyst which was subdivided in four smaller cysts with localized continuation from one part into the other. The cyst was filled with a yellowish cheesy mass.

Histologically, the wall of squamous epithelium was highly atrophic, on some places rests of sebaceous glands or granular calcifications could be observed. The content of the cyst mainly was amorphous with some cholesterin crystals. There were signs of increased intracranial pressure and midbrain compression with haemorrhage (Fig. 2).

Case 3 :

A 22 days old boy was born after unconspicuous pregnancy. Post partum, he showed increasing hydrocephalus internus. In computerized tomography, an intracerebral expansive process with bleeding was found. He died of shock. In autopsy, the brain weighed 420 g. In the right hemisphere, an orange-size well demarcated tumour with greyish-yellowish, finely cystic tissue and a recent bleeding displaced the central grey nuclei and neighbouring structures. The tumour was divided in two parts separated by a thin layer of connective tissue. Histologically, several cysts were lined by cuboidal or columnar epithelium with few mitotic figures. They were surrounded by a glial or fibrotic tissue. The strong bleeding made it impossible to investigate all parts of the tumour in a proper manner (Fig. 3).

(°) Institute of Neuropathology, Medizinische Hochschule Hannover, Konstanty Gutschow-Str. 8, D-3000 Hannover 61.

M. Chatel, F. Darcel and J. Pecker (eds.), Brain Oncology. ISBN-13: 978-94-010-8003-3

Case 4 :

A 62 years old man with an atypical state of somnolence was admitted to the hospital. Later an epileptic fit was followed by a slight hemiparesis of the left side. A median central expansion and an internal hydrocephalus were found. The psychomotoric unrest and the general confusion of the patient made the admission in a nursing home necessary. There the patient died of a pneumonia. In autopsy, the brain weighed 1350 g. The principal finding was a 20:10 mm large, solid, in part calcified suprasellar tumour. There was no intrasellar part of the tumour. The pituitary gland was macroscopically and histologically normal, the sellar diaphragm untouched. Histologically, the tumour was largely calcified. There was almost no epithelium left except one cone of squamous epithelium with microcysts exhibiting an adamantinomatous pattern and two thin cords of columnar cells. There were many keratin pearls and areas packed with cholesterin crystals surrounded by foreign body giant cells. The calcifications gave the tumour an almost stone-like appearance. The neighbouring brain tissue exhibited an impressive astrogliosis with many Rosenthal-fibres (Fig. 4).

DISCUSSION

It seems to be useful to suggest a more detailed classification of dysontogenetic brain tumours with attention for the special intracranial situation (Table I). Even in the classification of testis tumours, the WHO-classification and the different "British" classification are very often simultaneously used (3).

For the classification of germ cell tumours, I have tried to keep the known headings from the WHO-brain tumour classification: germinoma, embryonal carcinoma and choriocarcinoma. At the same time, it seemed necessary to subdivide these tumours because different prognoses and therapeutic approaches are linked to the diagnostic subdivisions. However, there are no real differences with the classification of tumours of the testis.

There are serious doubts that teratomas actually originate from germ cells (1). It may be that multipotential cells deriving from the neural crest are the stem cells for teratomas. At least in animals, the neural crest is able to differentiate also into mesenchymal cells (5).

On the other hand, germ cell tumours in the brain are — unlike the situation in the testis — certainly teratomas sensu lato. In the strict definition, teratomas are tumours which contain embryonic elements of all three primary germ layers. But it is easily thinkable that only one or two germ layers develop in a tumour following the same principles as in the development of tumours from all three germ layers, what I would call teratomas or teratoid tumours sensu lato. For practical reasons, the division in more or less malignant germ cell tumours and generally benign teratomas seems justified. The classical subdivision in monodermomas, didermomas and tridermomas originating from one, two or all three germinal layers enables the neuropathologist to establish a quite clear concept for the classification of a number of brain-specific

TABLE I

Proposed classification of dysontogenetic brain tumours and tumour-like lesions

A. Germ cell tumours

1. Germinoma
   a. Classical
   b. Spermatocytic
   c. Anaplastic
2. Embryonal carcinoma
   a. Classical
   b. Yolk-sac tumour (endodermal sinus tumour)
   c. Polyembryona
3. Choriocarcinoma
4. Mixed
   a. Germinoma with trophoblastic giant cells
   b. Teratocarcinoma
   c. Choriocarcinoma and any other type of germ cell tumour
   d. Other combinations.

B. Teratomas

1. Monodermomas
   a. Epidermoid cyst
   b. Enterogenous cyst
   c. Lipoma
   d. Craniopharyngioma
   e. (Rathke's cleft cyst)
2. Didermomas
   a. Dermoid cyst
3. Tridermoma
   a. Mature teratoma
   b. Immature teratoma (teratoids)
   c. Teratoma with malignant transformation.

C. Other malformative tumours and tumour-like lesions (neuroectodermal)

1. Cysts
   a. Arachnoidal cyst
   b. Ependymal-lined cyst
   c. Colloid cyst of the third ventricle
   d. Neuroglial-lined cyst
2. Choristoma (granular neuroma)
3. Hypothalamic neuronal hamartoma
4. Nasal glial heterotopia (nasal glioma).

D. Tumours of the phacomatoses

malformative lesions. For instance, epidermoid cysts as well as enterogenous cysts, or even brain lipomas can easily be regarded as unilaterally, dermoid cysts as bilaterally differentiated benign teratomas, whereas the mature teratoma sensu strictu shows parts of all germinal layers. In the present case 1, a teratoma sensu strictu (tridermoma) showed the macroscopic aspect of an epidermoid cyst. It is a typical case which provokes no problems of understanding if put into a teratological sequence (monodermoma-didermoma-tridermoma) as generally usual in teratology. The present case 2 is an example for a didermoma. Its tumorous attitude is impressive. In case 3, an inborn immature teratoma is presented. Its histological dignity is unsure, a clear recognition of the germinal layers is difficult. Therefore, the term immature teratoma or teratoid seems appropriate.

I have hesitated to include the craniopharyngioma and Rathke's cleft cyst in the teratomas sensu lato. But especially the so-called suprasellar craniopharyngioma calls in a number of questions, because quite often no intrasellar tumour portion can be found such as in the present case 4.

An origin from Rathke's pouch in those cases is very questionable, so that then the term "craniopharyngioma" simply would be wrong. An intrasellar occurrence of craniopharyngiomas or the occurrence of squamous cell nests in the pituitary glands are in my opinion no satisfactory arguments for an origin from Rathke's pouch (2, 4, 6). The vicinity to the origin of epidermoid cysts which may be situated everywhere in the brain, is evident. This might also be valid for Rathke's cleft cyst, though here a possible origin from Rathke's pouch seems to be more discussable. Therefore, I have put it in between brackets (Table I). However, the histological feature of craniopharyngioma, especially the resemblance with the embryonic enamel organ, is very distinct that it anyway has to be kept as entity (but within the teratomas), although the denomination remains questionable.

In the proposed classification, under the heading "other malformative tumours and tumour-like lesions" only remains a series of neuroectodermal malformations which do not have the character of teratomas sensu lato sive strictu.

SUMMARY

Clear-cut borders between different types of dysontogenetic brain tumours cannot always be drawn. Transitional cases between all forms of germ cell tumours may be found as well as transitional forms between teratomas and malformative tumour-like cysts.

Examples of transitional cases are given and an improved classification is suggested since the available classifications are neither detailed nor consistent enough.

KEY WORDS

Brain Tumours, Dysontogenetic tumours, Germ cell tumours, Teratomas, Malformative cysts, Classification.

REFERENCES

1. COLLINS (D.H.), PUGH (R.C.B.): The pathology of testicular tumours (Livingstone, 1964).
2. GOLDBERG (G.M.), ESHBAUGH (D.E.): Squamous cell nests of the pituitary gland as related to the origin of craniopharyngiomas. A study of their presence in the newborn and infants up to age four. Arch. Pathol. **70**: 293-299 (1960).
3. HEDINGER (C.): Pathologie der Hodentumoren. Pathologe, **1**: 179-187 (1980).
4. HUNTER (J.J.): Squamous metaplasia of cells of the anterior pituitary gland. J. Pathol. Bacteriol. **69**: 141-145 (1955).
5. LE DOUARIN (N.M.): The Neural Crest (Cambridge University Press, 1982).
6. LUSE (S.A.), KERNOHAN (J.W.): Squamous cell nests of the pituitary gland. Cancer, **8**: 623-628 (1955).
7. MOSTOFI (F.K.), SOBIN (E.H.) (eds.): Histological typing of testis tumours. International histological classification of tumours No. 16 (WHO, 1977).
8. RUBINSTEIN (L.J.): Tumors of the central nervous system. Atlas of Tumor Pathology, second series, fascile 6 (AFIP, 1972).
9. ZULCH (K.J.) (ed.): Histological typing of tumours of the central nervous system. International classification of tumours No 21 (WHO, 1979).

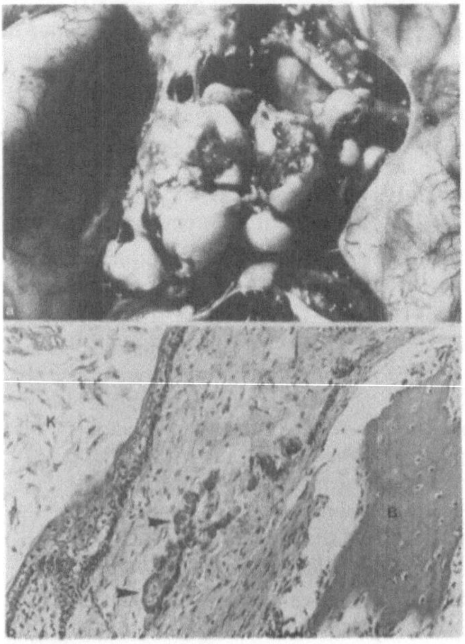

FIGURE 1:

a. Suprasellar teratoma with pearly appearance.

b. Squamous epithelial-lined wall of the tumour with bone (B) and undifferentiated glands (arrows). The cyst contains keratin lamellae (K). HE, 130x.

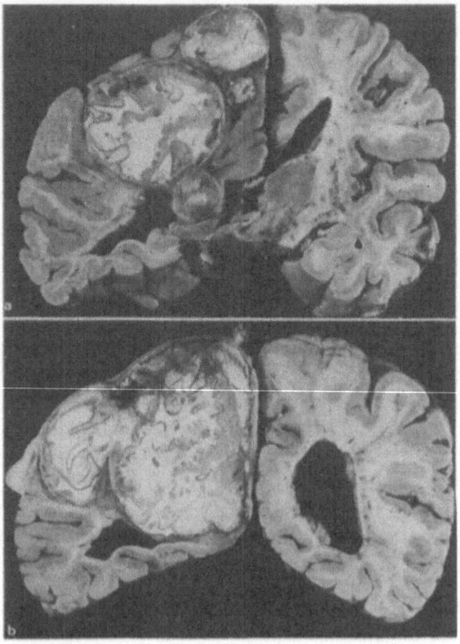

FIGURE 2:

Enormous dermoid cyst with partly multiolbular (a) and partly confluent (b) expansion.

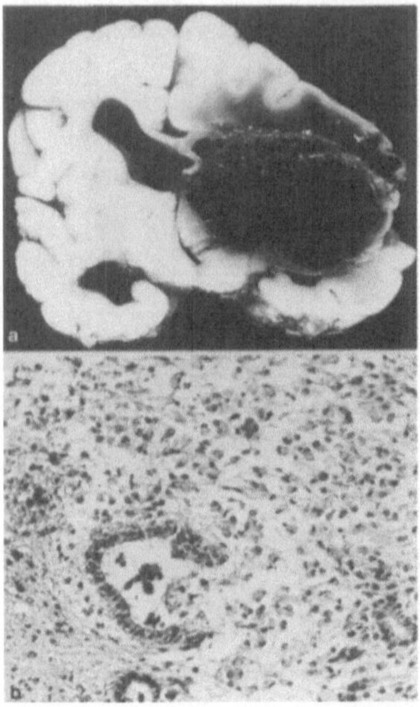

FIGURE 3:

a. Inborn immature teratoma with tumour bleeding.

b. Cysts lined with cuboidal epithelium. HE, 130x.

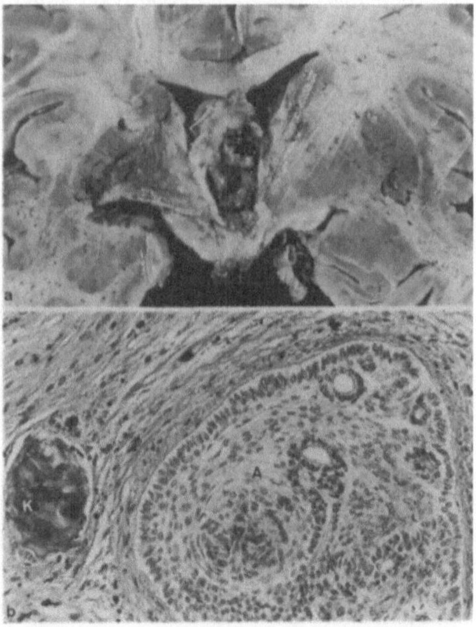

FIGURE 4:

a. Largely calcified suprasellar tumour.

b. Squamous epithelium with microcysts and adamantinomatous pattern (A) and keratin pearls (K) surrounded by gliotic tissue with Rosenthal-fibres. HE. 170 x.

Congenital intracranial tumors

J. BOHL (°), H.H. GOEBEL (°), S. AL-HAMI (°°), D. VOTH (°°), P. GUTJAHR (°°°).

INTRODUCTION

Tumors that are diagnosed already at birth or during the first or second week of life are called congenital tumors. They represent a special challenge to pediatric oncologists and to surgeons, and are relatively rare. From 1956 to August 1983 in the Pediatric Department of the University Hospital of Mainz, 1.027 children with tumors were observed and treated, 16 of them with congenital tumors. Among 479 tumor patients from 1956 to 1972 there was only one child with a congenital tumor; but from 1973 to 1983 there were 15 cases. Possibly, the absolute number of congenital tumors is increasing!

If, in addition, also those children are taken into consideration who presumably were born with such tumors but developed clinical signs only at a later stage, the total number of children is 18. Seven died, 11 survived without recurrences or metastases. Among these 18 children were only 8 with intracranial tumors: 1 teratoma, 1 craniopharyngeoma, 1 papilloma of the choroid plexus, 2 medulloblastomas, 1 astrocytoma, 1 spongioblastoma, and 1 hemangiopericytoma.

Over the recent 3 years, we observed three additional tumors: i.e., a meningeoma, a teratoma, and a ganglioneuroblastoma. Thus, we observed 11 such patients altogether between 1956 and to date.

Concerning congenital tumors and especially congenital intracranial tumors their prognosis is not only determined by histopathologic signs of malignancy; very often the localization and the operability alone are decisive. In this early period of life radiotherapy and chemotherapy bear a high risk of unfavorable late sequelae. Therefore, exclusive surgical intervention seems to be the most successful therapy and should be tried if possible. Several examples of congenital intracranial tumors are to elucidate and illustrate this complex of problems.

CASE HISTORIES

Patient 1: (KS 165/83).

The third pregnancy of a healthy mother was normal until the 33 rd week of gestation, when a sonographic examination showed an increased volume of the fetal head, corresponding to the 35th week of gestation. During the 37th week of gestation, slight uterine contractions commenced. The sonographic examinations now showed an enormous growth of the fetal head. The pregnancy had to be terminated operatively in the 42nd week of gestation by Caesarian section.

The mature male newborn showed a striking macrocephalus and a marked right exophthalmus. Widely opened fontanels and increasingly gaping cranial sutures indicated an elevated intracranial pressure. During the first days of life, the hydrocephalus internus enlarged. To determine type and grade of malignancy of the tumor, a biospy was taken from that part of the tumor, that was located in the right maxillary sinus.

Considering the poor prognosis no specific therapy was initiated and the child died 10 days after birth with clinical signs of impaired cardiac, circulatory and respiratory regulation of central origin.

The autopsy revealed a huge intracranial teratoma, replacing the entire right cerebral hemisphere, extending through osseous defects into the right orbita, and to the ocular bulbus, also filling the entire right maxillary sinus.

Histologically the tumor was a typical teratoma mainly with well differentiated tissue components derived from all three germ cell layers, but with a few less differentiated immature tissue components.

There were no other malformations.

(°) Division of Neuropathology, (°°) Department of Neurosurgery, (°°°) Department of Pediatrics, University of Mainz, Mainz/FRG - Allemagne.

M. Chatel, F. Darcel and J. Pecker (eds.), Brain Oncology. ISBN-13: 978-94-010-8003-3

Patient 2 (KS 183/82).
A healthy girl - 52 cm long and weighing 4000 g - was born at home one week before term. She was the second child of normal healthy parents, both 31 years of age. The child was brought to the hospital four days after birth because of an enlarging head and because of permanent shrilly crying. Sonographic and radiologic examinations (cranial CT) revealed a large intracerebral tumor, located supratentorially and extending from the brainstem into the cerebral hemispheres, mainly on the right side. The tumor showed many cystic areas, filled with fresh blood and had led to an occlusive hydrocephalus internus owing to an inhibited passage of cerebrospinal fluid.
Precise diagnosis of the tumor was not possible at this time (teratoma ?). As the prognosis seemed poor, the parents prohibited any therapy. The head further enlarged, she heavily vomited and had cerebral seizures. She died on the 46th day of life because of septicemia caused by Escherichia coli.
Histopathologically, the tumor was a widespread cystic astrocytoma, mainly of a subependymal giant cell astrocytoma type with large areas of necrosis, and remote and recent hemorrhages, as well as of circumscribed calcifications.
There were no signs of tuberous sclerosis.

Patient 3: (C.Y).
This little girl was 4 years old in 1983 when she had her first generalized seizure. Because of an increasing right-sided tremor, the child was examined for the second time in March 1985. A cranial CT revealed a large intracranial space occupying lesion on the left side. The E.E.G. showed pathologic features ; there was a papilledema of three diopters on both sides ; an X-ray of the skull demonstrated severely increased intracranial pressure.
In addition, the child showed a slight right hemiparesis, as well as a central paresis of the 5th cranial nerve. On April 4, 1985, a neurosurgical attempt was made to excise a well vascularized tumor from the right cerebral hemisphere. The tumor extended from the sphenoid wing to the occipital lobe and was adherent to the temporal base of the skull. Histopathological examination revealed a highly vascularized (angiomatous) meningeoma, mainly of the endotheliomatous type, with an unusual and rare variation of histologic patterns. Signs of malignancy could not be found. Postoperatively, there were no complications for the first 12 days ; but on the 13 th postoperative day a cerebral seizure produced severe hypoxic brain damage with subsequent edematous brain swelling and symptoms of downward cerebellar herniation.
Rapid neurosurgical decompression could not prevent brain death and the child died on April 26, 1985. An autopsy was not performed.

Patient 4: (K.W.).
Already a few days after the birth of this fullterm baby, her mother first noticed cerebral seizures. Every available technique (cranial CT, E.E.G., sonography, carotid angiography, A.E.H.P., and last not least craniotomy with biopsy) was employed to diagnose a large space occupying lesion with circumscribed calcifications and pathologic vascularization in the entire right cerebral hemisphere. Microscopically, the biopsy specimen showed a dysgenetic cerebral tissue mass with an uncertain blastomatous component like a gangliocytoma (Prof. Thomas, Edinger Institut, Frankfurt/Main). The main clinical symptoms were severe epileptic seizures often as persisting status epilepticus, that could not be suppressed by anti-epileptic drugs. In addition, the child had a left hemiparesis and weakness of her 5th and 6th cranial nerves, as well as muscle hypotonia. Her statomotor development was severely retarded. Her skull was asymmetric, larger on the right side.
The E.E.G. examinations showed highly abnormal patterns with polymorphous delta activity and irregular spike-potentials, with signs of a discontinuous bioelectric state.
On September 27, 1984 Prof. Voth, Mainz, performed subtotal hemispherectomy of the frontal and parietal lobes and part of the occipital lobe.
Only part of the right temporal lobe, medial and basal parts of the occipital lobe and the rostral basal ganglia remained. To everybody's great surprise postoperative development of the child was excellent. Neuropathological investigation of the surgical specimen by different neuropathologists led to similar or identical results: Dysplastic gangliocytoma (Prof. Goebel); ganglioneuroblastoma (Prof. Rubinstein); ganglion cell hamartoma (Prof. Burger); ganglioglioma (Prof. Scheithauer). Left hemiparesis and weakness of the 6th cranial nerve receded. Slight central weakness of the 5th cranial nerve persisted. Muscle tone also improved. The child seemed more awake and epilectic seizures had

subsided. Cranial CT controls in 1985 did not reveal recurrence of the tumor. E.E.G.-control findings also improved. All in all, the little girl showed encouraging development, although with marked retardation.

The latest clinical examination was on February 28, 1986. The left hemiparesis had persisted; there were no contractures. The spinal column showed an adjustable scoliosis, with right-sided convexity; a 2 cm difference in length between her legs, convergent strabism on the left, nystagmus and an uncertain weakness of her left 6th cranial nerve were noted. Pupillary activities were normal. She could sit without aid for a period of time. Her motor and mental developmental stage corresponded to that of a child less than 1 year old. Focal motor seizures with deviation of the eyes to the right and with an adversive component were observed in intervals of two or three days.

DISCUSSION

The congenital intracranial tumors recorded in this short communication are not directly comparable with those reported by other investigators. Concerning the incidence, the way of selection of cases and concerning the overall time of observation this study differs from others. Only primary congenital intracranial tumors of one hospital are considered and related to the total group of children afflicted with tumors. Obviously, the absolute frequency of congenital tumors had increased during the last 30 years in the region of this hospital, i.e., the Pediatric Department of the University Hospital in Mainz. There are no clues to possible etiologic factors in the history of our patients. The case of a congenital hemangiopericytoma (or of the hemangiopericytic type of a meningeoma) is exceptional to all others. No meningeomas were among primary CNS tumors of children with onset of symptoms during the first year of life observed between 1975 and 1980 by W. Jänisch. In our second patient with a presumable congenital meningeoma, clinical signs had started later.

In two patients of the tumor group discussed here an attempt of radical and complete tumor exstirpation proved unsuccessful because of extreme size of the tumor and severe technical difficulties.

In patient 4, a huge ganglioneuroblastoma could be successfully removed by subtotal hemispherectomy. Only this surgical therapy led to cessation of her permanent convulsions and her seizures receded to endurable frequency.

It is amazing that in this patient relatively little neurologic and psychologic deficits remained after neurosurgical intervention. Obviously, the excised brain areas had only few or no normal functional capacities.

This patients history illustrates the striking plasticity of the human brain in early childhood.

SUMMARY

In 1027 children with tumours observed between 1956 and 1983 only 16 had congenital neoplasms, 8 of which were of intracranial location. Since 1983 we observed 3 additional cases. The prognosis of congenital intracranial neoplasms is still worse than that of other congenital tumours. A complete excision would be the best therapy, but often the localization does not allow complete surgical removal. Four examples from our collection are demonstrated, e.g. an intracranial teratoma, an astrocytoma, a meningioma mixed with astrocytic components and a ganglio-neuroblastoma. This latter child was successfully treated by subtotal hemispherectomy and has now markedly improved.

REFERENCES

1. AL-HAMI (S.), VOTH (D.), GOEBEL (H.H.): Cranio-cerebrale Hemihypertrophie infolge kongenitalen dysplastischen Gangliocytoms. 37. Jahrestagung der Deutschen Gesellschaft für Neurochirurgie, Bonn, 4-7 Mai 1986.
2. BIGNAMI (A.), PALLADINI (G.), ZAPPELLA (M.): Unilateral megalencephaly with nerve cell hypertrophy. An anatomical and quantitative histochemical study. Brain Research, **9**: 103-114 (1968).
3. HANKO (E.): Konnatale Tumoren. Dissertation aus der Kinderklinik der J. Gutenberg-Universitat Mainz, 1983.
4. HAYASHI (K.), MIZOBUCHI (K.), TAGUCHI (K.), OHSUMI (S.), IKEHARA (I.), KOBAYASHI (K.): A case of cerebellar hamartoma suggesting abnormal cell migration. Acta Neuropathol (Berl), **69**: 283-287 (1986).
5. JÄNISCH (W.): Zur Epidemiologie der primären Geschwülste des Zentralnervensystems im ersten Lebensjahr. Arch. Geschwulstforsch., **55**: 489-494 (1985).

6. JÄNISCH (W.), SCHREIBER (D.), GERLACH (H.): Tumoren des Zentralnervensystems bei Feten und Säuglingen. Häufigkeit, Pathogenese, Pathomorphologie, Krankheitsverl äufe. (VEB Gustav Fischer Verlag Jena, 1980).

7. KIWIT (J.), SCHOBER (R.), LENARD (H.G.), BOCK (W.J.), WECHSLER (W.): Zur Klinik und Neuropathologie der Hemimegalencephalie. 37. Jahrestagung der Deutschen Gesellschaft für Neurochirurgie, Bonn, 4-7 Mai 1986.

8. KRETZSCHMAR (K.): Follow-up studies of brain tumours in infants and children. In: Tumours of the Central Nervous System in Infancy and Childhood. Edited by D. VOTH, P. GUTJAHR and C. LANGMAID, (Springer-Verlag, Berlin Heidelberg New York, 1982, pp. 130-141).

9. PASZTOR (A.), HARMAT (G.), KALMANCHEY (R.), DOBRONYI (I.): A rare case of infantile meningioma. Child's Nerv. Syst. **1**: 352-354 (1985).

10. PONTZ (B.F.), BOHL (J.), GUTJAHR (P.): Konnatales Astrocytom. der Kinderarzt, **15**: 777-781 (1984).

11. RUSSELL (D.S.), RUBINSTEIN (L.J.): Pathology of Tumours of the Nervous System (Edward Arnold, Publishers, 1977).

12. TOWNSEND (J.J.), NIELSEN (S.L.), MALAMUD (N.): Unilateral megalencephaly: Hamartoma or neoplasm ? Neurology, **25**: 448-453 (1975).

13. VOTH (D.), GUTJAHR (P.), LANGMAID (C.) (Editors): Tumours of the Central Nervous System in Infancy and Childhood. (Springer-Verlag, Berlin Heidelberg New York, 1982).

14. VOTH (D.), SCHRÖDER (J.M.), GUTJAHR (P.): Uber ein intrakranielles Hämangiopericytom beim Neugeborenen. Z. Kinderchir., **32**: 85-90 (1981).

KEY WORDS

Congenital intracranial neoplasms

TABLE
CONGENITAL INTRACRANIAL TUMORS (SINCE 1956)

N°	Name	Sex	Diagnosis at the age of	Localisation	Therapy	Histopathological diagnosis	Outcome
1	S.S.	m	2 1/4 years	sella turcica	operation	craniopharyngeoma	living
2	R.M.	f	2 months	right lateral ventricle	operation	papilloma of the choroid plexus	living
3	K.S.	m	7 weeks	fossa posterior cranil	operation and irradiation with Co60	medulloblastoma	death
4	P.C.	m	14 days	left hemisphere of the cerebellum	operation and ventriculo-peritoneal shunt	ependymoblastoma	living
5	B.M.	f	12 months	fronto-basal intracerebral	operation and chemotherapy	spongioblastoma	death
6	H.M.	m	10 days	temporo-parietal and occipital	operation	hemangiopericytoma	death
7	Z.S.	f	5 days	frontal	operation ventricular drainage	(teratoma : clinical diagnosis)	death
8	D.B.	m	37 weeks of gestation	right hemisphere of the brain	diagnostic biopsy	teratoma	death
9	A.S.	f	4 days	right hemisphere of the brain and central lobe	----	astrocytoma	death
10	C.Y.	f	6 years	left hemisphere of the brain	operation	meningeoma endotheliamatous	death
11	K.M.	f	13 days	right hemisphere of the brain	operation	ganglio-neuroblastoma	living and improved

FIGURE 1. Case 1 (in Table 1 no. 8: D.B.)
Congenital intracranial teratoma:

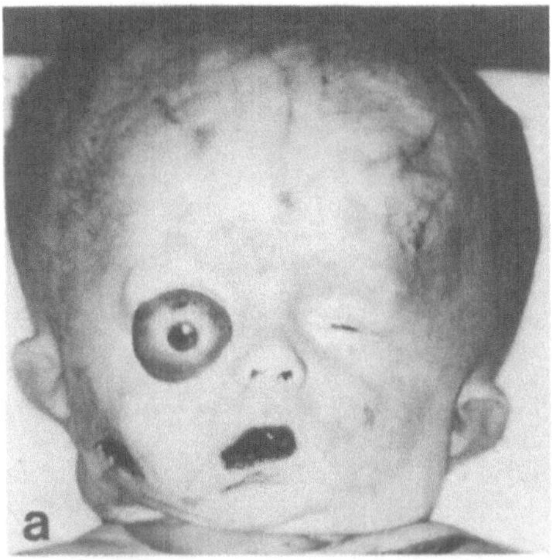

a) Newborn (male) showing a pronounced enlargement of the head and a marked exophthalmus on the right side.

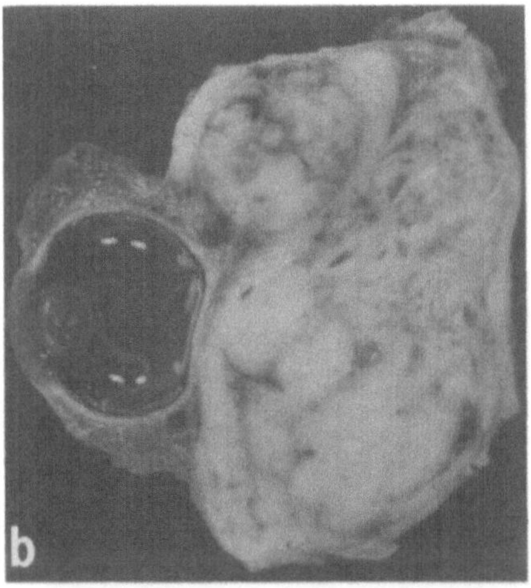

b) Right eye of the infant with a part of the tumor filling the entire orbita.

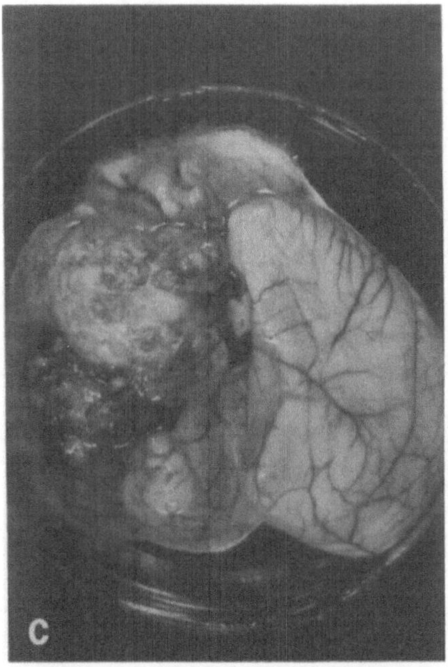

c) Base of the brain (without cerebellum). The right hemisphere is almost completely replaced by a huge polymorphous tumor: a teratoma.

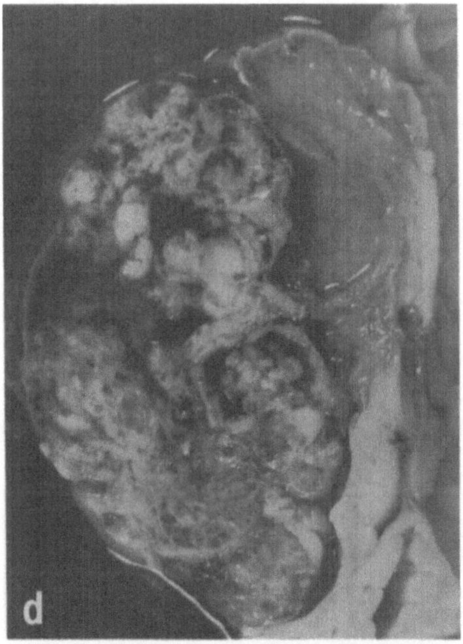

d) The gross section of the tumor shows different tissues. An occlusive hydrocephalus has developed in the other hemisphere.

FIGURE 2. Case 1 (in Table 1 no. 8: D.B.)
Congenital intracranial teratoma.
The histopathologic pattern of the tumor demonstrates a great variability with derivates of all three germ cell layers

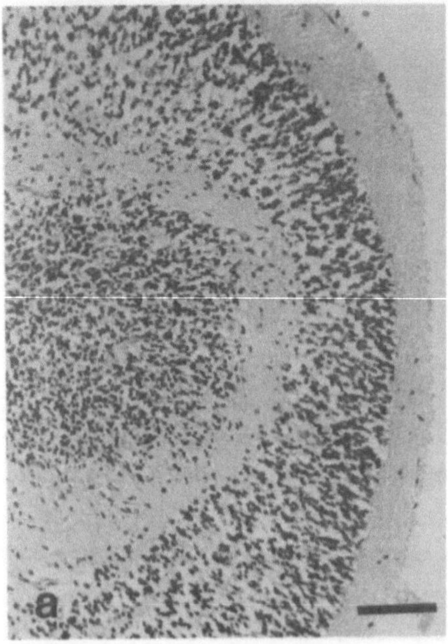

a) Cerebral tissue with an irregular stratification of cortical layers.

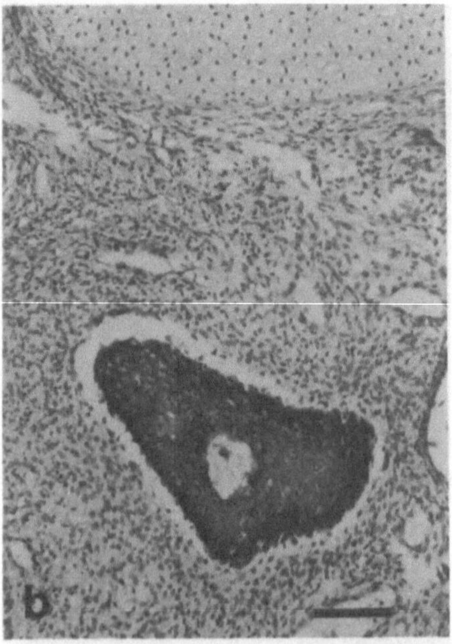

b) Connective tissue with cartilaginous and osseous components.

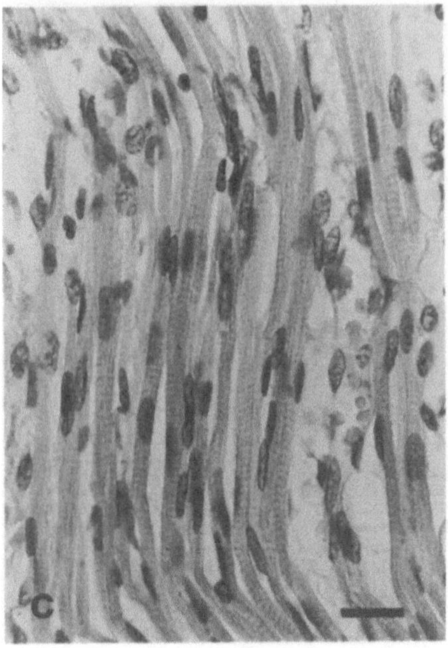

c) Skeletal muscle with typical cross-striations.

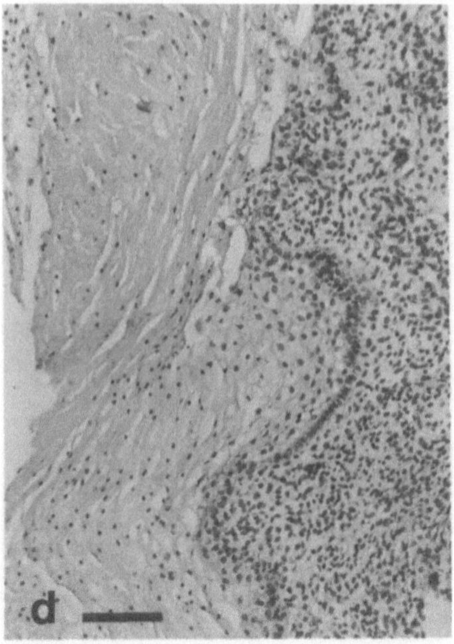

d) Epithelial tissue with a multilayered stratified epithelium. Formalin fixation, embedding in paraffin, H & E staining ; the scales represent 100 μm in a, b, and d, and 20 μm in c).

FIGURE 3. Case 2 (a and b) and Case 3 (c and d) (in Table 1 no. 9: A.S. and no. 10: C.Y.):

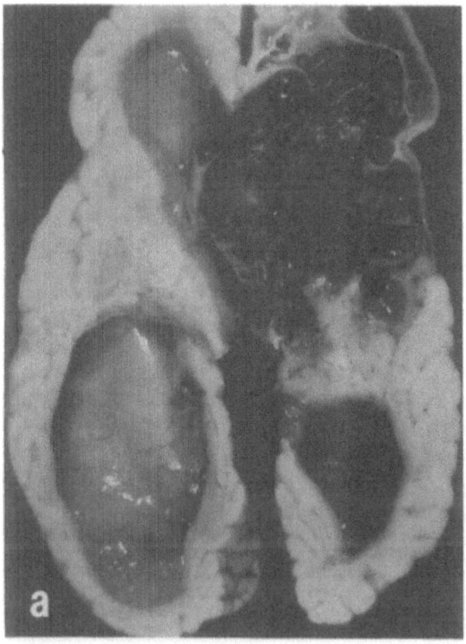

a) Gross section of both cerebral hemispheres. The right hemisphere is partly replaced by a huge cystic tumor with necrosis and many hemorrhagic foci.

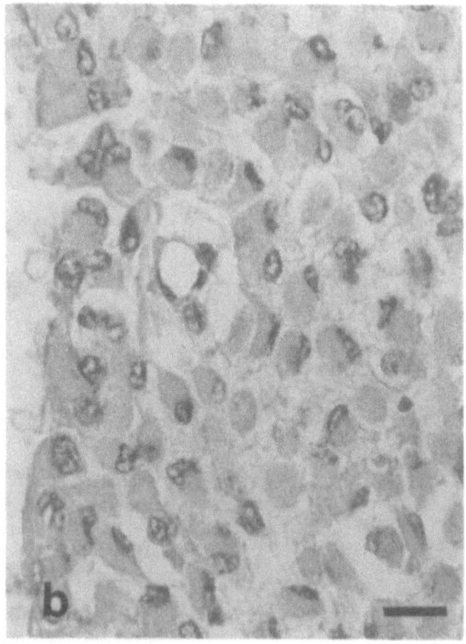

b) The histologic pattern shows an astrocytic tumor mainly composed of large cells with eccentric nuclei and homogeneous or granular cytoplasm. They are often positive with the anti-GFAP reaction.

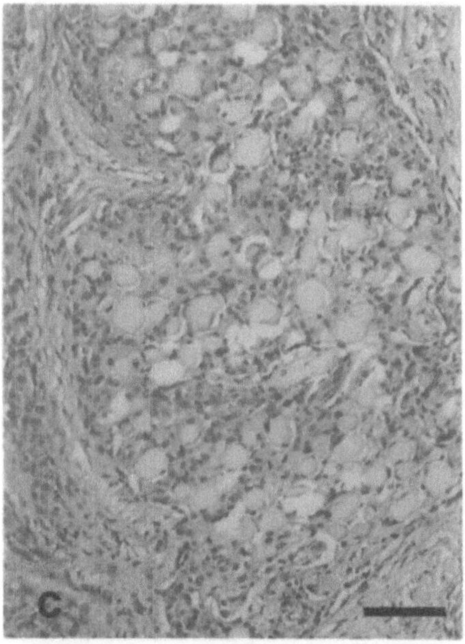

c) The histologic picture represents well differentiated parts of the meningeoma. Very often the tissue contains round and homogeneous corpuscules (negative with anti-GFAP). The tumor is positive with the anti-Vimentin reaction.

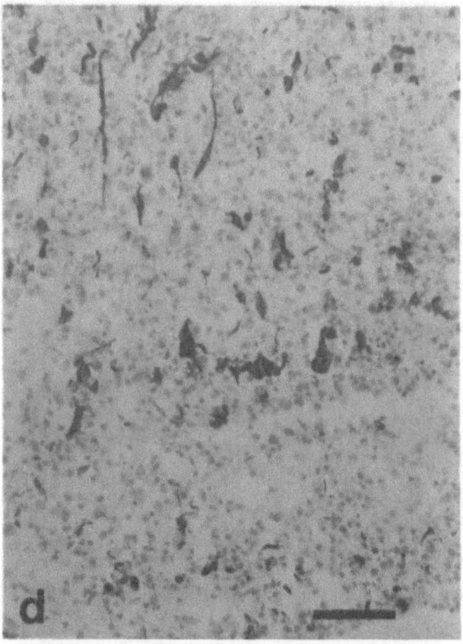

d) Among these typical tumor cells are some elongated irregular shaped cells, that are positive with the anti-GFAP reaction.
(b and c: Fixation in formalin, paraffin-embedding, H&E staining. d) Frozen section of fresh tissue, anti-GFAP). The scales represent 20 μm in b, and 100 μm in c and d.

FIGURE 4. Case 4 (in Table 1 no. 11: K.W.)
Cranial CT scans of a little girl before (a) and after (b) neurosurgery (right subtotal hemispherectomy). Note the obvious asymmetry of the skull and the brain

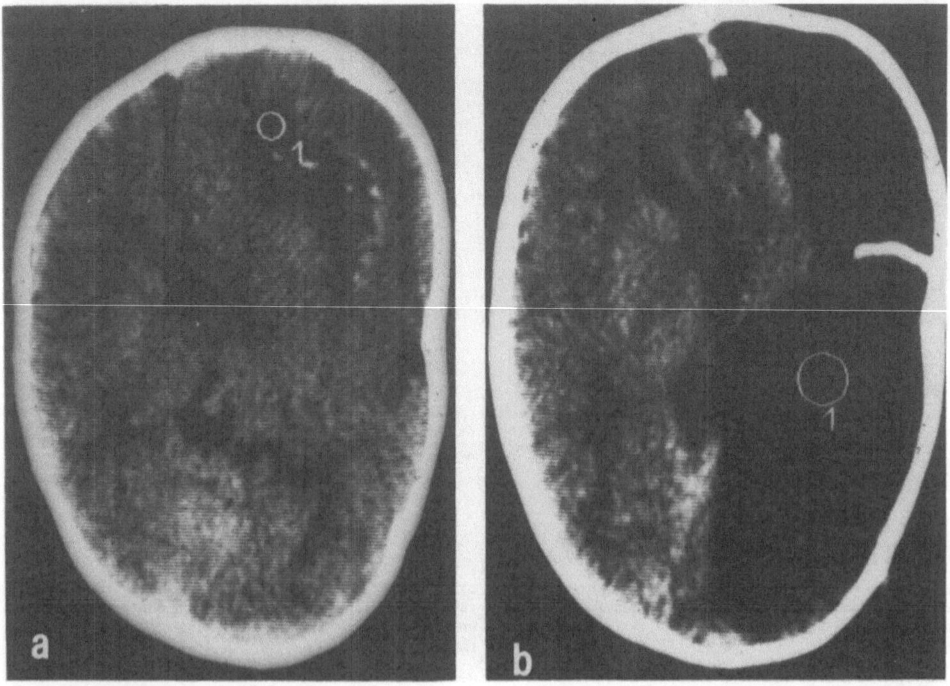

FIGURE 5. Case 4 (no. 11 in Table 1: K.W.):

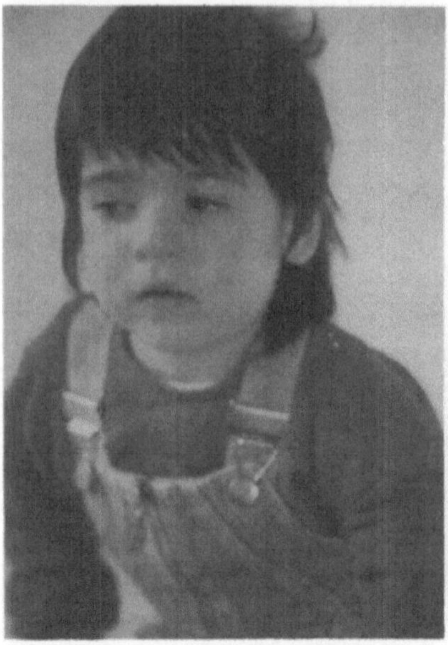

a) The young girl after the operation, about 2 years old.

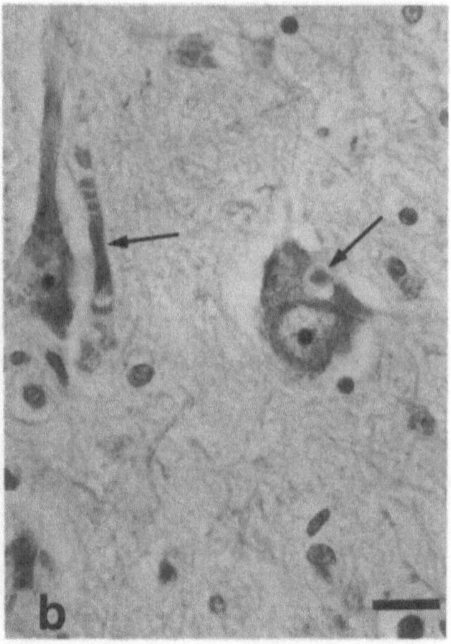

b) Typical histologic picture of a gangliocytoma. Some nerve cell bodies are in close vicinity to capillaries (arrows). Very often they are positive with the N.S.E. (Neurone Specific Enolase) reaction.

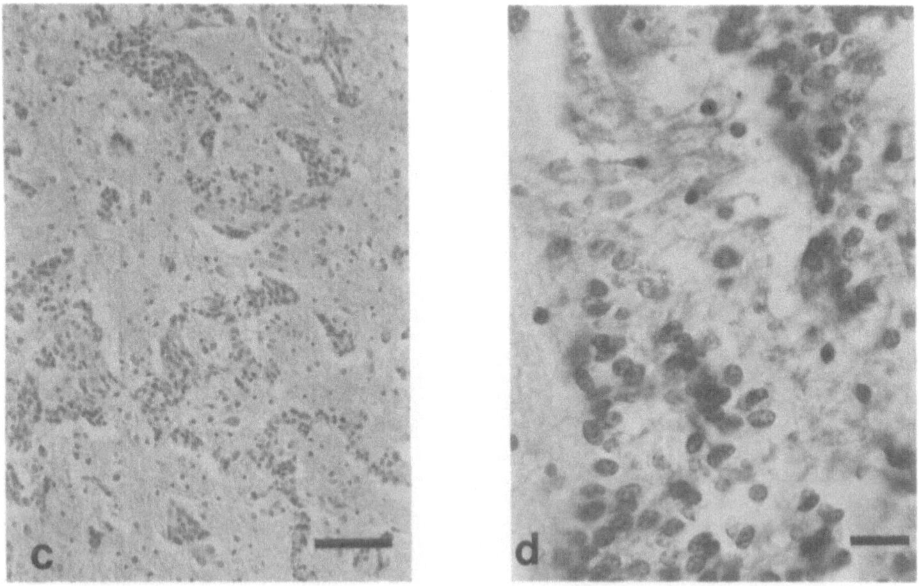

c) Other regions show an increase of small cells around blood vessels. They are positive with the S 100 reaction and are N.S.E.-negative. Many cells of the surrounding cerebral tissue are positive with anti-GFAP.

d) Higher magnification of a region from Fig. 5c.
(Formalin fixation, embedding in paraffin, H&E staining in c and d, Klüver-Barerra in b).
The black scales represent 20 μm in b and d, and 100 μm in c.

Meningiomas: the Value of Diagnostic Cytology by Tissue Imprints

U. SIMI (°), R. BUONAGUIDI (°°), F. FAGGIONATO (°°), G. GIACOMINI (°).

INTRODUCTION

The imprint technique is widely used in the cytopathologic diagnosis of several lesions and it is very useful in the correct histotyping of different neoplasias expecially lymphomas.

Imprint cytologic preparations combined with frozen sections of central nervous system neoplasias is a quite common procedure in various Pathology Laboratories all over the world (1, 2).

We have been using the imprint technique since 1984 in all cases of brain tumour which came to our observation. Among these we found 55 meningiomas and cytology really helped us in a better cytotyping of the neoplasias.

MATERIAL AND METHODS

Imprints have been prepared by touching a glass slide with fresh tissue and holding firmly this latter against the former.

Each preparation has been immediately fixed in 95° ethanol and carried to the Pathology Department. After 15-20 minutes of fixation the. slides were stained following the Papanicolaou technique.

If a rapid diagnosis was required, the smear preparations were fixed in 4% buffered formalin for 10-15 seconds and stained following a standard Hematoxylin-Eosin procedure. The tissue used for the imprints was fixed in 10% buffered formalin and routinely processed.

RESULTS

From the pure cytologic point of view we were able to classify meningiomas in eight subtypes:

1. Epithelioid meningioma. This subtype is mainly characterized by small layers of quite uniform cells with abundant eosinophilic granular cytoplasm (Fig. 1). The cells maintain a certain individuality.
2. Pseudosyncitial meningioma. It shows large clusters of benign cells merging together. The cytoplasmic borders are quite indefinite (Fig. 2).
3. Spindly meningioma. Most of the cells are spindle shaped with fusiform nucleus and faintly basophilic cytoplasm. They may be clustered or isolated (Fig. 3).
4. Whorly meningioma. The pattern is highly peculiar showing numerous benign whorls made by concentric layers of benign cells. The appearance is quite similar to a keratin pearl (Fig. 4).
5. Autolytic meningioma. The background shows numerous naked nuclei of various size (Fig. 5). They may be hyperchromatic and bring to mind the bipolar naked nuclei commonly found in the thin needle aspirates from benign lesions of the breast.
6. Psammomatous meningioma. Among clusters and layers reminiescent of the epithelioid and pseudosyncitial variants, numerous concentric concretions (calcospherites) are found (Fig. 6).
7. Angioblastic meningioma. The smear from this subtype may show arborizing blood vessels (Fig. 7). Meningioma cells may be found in layers, clusters and even isolated.
8. Xanthomatous meningioma. In this rare variant, histiocytoid cells with large granular cytoplasm and peripherally located, sometimes multiple, nuclei, are found scattered along the smear (Fig. 8).

(°) Servizio di Anatomia Patologica, Spedali S. Chiara, Pisa, I. (°°) Istituto di Neurochirurgia, Università di Pisa, Spedali S. Chiara, Pisa, I.

M. Chatel, F. Darcel and J. Pecker (eds.), Brain Oncology. ISBN-13: 978-94-010-8003-3

DISCUSSION

The squash and the imprint techniques are thought to be very helpful in the evaluation of nuclear details in meningiomas and to be a valuable adjunct to frozen examination (3). Both are particularly helpful in homogeneous highly cellular lesions with no whorls or psammoma bodies which may mimick metastatic carcinoma. In cytologic smears, cells from all subtypes of meningioma described above are generally uniform in size, shape and chromatin texture. Nucleoli are inconspicuous. Atypia may be found in all subtypes and by itself does not carry important implications on prognosis and on malignant behaviour (4).

In our material atypia was quite impressive in autolytic and angioblastic meningiomas. Few scattered atypical, sometimes multinucleated cells were found in almost all smears.

Then imprint cytology may be very useful in the correct histotyping of meningiomas but it may no help in the diagnosis of the malignant forms which require the counting of mitotic figures, possible only in histologic sections.

SUMMARY

Cytology can capture the finest cellular details which cannot be appreciated through frozen sections. Imprint smear preparations can be very valuable adjuncts in the intraoperative histotyping of meningiomas but may not be adequate to differentiate the malignant forms.

KEY WORDS

Meningioma, Imprint cytology, Diagnosis, Brain Tumors.

REFERENCES

1. BURGER (P.C.): Use of cytological preparations in the frozen section diagnosis of central nervous system neoplasia. Am J. Sur. Pathol. 9: 344-354 (1985).
2. ADAMS (J.H.), GRAHAM (D.J.), DOYLE (D.): Brain biopsy. The smear technique for neurosurgical biopsies (Chapman and Hall, 1981).
3. TAKAHASHI (M.): Color Atlas of Cancer Cytology (Igaku-Shoin, 1984).
4. WELLER (R.O.): Colour Atlas of Neuropathology (Oxford University Press, 1984).

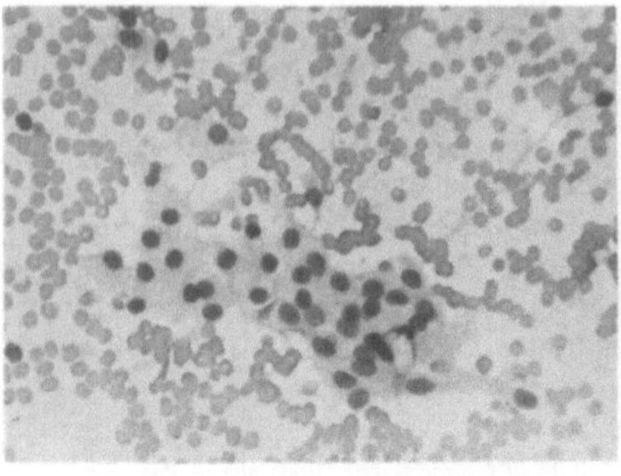

FIGURE 1. Epithelioid meningioma (Pap, 250x).

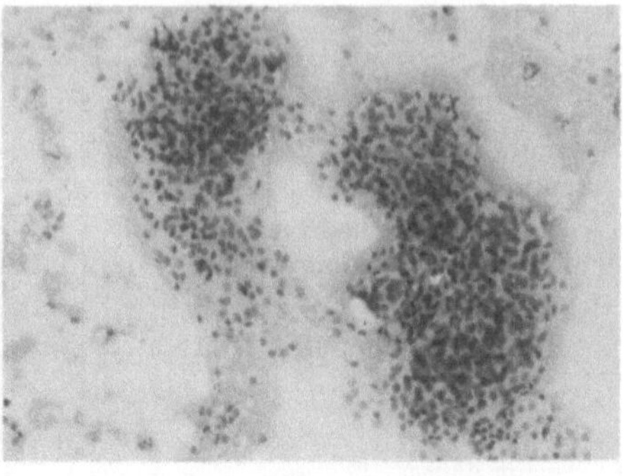

FIGURE 2. Pseudosyncitial meningioma (Pap, 100x).

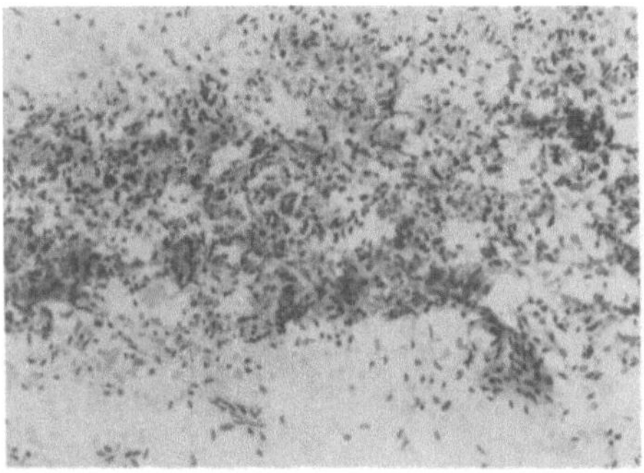

FIGURE 3. Spindly meningioma (Pap, 100x).

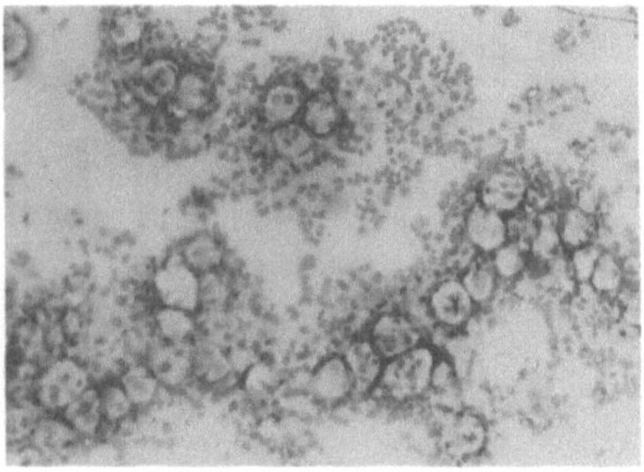

FIGURE 4. Whorly meningioma (Pap, 100x).

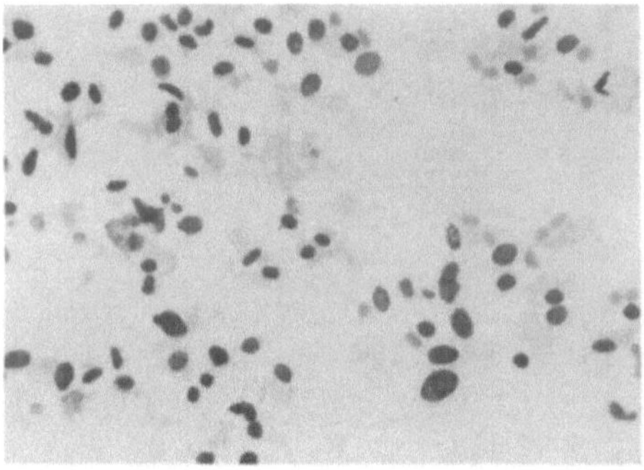

FIGURE 5. Autolytic meningioma (Pap, 400x).

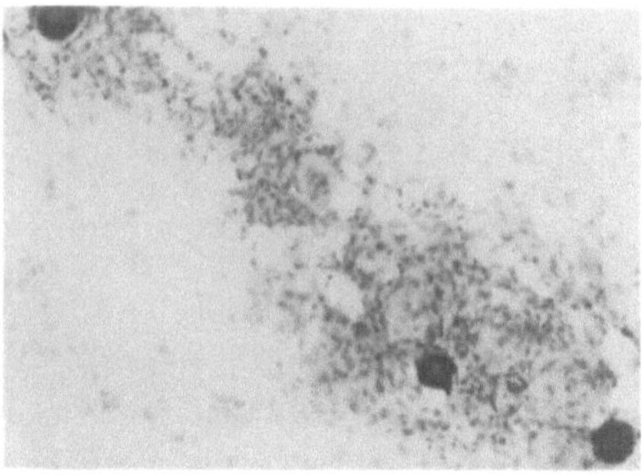

FIGURE 6. Psammomatous meningioma (Pap, 100x).

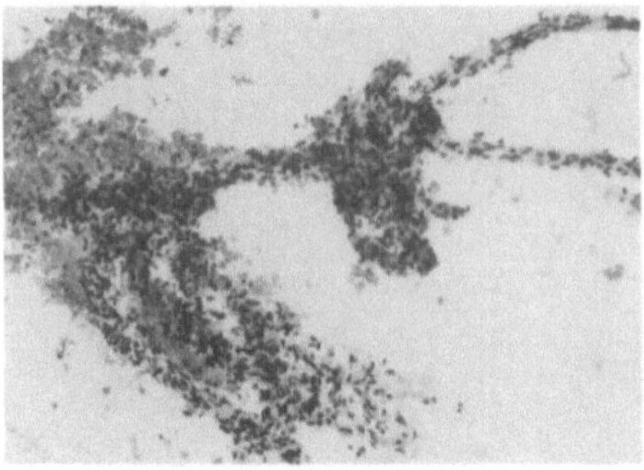

FIGURE 7. Angioblastic meningioma (Pap, 100x).

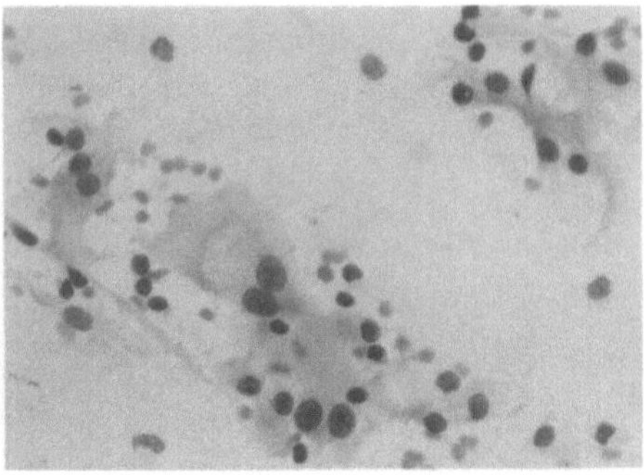

FIGURE 8. Xanthomatous meningioma (Pap, 400x).

PART III:
TUMORAL IMMUNOBIOLOGY AND ONCOBIOLOGY

Modulation of Class I and Class II Major Histocompatibility Complex Antigens in Gliomas

P. ZUBER (°), N. DE TRIBOLET (°).

INTRODUCTION

The concept of major histocompatibility complex (MHC) proposed by Gorer in 1937 (1) has been intensively developped in the last twenty years. Denoted H-2 in mice and HLA (Human Lymphocyte Locus A) in humans, it is a well defined locus on chromosome 17 in mice and on the short arm of chromosome 6 in humans. This system and its functions are present in all vertebrates (2). Following the physicochemical characteristics of proteins expressed by these genes, 3 families of MHC products have been defined and denoted class I, II and III (3). The first part of this chapter attempts to describe the main concepts associated with class I and II MHC antigens, especially their specific biological functions. We do not attempt to present class III products which correspond to proteins implicated in the complement system and do not seem to play a major role in the immune response directed against cancer.

1.1. Class I antigens

Class I products are glycoproteins (denoted H-2 K and D in mice and HLA-A, B and C in humans) expressed by all nucleated cells of a vertebrate organism (4). On the cell surface, this molecule is always associated non covalently with a shorter polypeptide, which does not belong to the MHC, β_2-microglobulin (3). In addition to their historical role of transplantation antigens (shared with the other classes of MHC), class I antigens are associated with numerous biological phenomena. Their most striking function observed in fundamental biology has been described first by Zinkernagel and Doherty (5). These authors have shown in mice that the specificity of cytotoxic T lymphocytes (CTL) on virally infected murine cells was not only defined by the infectious agent, but also by the H-2 K and D phenotype of the infected cells. It is now considered that during its maturation, a CTL is restricted to recognize viral (or any other cell surface) antigens in relationship with class I antigens of the sensitizing cell. In conclusion, MHC class I antigens are necessary for CTL activation.

1.2. Class II antigens

Class II products (denoted H-2 I in mice and HLA-DR, DC and SB in man) are composed of 2 polypeptidic chains non-covalently associated as well as of a number of carbon hydrates (6). These antigens are expressed on a limited number of normal cells, B and T lymphocytes, monocytes, macrophages, dendritic cells, Langerhans cells of epidermis and occasionally vascular endothelial cells. All these cells are able to function as accessory antigen presenting cells to helper T lymphocytes. They are responsible for lymphocyte activation in mixed lymphocyte culture (7) and generate CTL's (8). One praticularly striking feature of class II antigens is their association with the intensity of the immune response to defined antigens (9, 10). For this reason, they have also been denoted Ia (Immune response associated) antigens. They account for the class II restriction of helper T cells. In conclusion, MHC class II antigens modulate helper T cell activation.

2. Major histocompatibility complex and cancer

The function of the immune system is not only limited to recognition and elimination of foreign structures from the organism. It also plays an important role in detecting dedifferenciated cells which are likely to occur frequently in a multicellular organism. It has been demonstrated now that it was possible to detect on cultured tumoral cells antigens not expressed on the adult normal tissue from which these tumor cells originated. Such antigens have also been demonstrated in glioblastomas (11, 12, 13). An important objective of tumor immunology is to define the factors necessary for an antitumoral immune response. Recent works have demonstrated the major part played by MHC products in these responses.

(°) Neurosurgical Service, University Hospital, CH 1011 Lausanne, Switzerland.

M. Chatel, F. Darcel and J. Pecker (eds.), Brain Oncology. ISBN-13: 978-94-010-8003-3

2.1. Role of class I antigens in the control of tumor cell proliferation

Van der Eb et al (14, 15) reported a high tumorigenicity of Ad 12 adenovirus strain on rat cells and noted that Ad 12 infected cells dit not express class I antigens. In contrast, adenovirus strain Ad 5 infected cells strongly express these antigens and dot not produce any tumor. In this model the potential tumor development is inversely related to class I expression, cells carrying these markers are recognised and destroyed by the immune system and cannot be tumorigenic. Following this observation, Tanaka et al. (16) abolished the tumorigenicity of Ad 12 transformed mice cells. They transfected these cells with functionnal MHC gene which then expressed class I MHC antigens on the cell surface. After transfection, cells were reinjected into syngeneic mice. Survival of mice was directly related to the intensity of class I products expression in the different injected clones. These results show that class I gene expression in the MHC can suppress the tumoral potential in collaboration with the immune response.

2.2. Role of class II antigens on immune response to tumoral antigens

The association of accessory antigen presenting cell function and class II expression is already well described (17). Recently, Kern et al. (18) demonstrated the critical part played by these cells in the cell-mediated immune response against tumors. Their observations were centered on the CTL response (class I restricted) on a class II negative syngeneic erythroleukemia cell line (FBL). They studied the CTL activity of different spleen cells extracts against FBL cells. In spleen extracts free of helper T cells, CTL activity is abolished. Using a monoclonal antibody (MAB) directed specifically against a class II antigen, CTL activity of total spleen extracts is also repressed. When macrophages (class II positive) are added to accessory cell deprived samples, CTL activity is restored but if macrophage lysozomes are blocked by pretreating with choloroquine or NH4Cl, CTL activity is abolished again. These experiments demonstrate the critical part played by accessory antigen presenting cells in association with class II products for inducing the immune response to tumor associated antigens.

3. MHC antigen expression in non tumoral cerebral tissue

The first experiments evaluating the expression of MHC components were performed by absorbtion of specific antisera on tissue homogenates and evaluation of residual lymphocytotoxic activity (19). With this method, spleen expresses the strongest amount of class I antigen per gram of tissue followed by intestines, liver, lungs, kidneys... fat tissue and brain almost expressed nothing. More recently, a quantitative estimate of class I and II antigens distribution has been performed by absorbtion of a MAB. When compared to the spleen, brain fixation of anti class I MAB is only 1 % and anti-class II MAB'S are not fixed at all. This is very weak compared to kidneys (14 % and 90 %), liver (9 % and 19 %) or bone marrow (15 % and 2 %).

Immunohistology has facilitated the observation of this antigen distribution on the different cell types present in a single tissue. Thus, in normal brain, it is not possible to detect any class I antigen with these techniques on neural cells, astrocytes, oligodendrocytes, myelin or microglia. In contrast, blood vessels are strongly stained and account probably for the weak expression detected in homogenates (21, 22, 23). Class II antigens have also been studied with these techniques using anti-HLA-DR MAB'S. Only a few astrocyte like cells in white matter are positive (24, 25, 26). Frank et al. (27) demonstrated that these cells were also positive for glial fibrillary acidic protein in a double staining technique. They also showed a larger quantity of HLA-DR positive astrocytes in reactionnal tissue surrounding metastases and cerebral abscesses. Intracerebral blood vessels are also likely to fix these kinds of MAB'S (23). Finally, studies performed on fetal astrocytic cell lines from a 20 week old fetus, with radio-immunoassay, demonstrated the induction of class II antigens by treatment with interferon γ (γ IFN) (28).

4. MHC and gliomas

Natali et al (21) studied the expression of class I antigens on numerous tissues and their related tumors. In normal brain, they did not demonstrate any positive cells. A positive result was obtained in 1 out of 3 glioblastomas and in none of 4 astrocytomas. More recently. Lampson and Hickey (23) reported occasionally positive cell bodies for class I antigens in a malignant astrocytoma but not in low grade tumors. Class II antigens are present on a higher number of cells in tumoral than in normal tissue according to these authors. Piguet et al. (29) studied 11 gliomas, on 2 occasions no positive cell was detected, on the 9 other specimens 0.3 % to 40 % of cells were positive, without any correlation with histological grading. Bigner et al. (30) determined class I phenotype of 15 permanent cell lines of malignant gliomas between 54 and 612 passages. Personal observations on more than 45 glioblastoma cell lines with radioimmunassay always demonstrated a frankly positive (more than 6 times background) expression of these antigens. these observations are in contrast with the difficulty do detect class I antigens with immunohistology. These antigens could be induced in cell culture by factors present in the serum of the culture medium. Class II antigens, in contrast, are distributed very heterogeneously in tumor cell lines and clones. With cytotoxicity techniques, Carrel et al. (31) lysed 3 out of 8 glioma cell lines with anti HLA-DR D1-12 MAB and complement. This expression has also been confirmed by immunoprecipitation experiments (13). With a radioimmunoassay, Piguet et al. (32) found a positive expression of HLA-DR in 9 out of 22 cell lines, with 2 MAB'S directed against different epitopes of this molecule. The intensity of expression was similar for both MAB'S.

5. Modulation of class I and II antigen expression

Histocompatibility antigen expression is not fixed in a given tissue or cell line but is subjected to modulation by many factors. For instance, less than 1 % of mice brain cells are H-2 K positive with immunofluorescence. After intracerebral injection, of γ IFN, 50 % of these cells do express H-2 K (33). In addition, when cultivated, these cells are also H-2 K positive (34). Numerous normal and tumoral cell lines have already been studied in vitro for modulation of MHC products when cultivated with immunocompetent cells or cytokines called biological response modifiers (BRM). The role played by class I and II antigens in the intracerebral immune response has recently been pointed out by the works of Fierz et al. and Fontana et al. These authors studied the murine astrocyte as an accessory antigen-presenting cell. Fierz et al. (35) demonstrated the possible expression of class II antigens on rat astrocytes when cultivated with Con A stimulated spleen cell supernatant or murine γ IFN. Then they demonstrated that T cell proliferation in response to a given antigen was strongly stimulated in presence of these pretreated astrocytes and that this stimulating capacity was blocked by an anticlass II MAB. Fontana et al. (34) demonstrated that cultivated murine astrocytes were able to stimulate proliferation of haptene specific cytotoxic T lymphocytes restricted to a given H-2 K haplotype. This stimulation is blocked by a MAB directed against this class I haplotype. Thus, modulation of MHC products seems to be interesting in the field of cell mediated immune response to glial tumors because of the potential role of accessory cell played by astrocytes. We are going to describe a few biological response modifiers, their effect on cancers and especially gliomas. Among the numerous described cytokines, we shall limit our description to interferons and a new substance: Tumor Necrosis Factor (TNF).

Interferons are antivirally active proteins acting nonspecifically inside cells homologous to those which synthesize them. Historically, it is because of their viral replication inhibitory function that they have been identified in 1957. Two major kinds of interferons a· e described today, types I and II.

Type I IFN's (or viral IFN's) are α and β IFN's. They share a common cellular receptor and are both encoded by chromosome 9 in man. α IFN is produced by leucocytes stimulated by some viruses. β IFN is produced by fibroblasts in presence of RNA or of polymers ressembling RNA (36, 37).

Type II IFN (or immune IFN) is γ IFN. It possesses a receptor distinct from that of type I IFNs; it is coded on chromosome 12 and produced by some T cells in response to an immune stimulus. In vitro, it's biosynthesis can be stimulated in lymphocytes cultures by phytohemaglutinine or Con A. IFN's can also inhibit cell division in vivo and in vitro. They increase membrane density and membrane proteine/lipid ratios, decrease cell motility, and increase cellular negative charge. They modulate, as will be discussed, MHC antigen expression. Finally, they considerably increase NK cell cytotoxicity (38). δ IFN is also able to induce myelomonocytic cells, to influence differenciation of B cells and antibody production and to induce the expression of class II antigens.

Endotoxin stimulated BCG immunized mouse serum is able to necrotize tumors grafted subcutaneously in « nude » mice (41). The factor responsible for this effect has been isolated (42) and cloned in mice (43) and man (44, 45). It is a monokine a structure similar to lymphotoxin denoted **Tumor Necrosis Factor.** TNF has a cytotoxic and even cytolytic effect in vitro on a number of tumoral cell lines (46, 47). Its identity with cachectin has been demonstrated recently after demonstration of its pyrogenic effect as well as IL-1 biosynthesis inducer, prostaglandin E2 production stimulator, neutrophil and eosinophil activator and lipoproteine lipase activator (48, 49).

5.1. Effect of biological response modifiers on MHC gene products of normal and tumoral cells.

Several authors reported an increase of class I antigens on a large panel of murine and human cells in the presence of α IFN (50, 51, 52, 53). γ IFN acts more specifically on class II antigen expression and associated immune response. Pober et al. (54) demonstrated the proportionality between CTL induction amplitude against human endothelial and fibroblastic cells and HLA-DR expression. A MAB directed against the HLA-DR molecule inhibited this response. Basham and Merigan (55) demonstrated that human recombinant γ IFN increased HLA-DR expression on HLA-DR positive melanoma cell lines whereas α IFN was not active. Carrel et al. (56) even demonstrated a possible induction of this marker on DR negative melanoma cell lines. In summary, α and β IFN's increase class I antigens expression but at higher concentrations than γ IFN. Additionally, γ IFN induces selectively class II antigens expression.

Recently, Collins et al. (57) reported a specific increased expression of class I products when human fibloblasts or umbilical endothelial cells were incubated with TNF. They also showed that TNF increased intracellular expression of class I associated mRNA.

5.2. Biological response modifiers and gliomas.

We have tested α and γ IFNs effects on several glioma cell lines as well as on a line of fetal astrocytes (32). We observed that recombinant human α IFN was able to increase the spontaneous expression of class I antigens on 3 out of 6 cell lines tested but never influenced HLA-DR expression. Recombinant human γ IFN in contrast was able to increase spontaneous class I expression in 7 out of 10 cell lines but also increased the expression of HLA-DR in 3 spontaneously positive lines. γ IFN has even induced the expression of class II antigens in 3 out of 7 spontaneously negative cell lines. In another report we have studied HLA-DR expression on 2 glioma cell lines and their clones (58). One of these lines (LN 340) has been induced by γ IFN to express HLA-DR as did the tumor from which this line originated. In addition, every clone and subclone produced from this line has been induced to express HLA-DR with γ IFN but not with α IFN. The other cell line was not modulated by γ IFN but 4 out of 7 clones have been induced to express HLA-DR. These results show that among a particular glioma cell line, there is a heterogeneous population of cells some of these being able to express class II antigens when stimulated by γ IFN. γ IFN also had a heterogeneous effect on cell growth since only 5 out of 9 cell lines have been inhibited. These results have been confirmed by others (59). Many clinical trials have been attempted in glioma patients with both α and β IFN, they have been recently reviewed (60). A few positive responses have been reported which are not convincing yet.

Preliminary data from our laboratory show that TNF allows a selective modulation of class I antigens on glioma cell lines and clones. Class II antigens as well as tumor associated antigens are not influenced by this monokine. The first results of clinical trials with TNF have not been published yet.

CONCLUSION

The works we have briefly reviewed point out the part played by class I and II MHC gene products in the cellular immune response to cancer. In vitro models demonstrate a possible modulation or induction of these markers with biological response modifiers.

There is a potential interest for immunotherapy of human gliomas if we consider a possible in vivo modulation with these cytokines. Recent experiments have demonstrated a cytotoxic activity of IL-2 activated lymphocytes (LAK cells) againts glioma cell lines (61). Positive clinical responses have been reported with this kind of cells on other types of cancer (62). A combination of MHC antigens modulation and of specifically activated cytotoxic T lymphocytes could be the next step in the fight against malignant gliomas.

KEY WORDS

Gliomas, HLA Typing, Immunomodulation.

REFERENCES

1. GORER (P.A.): Genetic and antigenic Basis of Tumour Transplantation. J. Pathol. Bacteriol., **44**: 691-697 (1937).
2. HOOD (L.E.), WEISSMANN (I.L.), WOOD (W.B.), WILSON (J.H.): Immunology (The Benjamin/Cummings, 1984).
3. KLEIN (J.): The Major Histocompatibility Complex of the Mouse, Science, **203**: 516-521 (1979).
4. DAUSSET (J.): The Major Histocompatibility Complex in Man. Science, **213**: 1469-1474 (1981).
5. ZINKERNAGEL (R.M.), DOHERTY (P.C.): H-2 Compatibility Requirements for T-cell Mediated Lysis of Target Cells Infected with Lymphocytic Choriomeningitis Virus. Different Cytotoxic T-cell Specificities Are Associated with Structures Coded for in H-2 K or H-2 D. J. Exp. Med., **141**: 1427-1436 (1975).
6. CULLEN (S.E.), FREED (J.H.), NATHENSON (S.G.): Structural and Serological Properties of Murine Ia Alloantigens. Transplant, Rev., **30**: 236-270 (1976).
7. MEO (T.), DAVID (C.S.), NABHOLZ (M.): Demonstration by MLR Test of a Previously Unsuspected Intra H-2 Crossover. Transplant. Proc., **54**: 1339-1350 (1973).
8. KLEIN (J.): Genetics of Cell-Mediated Lymphocytotoxicity in the Mouse. Springer Seminars in Immunopathol., **1**; 31-49 (1978).
9. Mc DEVITT (H.O.), CHINITZ (A.): Genetic Control of the Antibody Response: Relationship between Immune Response and Histocompatibility (H-2) Type. Science, **167**: 1207-1208 (1969).
10. Mc DEVITT (H.O.), DEAK (B.D.), SHREFFLER (D.C.), KLEIN (J.), STIMPFLING (J.H.), SNELL (G.D.): Genetic Control of the Immune Response: Mapping of the Ir-1 Locus. J. Exp. Med., **135**: 1259-1277 (1972).
11. BOURDON (M.A.), WIKSTRAND (C.T.), FURTHMAYR (H.), MATTHEWS (T.J.), BIGNER (D.D.): Human Glioma Mensenchymal Extracellular Matrix Antigen Defined by Monoclonal Antibody. Cancer Res., **43**: 2796-2805 (1983).
12. COAKHAM (H.B.), GARSON (J.A.), BROWNELL (B.), KEMSHEAD (J.T.): Monoclonal Antibodies as Reagents for Brain Tumour Diagnostic: A Review. Journal of the Royal Society of Medicine, **77**: 780-787 (1984).
13. DE TRIBOLET (N.), CARREL (S.), MACH (J.P.): Brain Tumor-Associated Antigens. Prog. Exp. Tumor Res., **27**: 118-131 (1984).
14. SCHRIER (P.I.), BERNARDS (R.), VAESSEN (R.T.M.J.) HOUWELING (A.), Van der EB (A.J.): Expression of Class I Major Histocompatibility Antigens Switched off by Highly Oncogenic Adenovirus 12 in Transformed Rat Cells. Nature, **305**: 771-775 (1983).
15. BERNARDS (R.), SCHREIER (P.I.), HOUWELING (A.), BOS (J.L.), Vand der EB (A.J.): Tumorigenicity of Cells Transformed by Adenovirus Type 12 by Evasion of T-Cell Immunity. Nature, **305**: 776-779 (1983).
16. TANAKA (K.), ISSELBACHER (K.J.), KHOURY (G.), JAY (G.): Reversal of Oncogenesis by the Expression of a Major Histocompatibility Complex Class I Gene. Science, **228**: 26-30 (1985).
17. UNANUE (E.R.), BELLER (D.I.), LU (C.Y.), ALLEN (P.M.): Antigen Presentation: Comments on its Regulation and Mechanism. J. Immunol., **132**: 1-5 (1984).
18. KERN (D.E.), KLARNET (J.P.), JENSEN (M.C.V.), GREENBERG (P.D.): Requirement for Recognition of Class II Molecules and Processed Tumor Antigen for Optimal Generation of Syngeneic Tumor-Specific Class I Restricted CTL. J. Immunol., **136**: 4303-4311 (1986).
19. BERAH (M.), HORS (J.), DAUSSET (J.): A Study of HLA Antigens in Human Organs. Transplantation, **9**: 185-192 (1970).
20. WILLIAM (K.A.), HART (D.N.J.), FABRE (J.W.), MORRIS (P.J.): Distribution and Quantitation of HLA-ABC and DR (Ia) Antigens on Human Kidney and other Tissues. Transplantation, **29**: 274-279 (1980).
21. NATALI (P.G.), BIGOTTI (A.), NICOTRA (M.R.), VIORA (M.), MANFREDI (D.), FERRONE (S.): Distribution of Human Class I (HLA-ABC) Histocompatibility Antigens in Normal and Malignant Tissues of Nonlymphoid Origin. Cancer Res., **44**: 4679-4684 (1984).
22. DAAR (A.S.), FUGGLE (S.V.), FABRE (J.W.), TING (A.), MORRIS (P.J.): The Detailed Distribution of HLA-ABC Antigens in Normal Human Organs. Transplantation, **38**: 287-292 (1984).
23. LAMPSON (L.A.), HICKEY (W.F.): Monoclonal Antibody Analysis of MHC Expression in Human Brain Biopsies: Tissue Ranging from « Histologically Normal » to that Showing Different Levels of Glial Tumor Involvement. J. Immunol., **136**: 4054-4062 (1986).
24. de TRIBOLET (N.), HAMOU (M.F.), MACH (J.P.), CARREL (S.), SCHREYER (M.): Demonstration of HLA-DR Antigens in Normal Human Brain. J. Neurol., Neurosurg. and Psy., **47**: 417-418 (1984).
25. NATALI (P.G.), de MARTINO (C.), QUARANTA (V.), NICOTRA (M.R.), FREZZA (F.), PELLEGRINO (M.A.), FERRONE (S.): Expression of Ia-like Antigens in Normal Human Nonlymphoid Tissues. Transplantation, **31**: 75-78 (1981).
26. DAAR (A.S.), FUGGLE (S.V.), FABRE (J.W.), TING (A.), MORRIS (P.J.): The Detailed Distribution of MHC Class II Antigens in Normal Human Organs. Transplantation **38**: 293-298 (1984).

27. FRANK (E.), PULVER (M.), de TRIBOLET (N.): Expression of Class II Major Histocompatibility Antigens on Reactive Astrocytes and Endothelial Cells within the Gliosis Surrounding Metastases and Abscesses. J. Neuroimmunol. **12**: 29-36 (1986).

28. PULVER (M.), CARREL (S.), MACH (J.P.), de TRIBOLET (N.): Cultured Human Fetal Astrocytes Can be Induced by IFN δ to Express HLA-DR. J. Neuroimmunol., (in press).

29. PIGUER (V.), CARREL (S.), de TRIBOLET (N.): Modulation of HLA-DR Expression and Growth Inhibition on Glioma Cells: Heterogeneous Responses to Interferon δ. J. of Neurooncology, **(in press).**

30. BIGNER (D.D.), BIGNER (S.H.), PONTEN (J.), WESTERMARK (B.), MAHALEY (M.S.) Jr., RUOSLAHTI (E.), HERSCHMAN (H.), ENG (L.F.), WIKSTRAND (C.J.): Heterogeneity of Genotypic and Phenotypic Characteristics of Fifteen Permanent Cell Lines Derived from Human Gliomas. J. Neuropathol. Exp. Neurol., **15**: 201-229 (1981).

31. CARREL (S.), de TRIBOLET (N.), GROSS (N.): Expression of HLA-DR and Common Acute Lymphoblastic Leukemia Antigens on Glioma Cells. Eur. J. Immunol., **12**: 354-357 (1982).

32. PIGUET (V.), Diserens (A.C.), CARREL (S.), MACH (J.P.), de TRIBOLET (N.): the Immunobiology of Human Gliomas. Springer Semin. Immunopathol., **8**: 111-127 (1985).

33. WONG (G.H.), BARTLETT (P.F.), CLARK-LEWIS (I.), BATTYE (F.), SCHRADER (J.W.): Inducible Expression of H-2 and Ia Antigens on Brain cells. Nature, **310**: 688-691 (1984).

34. FONTANA (A.), ERB (P.), PIRCHER (H.), ZINKERNAGEL (R.), WEBER (E.), FIERZ (W.): Astrocytes as Antigen-Presenting Cells. Part II: Unlike H-2k-Dependent Cytotoxic T cells, H-2 Ia-Restricted T cells are only Stimulated in the Presence of Interferon- δ. J. Neuroimmunol., **12**: 15-28 (1986).

35. FIERZ (W.), ENDLER (B.), RESKE (K.), WEKERLE (H.), FONTANA (A.): Astrocytes as Antigen Presenting Cells. I. Induction of Ia Antigen Expression on Astrocytes by T Cells via Immune Interferon and its Effect on Antigen Presentation. J. Immunol., **134**: 3785-3793 (1985).

36. HIGGINS (P.G.): Interferons. J. Clin. Pathol., **37**: 109-116 (1984).

37. WALSH (J.P.): The Interferons. Medical Laboratory Sciences, **42**: 346-351 (1985).

38. BLOOM (B.R.): Interferons and the Immune System. Nature, **284**: 593-595 (1980).

39. TRINCHIERI (G.), PERUSSIA (B.): Immune Interferon: A Pleiotropic Lymphokine with Multiple Effects. Immunology Today, **6**: 131-136 (1985).

40. DOHERTY (P.C.): Cell-Mediated Immunity and the CNS a Key Role for δ Interferon. TINS, 41-42 (1985).

41. CARSWELL (E.A.), OLD (L.J.), KASSEL (R.L.), GREEN (S.), FIORE (N.), WILLIAMSON (B.): An Endotoxin-Induced Serum Factor that Causes Necrosis of Tumors. Proc. Nat. Acad. Sci. USA, **72**: 3666-3670 (1975).

42. AGGARWAL (B.B.), KOHR (W.L.), HASS (P.E.), MOFFAT (B.), SPENCER (S.A.), HENZEL (W.L.), BRINGMAN (T.S.), NEDWIN (G.E.), GOEDDEL (D.W.), HARKINS (R.N.): Human Tumor Necrosis Factor: Production, Purification and Characterization. J. Biol. Chem, **260**: 2345-2354 (1985).

43. PENNICA (D.), HAYFLICK (J.S.), BRINGMAN (T.S.), PALLADINO (M.A.), GOEDDEL (D.V.): Cloning and Expression in Escherichia Coli of the cDNA for Murine Tumor Necrosis Factor. Proc. Natl. Acad. Sci. USA, **82**: 6060-6064 (1985).

44. MARMENOUT (A.), FRANSEN (L.), TAVERNIER (J.), Van der HEYDEN (J.), TIZARD (R.), KAWASHIMA (E.), SHAW (A.), JOHNSON (M.J.), SEMON (D.), MULLER (R.), RUYSCHAERT (M.R.), Van VLIET (A.), FIERS (W.): Molecular Cloning and Expression of Human Tumor Necrosis Factor and Comparison with Mouse Tumor Necrosis Factor. Eur. J. Biochem. **152**: 515-522 (1985).

45. SHIRAI (T.), YAMAGUCHI (H.), ITO (H.), TODD (C.W.), WALLACE (R.B.): Cloning and Expression in Escherichia Coli of the Gene for Human Tumor Necrosis Factor. Nature, **313**: 803-806 (1985).

46. WATANABE (N.), NIITSU (Y.), NEDA (H.), SONE (H.), YAMAGUCHI (N.), UMETSU (T.), URUSHIZAKI (I.): Antitumor Effect of Tumor Necrosis Factor against Various Primarily Cultured Human Cancer Cells. Jpn. J. Canc. Res. (Gann), **76**: 1115-1119 (1985).

47. FRANSEN (L.), Van der HEYDEN (J.), RUYSSCHAERT (R.), FIERS (W.): Recominant Tumor Necrosis Factor: Its Effect and its Synergism with Interferon- δ on a Variety of Normal and Transformed Human Cell Lines. Eur. J. Clin. Oncol., (1986).

48. BEUTLER (B.), CERAMI (A.): Cachectin and Tumor Necrosis Factor as Two Sides of the Same Biological Coin. Nature **320**, 584-588 (1986).

49. DINARELLO (C.A.), CANNON (J.C.), WOLFF (S.M.), BERNHEIM (H.A.), BEUTLER (B.), CERAMI (A.), FIGARI (I.S.), PALLADINO (M.A.), O'CONNOR (J.V.): Tumor Necrosis Factor (Cachectin) is an Endogenous Pyrogen and Induces Production of Interleukin 1. J. Exp. Med., **163**: 1433-1450 (1986).

50. LINDAHL (P.), LEARY (L.), GRESSER (I.): Enhancement by Interferon of the Expression of Surface Antigens on Murine Leukemia L 1210 Cells. Proc. Natl. Acad. Sci. USA, **69**: 721-723 (1972).

51. HERON (I.), HOKLAND (M.), BERG (K.): Enhanced Expression of β 2-microglobulin and HLA Antigens on Human Lymphoid Cells by Interferon. Proc. Natl. Acad. Sci. USA, **75**: 6215-6219 (1978).

52. FELLOUS (M.), KAMOUN (K.), GRESSER (I.), BONO (R.): Enhanced Expression of β2-microglobulin on Interferon-Treated Human Lymphoid Cells. Eur. J. Immunol., **9**: 446-449 (1979).

53. KELLEY (V.E.), FIERS (W.), STROM (T.B.): Cloned Interferon δ but not Interferon α or β induces Expression of HLA-DR Determinants by Fetal Monocytes and Myeloid Leukemic Cell Lines. J. Immunol., **132**: 240-245 (1984).

54. POBER (J.S.), COLLIONS (T.), GIMBRONE Jr (M.A.), COTRAN (R.S.), Gitlin (J.D.), FIERS ((W.), CLAYBERGER (C.), KRENSKY (A.M.), BURAKOFF (S.J.), REISS (C.S.): Lymphocytes Recognize Human Vascular Endothelial and Dermal Fibroblast Ia Antigens Induced by Recombinant Immune Interferon. Nature, **305**: 726-729 (1983).

55. BASHAM (T.Y.), MERIGAN (T.C.): Recombinant Interferon- δ Increases HLA-DR Synthesis and Expression. J. Immunol., **130**: 1492-1494 (1983).

56. CARREL (S.), SCHMIDT-KESSEN (A.), GIUFFRE (L.): Recombinant Interferon- δ Can Induce the Expression of HLA-DR and -DC or DR-negative Melanoma Cells and Enhance the Expression of HLA-ABC and Tumor Associated Antigens. Eur. J. Immunol., **15**: 118-123 (1985).

57. COLLINS (T.), LAPIERRE (L.A.), FIERS (W.), STROMINGER (J.L.), POBER (J.S.): Recombinant Human Tumor Necrosis Factor Increases mRNA Levels and Surface Expression of HLA-AB Antigens in Vascular Endothelial Cells and Dermal Fibroblasts in Vitro. Proc. Natl. Acad. Sci. USA, **83**: 446-450 (1986).

58. PIGUET (V.), CARREL (S.), DISERENS (A.C.), MACH (J.P.), de TRIBOLET (N.): Heterogeneity of the Induction of HLA-DR Expression by Human Immune Interferon on Glioma Cell Lines and Their Clones. JNCI, **76**: 223-228 (1986).

59. TAKIGUCHI (M.), TING (J.P.Y.), BUESSOW (S.C.), BOYER (C.), GILLESPIE (Y.), FRELINGER (J.A.): Response of Glioma Cells to Interferon-gamma: Increase in Class II RNA, Protein and Mixed Lymphocyte Reaction-Stimulating Ability. Eur. J. Immunol., **15**: 809-814 (1985).

60. MAHALEY (M.S.), URSO (M.B.), WHALEY (R.A.), BLUE (M.), WILLIAMS (T.E.), GUASPARI (A.), SELKER (R.G.): Immunobiology of Primary Intracranial Tumors. Part 10: Therapeutic Efficacy of Interferon in the Treatment of Recurrent Gliomas. J. Neurosurg., **63**: 719-725 (1985).

61. JACOBS (S.K.), WILSON (D.J.), KORNBLITH (P.L.), GRIMM (E.A.): In Vitro Killing of Human Glioblastoma by Interleukin-2 Actived Autologous Lymphocytes. J. Neurosurg., **64**: 114-117 (1986).

62. ROSENBERG (S.A.), LOTZE (M.T.), MUUL (L.M.), LEITMANN (S.), CHANG (A.E.), ETTINGHAUSEN (S.E.), MATORY (Y.L.), Skibber (J.M.), SHILOMI (E.), VETTO (J.T.), SEIPP (C.A.), SIMPSON (C.), REICHERT (C.M.): Observations on the Systemic Administration of Autologous Lymphokine-Activated Killer Cells and Recombinant Interleukin-2 to Patients with Metastatic Cancer. N. Engl. J. Med., **313**: 1485-1492 (1985).

Isolation, Functional Properties and Clonal Analysis of Tumor-Infiltrating Lymphocytes from Human Brain Tumors

S. MIESCHER, Th. L. WHITESIDE, V. von FLIEDNER, N. de TRIBOLET.

INTRODUCTION

Despite the numerous reports of decreased or defective systemic cell mediated immunity in glioma patients (1-7) there is evidence of a local immune response to the tumor. Thus mononuclear cell (MNC) infiltrates have been demonstrated within the parenchyma of human glial tumors in 30-60 % of cases reported in the literature (8, 9). Other studies have correlated the intensity of MNC infiltrates with tumor histology and survival in glioma patients (10-12). Von Hanwehr and co-workers (9) found that T lymphocytes constituted the major fraction of the infiltrates in gliomas. However the nature and functional capabilities of these cells and their potential cytolytic role in preventing tumor growth remain poorly understood. To resolve these questions it is necessary to isolate the tumor infiltrating lymphocytes (TIL) from the tumor tissue. To this end TIL from 7 human brain tumors were isolated using enzyme digestion and density gradient centrifugation. The resulting TIL fractions were then cloned in a limiting dilution assay (13) that allows virtualy all peripheral blood resting T cells to undergo clonal expansion. The frequency of proliferating T lymphocyte precursors (PTL-P) can then be calculated thus giving an indication of immunocompetent T cells present in the original infiltrate compared to patient and normal peripheral blood. In addition the clones obtained can be expanded to allow for functional assays in vitro. This report demonstrates that TIL cloned from human gliomas and grown in the presence of interleukin-2 do exhibit cytolytic activity in vitro in both allogeneic and autologous systems.

MATERIALS AND METHODS

Tumor tissues

Surgical biopsies were obtained from nine patients with brain tumors (6 glioblastomas, 3 low grade gliomas) undergoing surgery for therapeutic reasons. Tissues were collected into sterile medium (RPMI 1640) containing antibiotics and nystatin (all from Gibco, Basel, Switzerland) and subjected to enzyme digestion followed by density gradient centrifugation as previously described (14).

TIL + PBL preparations

Lymphocyte numbers in the TIL fractions were determined from May-Grünwald-Giemsa (MGG) smears, and T11+ lymphocytes were quantitated by immunofluorescence as described earlier (14). Peripheral blood was obtained from normal volunteers and patients at the time of surgery, and mononuclear cells separated on Ficoll-Hypaque gradients.

Microcultures of TIL

A limiting-dilution microculture system described by Moretta et al. (13) was used. PBL were plated at 1, 2 and 5, while TIL were plated at 20, 50, 100 or 200 T11+ cells per well in 96-well Costar plates and grown as described before (14). Minimal estimates of the proliferating T lymphocyte precursors (PTL-P) were obtained by the minimum X^2 method from the Poisson distribution relationship between cell number and the logarithm of the percentage of non-responding (negative) microcultures (15).

Ludwig Institute for Cancer Research, Lausanne Branch, Epalinges Switzerland and Department of Neurosurgery, CHUV, Lausanne. Switzerland.

M. Chatel, F. Darcel and J. Pecker (eds.), Brain Oncology. ISBN-13: 978-94-010-8003-3

Assays of cytolytic activity

Cytolytic activities of individual microcultures obtained from TIL plated under limiting-dilution conditions were tested against two or more different types of ^{51}Cr-labeled target cells. Target cells labeled with ^{51}Cr were placed in wells of V-bottomed microtiter trays (5×10^3/well). The microculture suspension was added to each well, making a final volume of 200 μl per well. Microplates with target cell-lymphocyte mixtures were centrifuged at 100 g for 5 min and then incubated for 4 hrs at 37 °C. The plates were then centrifuged again (200 g for 5 min), and 100 μl of supernatant was removed for measurement of ^{51}Cr release in a gamma counter. Specific lysis was calculated according to the formula :

$$\text{Percent specific lysis} \quad \frac{\text{Experimental release} - \text{spontaneous release}}{\text{Maximum release} - \text{spontaneous release}} \times 100$$

Spontaneous release was determined in control microcultures containing ^{51}Cr-labeled target cells in culture medium, but no responder cells, and incubated in the same way as experimental microcultures. Maximum release was determined by lysing ^{51}Cr-labeled cells with 0.1 N HCl. Cultures in which ^{51}Cr release exceeded the mean spontaneous release by more than 3 standard deviations (3SD) were considered positive for cytolytic activity.

Target cells

The following cells and cell lines were labeled with ^{51}Cr and used as target cells in assays of cytolytic activity: (a) K562 human erythroleukemia cells which allow the detection of NK-like activity; (b) autologous tumor cells established and maintained in culture (16); (c) allogeneic glioma cell lines G215, 992b and 340 established from fresh surgical specimens (16). Cells to be used as targets were washed 3 times after trypsin EDTA treatment and then incubated in medium for 1 hr at 37 °C before labeling with ^{51}Cr.

Proliferative responses of TIL and PBL

Lymphocytes were plated according to the number of T11+ cells in 96-well round-bottom microtiter plates (n° 3799, Costar, Cambridge, MA). Each well contained from 2.5×10^4 to 5×10^4 T cells in 100 μl of culture medium. Phytohemagglutinin (PHA; Gibco, Grand Island, NY) was added in 100 μl of medium/well at a final 1 % (vol/vol) concentration. Cultures were set up in triplicate and incubated at 37 °C in 5 % atmosphere of CO_2 for 60 hours. Twelve hours before harvest, ^3H-thymidine (Amersham, specific activity 6.7 Ci/mmol) was added (1 μCi/well). Cells were harvested and washed on Whatmann filters (934-AH, Reeve Angel) using a Dynatech Titertek harvester. Triplicate samples were counted for 1 min/sample in a liquid scintillation counter.

RESULTS

Recovery of lymphocytes from gliomas

The recovered TIL fractions contained from 0.6 to 7-9 x 10^5 cells per wet gm of tumor of which $T11^+$ lymphocytes constituted from 10-50 %. Granulocytes, basophils and macrophages constituted the rest with very few if any B lymphocytes. The T lymphocytes ($T11^+$, $T3^+$) were small, non blastic, HLA-DR^- and did not express the receptor for IL-2.

Interestingly in 2 cases (L.M. and W.S.) a significant proportion (10 %) of large granular lymphocytes (IGL), in addition to small lymphocytes were recovered which also reflected in the functional assays in that many clones tested from these 2 patients demonstrated NK-like activity.

Proliferative responses of glial lymphocytes (Table 1)

The TIL populations obtained from glial tumors did not respond or only marginally to PHA. In contrast the autologous PBL responded within the range found for normal PBL. Control normal PBL remained fully responsive to PHA even after incubation with the same enzyme mixture used for digestion of the tumor biopsies.

TABLE 1

Comparative PHA responses and frequencies of proliferating T lymphocyte precursors (PTL-P) among the peripheral blood lymphocytes (PBL) and tumor-infiltrating lymphocytes (TIL) of patients with glial tumors

Tumor patient	PHA response (cpm x 10^{-3})				Frequency (95 % confidence limits)	
	PBL		TIL		PBL	TIL
	—	PHA	—	PHA		
1. L.M.	0.6 ± 0.1	60.8 ± 5	0.8 ± 0.3	10.4 ± 0.8	0.5 (0.4 - 0.6)	0.05 (0.04 - 0.06)
2. B.A.	0.6 ± 0.2	20.6 ± 0.8	0.3 ± 0.02	0.2 ± 0.01	0.12 (0.09 - 0.16)	0.01 (0.008 - 0.01)
3. W.S.	1.3 ± 0.3	28.4 ± 8	0.7 ± 0.1	1.8 ± 0.4	0.46 (0.4 - 0.56)	0.01[a]
CONTROLS						
PBL :						
1.	2.0 ± 0.5	64.2 ± 1.8			1.0 (0.61 - 1.4)	
2.	3.0 ± 0.1	83.0 ± 0.7			0.56 (0.44 - 0.68)	
PBL + enzymes						
1.	1.8 ± 0.1	70.0 ± 3			0.79 (0.55 - 1.11)	
2.	1.8 ± 0.2	38.0 ± 2			0.53 (0.38 - 0.66)	

[a] Less than 1 cell in 100 with proliferative capacity.

Comparison of proliferating T lymphocyte precursor (PTL-P) frequencies in TIL and autologous PBL from patients with glial tumors (Table 1)

The frequency of PTL-P was determined by limiting dilution analysis. The TIL populations all demonstrated much lower PTL-P frequencies (range 0.05 to 0.01) compared to their autologous PBL (range 0.12-0.5) or normal control PBL (range 0.53-1.0). Furthermore the enzyme treatment did not significantly alter the proliferative ability of normal PBL in this system and does not account for the low PTL-P frequencies found in these glial tumors. Thus it can be seen that the TIL population had depressed responses at both the population level (as evidenced by the PHA response) and at the single cell level (as evidenced by the PTL-P frequencies).

Cytolytic activity of cloned TIL from glial tumors

The proliferating microcultures obtained from the limiting dilution assay were expanded and tested in ^{51}Cr-release assays against different tumor cell targets. Two TIL fractions were assessed in detail. For example in patient L.M. 19 of 20 microcultures tested demonstrated NK-like activity as evidenced by lysis of K562 cells, several lysed allogeneic tumor cells, G215, 992b and 340 and one out of 38 exhibited a high specific lysis of 74 % against autologous tumor cells established and maintained in culture from the original biopsy. However in patient B.A. only 10 of 24 microcultures tested had NK-like activity, many more lysed allogeneic cultured glioma cells and 3 lysed the autologous tumor cells again demonstrating high specific lysis of 57 %, 79 % and 150 % respectively. These clones were phenotyped and two expressed the T8 (cytolytic) surface marker whereas the third contained a mixture of $T4^+$ (helper) and $T8^+$ cells. A third patient (W.S.) showed 7 of 10 microcultures with NK-like activity correlating with the presence of large granular lymphocytes found in the infiltrate after enzyme digestion. Phenotypic analysis revealed 3 $T4^+$, 3 $T8^+$ and 1 mixture of $T4^+$ and $T8^+$ cells expressing NK-like activity.

DISCUSSION

The results presented here demonstrate that despite the small infiltrates seen in human brain tumors by immunohistology (data not shown) the T lymphocytes can be isolated, enriched and expanded in vitro in the presence of interleukin-2. Indeed a significant enrichment is obtained as the digest of these tumor tissues in general contained less than 1 % of lymphocytes prior to separation on density gradients. These T lymphocytes bore no evidence of activation in situ, as suggested for infiltrating lymphocytes in other tumor types (17, 18). Thus T lymphocytes from glial tumors were small non-blastic cells expressing the T3 and T11 antigens but were negative for the activation antigens (HLA-DR and the IL-2 receptor). The proliferative response to PHA was found to be depressed in these TIL compared to autologous PBL and normal PBL controls, in agreement with results reported earlier for TIL derived from other human solid tumors (19). On a population level this poor responsiveness to lectins could be explained by the presence of tumor cells especially as our TIL preparations frequently contained less than 30% T11$^+$ lymphocytes and that the major contaminant was tumor cells. There are many reports describing immunoinhibitory factors produced by tumor cells (20, 21) including human glioblastoma cells (22). It may be that the depressed responses of TIL seen in vitro are accounted for by a factor-induced inhibition in vivo. Furthermore even on a single cell level in a limiting dilution assay the TIL population was depressed as evidenced by the decreased frequency of PTL-P in TIL compared to the autologous PBL and normal PBL.

The limiting-dilution assay employed allowed expansion of the cloned TIL for functional assessment. Interestingly the majority of proliferating clones demonstrated cytolytic activity although there was a very heterogeneous cytolytic profile that varied with individual glial tumors. Thus NK-like activity was noticeably present in 2 tumors. Many clones showed allogeneic cytolytic activity and of note auto-cytolytic activity with high specific lysis values was demonstrated. These cytolytic clones could be maintained for up to 2 months in recombinant IL-2. Further efforts are required to try and define the nature and specificity of these auto-cytolytic clones and to develop means of bulk expansion with a view to immunotherapy.

SUMMARY

Tumor-infiltrating lymphocytes (TIL) were isolated from surgical biopsies (6 glioblastomas, 3 low grade gliomas) by enzyme digestion followed by differential density-gradient centrifugation. These TIL-enriched fractions contained from 10-50 % non-blastic T lymphocytes (T11$^+$, T3$^+$, HLA-DR$^-$, IL-2 receptor$^-$) which showed depressed proliferative responses to lectin stimulation compared to autologous and normal circulating lymphocytes. The TIL were cloned by limiting dilution and the resulting frequency of proliferating T-lymphocyte precursors was also depressed in TIL ($\leq$ 0.05) compared to autologous (0.12-0.5) or normal (0.56-1.0) blood. Clonal analysis of 3 glioblastomas revealed a heterogeneous cytolytic pattern with activity against the tumor targets K562 (NK-like activity), allogeneic and autologous glioma tumor targets. Indeed, virtually all clones obtained and expanded in vitro displayed cytolytic activity and this would seem to indicate a selective accumulation of effector cells at the tumor site.

KEY-WORDS

Tumor-infiltrating lymphocytes, limiting dilution analysis, cytolytic activity.

REFERENCES

1. BROOKS (W.H.), NETSKY (M.G.), NORMANSELL (D.E.), HORWITZ (D.A.): Depressed cell-mediated immunity in patients with primary intracranial tumors, J. Exp. Med., 136 (1972) 1631-1647.
2. BROOKS (W.H.), CALDWELL (H.D.), MORTARA (R.H.): Immune responses in patients with gliomas, Surg. Neurol. 2 (1974) 419-423.
3. KASZUBOWSKI (P.A.), HUSBY (G.), TUNG (K.S.K.) et al.: T-lymphocyte subpopulations in peripheral blood and tissues of cancer patients. Cancer Res., 40 (1980) 4648-4657.
4. MENZIES (C.B.), GUNAR (M.T.), BEHAN (P.D.): Impaired thymus-derived lymphocyte function in patients with malignant brain tumor. Clin. Neuro. Neurosurg. 82 (1980) 157-168.
5. ROSZMAN (T.L.), BROOKS (W.H.), ELLIOTT (L.H.): Immunobiology of primary intracranial tumors. Suppressor cell function and lectin-binding lymphocyte subpopulations in patients with cerebral tumors. Cancer, 50 (1982) 1273-1279.

6. THOMAS (D.G.T.), LANNINGEN (C.B.), BEHAN (P.D.): Impaired cell-mediated immunity in human brain tumors. Lancet II (1975) 1389-1390.

7. YOUNG (H.F.), SALAKAS (R.), KAPLAN (A.M.): Inhibition of cell-mediated immunity in patients with brain tumors. Surg. Neurol. 5 (1976) 19-23.

8. TAKEUCHI (J.), BARNARD (R.D.): Perivascular lymphocytic cuffing in astrocytomas. Acta Neuropathol., 35 (1976) 265-271.

9. VON HANWEHR (R.I.), HOFMAN (F.M.), TAYLOR (C.R.), APUZZO (M.L.J.): Mononuclear lymphoid populations infiltrating the microenvironment of primary CNS tumors. Characterization of cell subsets with monoclonal antibodies. J. Neurosurg. 60 (1984) 1138-1147.

10. BROOKS (W.H.), MARKESBERY (W.R.), GUPTA (G.D.) et al.: Relationship of lymphocyte invasion and survival of brain tumor patients. Ann. Neurol. 4 (1978) 219-224.

11. PALMA (L.), DILORENZO (N.), GUIDETTI (B.): Lymphocytic infiltrates in primary glioblastomas and recidivous gliomas. Incidence, fate and relevance to prognosis in 228 operated cases. J. Neurosurg., 49 (1978) 854-861.

12. RIDLEY (A.), CAVANAGH (J.B.): Lymphocytic infiltration in gliomas, Evidence of possible host resistance. Brain 94 (1971) 117-124.

13. MORETTA (A.), PANTALEO (G.), MORETTA (L.), CEROTTINI (J.C.), MINGARI (M.C.): Direct demonstration of the clonogeneic potential of every human peripheral blood T cell. Clonal analysis of HLA-DR expression and cytolytic activity. J. Exp. Med., 157 (1983) 743-754.

14. WHITESIDE (T.L.), MIESCHER (S.), HURLIMANN (J.), MORETTA (L.), VON FLIEDNER (V.): Separation, phenotyping and limiting-dilution analysis of T lymphocytes infiltrating human solid tumors. Int. J. Cancer 37 (1986) 803-811.

15. TASWELL (C.): Limiting dilution assays for the determination of immunocompetent cell frequencies. I. Data analysis. J. Immunol. 126 (1981) 1614-1620.

16. STUDER (A.), TRIBOLET (N. de), DISERENS (A.C.), GAIDE (A.C.), MATTHIEU (J.M.), CARREL (S.), STAVRON (D.): Characterization of four human malignant glioma cell lines. Acta Neuropathol., 66 (1985) 208-217.

17. KLEIN (E.), VANKY (F.), GALILI (V.), VOSE (B.M.), and FOOP (M.): Separation and characteristics of tumor-infiltrating lymphocytes in man. In: M.G. Hanna and I.P. Witz (eds.), Contemporary topics in immunobiology, vol. 10 pp. 79-107, Plenum, New York (1980).

18. POPPEMA (S.), BROCKER (E.B.), LEU (L. de), TERBRACK (D.), VISSCHER (T.), TERHAAR (A.), MACHER (E.), THE (T.H.), and SORG (C.): In situ analysis of the mononuclear cell infiltrate in primary malignant melanoma of the skin. Clin. Exp. Immunol., 51, 77-82 (1983).

19. MIESCHER (S.), WHITESIDE (T.L.), CARREL (S.), VON FLIEDNER (V.): Functional properties of tumor-infiltrating and blood lymphocytes in patients with solid tumors: effects of tumor cells and their supernatants on proliferating responses of lymphocytes. J. Immunol. 136 (1986) 1899-1907.

20. PUTNAM (J.B.), ROTH (J.A.): Identification and characterization of a tumor-derived immunosuppressive glycoprotein from murine melanoma K-1735. Clin. Immunol. Immunother., 19 (1985) 90-100.

21. RENK (C.M.), GUPTA (R.J.), MORTON (D.L.): Inhibition of normal allogeneic lymphocyte mitogenesis by a factor released from human tumor cells in culture. Cancer Immunol. Immunother., 11 (1981) 7.

22. FONTANA (A.), HENGARTNER (H.), TRIBOLET (N. de), WEBER (E.): Glioblastoma cells release interleukin-1 and factors inhibiting interleukin-2 mediated effects. J. Immunol., 4 (1984) 1837-1844.

The Applications of Monoclonal Antibodies in Neuro-Oncology

E.V. COLAPINTO, (°) [1] - Y.S. LEE, [1] - R.E. McLENDON, [1] -
P.A. HUMPHREY, [1] - M.R. ZALUTSKY, [3, 1] - H.S. FRIEDMAN, [1] -
C.N. PEGRAM[1] - S.H. BIGNER, [1] - D.E. BULLARD, [2, 1] - C.J. WIKSTRAND, [1] -
D.D. BIGNER [1, 2].

INTRODUCTION

Central nervous system (CNS) malignancies represent one of the most devastating forms of cancer. Malignant gliomas, the most commonly occurring primary tumor of the CNS, have a particularly bleak prognosis despite surgery and combined radiation and chemotherapy (1, 2). Immunological approaches to diagnosis and treatment have seemed attractive, but in the past have been frustrated by technological limitations (3, 4). Monoclonal antibody methodology offers major advantages over conventional methods of antiserum production: a practically unlimited source of homogeneous, highly specific reagent which may be prepared using impure or complex antigens. This has led to a new age in neuroimmunology and neuro-oncology, with the potential for better understanding of the basic cell biology of CNS neoplasia, and for improvement in diagnosis, imaging, and therapy.

MATERIALS AND METHODS

The production and characterization of monoclonal antibodies have been described in reports from this laboratory (5, 9), as have the immunohistochemical techniques using monoclonal antibodies for **in vitro** neuropathological diagnosis (6, 7). The methodology of localization and imaging studies has been detailed (10, 11).

RESULTS AND DISCUSSION

Monoclonal antibodies can serve as biological probes for previously biochemically defined nervous system antigens, such as glial fibrillary acidic protein (GFAP), the intermediate filament protein of glial cells. Pegram et al. of this laboratory reported the characterization of four monoclonal antibodies which recognized the same, or spatially close, epitopes specific to GFAP in a number of different animal species. Furthermore, these monoclonal antibodies were reactive with normal, reactive, and neoplastic astrocytes following various methods of fixation (5).

A study from this laboratory has described the use of three of these GFAP-specific monoclonal antibodies combined in a "cocktail" preparation to stain formalin-fixed, paraffin-embedded normal and neoplastic brain tissues and compared the results to a reference polyvalent anti-GFAP antiserum (6). The quality of the immunohistochemical detection of GFAP by the monoclonal "cocktail" closely approached that of the high titre polyclonal antisera. McLendon et al. note that a monoclonal "cocktail" represents an excellent reagent for large multi-institutional studies and for studies of extended duration because of the unlimited supply and the well defined nature of such a "cocktail", in contrast to the limited shelf life and biological variation inherent in the generation of polyclonal antisera (6).

There are important applications of monoclonal antibodies in the diagnosis of cytologic specimens obtained from cerebrospinal fluid and from fine needle aspirates of intracranial masses. Vick et al. (7) employed a panel of four monoclonal antibodies: UJ13A, which stains most neoplastic and non-neoplastic cells of neuroectodermal origin; a "cocktail" composed of three anti-GFAP antibodies (α-GFAP); B72.3, which reacts with most carcinomas; and 2D1, a pan leukocyte marker

(°) Preuss Laboratory For Brain Tumor Research, Anal - 1. Departments of Pathology - 2. Surgery (Neurosurgery) -and 3. Radiology, Duke University Medical Center. Durham, North Carolina, USA 27710.

M. Chatel, F. Darcel and J. Pecker (eds.), Brain Oncology. ISBN-13: 978-94-010-8003-3

(Table I summarizes the antibody reactivity patterns). In 53 specimens (21 cerebrospinal fluids, one ventricular fluid, two brain cyst fluids, 12 needle washings, 15 imprints, one subdural fluid, and one post-shunt fluid) this panel accurately differentiated between primary brain tumors, metastases, leukemias and lymphomas. However, no monoclonal antibodies are presently available which will identify the tissue of origin of a metastasis, distinguish reactive gliosis from astrocytoma, nor differentiate between glial tumors of astrocytic, oligodendroglial or ependymal origin.

TABLE I*

Summary of Antibody Reactivity Patterns

	UJ13A	α-GFAP	B72.3	2D1
Gliomas	+	+	—	+/—
Normal brain fragments	+	+	—	—
Non-glial primary CNS tumors	+	—	—	—
Small cell undifferentiated carcinoma and embryonal rhabdomyosarcoma	+	—	—	—
Non-small cell carcinoma	—	—	—	—
Melanoma	—	—	—	—
Lymphoma-Leukemia	—	—	—	+
Inflammation	—	—	—	+

* From Vick, W.W., Bigner, S.H., Wikstrand, C.J., Bullard, D.E., Kemshead, J.T., Coakham, H.B., Schlom, J., Johnston, W.W., Bigner, D.D.: The use of a panel of monoclonal antibodies in the evaluation of cytologic specimens from the central nervous system. In press, Acta Cytologica (1986).

Monoclonal antibodies with operational specificity, that is, antibodies reactive with glioma-associated antigens but not normal adult brain tissue include 81C6, C12, D12 and E9 produced by this laboratory. Monoclonal antibody 81C6 defines a novel human glioma-associated extracellular matrix glycoprotein (GMEM) found in human anaplastic gliomas but not in normal human brain tissue (8). C12 and D12 were derived by immunization of Balb/c mice with human glioma cell line D-54 MG, and define membrane proteins of 180kDa and 88kDa size (9). E9 was also derived after immunization of mice with D-54, and recognizes an epitope expressed by the extracellular matrix of cultured human glioma cells and glioma biopsies (10).

In addition to **in vitro** reactivity with human glioma antigens, these monoclonal antibodies have demonstrated **in vivo** localization as well. In paired label studies, radiolabelled 81C6 has been shown to specifically localize in D-54 MG subcutaneous and intracranial xenografts in athymic mice (11). In another study from this laboratory, C12, D12, and E9 were demonstrated to specifically localize in D-54 xenografts in athymic mice (10).

The promise of such specific antibodies in neuro-oncology is their potential for use as imaging agents and as agents to selectively deliver therapeutic substances. A study using D-54 MG intracranial xenografts in athymic rats showed that radiolabelled 81C6 did localize to the intracranial tumor and that the degree of localization was sufficient to allow imaging of tumors as small as 20 mg. Only tumors exceeding 300 mg could be imaged with non-specific radiolabelled control antibody (12).

Therapeutic studies have been carried out in this laboratory using athymic rats bearing intracranially transplanted D-54 MG tumors. Administration of radiolabelled monoclonal antibody 81C6 early in the course of tumor growth significantly prolonged survival and yielded approximately a 20% cure rate (unpublished data).

Our laboratory, in addition to developing new monoclonal antibodies, is working on methods to improve their localization and delivery. One method being currently investigated is the use of enzymatically prepared immunoglobulin fragments, such as Fab and F(ab')2, which offer certain theoretical advantages over intact antibody as agents for localization. Fragments are more rapidly cleared from tissues resulting in reduction in background activity and reduced radiation dose to tissues; the smaller fragments may pass the blood brain barrier more easily and so access brain tumors better; the lack of a Fc region may reduce immunogenicity of murine protein in humans, and may also result in less non-specific binding mediated by Fc receptors. Other avenues of investigation include the assessment of the potential advantages of intracarotid over intravenous administration of monoclonal antibodies, and the possible benefits of blood brain barrier disruption to improve monoclonal antibody localization.

Early Phase 1 imaging studies have been carried out by investigators with various monoclonal antibodies: de Tribolet with Mel-14, Coakham with UJ13A, and in collaboration with Coakham, in three patients with 81C6. Early results show little to no toxicity in human subjects, and have demonstrated specific localization in intracranial tumors with the generation of diagnostic images. Monoclonal antibodies with localizing potential in humans are displayed in Table II. Future work will determine the optimum dosages, the best route of administration, the necessity of blood brain barrier disruption, and the role of antibody fragments. Dosimetry calculations from these Phase 1 biodistribution studies will determine the feasibility of therapeutic trials with higher doses of radioactivity.

TABLE II

Monoclonal Antibodies Presently Near Phase I Clinical Trials in Brain Tumor Patients (adapted from Davies et al., 1986)

Monoclonal Antibody	Antigen	Antigen Locus	Nervous System Tumor Type	Reference
UJ13A	Pan neuroectoderm ? glycolipid	Cell Surface	All neuroectodermal	Allan et al., 1983
81C6	220kDa glycoprotein	Extracellular matrix	Gliomas, melanoma	Bourdon et al., 1983
UJ181.4	Embryonic and neoplastic neuronal cells	Cell surface	Neuroblastomas Medulloblastomas	Coakham et al., 1985
Mel-14	Chondroitin Sulfate Proteoglycan	Cell surface and matrix	Melanomas Gliomas	Carrel et al., 1980
C12	180kDa protein	Cell surface	Gliomas	Wikstrand et al., 1986
D12	88kDa protein	Cell Surface and Extracellular Matrix	Gliomas	Wilkstrand et al., 1986
E9	?	Extracellular Matrix	Gliomas	Wikstrand et al., 1986

SUMMARY

Malignant gliomas have a grave prognosis despite current therapy. Monoclonal antibody technology provides a powerful new biochemical tool that has the potential to improve this situation. The ***in vitro*** *diagnosis of central nervous system neoplasia has benefited from the application of monoclonal antibodies in immunohistochemistry. Monoclonal antibodies reactive with human glioma-associated antigens have demonstrated specific localization in human glioma xenografts and have shown efficacy in imaging and therapeutic studies in animal models. Early clinical studies with monoclonal antibodies in brain tumor patients are providing some encouraging preliminary results, with no significant toxicity encountered to date.*

KEY WORDS

Monoclonal antibody, glioma, glioma-associated antigen, xenograft.

REFERENCES

1. GREEN (S.B.), BYAR (D.P.), WALKER (M.D.), et al.: Comparisons of carmustine, procarbazine, and high dose methylprednisolone as additions to surgery and radiotherapy for the treatment of malignant glioma. Cancer Treat Rep, **67**: 121-132 (1983).
2. WALKER (M.D.), ALEXANDER (E.), HUNT (W.E.), MacCARTY (C.S.), MAHALEY (M.S.), NORREL (H.A.), OWENS (G.), RANSAHOFF (J.), WILSON (C.B.), GEHAN (E.A.), STRIKE (T.A.): Evaluation of BCNU and/or radiotherapy in the treatment of anaplastic gliomas. J. Neurosurg., **43**: 333-343 (1978).

3. MAHALEY (M.S.), MAHALEY (J.L.), DAY (E.D.): Localization of radioantibodies in human brain tumors II. Radioautography. Cancer Res., **2**: 779-793 (1965).

4. MAHALEY (M.S.), DAY (E.D.), BIGNER (D.D.): Problems inherent to the **in vivo** localization of anti-brain tumor antibodies. Ann NY Acad. Sci., **159**: 451-460 (1969).

5. PEGRAM (C.N.), ENG (L.F.), WIKSTRAND (C.J.), McCOMB (R.D.), LEE (Y.L.), BIGNER (D.D.): Monoclonal antibodies reactive with epitopes restricted to glial fibrillary acidic protein of several species. Neurochem. Pathol., **3**: 119-138 (1985).

6. McLENDON (R.E.), BURGER (P.C.), PEGRAM (C.N.), ENG (L.F.), BIGNER (D.D.): The immunohistochemical application of three anti-GFAP monoclonal antibodies to formalin-fixed paraffin-embedded normal and neoplastic brain tissues. J. Neuropathol. Exp. Neurol., **45**: 692-703 (1986).

7. VICK (W.W.), BIGNER (S.H.), WIKSTRAND (C.J.), BULLARD (D.E.), KEMSHEAD (J.), COAKHAM (H.G.), SCHLOM (J.), JOHNSTON (W.W.), BIGNER (D.D.): The use of a panel of monoclonal antibodies in the evaluation of cytologic specimens from the central nervous system. In press, Acta Cytol (1986).

8. BOURDON (M.A.), WIKSTRAND (C.J.), FURTHMAYR (H.), MATTHEWS (T.J.), BIGNER (D.D.): Human glioma-mesenchymal extracellular matrix antigen defined by monoclonal antibody. Cancer Res., **43**: 2796-2805 (1983).

9. WIKSTRAND (C.J.), McLENDON (R.E.), BULLARD (D.E.), FREDMAN (P.), SVENNERHOLM (L.), BIGNER (D.D.): Production and characterization of two human glioma xenograft-localizing monoclonal antibodies (Mabs). Cancer Res., **46**: 5933-5940 (1986).

10. WIKSTRAND (C.J.), McLENDON (R.E.), CARREL (S.), KEMSHEAD (J.T.), MACH (J.P.), COAKHAM (H.B.), TRIBOLET (N. de), BULLARD (D.E.), ZALUTSKY (M.R.), BIGNER (D.D.): Comparative localization of glioma reactive-monoclonal antibodies in vivo in an athymic mouse human glioma xenograft model. In press, J. Neuroimmunol. (1986).

11. BOURDON (M.A.), COLEMAN (R.E.), BLASBERG (R.G.), GROOTHUIS (D.R.), BIGNER (D.D.): Monoclonal antibody localization in subcutaneous and intracranial human glioma xenografts: paired label and imaging analysis. Anticancer Res, **4**:133-140 (1984).

12. BULLARD (D.E.), ADAMS (C.J.), COLEMAN (R.E.), BIGNER (D.D.): **In vivo** imaging of intracranial human glioma xenografts comparing specific with nonspecific radiolabeled monoclonal antibodies. J. Neurosurg., **64**: 257-262 (1986).

13. ALLAN (P.M.), GARSON (J.A.), HARPER (E.L.), ASSER (U.), COOKHAM (H.B.), BROWNELL (B.), KEMSHEAD (J.T.): Biological characterization and clinical application of a monoclonal antibody recognizing an antigen restricted to neuro-ectodermal tissues. Int. J. Cancer **31**: 591-598 (1983).

14. CARREL (S.), ACCOLA (R.S.), KARMEYOLA (A.L.), MACH (J.P.): Common human melanoma associated antigen (s) detected by monoclonal antibodies. Cancer Res **40**: 2523-2528 (1980).

15. COAKHAM (H.B.), GARSON (J.A.), ALLAN (P.M.), HARPER (E.L.), BROWNELL (B.), KEMSHEAD (J.T.), LANE (E.B.): Immunohistological diagnosis of central nervous system tumors using a monoclonal antibody panel. J. Clin Path **38**: 165-173 (1985).

16. DAVIES (A.G.), RICHARDSON (R.B.), BOURNE (S.P.), KEMSHEAD (J.T.), COAKHAM (H.B.): Immunolocalisation of human brain tumours. In Bleehan N (E.D.) Tumours of the Brain (Springer-Verlag, 1986).

In-vivo-localization of Radiolabelled Monoclonal Antibody in Human Gliomas

J. BEHNKE, J.P. MACH, F. BUCHEGGER, S. CARREL,
B. DELALOYE, N. de TRIBOLET (°).

INTRODUCTION

Monoclonal antibodies can act as carriers for radionuclides. The radiolabelling of monoclonal antibodies directed against tumor antigens and the radioimmunodetection by means of external scanning or direct measurement of radioactivity in the tumor and different tissues is a prerequisite for estimating the enrichment of the antibody in the tumor. The paired-label technique described by Pressmann et al. (1) permits to measure directly the intratumoral enrichment of the tumor directed antibody due to its binding to the target cell over the nonspecific accumulation. It allows, by help of the specificity index (2), to define specific antibody uptake excluding factors like vascularity, necrosis, extracellular space, in-vivo radiolysis, binding through the Fc-portion (3) and uptake into the reticulo-endothelial system since these factors apply equally to the control-antibody and to the tumor directed antibody.

In the following, results are presented concerning the radioimmunolocalization of gliomas using the antimelanoma monoclonal antibody Mel-14. It recognizes a neuroectodermal antigen present on the majority of gliomas. Carrel et al. (4) have raised it after immunization of mice with a melanoma cell line. Mel-14 is an IgG2 antibody (5) and recognizes a 230 kd polypeptide (6). It bound in antibody binding radioimmunoassay to all melanoma cell lines tested without any significant reactivity to control non-melanoma cell lines (4). In further studies (5, 6, 7, 8) Mel-14 was found to be reactive with half of the glioma cell lines as well as with two of the three neuroblastoma and medulloblastoma cell lines tested. 132 brain tumors have been tested for reactivity with Mel-14 in immunohistochemistry on frozen sections (9) and using the avidin-biotin-immunoperoxidase method. Mel-14 bound to tumor endothelial cells of 75 % of the 35 glioblastomas tested and the proportion of positive endothelial cells within the positive glioblastomas was 80 %. Normal brain was not found to be stained. Wikstrand et al. (10) studied the immunolocalization in nude mice xenografted subcutanously with human gliomas. Using the paired label method, they found evidence for specific uptake of Mel-14 into the tumor with specificity indices ranging from 2 to 5 relative to the blood pool.

METHODS

The patients who were scheduled for surgical resection of a glioblastoma preoperatively received radiolabelled monoclonal antibody Mel-14 for in-vivo localization of the antibody in the tumor. F (ab') 2-fragments of Mel-14 were labelled with I-123 and I-125 and as a control F (ab') 2-fragments of an irrelevant IgG were labelled with I-131 using the iodogen method and filtered on a Sephadex-G-25 column equilibrated in pyrogen free 0.15 M saline. The I-123 has a physical half life of 13 hours and was used only for external scanning, whereas labelling with I-125 allowed later measurement of radioactivity in tissues specimens. The patients had no personal history of allergy and received 2 mg clemastine p.o. and 100 mg prednisolon i.v. 1 h before the injection, and 400 mg perchlorate on the day of the injection. 10 drops Lugol 5 % iodine solution p.o. every day for 5 days beginning on the day before the injection were also given. The mixture of I-125 and I-123 labelled F (ab) 2-fragments of Mel-14 and I-131-F (ab) 2-fragments of an irrelevant IgG was diluted in

(°) Neurosurgical Service and Devision of Nuclear Medicine CHUV, CH-1011 Lausanne and Ludwig Institute of Cancer Research, CH-1066 Epalinges.

M. Chatel, F. Darcel and J. Pecker (eds.), Brain Oncology. ISBN-13: 978-94-010-8003-3

100 ml 0.9 % NaCl solution. In case 1, the mixture was injected intravenously over 30 min. and in case 2 intracarotidally. Cases 3 and 4 concern double label studies with Mel-14 in which the radiolabelled antibody was injected intravenously. The patients were tested by computerized tomoscintigraphy at 6 and 24 hours after injection. Two days after injection, the operation was performed. Activities of I-125 and I-131 were counted at later time points in tumor and normal tissues. Tumor material in cases 1 and 2 was used for immunohistochemistry with Mel-14 using the biotin-avidin-peroxidase method and was also cultured in monolayer in order to obtain cells for an antibody binding radioimmunoassay with Mel-14. Cells in case 1 were obtained after the second passage at 6 weeks, in case 2 after the second passage at 5 weeks.

RESULTS

In case 1, the immuno histochemistry of the tumor with Mel-14 showed in the whole tumor typical positive endothelial cells. More than 95 % were found to bind Mel-14. In the antibody binding radioimmunoassay, the activity bound to cells of this tumor obtained from the monolayer culture was 15 times greater than that of the control, resulting in a binding ratio of 15, which is considered to be strongly positive. The activity per gram bound to the specific antibody fragment was 13.95 times higher in the tumor than in resected normal brain, whereas the activity bound to the control was 5.51 times higher in tumor than in normal brain, resulting in a specificity index of localization of 2.53 (see TABLE). The same ratios for tumor and blood gave values of 2.29 for the isotope of the specific antibody fragment and 0.42 for the isotope of the control, resulting in a specificity index of 5.39. The values were obtained by taking an average of two different tumor specimens. Following values were obtained with a tumor specimen which was rich in blood vessels. The tumor to brain ratio for the activity per gram bound to specific antibody fragment was 18.45 and for that bound to the control 5.87, resulting in a specificity index of 3.15. The specificity index relative to blood was 6.69 for the vessel rich part. The external scanning of the tumor by tomoscintigraphy showed a strong accumulation of activity in the skull, behind which the localization of the tumor was possible but difficult.

TABLE

Accumulation of antibody fragment versus control in tumor of case 1 as compared whith normal tissues. The values refer to an average of two specimens.

Comparison with normal tissue	Antibody fragment uptake*	Control uptake **	Specificity index ***
Normal brain	13.95	5.51	2.53
CSF	84.39	37.38	2.26
Blood	2.29	0.42	5.39
Plasma	1.46	0.26	5.61
Muscle	2.92	1.55	1.88

(*) Activity of the antibody-fragment bound isotope per gram tumor divided by the activity of the same isotope per gram normal tissue.
(**) Activity of the control bound isotope per gram tumor divided by the activity of the same isotope per gram normal tissue.
(***) Antibody uptake divided by control uptake.

In case 2, the immunohistochemistry with Mel-14 showed different pictures: a small portion with highly malignant glioma cells and capillary proliferations was strongly positive for Mel-14 on the endothelial cells, while the main part of the tumor was a low grade glioma and did not react with Mel-14. In the antibody binding radioimmunoassay, the activity bound to the tumor cells obtained from a monolayer culture was 7 times greater than the background activity, resulting in a binding ratio of 7, which is considered as moderately positive In the tissue counting, the activity per gram bound to the antibody fragment was in the highly malignant portion of the tumor 4.87 times higher than in normal brain, whereas the activity per gram bound to the control was 3.15 times higher than in normal brain, resulting in a specificity index of localization of 1.66. The corresponding specificity index of the less malignant tumor part was 1.46. The same ratios of tumor and blood in the highly malignant part were 0.59 for the specific antibody fragment and 0.22 for the control, resulting in a specificity index of 2.7. The corresponding specificity index in the less malignant part was 2.36. In the highly malignant part, the same ratios for tumor and bone marrow gave 1.24 for the antibody fragment and 2.19 for the control resulting in a specificity index of 0.57. The corresponding specificity index was 0.50 in the less malignant tumor part. The in vivo localization of the tumor by means of external scanning was not possible. The specificity index relative to the blood was 4.81 in case 3 and 4.28 in case 4. The specificity indices relative to bone marrow were 2.60 in case 3 and 3.59 in case 4. An in-vivo localization was also doubtful in these two cases.

DISCUSSION

The immunohistochemistry of the tumors obtained in cases 1 and 2 and the antibody binding radioimmunoassays with cells obtained from their monolayer cultures indicate that Mel-14 binds to cytoplasmatic antigens of endothelial cells and to the surface of the tumor cells in both tumors. The specificity indices relative to the blood ranged between 2.36 (less malignant part in case 2) and 6.69 (vessel rich tumor part in case 1) and the results are comparable, in this respect, with results obtained with Mel-14 in the nude mouse system (10). Mach et al. (11) obtained specificity indices between 2.76 and 7.0 relative to serum with an average of 4.7 in three patients suffering from colorectal cancer using a whole monoclonal antibody against colon carcinoma. The counting of different tumor specimens in cases 1 and 2 indicates that the uptake of the specific antibody is not uniform and differs dependent on the tumor part, an observation which Pressmann et al. (1) already had made. In case 1, the tumor part which showed higher specific antibody enrichment as indicated by higher specificity indices had a higher vascularization as shown macroscopically. In case 2, the tumor part with higher specific antibody uptake corresponded to an area with higher vascularization, more malignant tumor cells and, in constrast to the other part, Mel-14 positive endothelial cells. Moshakis et al. (12) have shown in autoradiography that the specific antibody mostly enriches in areas of high vascularity. The increased specificity indices in the vessel rich tumor parts cannot be due to higher blood content or accumulation of interstitial fluid in the tumor, because any increase of blood or serum in the tumor would also increase the accumulation of activity bound to the control and would lead to a decreased specificity index. Whether the better values for the vessel rich part are due to increased binding to the more numerous endothelial cells or to the more malignant tumor cells or to a better clearance caused by a higher blood to tumor transport rate with consequent specific binding to tumor cells, cannot be decided here.

The lowest specificity indices were obtained in case 2. Different reasons can be discussed. Since the main tumor part corresponded to a low grade glioma with only few vessels, which all were negative for Mel-14 in immunhistochemistry, the mechanisms discussed above could be involved. The antibody binding radioimmunoassay with only half the binding ratio as compared to case 1 suggests that in this case less target antigens were available for binding the specific antibody. It should be considered that the cells obtained from the monolayer culture are not representative of the whole tumor and that probably only the more malignant small part of the tumor contributed some tumor cells for culture. An other reason could be the active enrichment of specific antibody in the bone marrow as indicated by the specific index of tumor localization of 0.57 relative to bone marrow. The high antibody uptake in the bone marrow could have reduced the amount of antibody available for binding to the tumor. The specificity indices relative to bone marrow greater than 1 in cases 3 and 4 with corresponding better indices relative to other tissues could confirm this argument. The specific enrichment in the bone marrow occured although the specific antibody was injected intracarotidally, indicating that the first passage through the brain was not effective enough to reduce the amount of specific antibody capable to bind elsewhere. Bullard et al. (13) could not see any difference between the antibody uptake following intracarotid or intravenous infusion of monoclonal antibodies in an experimental model.

In each of the present cases, the external detection of tumor by tomoscintigraphy was difficult because of accumulation of antibody fragments in the skull. Whether the antibody accumulation in the bone is unspecific and due to uptake by the reticulo-endothelial system or specific as shown in case 2 cannot be decided here. The specificity indices for tumor localization relative to bone marrow in cases 3 and 4 were high, but blood, which is not reproducibly to remove from the bone marrow, could have increased the specificity indices in the cases 3 and 4.

The results indicate that there is some accumulation of specific antibody fragment and control in the tumors but there is also a definitely higher uptake of the antibody fragment due to its specificity. A better occupation of the tumor cell surface with antibodies could improve the results. It could be achieved by combining different monoclonal antibodies binding to different tumor target antigens.

SUMMARY

F(ab')2-fragments of the antimelanoma monoclonal antibody MeI-14 were labelled with I-123 for external scanning and with I-125 for in-vitro measurement and injected intravenously into patients scheduled for surgical resection of a glioma. The paired-label study was performed by injecting simultaneously I-131-labelled control F(ab')2-fragments. The patients were tested by computerized tomoscintigraphy. After surgery, the activities of I-125 and I-131 were counted in tumor and normal tissue. The results indicate that there is a definite uptake of the antibody in the tumor due to its specificity. The external detection was difficult because of accumulation of antibody fragments in the skull.

KEY WORDS

Monoclonal Antibodies, Imaging, Gliomas.

REFERENCES

1. PRESSMANN (D.), DAY (E.), BLAU (M.): The use of paired labeling in the determination of tumor-localizing antibodies. Cancer Res. **17**, 845-850 (1957).
2. MACH (J.P.), CARREL (S.), MERENDA (C.), SORDAT (B.), CEROTTINI (J.C.): In vivo localization of radiolabelled antibodies to carcinoembryonic antigen in human colon carcinoma grafted into nude mice. Nature, **248**, 704-706 (1974).
3. HOPF (U.), MEYER ZUM BUSCHENFELDE (K.H.), DIETRICH (M.P.): Demonstration of binding sites for IgG Fc and the third complement (C3) on isolated hepatocytes. J. Immunol., **117**, 639-645 (1976).
4. CARREL (S.), ACCOLLA (R.S.), CARMAGNOLA (A.L.), MACH (J.P.): Common human melanoma-associated antigen(s) detected by monoclonal antibodies. Cancer Res, **40**, 2523-2528 (1980).
5. CARREL (S.), TRIBOLET (N. de), MACH (J.P.): Human melanoma- and glioma-associated antigen(s) identified by monoclonal antibodies. In : BUSCH (H.), YEOMAN (L.): Methods in Cancer Research, Vol. XX: Tumor Markers (Orlando 1982) 317-354.
6. CARREL (S.), SCHREYER (M.), SCHMIDT-KESSEN (A.), MACH (J.P.): Reactivity spectrum of 30 monoclonal antibodies to a panel of 28 melanoma and control cell lines. Hybridoma, **1**, 387-397 (1982).
7. CARREL (S.), TRIBOLET (N. de), MACH (J.P.): Expression of neuroectodermal antigens common to melanomas, gliomas, and neuroblastomas. Acta Neuropathol. (Berl), **57**, 158-164 (1982).
8. MURALT (B. de), TRIBOLET (N. de), DISERENS (A.C.), STAVROU (D.), MACH (J.P.), CARREL (S.): Phenotyping of 60 cultured human gliomas and 34 other neuroectodermal tumors by means of monoclonal antibodies against glioma, melanoma and HLA-DR antigens. Eur. J. Cancer, Clin. Oncol., **21**, 207-216 (1985).
9. BEHNKE (J.), CARREL (S.), TRIBOLET (N. de): Immunohistochemical localization of a neuroectodermal antigen in human brain tumors with the antimelanoma monoclonal antibody MeI-14. In preparation.
10. WIKSTRAND (C.J.), McLENDON (R.E.), KEMSHEAD (J.), COAKHAM (H.), MACH (J.P.), CARREL (S.), TRIBOLET (N. de), BULLARD (D.E.), BIGNER (D.D.): Comparative localization of glioma-reactive monoclonal antibodies in vivo in an athymic mouse human glioma xenograft model. J. Neuroimmunol. (in press).
11. MACH (J.P.), CHATAL (J.F.), LUMBROSO (J.D.), BUCHEGGER (F.), FORNI (M.), RITSCHARD (J.), BERCHE (C.), DOUILLARD (J.Y.), CARREL (S.), HERLYN (M.), STEPLEWSKI (Z.), KOPROWSKI (H.): Tumor localization in patients by radiolabeled monoclonal antibodies against colon carcinoma. Cancer Res., **43**, 5593-5600 (1983).
12. MOSHAKIS (V.), McILHINNEY (R.A.J.), NEVILLE (A.M.): Cellular distribution of monoclonal antibody in human tumours after i.v. administration. Br. J. Cancer, **44**, 663-669 (1981).
13. BULLARD (D.E.), BOURDON (M.), BIGNER (D.D.): Comparison of various methods for delivering radiolabeled monoclonal antibody to normal rat brain. J. Neurosurg., **61**, 901-911 (1984).

Levels of Polyamine Biosynthetic Decarboxylase Activities as Indicators of the Degree of Malignancy of Human Primary Central Nervous System Tumors

G. LUCCARELLI (°), M.E. FERIOLI (°°), G. BROGGI (°) and G. SCALABRINO (°°).

The polyamines, putrescine, spermidine and spermine, which are ubiquitous organic cations of low molecular weight in all living organisms, are distributed in the different areas of mammalian central nervous system (CNS) (1-8). The levels of polyamines vary markedly between brain regions (9, 10). Areas with considerable white matter contain higher levels of spermidine, although this correlation with white matter is by no means perfect (10-12). These polyamines are known to be synthesized in human nervous tissues, because the presence of the four enzymes of the biosynthesis pathway of polyamines, i.e., L-ornithine decarboxylase (EC 4.1.1.17) (ODC), S-adenosyl-L-methionine decarboxylase (EC 4.1.1.50) (AMD), spermidine synthase (EC 2.5.1.16) and spermine synthase (EC 2.5.1.—) in mammalian CNS in now well documented (9, 13, 14). These polyamines can diffuse from human nervous tissues into cerebrospinal fluid (CSF) (15). It has been demonstrated that interconversion of polyamines can also take place in mammalian CNS (8, 16, 17). Although the physiological function of these amines is still not well understood at the molecular level, an abundant literature suggests that the concentrations of polyamines inside the eukaryotic cells are highly regulated and that polyamines play essential roles in cellular growth (whether normal or neoplastic) and differentiation (for review see 18, 19).

There is mounting interest in a variety of biochemical and/or immunologic molecules as potential markers for human CNS tumors. These molecules can be detected in neoplastic cells from which they may leak out into the CSF and can be detected there (20-22). Polyamines are widely considered, despite some limitations, as helpful markers in the diagnosis of human brain tumors and in the evaluation of the degree of tumor malignancy and of effectiveness of therapy (20, 23-25).

High levels of putrescine and spermidine have been found in the CSF of untreated patients with different types of malignant brain tumors, such as glioblastoma multiforme (grade IV astrocytoma), anaplastic astrocytoma (grade III astrocytoma), medulloblastoma, ependymoma and pituitary tumors (26-30). Interestingly enough, there is good correlation between patient status and CSF levels of putrescine and sometimes of spermidine for patients with medulloblastoma, although some few false-negative results have been reported (27, 28). More importantly, in patients with these types of cancer, an elevation in CSF putrescine level may be the earliest indicator of tumor recurrence (27, 28). The correlation between clinical status of the cancer patients and the CSF levels of polyamines (especially putrescine) was not always so good for patients with glioblastoma multiforme or with anaplastic astrocytoma, particularly when these CNS tumors were localized within the cerebral hemispheres (29, 31). While polyamines might, therefore, reflect the cell growth activity of brain tumors, the diagnostic usefulness is limited when the compounds can not reach the CSF. Studies of brain diffusion and capillary permeability of putrescine substantiate this (31). Furthermore, the CSF levels of putrescine and spermidine frequently declined in patients with medulloblastomas or astrocytomas during favorable responses to therapy followed by a clinical improvement and, in some instances, these levels become very close to those seen in reference patients with various non neoplastic CNS diseases (26). However, increases in the CSF polyamine levels, albeit to a lesser degree than in patients with primary CNS tumors, have been found in patients with a variety of non-neoplastic CNS diseases, such as infectious diseases, degenerative diseases and vascular

(°) Neurological Institute "C. Besta", (°°) Institute of General Pathology and C.N.R. Centre for Research in Cell Pathology, University of Milano, via Mangiagalli, 31, 20133 Milano (Italy).

M. Chatel, F. Darcel and J. Pecker (eds.), Brain Oncology. ISBN-13: 978-94-010-8003-3

diseases (26, 27). Therefore, it has become quite clear that an increased CSF polyamine levels is by itself not strictly specific for tumor patients and it might be due either to rapid growth of cells or to necrosis of cells, both of which are accompanied by a high leakage of polyamines.

Attempts to correlate the CSF polyamine levels with the degree of malignancy of the different primary brain tumors and to the tumor size have also failed to fully materialize, which is the major reason why determination of the CSF polyamine levels has never become an useful routine procedure for diagnosis and monitoring of primary human brain tumors.

Much more promising are the few studies in which polyamine contents of human brain neoplastic tissues from untreated patients have been assayed. All the data available agree that these tumors generally have higher putrescine concentrations than those in normal human brain (9, 32). Furthermore, the extent of this elevation in putrescine has been found to be a reliable indicator of the degree of malignancy (by conventional histopathological criteria) of brain tumors of the astrocytoma group (32). Therefore, all the data available about polyamine contents in CSF of patients with CNS tumors or in brain neoplastic tissues concur that the putrescine level is the most reliable and is the only one which may be of some usefulness in clinical oncology of patients with primary CNS tumors.

Because of all the doubts about the significance of polyamine determinations in CSF from cancer patients and because of the small numbers of patients screened for polyamine content in brain tumors, we decided to measure the activities of the two polyamine biosynthetic decarboxylases, namely ODC and AMD in different types of primary human CNS tumor tissues surgically excised from untreated patients and to correlate the levels with the degree of malignancy by conventional histopathological criteria (33). Whenever possible, we studied primary CNS tumors with well-defined growth rates and grades of malignancy according to conventional histopathological criteria. The number of patients with each type of primary CNS tumors was large enough for the results to be evaluated by suitable statistical tests.

In experimental oncology research with Morris rat hepatomas with vastly different growth rates (34), and with chemical carcinogenesis in mouse skin (35, 36), it has been found that the degree of ODC enhancement can be a useful biochemical indicator of neoplastic growth. Furthermore, a previous study in our laboratory (37) demonstrated that the extent of the increases in the activities of ODC and AMD in the epidermis of human epitheliomas was directly proportional to the neoplasm's growth rate and therefore correlated well with the tumor's malignancy.

Our major finding was a correlation between the activities of polyamine biosynthetic decarboxylases (particularly ODC) and the growth rate and degree of malignancy of the neoplasm for most of the primary CNS tumors we tested. The ODC activity in the astrocytoma group significantly and progressively increased from infratentorial pilocytic astrocytoma (grade I) to supratentorial glioblastoma multiforme (grade IV) through supratentorial astrocytoma of grades II and III (33). It is well known that the growth rate is much slower for low-grade, well differentiated astrocytomas than for the high-grade, malignant gliomas, including glioblastoma multiforme (38). More importantly, medulloblastoma, a highly malignant brain tumor, had the highest level of ODC activity among all the primary CNS tumors of whatever histogenetic origin we tested (33).

The activity of AMD in the same types of brain tumors significantly and progressively increased from the infratentorial pilocytic grade I astrocytoma to the supratentorial grade III astrocytoma, so that it, as well as ODC, paralleled quite well the degree of histopathological malignancy (33). However, there was no further increase in AMD activity from supratentorial grade III astrocytoma to glioblastoma multiforme (grade IV). Therefore, the increase in AMD activity in the astrocytoma group tumors was not entirely similar to that in ODC activity. The surprising finding was, however, that in medulloblastomas there is a clear dichotomy between the levels of the two polyamine biosynthetic decarboxylases, with the highest ODC levels and the lowest AMD levels of any of the human brain tumors of neuroepithelial tissue we have tested (33). We also wish to emphasize our results for various types of human meningiomas. When, as suggested by Rubinstein (39), we divided the meningiomas into atypical and typical forms on the basis of the presence or absence of mitotic figures, regardless of histologic variants, we found that ODC levels in the atypical forms were significantly higher than those in the typical forms, without corresponding significant differences in the AMD levels (33). It should be recalled that it has been claimed that the incidence of mitotic figures in tumors of meningeal tissues is an important criterion for assessment of the likelihood of recurrence and a rough prognosticator for rapid growth (32, 40).

When we compare the usefulness of polyamine contents in CSF and CNS tumor specimens with that of activity of the polyamine biosynthetic decarboxylases in CNS tumors after their surgical removal, for diagnosis and, even more importantly, prognosis in the clinical oncology of CNS primary tumors, we feel that: (1) measurements of CSF polyamine levels can be useful for short-time evaluation of a specific course of therapy and for detection of remission or relapse of the neoplastic disease, but are of little or no use for evaluating the degree of malignancy of the tumor, particularly when used without other CNS tumor markers and (2) the activities of the polyamine biosynthetic decarboxylases, especially ODC, are by far better indicators of the degree of malignancy of the tumor, but are of no use for evaluating the effectiveness of the therapy, because, obviously, repeated samples can not be obtained.

Therefore, the two polyamine biosynthetic decarboxylases, especially ODC, are important tools to use for study not only of the CNS ontogeny (13, 41-47) but also of human CNS tumors. It is important to mention here that mammalian CNS shows a peculiar ontogenic pattern of the activities of the two polyamine biosynthetic decarboxylases, because only ODC is very active during embryonal life and only AMD is very active during adult life (13, 41, 42, 48, 49). From the point of view of the levels of the polyamine biosynthetic decarboxylase activities, medulloblastoma, which shows a very high level of ODC activity and a very low level of AMD activity, is confirmed to be a typical embryonic tumor of CNS.

SUMMARY

We measured the levels of ornithine decarboxylase (ODC) and S-adenosylmethionine decarboxylase (AMD) activities in various types of primary human tumors of the central nervous system (CNS). In astrocytomas ODC levels increased progressively from infratentorial pilocytic astrocytoma (grade I) to glioblastoma multiforme (grade IV) and correlated well with the degree of histologic malignancy of the tumor. AMD activity levels, however, correlated with tumor malignancy only up to grade III astrocytoma. Medulloblastoma had the highest ODC activities of all the CNS tumors tested but had low AMD activities. No significant differences in either of the polyamine biosynthetic decarboxylase levels were observed among the several variants of meningiomas tested. However, atypical forms of meningiomas, i.e., those with mitotic figures, whatever the histologic variants, had higher levels of ODC, but not of AMD, than the typical forms, i.e., those without mitotic figures.

KEY WORDS

Polyamines, Brain Tumors, Gliomas.

REFERENCES

1. KREMZNER (L.T.): Metabolism of polyamines in the nervous system. Fed. Proc., **29**: 1583-1588 (1970).
2. RUSSELL (D.H.), MEDINA (V.J.), SNYDER (S.H.): The dynamics of synthesis and degradation of polyamines in normal and regenerating rat liver and brain. J. Biol. Chem., **245**: 6732-6738 (1970).
3. SHASKAN (E.G.), SNYDER (S.H.): Polyamine turnover in different regions of rat brain. J. Neurochem., **20**: 1453-1460 (1973).
4. SHAW (G.G.), PATEMAN (A.J.): The regional distribution of the polyamines spermidine and spermine in brain. J. Neurochem., **20**: 1225-1230 (1973).
5. HARIK (S.I.), SNYDER (S.H.): Putrescine: regional distribution in the nervous system of the rat and the cat. Brain Res., **66**: 328-331 (1974).
6. SEILER (N.), LAMBERTY (U.): Interrelations between polyamines and nucleic acids: changes of polyamine and nucleic acid concentrations in the developing rat brain. J. Neurochem., **24**: 5-13 (1975).

7. SEILER (N.), SCHMIDT-GLENEWINKEL (T.): Regional distribution of putrescine, spermidine and spermine in relation to the distribution of RNA and DNA in the rat nervous system. J. Neurochem., **24**: 791-795 (1975).

8. HALLIDAY (C.A.), SHAW (G.C.): The distribution and metabolism of putrescine, spermidine and spermine injected into the cerebral ventricles of rabbits. J. Neurochem., **26**: 1199-1205 (1976).

9. KREMZNER (L.T.), BARRETT (R.E.), TERRANO (M.J.): Polyamine metabolism in the central and peripheral nervous system. Ann. N.Y. Acad. Sci., **171**: 735-748 (1970).

10. SNYDER (S.H.) SHASKAN (E.G.), HARIK (S.I.): Polyamine disposition in the central nervous system. In: Polyamines in Normal and Neoplastic Growth. Ed. D.H. Russell, Raven Press, New York, pp. 199-213 (1973).

11. SHIMIZU (H.), KAKIMOTO (Y.), SANO (I.): The determination and distribution of polyamines in mammalian nervous system. J. Pharmac. Exp. Ther., **143**: 199-204 (1974).

12. KREMZNER (L.T.): Polyamine metabolism in normal and neoplastic neural tissue. In : Polyamines in Normal and Neoplastic Growth. Ed. D.H. Russell, Raven Press, New York, pp. 27-40 (1973).

13. SHASKAN (E.G.), HARASZTI (J.H.), SNYDER (S.H.): Polyamines: developmental alterations in regional disposition and metabolism in rat brain. J. Neurochem., **20**: 1443-1452 (1973).

14. RAINA (A.), PAJULA (R.L.), ELORANTA (T.): A rapid assay method for spermidine and spermine synthases. Distribution of polyamine-synthesizing enzymes and methionine adenosyltransferase in rat tissues. FEBS Lett., **67**: 252-255 (1976).

15. SHAW (G.G.): The polyamines in the central nervous system. Biochem. Pharmacol., **28**: 1-6 (1979).

16. STURMAN (J.A.), INGOGLIA (N.A.), LINDQUIST (T.D.): Interconversion of putrescine, spermidine and spermine in goldfish and rat retina. Life Sci., **19**: 719-724 (1976).

17. SEILER (N.), BOLKENIUS (F.N.): Polyamine reutilization and turnover in brain. Neurochem. Res., **10**: 529-544 (1985).

18. SCALABRINO (G.), FERIOLI (M.E.): Polyamines in mammalian tumors. Part I. Adv. Cancer Res., **35**: 151-268 (1981).

19. SCALABRINO (G.), FERIOLI (M.E.): Polyamines in mammalian tumors. Part II. Adv. Cancer Res., **36**: 1-102 (1982).

20. SEIDENFELD (J.), MARTON (L.J.): Biochemical markers of central nervous system tumors measured in cerebrospinal fluid and their potential use in diagnosis and patient management: a review. J. Natl. Cancer Inst., **63**: 919-931 (1979).

21. TRIBOLET (N. de), CARREL (S.): Human glioma tumour-associated antigens. Cancer Immunol. Immunother., **9**: 207-211 (1980).

22. WICKSTRAND (C.J.), BIGNER (D.D.): Immunobiologic aspects of the brain and human gliomas. Am. J. Pathol., **98**: 515-567 (1980).

23. MARTON (L.J.): Polyamines and brain tumors. Natl. Cancer Inst. Monogr., **46**: 127-131 (1977).

24. MARTON (L.J.): Polyamines and brain tumors: relationship to patient monitoring and therapy. Adv. Polyamine Res., **3**: 425-430 (1981).

25. MARTON (L.J.): CSF polyamines. Potential as brain tumor markers. Arch. Neurol., **38**: 73-74 (1981).

26. MARTON (L.J.), HEBY (O.), LEVIN (V.A.), LUBICH (W.P.), CRAFTS (D.C.), WILSON (C.B.): The relationship of polyamines in cerebrospinal fluid to the presence of central nervous system tumors. Cancer Res., **36**: 973-977 (1976).

27. MARTON (L.J.), EDWARDS (M.S.), LEVIN (V.A.), LUBICH (W.P.), WILSON (C.B.): Predictive value of cerebrospinal fluid polyamines in medulloblastoma. Cancer Res., **39**: 993-997 (1979).

28. MARTON (L.J.), EDWARDS (M.S.), LEVIN (V.A.), LUBICH (W.P.), WILSON (C.B.): CSF polyamines: a new and important means of monitoring patients with medulloblastoma. Cancer, **47**: 757-760 (1981).

29. FULTON (D.S.), LEVIN (V.A.), LUBICH (W.P.), WILSON (C.B.), MARTON (L.J.): Cerebrospinal fluid polyamines in patients with glioblastoma multiforme and anaplastic astrocytoma. Cancer Res., **40**: 3293-3296 (1980).

30. FULTON (D.S.), MARTON (L.J.), LUBICH (W.P.), WILSON (C.B.): Polyamine levels in CSF from patients with pituitary tumors or nonneoplastic pituitary disease. Arch. Neurol., **39**: 47-48 (1982).

31. PIERANGELI (E.), LEVIN (V.A.), SEIDENFELD (J.), MARTON (L.J.): Putrescine diffusion in cat brain and capillary permeability in rat brain: relation to CSF putrescine levels in brain tumor patients. Eur. J. Cancer, **17**: 143-147 (1981).

32. HARIK (S.I.), SUTTON (C.H.): Putrescine as a biochemical marker of malignant brain tumors. Cancer Res., **39**: 5010-5015 (1979).

33. SCALABRINO (G.), MODENA (D.), FERIOLI (M.E.), PUERARI (M.), LUCCARELLI (G.): Degrees of malignancy in human primary central nervous system tumors: ornithine decarboxylase levels as better indicators than adenosylmethionine decarboxylase levels. J. Natl. Cancer Inst., **68**: 751-754 (1982).

34. WILLIAMS-ASHMAN (H.G.), COPPOC (G.L.), WEBER (G.): Imbalance in ornithine metabolism in hepatomas of different growth rates as expressed in formation of putrescine, spermidine and spermine. Cancer Res., **32**: 1924-1932 (1972).

35. O'BRIEN (T.G.): The induction of ornithine decarboxylase as early, possibly obligatory, event in mouse skin cancerogenesis. Cancer Res., **36**: 2644-2653 (1976).

36. BOUTWELL (R.K.), O'BRIEN (T.G.), VERMA (A.K.), WEEKES (R.G.), YOUNG (L.M. de), ASHENDEL (C.L.), ASTRUP (E.G.): The induction of ornithine decarboxylase activity and its control in mouse skin epidermis. Adv. Enzyme Regul., **17**: 89-112 (1979).

37. SCALABRINO (G.), PIGATTO (P.), FERIOLI (M.E.), MODENA (D.), PUERARI (M.), CARU (A.): Levels of activity of the polyamine biosynthetic decarboylases as indicators of degree of malignancy of human cutaneous epitheliomas. J. Invest. Dermatol., **74**: 122-124 (1980).

38. STELL (G.G.): Growth kinetics of brain tumours. In: Brain Tumors. Eds. D.G.T. Thomas, D.I. Graham, Butterworths, London, pp. 10-20 (1980).

39. RUBINSTEIN (L.J.): Tumors of the central nervous system. In: Atlas of Tumor Pathology, 2nd Series, Fascicle 6. Armed Forces Inst. of Pathology, Washington D.C., pp. 169-190 (1972).

40. CROMPTON (M.R.), GAUTIER-SMITH (P.C.): The prediction of recurrence in meningiomas. J. Neurol. Neurosurg. Psychiat., **33**: 80-87 (1970).

41. ANDERSON (T.R.), SCHANBERG (S.M.): Ornithine decarboxylase activity in developing rat brain. J. Neurochem., **19**: 1471-1481 (1972).

42. SCHMIDT (G.L.), CANTONI (G.L.): Adenosylmethionine decarboxylase in developing rat brain. J. Neurochem., **20**: 1373-1385 (1973).

43. STURMAN (J.A.), GAULL (G.E.): Polyamine biosynthesis in human fetal liver and brain. Pediat. Res., **8**: 231-237 (1974).

44. GILAD (G.M.), KOPIN (I.J.): Neurochemical aspects of neuronal ontogenesis in the developing rat cerebellum: changes in neurotransmitter and polyamine synthesizing enzymes. J. Neurochem., **33**: 1195-1204 (1979).

45. SLOTKIN (T.A.): Ornithine decarboxylase as a tool in developmental neurobiology. Life Sci., **24**: 1623-1630 (1979).

46. LAITINEN (S.I.), LAITINEN (P.H.), HIETALA (O.A.), PAJUNEN (A.E.I.), PIHA (R.S.): Developmental changes in mouse brain polyamine metabolism. Neurochem. Res., **7**: 1477-1485 (1982).

47. RUEL (J.), CHÉNARD (C.), COULOMBE (P.), DUSSAULT (J.H.): Thyroid hormones modulate ornithine decarboxylase in the immature rat cerebellum. Can. J. Physiol. Pharmacol., **62**: 1279-1283 (1984).

48. ANDERSON (T.R.), SCHANBERG (S.M.): Effect of tyroxine and cortisol on brain ornithine decarboxylase activity and swimming behavior in developing rat. Biochem. Pharmacol., **24**: 495-501 (1975).

49. GRILLO (M.A.), FOSSA (T.), DIANZANI (U.): Arginase, ornithine decarboxylase and S-adenosylmethionine decarboxylase in chicken brain and retina. Int. J. Biochem., **15**: 1081-1084 (1983).

Red Blood cell Polyamines in the Long Term Follow-up of Malignant Gliomas

J. Ph. MOULINOUX (°), V. QUEMENER (°),
F. DARCEL (°°), J. FAIVRE (°°°), M. CHATEL (°°).

Although they were first detected at the end of the 18th century by the famous chemist A. Vauquelin (1), who, among other achievements, first formulated the concept of the amino acid, the true significance of polyamines did not become apparent until the second half of the 20th century. For a long time they were erroneously considered to be "simple" end products of degradation, a view which is reflected in the names which were attached to them (putrescine, cadaverine, spermidine, spermine), before their finely regulated metabolism and their relationship with the cell cycle came to be studied (2).

The biological importance of polyamine metabolism stems mainly from the observation that this seems to be closely associated with cell proliferation and that polyamines and some of their derivatives and also various drugs which affect polyamine metabolism can influence cell division and sometimes also cell differentiation (Fig. 1).

From a clinical viewpoint, this metabolism has an obvious diagnostic potential, especially in cancerology. Since the polyamines synthesized by proliferating cells can be measured qualitatively in biological fluids (blood, urine, CSF), these molecules are possible markers of cancer.

$NH_2 — (CH_2)_4 — NH_2$ .... Putrescine
$NH_2 — (CH_2)_3 — NH — (CH_2)_4 — NH_2$ .... Spermidine
$NH_2 — (CH_2)_3 — NH — (CH_2)_4 — NH — (CH_2)_3 — NH_2$ .... Spermine

The first study which tried to evaluate the clinical importance of measuring polyamines in the urine of cancer patients was carried out by D.H. Russell in 1971 (3). Measurements in urine, and similary measurements made in whole blood, plasma or serum from cancer patients, did not show a very satisfactory correlation between the concentration of polyamines and the stage of tumour evolution (4).

In contrast, in 1974, Marton et al. (5) showed that the presence of a malignant brain tumour was always accompanied by an abnormally high level of putrescine in the cerebrospinal fluid. The same group later demonstrated that monitoring of polyamines in CSF allowed a better management of children suffering from medulloblastoma (6, 7).

(°) Unité fonctionnelle de Biologie Cellulaire. (°°) Service de Neurologie. (°°°) Service de Neurochirurgie, Centre Hospitalier Universitaire de Rennes, Rennes, France.

M. Chatel, F. Darcel and J. Pecker (eds.), Brain Oncology. ISBN-13: 978-94-010-8003-3

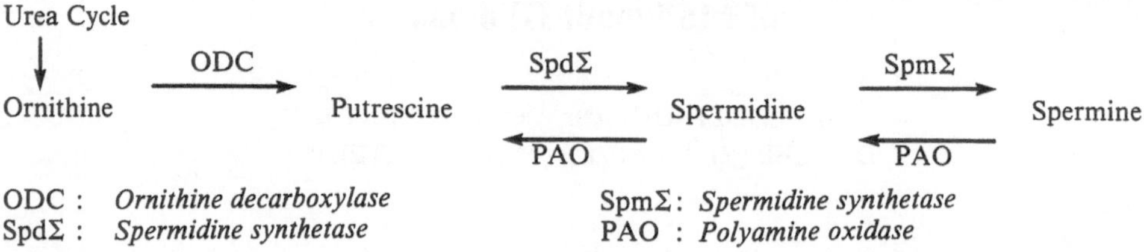

FIGURE 1.

Since nearly all the free circulating polyamines are transported by red blood cells, we were particularly interested in this cellular compartment (8). Knowing that polyamines are not metabolized to any great extent in erythrocytes and that these cells actively accumulate spermidine and spermine (8) we began to study changes in levels of these two molecules within red cells during periods of cell division: on one hand a regulated proliferation such as experimental liver regeneration in the rat (9), and on the other hand uncontrolled division in the 3 LL Lewis lung carcinoma (10). In both these animal models we observed that the spermidine levels varied in parallel with the level of cell proliferation.

These experimental results led us to investigate the clinical relevance of an estimation of red blood cell polyamine levels as a circulating biochemical marker of cell proliferation in patients with neoplastic disease of different histological types. In particular, we studied broncho-pulmonary tumours (10), hepatocarcinoma (11), acute Leukemia (12) and malignant brain tumours (13, 14, 15, 16).

We became especially interested in patients with malignant brain tumours for many reasons. These included the fact that the mitotic index is extremely low or zero in normal brain tissue and thus the markers of cell proliferation, that is, the polyamine levels, may be considered as true tumour markers in this type of lesion. In addition, taking a blood sample to measure red cell polyamine levels present less risk to the patient, already suffering from an expanding intra-cranial mass, than the lumbar puncture necessary to measure CSF polyamines.

Thus, in the first stage of this study we chose patients undergoing neurosurgery, for whom we could obtain samples of tumour, CSF and blood at the same time, and studied the distribution of polyamines in these three tissues. The measurement of polyamines were carried out by HPLC, as previously described (10-16).

The normal levels of polyamines in red blood cells are (mean $\pm$ standard deviation, $n = 45$), 8.0 ± 3.1 nmoles/8.10^9 cells for spermidine, and 6.2 ± 2.1 nmoles/8.10^9 cells for spermine. The physiological levels of putrescine and spermidine in CSF are (mean $\pm$ standard deviation, $n = 10$) 160 ± 85 pmoles/ml and 82 ± 6 pmoles/ml respectively.

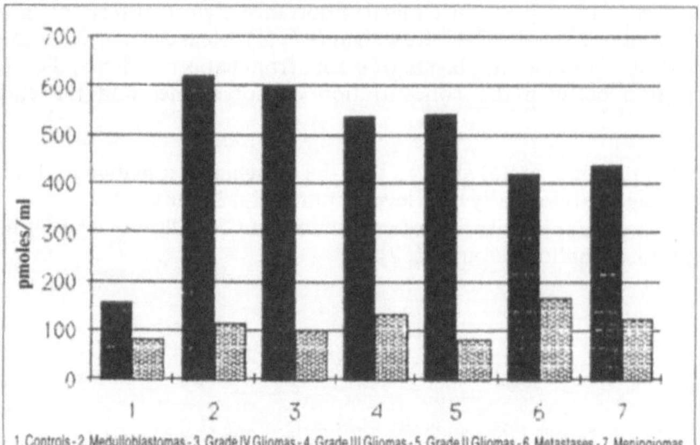

FIGURE 2. Putrescine ■ and spermidine □ levels in the CSF of patients with brain tumours.

This vertical study involving 73 patients with neuro-epithelial tumours (17 grade IV gliomas, 16 grade III gliomas, 5 grade II gliomas, 8 medulloblastomas, 7 meningiomas and 8 metastatic tumours) first of all allowed us to confirm the hypothesis that, as a general rule, the presence of a brain tumour is accompanied by a significant increase in the polyamine levels: in the CSF, and particularly the putrescine level, regardless of the histological type (Fig. 2).

In contrast, we did not see a significant increase in the red cell levels of polyamines, except in the patients with grade IV glioma, as is shown in Figure 3; although the highest intra-tumoral concentrations of polyamines were observed in medulloblastomas (Fig. 4).

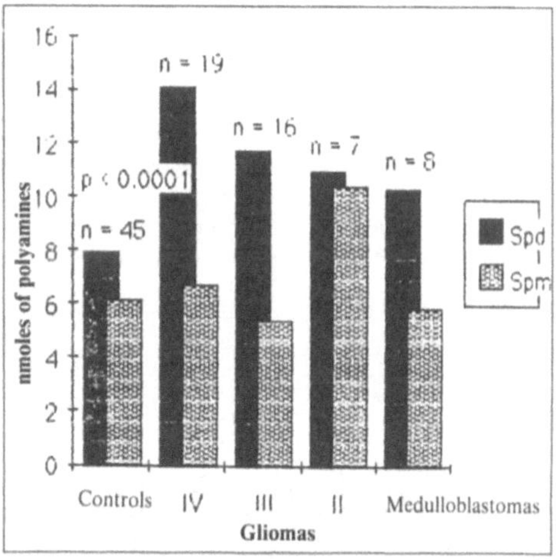

FIGURE 3. Pre-operation levels of RBC Polyamines. The results are expressed as nmoles polyamines / 8 × 10^9 red cells. n = number of patients.

Although the brain tumours were all accompanied by an unusually high level of CSF polyamines, there was no statistically significant correlation between the concentration of putrescine present in the tumour and that present in the CSF, except in the case of medulloblastoma. This latter type of tumour is known to possess a particularly high ornithine decarboxylase activity (17) which may be one factor contributing to the elevated polyamine levels, another factor being the proximity of most of these tumours to the fourth ventricle.

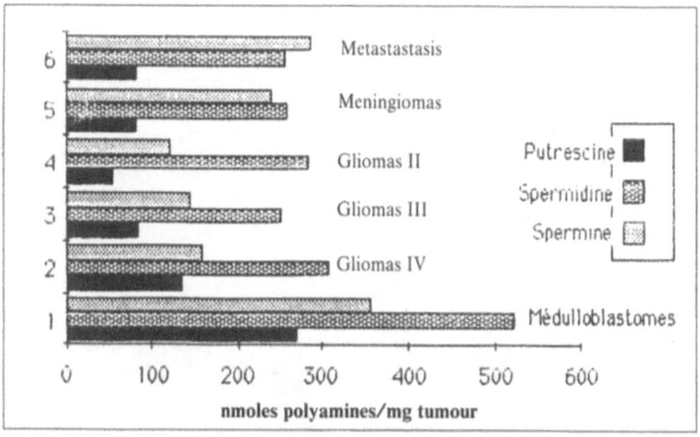

FIGURE 4. Intratumoral polyamines levels

In contrast, in malignant glioma, tumours which are generally situated deep within the brain, the secretion of tumour derived polyamines takes place mainly by way of the blood, which might explain the significant correlation observed between the spermidine/spermine ratios in red blood cells and in tumours (13). As we will see below, a very precise relationship exists between the RBC levels of spermidine and of spermine and this has a definite diagnostic value during the post-operative management of patients suspected to have recurring malignant glioma.

In the second stage of the study, we tried to evaluate the clinical relevance of estimating the RBC polyamine levels during the post-operative period in patients suffering from supratentorial malignant glioma.

This was an horizontal study carried out on 47 patients with malignant glioma classified according to the histological grade of the disease (WHO classification), studied for periods between 2 and 28 months (average = 11 months). The group consisted of 21 grade IV gliomas, 24 grade III gliomas and 2 grade II gliomas. The patients were examined at intervals of 4 weeks on average and X-ray tomography scans (CT) were carried out every three months. In all cases a diagnosis of recurrence was based solely on clinical criteria and the CT Scan. 360 polyamine determinations were carried out, and each patient was the subject of from 5 to 31 measurements (mean = 10). This cancer patient group was compared with two control groups, one of 45 healthy subjects without any detectable neoplastic disease and the other of 67 patients with non-neoplastic diseases (Table I).

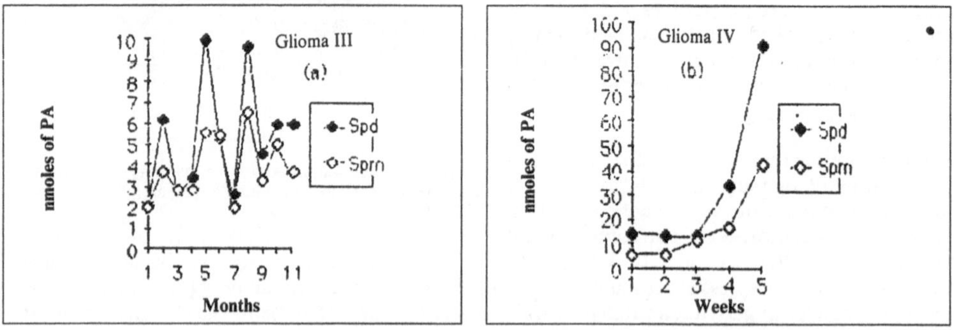

FIGURE 5. Examples of Variations in RBC Polyamine Levels: a) In remission; b) During recurrence.

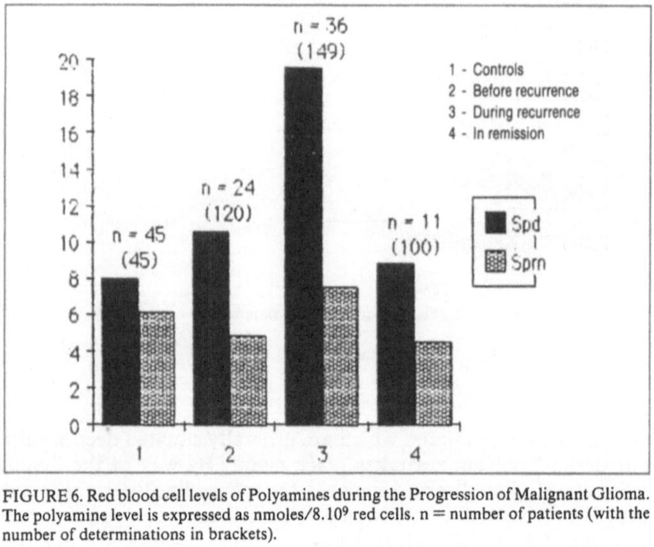

FIGURE 6. Red blood cell levels of Polyamines during the Progression of Malignant Glioma. The polyamine level is expressed as nmoles/8.10^9 red cells. n = number of patients (with the number of determinations in brackets).

As an example, in Figure 5, we show the post-operative variations observed over an extended period in two patients, one treated for grade III glioma and the other for grade IV glioma.

TABLE I

Non-Neoplastic Brain Disease	Spermidine	Spermine
	nmoles/8.10^9 red cells	
Multiple sclerosis n = 15	10.9 (2.2)	6.3 (4.1)
Cerebral vascular disease n = 13	13.5 (1.6)	5.0 (0.7)
Polyneuritis n = 11	14.6 (1.7)	7.4 (1.7)
Meningitis n = 3	10.7 (8.1)	8.0 (5.6)
Hydrocephaly n = 3	12.4 (6.6)	4.5 (2.3)
Myasthenia Gravis n = 3	15.0 (2.8)	5.2 (1.4)
Spino-cerebellar degeneration n = 2	7.7	4.7
Migraine n = 2	6.1	3.5
Encephalomyelitis n = 2	17.1	3.2
Miscellaneous n = 10	15.7 (7.5)	6.9 (2.6)

n = number of patients (standard error of the mean)

Firstly, the study revealed that the variations in the levels of polyamines in red blood cells were generally correlated with changes in the clinical condition and in the CT Scans. Clinical deterioration, measured objectively by the reduction in Karnofsky's index, was accompanied, in most cases, by an increase of the RBC levels of spermidine.

In Figure 6 we give the mean levels of RBC polyamines in patients before recurrence and during recurrence, together with values from those patients who did not recur during the course of the study. Presented in this way the level of spermidine in the red cells during recurrence was significantly increased ($p < 10^{-6}$) compared with that observed before recurrence or in the absence of recurrent disease.

In addition, when we looked at the polyamine profiles of each individual patient who experienced tumour recurrence during the study, we noted that, in every case, this was accompanied by an abnormal level of polyamines (before and/or during the relapse).

Thus, in 100% of cases of grade II and III glioma and in 90% of grade IV glioma patients, tumour recurrence is associated with spermidine levels of over 14 nmole/8.10^9 red cells (two standard deviations above the mean). Similary, 66% of the stage IV gliomas and 20% of the grade III gliomas showed a link between tumour progression and unusually low levels of spermine, i.e. less than 2 nmoles/8.10^9 cells, two standard deviations below the mean. The normal levels of polyamines (mean ± 2 standard deviations) are 2-14 nmoles/8.10^9 cells for spermidine and 2-10 nmoles/8.10^9 cells for spermine, and, in our recurrent patients, a spermine level above 10 nmoles/8.10^9 cells was always associated with a spermidine level greater than 14 nmoles/8.10^9 cells; thus we considered a spermidine concentration higher than 14 nmoles/8.10^9 cells or a spermine concentration lower than 2 nmoles/8.10^9 cells to be abnormal.

According to these criteria, regardless of the histological grade of the disease, 100% of the patients with recurrence presented with an abnormal level of polyamines at least once during the study. 3 patients surgically treated for grade III malignant glioma did not develop recurrent disease during the study, although their spermidine and spermine level were abnormal accorded to the criteria. These three defined above false positive results should be considered as 'relative', since these patients are still alive (which is not the case for the other patients showing abnormal polyamine levels and recurrence). As is shown in Table I, the development of non-neoplastic brain disease may nevertheless, be accompanied by abnormal levels of RBC polyamines.

It should be emphasized that, in 30% of the cases, the abnormal polyamine level preceded the first clinical signs of recurrence and a positive CT scan by between 1 and 5 months. Furthermore, we have observed that when the red cell levels of spermidine and spermine are normal, any clinical or scanner-derived evidence of recurrence should be reconsidered. In fact, in 3 patients with normal polyamine levels, CT images which suggested recurrence of the tumour were later shown to represent the formation of scar tissue.

In order to follow tumour proliferation more closely from the measurement of circulating polyamines, we first checked that there was a highly significant correlation ($r \neq 1$) between the levels of spermidine and spermine in the red blood cells. We then calculated the constants (a and b) for regression lines relating the corresponding values of spermidine and spermine measured within the three groups of patients, that is before and during recurrence, and in remission (Table II). As can be seen from this Table, although there is no significant correlation between the levels of spermidine and spermine measured in healthy controls ($r = 0.4$), the situation is completely different in patients before and during recurrence.

It is also noteworthy that patients who have not gone into regression, but nevertheless show abnormal levels of polyamines, have a close correlation between their spermidine and spermine concentrations ($r = 0.80$, $p < 10^{-3}$), as do the patients before ($r = 0.70$) or during ($r = 0.80$) recurrence; whereas for patients in remission with normal levels of polyamines the correlation is much weakes ($r = 0.48$, $p < 5.10^{-2}$).

TABLE II

Patients	r	Equation
Before recurrence (n = 24, 120 determinations)	0.70 (*)	y = 1.82 × +1.6
During recurrence (n = 36, 149 determinations)	0.80 (*)	y = 1.64 × +7.16
In remission:		
— with abnormal polyamine levels (n = 6, 50 determinations)	0.80 (*)	y = 1.18 × +5.15
— with normal polyamine levels (n = 5, 50 determinations)	0.48 (**)	y = 0.69 × +3.50
During radio-necrosis (n = 3, 18 determinations)	0.83 (*)	y = 0.50 × +4.25
Controls (n = 45, 45 determinations)	0.40 (NS)	y = 0.53 × +4.68

r = correlation coefficient. (*) $p < 10^{-3}$. (**) $p < 5.10^{-2}$. (NS) not significant.
Equation: y (nmoles spermidine) = a . x (nmoles spermine) + b.

In a previous study in which we followed a small number of patients (14), we observed that the gradient (a) of the regression line changed with time so as to be inversely proportional to the Karnofsky index.

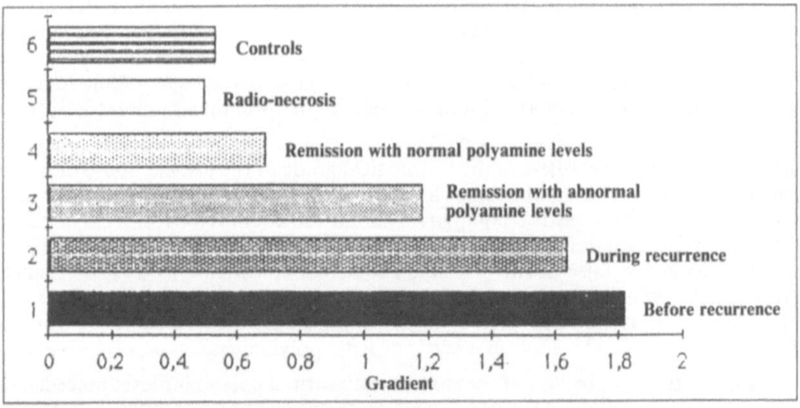

FIGURE 7. Gradients of the regression lines calculated from pairs of values for spermidine and spermine levels. In patients before and during recurrence, and in patients in remission or undergoing radio-induced necrosis. The number of patients (and the number of determinations) are the same as those shown in Table II.

Thus, during the course of the disease, a reduction in the value of Karnofsky's index is usually accompanied by an increased slope in the regression line. From a statistical point of view (Fig. 7), the gradient seems to be related to the proliferative state of cells in the cranial cavity. We have noted a statistically significant difference between two groups of subjects ($p < 10^{-6}$); one group consisting of healthy controls, patients undergoing radionecrosis and those in remission with normal levels of polyamines and the other containing patients in remission but with abnormal levels of polyamines and patients before and during recurrence.

We wish to emphasize that we have also found a statistically significant difference ($p < 10^{-3}$) between two sub-populations of patients, those in whom remission was associated with normal levels of polyamines and those who were in remission but presented abnormal polyamine levels. This latter group seems to be comparable to patients before and during recurrence, at least from a statistical point of view. This provides a possible explanation for the 'relative' false positives, the patients in clinical remission with normal CT scans presenting with abnormal levels of spermidine and spermine (which bring about an increase in the gradient of the regression line). They might be considered to be in a phase of 'biological recurrence', and the levels of RBC polyamines might thus act as a useful marker to predict tumour recurrence.

In order to make the clinical application of these results easier, we have defined a critical range spermidine and spermine concentrations based on the levels of the two polyamines observed in patients shown to have recurrent disease by clinical criteria and by CT scanning. With the aid of this graphical representation (shown in Fig. 8), it is possible to identify (with a statistical error of less than 5%) subjects in which cell proliferation in the brain has restarted and where, in consequence, a tumour will recur, simply by taking account of the red blood cell levels of spermidine and spermine measured in the patient.

Although the biological mechanism underlying these changes is not yer clear, this sort of analysis has an obvious diagnostic value during the post-operative management of patients suspected to have recurrent malignant supra-tentorial glioma. By allowing a precise estimation of the cell proliferative activity within the brain, the determination of polyamine levels in red blood cells will be an important therapeutic tool in the future. In theory, a patient could be treated for recurrence before any clinical or CT signs appear, that is, before a solid tumour develops. It would seem to be advisable to commence anti-proliferative therapy as soon as these first biological signs of intra-cranial cell division appear, and to modifiy this treatment as a function of the level of brain hyperplasia, as estimated from the red cell polyamine levels.

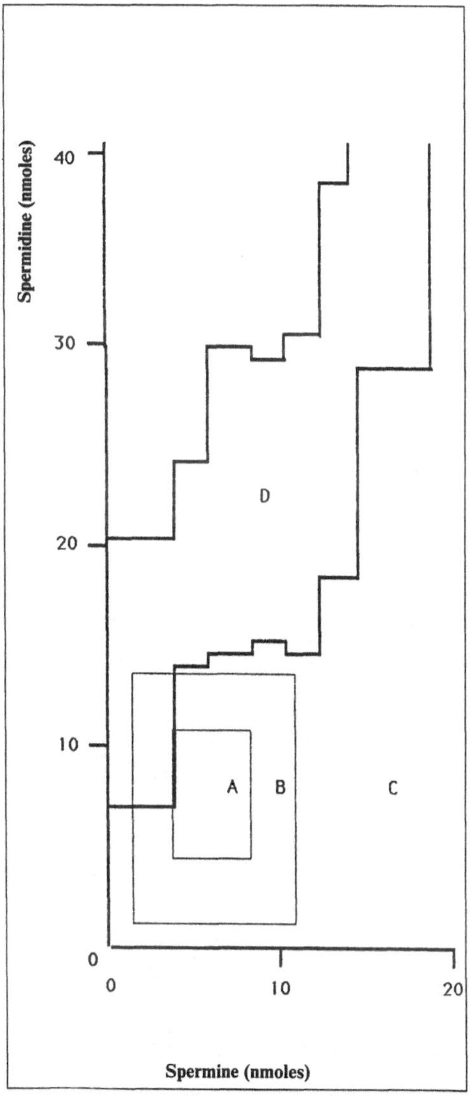

FIGURE 8. Theoretical region in which intra-cranial cell proliferation occurs, calculated from pairs of spermidine and spermine concentrations in patients with recurrent malignant supra-tentorial glioma (± 2 standard deviations). Pairs of values of spermidine and spermine measured in normal subjects (A) ± standard deviation, (B) ± 2 standard deviations, (C) Region corresponding to pairs of polyamine levels found during radio-necrosis.

SUMMARY

Preliminary data have suggested that Red Blood Cell Polyamine levels were correlated with the clinical and T.D.M. evolutions.
From the monitoring (2 to 28 months) of the post-operative treatment of gliomas grade IV (n=14), III (n=18), II (n=2), patients, it could be noticed that:
1°/ 100 % of patients whose tumor recurred, showed at least one time abnormal RBC SPD (> 14 nmoles/8.10⁹ RBC, mean + 2 S.D.) and/or SPM (< 2 nmoles/8.10⁹ RBC, mean - 2 S.D.) values.
2°/ 30 % of patients who recurred had abnormal RBC polyamines concentrations one to six months before any clinical or TDM sign of tumor progression.
3°/ in the presence of a patient with normal values of RBC polyamines levels, clinical or TDM arguments of tumor progression have to be reconsidered.
4°/ during individual follow-up, and only in case of tumor progression, RBC SPD levels of each patients are in a general manner significantly correlated to those of SPM (r = 0.9), and the slope of their straight regression line (SRL) are related to the importance of the intracranial cell proliferation.
We propose a graphic model including a "Space of Proliferative Activity" corresponding to RBC SPD and SPM levels in case of tumour recurrence (p < 10-3), which can be routinely used during the post-operative follow up of these patients.

KEY WORDS

Polyamines, Malignant Gliomas.

ACKNOWLEDGMENTS

This work was supported by CNRS (Contract RL 69, No. 866 ONO 315), the Ligue Française Contre le Cancer and the Fondation Jean Langlois. We should like to thank Mr. Christian Martin and Mr. René Havouis for their technical assistance.

REFERENCES

1. VAUQUELIN (A.): Expériences sur le sperme humain. Ann. Chim., **9**, 64-80 (1791).
2. HEBY (O.): Roles of polyamines in the control of cell proliferation and differenciation, Differentiation, **19**, 1-20 (1981).
3. RUSSEL (D.H.): Increased polyamines concentrations in the urine of human cancer patients, Nature, **233**, 144-145 (1971).
4. SCALABRINO (G.), FERIOLI (M.E.): Polyamines in mammalian tumors. Adv. in Cancer Res., Vol. 35 (Part I), Vol. 36 (Part II), Academic Press, Inc. (1982).
5. MARTON (L.J.), HEBY (O.), WILSON (C.B.): Increased polyamine concentrations in the CSF of patients with brain tumors. Int. J. Cancer, **14**, 731-735 (1974).
6. MARTON (L.J.), EDWARDS (M.S.), LEVIN (V.A.), LUBICH (W.P.), WILSON (C.B.): The relationship of polyamines in the CSF to the presence of central nervous system tumors, Cancer Res., **39**, 993-997 (1979).
7. MARTON (L.J.), EDWARDS (M.S.), LEVIN (V.A.), LUBICH (W.P.), WILSON (C.B.): CSF polyamines: a new and important means of monitoring patients with medulloblastoma. Cancer, **47**, 757-760 (1981).
8. MOULINOUX (J.-Ph.), QUEMENER (V.), QUASH (G.A.): In vitro studies on the entry of polyamines into normal red blood cells, Biochimie, **66**, 385-393, (1984).
9. MOULINOUX (J.-Ph.), QUEMENER (V.), CHAMBON (Y.): Evolution of red blood cell polyamine levels in partially hepatectomized rat. Eur. J. Cancer, in press (1986).
10. MOULINOUX (J.-Ph.), QUEMENER (V.), LARZUL (J.J.), ROCH (A.M.), TOUJAS (L.), QUASH (G.A.): Red blood cell polyamines in mice bearing the Lewis lung carcinoma (3LL) and in patients with bronchopulmonary cancers, Int. J. Cancer, **34**, 277-281 (1984).
11. MOULINOUX (J.-Ph.), DELAMAIRE (D.), BEAU (B.), QUEMENER (V.), BRISSOT (P.), LE CALVE (M.), DEUGNIER (Y.), CHAMBON (Y.), BOUREL (M.): Diagnosis value of erythrocyte polyamines and histaminemia in malignant hepatic tumors and in liver cirrhosis, Clin. Chim. Acta, **145**, 77-87 (1985).
12. QUEMENER (V.), LE GALL (E.), EDAN (C.), MOULINOUX (J.-Ph.): Red blood cell polyamine levels in children with acute leukemia: their clinical interest in desease staging and monitoring of therapy efficiency. Cancer J., **1** (4), 174-180 (1986).
13. MOULINOUX (J.-Ph.), QUEMENER (V.), CHATEL (M.), DARCEL (F.): Polyamines in human brain tumors: a correlative study between tumor, CSF and red blood cell free polyamines levels, J. Neuro-Oncology, **2**, 153-158 (1984).
14. MOULINOUX (J.-Ph.), QUEMENER (V.), HERCOUET (H.), DARCEL (F.), CHATEL (M.): Red blood cell polyamines in malignant glioma patients. Spermidine and spermine blood levels and tumour evolution, Biology of Brain Tumour, MD Walker and DGT Thomas (eds), Martinus Nijhoff Publishers, Boston, 67-74 (1986).
15. CHATEL (M.), DARCEL (F.), QUEMENER (V.), MOULINOUX (J.-Ph.): Red blood cell polyamines as biochemical markers of supratentorial malignant gliomas. J. Anticancer Res., in press (1986).
16. PECKER (J.), CHATEL (M.), MOULINOUX (J.-Ph.), DARCEL (F.): Intérêt du dosage des polyamines dans la surveillance évolutive des tumeurs neuro-épithéliales de l'encéphale, Bull. Acad. Nat. Méd., **168**, 626-634 (1984).
17. SCALABRINO (G.), MODENA (D.), FERIOLI (M.E.), PUERARI (M.): Degrees of malignancy in human primary CNS tumors: ODC levels as better indicators than adenosyl-methionine decarboxylase levels, JNCI, **68**, 751-754 (1982).

The Selective Release of Polypeptides from Human Glioma Cell Cultures and their Modification by Dexamethasone

D.E. BATEMAN (°), J.R. McDERMOTT (°°), D. HUGHES (°°), J.A. EDWARDSON (°°).

Human and animal glioma cell cultures release a number of products (1, 2) some of which have biological activity, eg endothelial proliferation factor (3). In the case of animal glioma cultures the release of these products is modified by steroids such as hydrocortisone (4).

The release of products by gliomas may be involved in the genesis of some of the pathophysiological effects of human gliomas. Endothelial proliferation is a prominent histological feature of some gliomas and this may be related to the production of endothelial proliferation factor by glioma cells. Autoradiographic studies have shown increased capillary permeability in normal blood vessels adjacent to animal gliomas, which may be caused by a soluble factor released from glioma cells (5).

Steroids have a major role in the medical management of patients with gliomas, rapidly improving the neurological deficit and relieving the symptoms of raised intracranial pressure, although the precise mechanism of their action is unknown. However, since steroids are capable of modifying the release of products from animal gliomas (4), the beneficial action of dexamethasone in the treatment of human gliomas may be partly due to effects on the release of biologically active products from gliomas.

We have, therefore, examined the release of polypeptides by human glioma cell cultures and the effect of dexamethasone on the amount and nature of released material.

MATERIALS AND METHODS

Glioma cell cultures

The procedure was essentially as described by Freshney (6). Glioma biopsy specimens collected in medium (DMEM) at the time of removal from the patient, were rinsed three times in medium and then chopped into one mm pieces using crossed scalpel blades. About a hundred pieces were transferred to a 25 cm^3 flask (Costar) containing 5 ml of medium and 200 units/ml of collagenase (Sigma) for 24-48 hours. The cells were then spun down, the medium removed and the pellet dispersed in medium using a Pasteur pipette. Quadruplicate or triplicate cultures were set up for each biopsy specimen if possible.

When two cultures from the same biopsy specimen were confluent the medium was changed to RPMI 1640 in the presence or absence of dexamethasone (from stock solution 5 mg/ml in ethanol) one culture receiving dexamethasone (10 μg/ml or 200 ng/ml) and the other an equivalent volume of ethanol. This medium was changed daily for three consecutive days. On the final day the medium was taken off, the culture washed three times in Hanks and replaced with 1 ml of RPMI 1640 ($\pm$ dexamethasone) containing 25 μCi of each of the following five amino acids: ^{3}H leucine, ^{3}H lysine, ^{3}H proline, ^{3}H arginine and ^{3}H valine (Amersham). After six hours incubation the medium of each culture was removed and centrifuged to remove any loose cells. 5 ml of 0.1 M-HC1 were added to the culture flask and the cells were scraped off using a plastic Costar cell scraper. The cells were then homogenised, and centrifuged to remove cell debris. The medium and cell extract were stored at -20°C until further use.

(°) Wessex Neurological Centre, Southampton General Hospital, (°°) MRC Neuroendocrinology Unit, Newcastle upon Tyne.

M. Chatel, F. Darcel and J. Pecker (eds.), Brain Oncology. ISBN-13: 978-94-010-8003-3

Removal of non-incorporated labelled amino acids

The free labelled amino acids were removed from the medium and extract by elution from ODS cartridges (Sep-Pak C18, Waters Associates), The cartridges were wetted with 2 ml 80 % methanol, followed by 5 ml 2 % acetonitrile containing 0.1 % trifluoroacetic acid (TFA). The medium and extract were put onto the Sep-Pak and washed extensively (5 ml × 10) with 2 % acetonitrile + 0.1 % TFA . The radio-labelled material was eluted from the Sep-Pak with 2 ml of 70 % acetonitrile + 0.1 % TFA. A sample (10 μl) was added to liquid scintillant (fisofluor 1) and radioactivity determined in a counter. The rest was divided into 0.5 ml aliquots and dried in a Vortex evaporator.

Gel electrophoresis

Sodium dodecyl sulphate (SDS) polyacrylamide gel electrophoresis was carried out in a Protean cell (Bio-Rad) using the Laemmli buffer system as described below.

10 % acrylamide separating gels were prepared in 40 ml lots by the addition of 13.33 ml acrylamide stock (29.2 g acrylamide plus 0.8 g N.N'-methylenebisacrylamide in 100 ml) to 10 ml of Tris-HCl buffer, pH 8.8 containing 0.4 % SDS (Laemmli 1970) and 16.67 ml distilled water. The solution was then filtered through grade 542 filter paper (Whatman) and 133 μl of ammonium persulphate and 40 μl of N, N, N'.N'-tetramethylethylenediamine (TEMED) were added to the solution which was then poured between the glass plate sandwich, overlayered with distilled water and left to polymerise overnight. The following morning the water overlayer was removed and replaced with the 4.5 % acrylamide stacking gel (consisting of 1.5 ml 30 % acrylamide stock, 2.5 ml Tris-HCl buffer, pH 6.8 containing 0.4 % SDS/ 6 ml water, 30 μl ammonium persulphate and 10 μl TEMED).

The Vortex-dried samples were treated by adding 100 ml of the sample buffer described by Laemmli (1970), which contained 2/3 % SDS and 5 % 2-mercaptoethanol. The samples, along with a 1:1 dilution of 0.5 % aqueous bromophenol blue/sample buffer mixture, were then vortexed and heated at 100 °C for 15 min in polypropylene tubes. The samples were then loaded on top of the stacking gel, overlayered with running buffer (0.025 M Tris/0.192 M glycine/0/1 % SDS) and electrophoresed at a current of 20 mA/gel until the bromophenol blue marker dye had reached the top of the separating gel (approximately lhr) and then electrophoresed at a current of 40 mA/gel until the bromophenol blue dye reached the bottom of the gel (approximately 2 further hours).

After electrophoresis the gels, which were 1.5 mm thick, were fixed in a solution of 50 % ethanol/10 % glacial acetic acid for not less than 1 hr. The gels were then rehydrated in distilled water overnight and silver-stained using the ammoniacal-silver method of Oakley et al (1980) with the additional use of the dithiothreitol sensitisation step of Morrissey (1981).

Following staining of the gels each lane was cut into 2 mm alices and the individual alices dissolved by boiling in 200 μl hydrogen peroxide (100 vol) for 5-6 hours. Scintillant (Fiso Fluor 1) was then added and the radioactivity determined in a counter.

Characterisation of cultures by immunofluorescence

After passage, cells from each culture were plated out in tissue culture chamber alides (Lab-Tek) and grown in normal medium for three days. The cultures were then fixed in formol calcium for 20 mins. After three washes in PBS/0.2 % Triton one of the following antisera were placed in one of the chamber cells: GFAP (Dako) 1:100, fibronectin (Sera Laboratories) neat; factor VIII (Dako) 1:50 for 30 mins. Following three further washes the appropriate FITC antibody (Miles) 1:20 was added for 30 mins. The slides were washed twice in PBS/0.2 % Triton, given a final wash in PBS and mounted in PBS/glycerol and the coverslip sealed with nail varnish. The slides were then viewed under the fluorescence microscope and the proportion of positive cells counted.

RESULTS

The immunofluorescence study showed that three cell cultures were positive for GFAP, the remainder being negative. None of the cultures were positive for fibronectin or factor VIII (Table I).

Comparison of the gel electrophoresis profile of radiolabelled material in the extract and the medium showed considerable differences (Fig. 1) with selective release of some proteins. The results show that there was wide variation in the percentage of released material between the different cultures (Table 2). The three separate results for the culture GCCM were very similar (3 - 5 % released).

The effect of dexamethasone was inconsistent. At the low dose of dexamethasone (200 ng/ml) there was no effect of dexamethasone on the percentage of released material for the culture GCCM, but there was considerable suppression for the culture Rudd. At the higher dose (10 μg/ml) in the cultures GCCM and Hall, the percentage of released material was increased by dexamethasone, and in the other case (Little) suppression of the release of radiolabelled material was seen.

No differences in the profile of released material was seen with the cultures, Rudd and Little (Fig. 2; Fig. 3) in the presence of dexamethasone but with Hall (Fig. 4) there was a considerable increase in the 52K polypeptide (gel slice 28) and reduction in the 66K polypeptide (gel slice 19) in the presence of dexamethasone.

DISCUSSION

Comparison of the gel profiles of released material from the medium and extract of the same culture shows that the material in the medium is selectively released from the cells (Fig. 1). The proportions of the individual peaks in the medium and extract are considerably different indicating that cell lysis cannot explain the appearance of radiolabelled material in the medium.

Five separate experiments were done using the culture GCCM. The results of these experiments are all in close agreement with the percentage of release material varying between 3-7 % irrespective

TABLE I

Immunofluorescent Markers in Human Glioma Cultures

Culture	GFAP	Fibronectin	Factor VIII
Rudd	++ 50 %	—	—
Hall	—	—	—
Little	—	—	—
GCCM	—	—	—
Parker	+ 10 %	—	—
Jones	+ 10 %	—	—
Walker	—	—	—
Dickinson	—	—	—

The figures show the percentage of positive cells.

TABLE II

Radioactivity (dpm) incorporated into polypeptides from human glioma cells in culture: Effect of Dexamethasone

		CONTROL				DEXAMETHASONE		
Culture	Passage No	Dose of Dex/ml	Medium (dpm)	Extract (dpm)	% Release	Medium (dpm)	Extract (dpm)	% Release
Walker	1	—	222020	1540340	14			
Dickson	1	—	252175	2001179	13			
Jones	1	—	220860	897840	24			
Parker	1	—	192110	943850	20			
Parker	2	—	159360	934230	17			
GCCM*	18	—	134950	2891370	5			
GCCM	18	200 ng	285080	9864005	3	172540	6776035	3
GCCM	18	10 μg	139560	3805470	4	181740	2711640	7
Rudd	1	200 ng	352290	1399182	25	429703	2925455	15
Hall	1	10 μg	249727	2096273	12	246251	1294932	19
Little	1	10 μg	236188	1594489	15	170436	1665291	10

Mean % release (excluding GCCM) = 14 % ± 7.

(*) The glioma cell line GCCM a kind gift of Dr R I Freshney.

Cultures were incubated with ^{3}H amino acids in the presence or absence of dexamethasone. Labelled polypeptides in the medium and cell extracts were isolated using C18- Sep Paks.

FIGURE 1

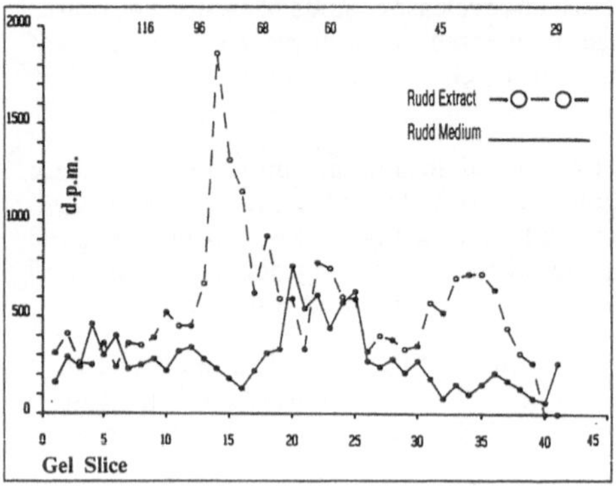

FIGURE 2

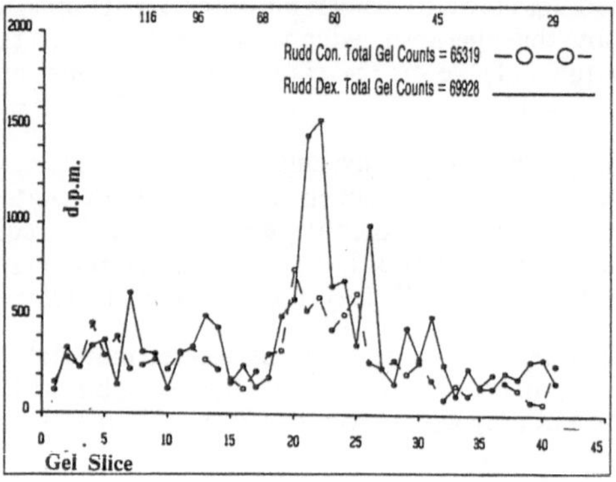

FIGURE 3

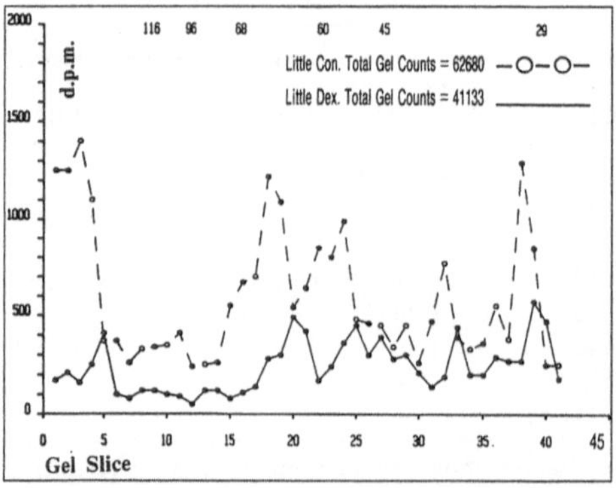

FIGURE 4

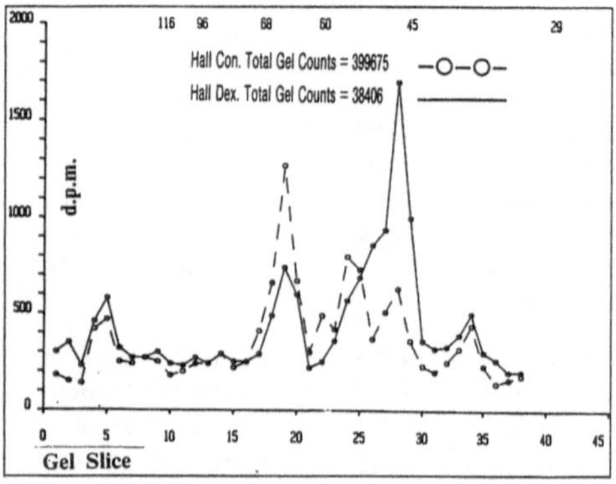

FIGURE 1-4. Show the gel profiles of released polypeptides with standard molecular weight markers (116 ....96).

of treatment with dexamethasone. The consistency of these results using the same culture demonstrates the reliability and reproducibility of the technique.

All the cultures studied showed release of rapidly synthesised proteins. The percentage of released material was variable from 3-25 %. If the glioma cell line GCCM which showed a very low percentage release is excluded, the mean percentage of released material is 17 % ± 5.1. Previous reports of the release of radiolabelled material from animal glioma cultures demonstrated that as much as 40 % of the material may be released (8) so the figures obtained in these experiments are of the same order of magnitude.

The higher dose of dexamethasone (10 μg/ml) was chosen to correspond to the probable maximum tissue concentration using an effective clinical dose (16 mg daily) (R I Freshney, personal communication), though considerably higher doses of dexamethasone (64 mg daily) are used in some situations to treat gliomas. Some of the experiments were also done at 200 ng/ml to avoid the criticism that only the effect of a maximum dose of dexamethasone was being evaluated.

Although the effect of dexamethasone was inconsistent , the experiments clearly show that it is capable both of modifying the total amount and the profile of released polypeptide material. If the glioma cell line GCCM is excluded from consideration on the basis that it is atypical in terms of passage number and small percentage of released material, dexamethasone considerably suppressed the amount of released material in the two cultures Rudd and Little. Although there was overall increase in the amount of released material in the culture Hall in response to dexamethasone, release of the 66K polypeptide was suppressed.

These experiments have demonstrated that generally there is considerable release of rapidly synthetized polypeptides by gliomas. Until the precise effects of these polypeptides are known, it is not possible to directly implicate them in the pathophysiological effects of gliomas. However, some known glial products are trophic (9) (eg nerve growth factor) and gliomas have been shown to produce endothelial proliferation factor (3), which is likely to be pathophysiologically important since endothelial proliferation can be a prominent feature of some gliomas. It would not be surprising, therefore, if some of these polypeptides were capable of reversibly depressing surrounding neuronal function and altering the permeability of endothelial cells thereby causing some of the pathophysiological effects of gliomas.

The experiments also show that, in some cases, dexamethasone, at a clinically effective dose, is capable of altering both the amount and the proportions of the released polypeptides; this may be relevant to its mechanism of action in improving the neurological deficit and ameliorating the oedema associated with gliomas. Further experiments are required to assess this possibility.

The profiles of released material were very similar in all the cultures studied. If these products were released into the circulation, it might be possible to use them as tumour markers by raising monoclonal antibodies. However, it would be necessary to demonstrate that these proteins differed from those released by normal glia or were produced in considerably greater amounts by gliomas.

SUMMARY

Human glioma cell cultures are known to release a selective pattern of proteins. However, release of smaller molecular weight substances by gliomas are possibly more likely to be involved in their pathophysiological effects by a local neuromodulatory or circulatory action. We have therefore studied the release of polypeptides/peptides by human glioma cell cultures and the effect of dexamethasone on the amount and profile of released material.

Duplicate human glioma cell cultures were derived from glioma biopsy specimens and grown in serum free medium after confluence ± dexamethasone. Tritiated amino acids were added to the incubation medium for 6 hours and the proportion of released material determined by comparison of the amount of radiolabelled polypeptides in the medium and cellular extract. The profile of released material was determined by gel electrophoresis.

The mean percentage of released material was 17 % ± 5.1. The profile of released material was similar for all three glioma cell cultures studied. The effect of dexamethasone on the amount and pattern of released material was variable, though possibly more experiments may demonstrate a more consistent effect.

The results confirm that glioma cell cultures release considerable amounts of polypeptides/peptides. The profile of released material was similar to all three cultures, suggesting that if they enter the circulation they could be used as tumour markers enabling better diagnosis and assessment of treatment.

Dexamethasone is capable of modifying the amount and pattern of released material and this may be related in part to its beneficial action in the treatment of patients with gliomas. Further experiments are required to determine whether the released material has local neuromodulatory or circulatory effects.

KEY WORDS

Polypeptides, Glioma Culture, Dexamethasone.

REFERENCES

1. McKEEVER (P.E.), QUINDLEN (E.), BANKS (M.A.), WILLIAMS (V.), KORNBLITH (P.L.), LAVERSON (S.), GREENWOOD (M.A.), SMITH (B.): Biosynthesised products of cultured neuroglial cells; 1 Selective release of proteins by cells from human astrocytomas. Neurology 1981, 31, 1445-1452.
2. ARENANDER (A.T.), VELLIS (J. de): Glial released proteins: 111 Influence on neuronal morphological differentiation. Brain Res 1981, 224, 117-127.

3. SUDDITH (R.L.), KELLY (P.J.), HUTCHISON (H.T.), MURRAY (E.A.), HABER (B.): In vitro demonstration of an endothelial proliferative factor produced by neural cell lines. Science 1975, 190, 682-684.

4. ARENANDER (A.T.), VELLIS (J. de): Glial released proteins in clonal cultures and their modulation by hydrocortisone. Brain Res 1980, 200, 401-409.

5. MOLNAR (P.), BLASBERG (R.G.), HOROWITZ (M.), SMITH (B.), FENSTERMACHER (J.): Regional blood to tissue transport in RT - 9 brain tumours. J. Neurosurg. 1983a, 58, 874-884.

6. FRESHNEY (R.I.): Tissue culture of glioma of the brain in Brain Tumors eds D.G.T. Thomas and D.I. Graham Butterworths 1980, 42-47.

7. LAEMMLI (U.K.): Cleavage of structural proteins during the assembly of the head of bacteriophage T4, Nature, 1970, 227, 680-685.

8. SHITARA (N.), McKEEVER (P.E.), SMITH (B.H.), PLEASANTS (R.E.), BANKS (M.A.), KORNBLITH (P.L.): Products of neuroglial cells III, J. Neurochem. 1982, 39, 948-953.

9. NORRGREN (G.), EBENDAL (T.), BELEW (M.), JACOBSON (C.O.), PORTH (J.): Release of nerve growth factor by human glial cells in culture. Exp. cell Res. 1980, 130, 31-39.

Preliminary Assessment of the Correlation between Clinicopathological Features of Intracranial Tumours and the Amount of Extractable Angiogenic Activity: High and Low M_r factors

J. VAFIDIS, J.E. MEATS, H. REID, R.H. LYE, J.B. WEISS (°).

INTRODUCTION

An adequate blood supply is essential to the continued growth of an intracranial neoplasm (1). Tumour factors capable of inducing host endothelial cells to proliferate, form capillaries and so migrate towards a neoplasm have been described (2,3). These factors are broadly grouped into high (approx. 20,000) and low (300-600) molecular mass (M_r) categories (2, 4, 5, 6, 7). Angiogenic activity has been demonstrated in cell cultures of meningiomas (7).

In this investigation we obtained tumour extracts of high and low M_r from four patients with meningiomas. Both types of extract stimulated endothelial cell proliferation — a prerequisite for angiogenic activity (8). For each tumour, an attempt was made to compare the degree of contrast enhancement on CT scans, the 'vascular blush' on angiography and a histopathological 'vascularity index' with angiogenic activity expressed as a measure of induction of endothelial cell proliferation.

MATERIALS AND METHODS

Tumour samples from four patients with histologically proven meningiomas were examined. Before operation each patient underwent CT scanning. In those cases where the software was available, the increase in Hounsfield number of a designated tumour area following intravenous contrast enhancement was noted and the expression:

$$\frac{\text{Post contrast Hounsfield No.}}{\text{Pre contrast Hounsfield No.}}$$

was used to quantify this change. Earlier cases were graded as + moderate enhancement and ++ marked enhancement.

A digital intravenous angiogram (DIVA) was obtained on each patient pre-operatively and the degree of 'tumour blush' was defined on an ordinal scale which showed little inter-observer variability (Table I).

At operation the surgeon was asked to comment independently on the vascularity or otherwise of the tumour, rating this as 'avascular, moderately vascular or very vascular', according to whether there was no haemorrhage, obvious tumour vessels present but easily controlled haemorrhage during removal, or heavy bleeding from the tumour and its capsular vessels respectively.

TABLE I

Tumour 'Vascularity' on DIVA examination

Grade	Tumour Blush
0	None
I	Faint blush - no abnormal vessels seen.
II	Moderate, well defined blush
III	Marked blush with prominent abnormal tumour vessels visible

(°) Departments of Neurosurgery, Neuropathology and Medical Biochemistry, University of Manchester, U. K.

M. Chatel, F. Darcel and J. Pecker (eds.), Brain Oncology. ISBN-13: 978-94-010-8003-3

An experienced neuropathologist examined haematoxylin and eosin preparations of tumour samples to assess vascularity according to a standard 'vascularity index' (MAGS (9)).

Independently, tumour samples from the same specimens were cooled to -20 °C immediately after excision and then processed according to the flow diagram in figure 1.

a) Preparation of extractable angiogenic activity

Under constant temperature conditions (4 °C) tumour was homogenised in MEM culture medium (Gibco, Scotland), centrifuged and passed through a YM5 membrane. The filtrate in some instances was applied to a Biogel P_2 column (1.6 × 80 cm) in 10 % propan — 2 ol v/v (M_r 200-1000) and the fractions obtained, tested on the CAM assay (10). Both filtrate and retentate were tested for angiogenic activity by thymidine uptake in capillary endothelial cells and the retentate was also tested on the CAM.

b) Endothelial Cell Proliferative Assay

Collagen gels were prepared one week prior to use in the assay. Type I collagen were obtained from rat tail tendon (final collagen solution concentration = 1.3 mg/ml). Aliquots of 50 µl of collagen solution were placed in separate perspex wells and incubated at 37 °C for 20 minutes. The plates were then washed in autoclaved distilled water and dried overnight in a flow hood.

On day 1 of the endothelial cell proliferation assay the collagen gels on microwell plates were reconstituted with 200 µl of minimal essential medium (MEM) for 2-3 hours. Surplus MEM was then removed and replaced with 100 µl of fresh MEM containing 15 % foetal calf serum (FCS) HI. Approximately 5000 adrenal capillary endothelial cells, prepared by the method of Folkman, were seeded into each microwell in 100 µl of MEM + 15 % FCS (HI) and incubated at 37 °C overnight.

On day 2 excess media was removed from the microwells and samples of crude tumour extract (high and low M_r range) in 100 µl of MEM in 2 % FCS (HI) were added to each well.

c) Endothelial Cell Proliferative Assay

On day 4, 0.4 µCi of ^{3}H thymidine were added to each well, thus labelling the cells. Incubation at 37 °C continued until days when the cells were washed three times with phosphate buffer saline. 70 µl of 0.01 % bacterial collagenase were added to each cell and incubated at 37 °C for 20 minutes. Using a cell harvester the cells were collected and radioactivity was measured by liquid scintillation. An example is shown in Table II.

RESULTS

Low M_r fractions gave positive results on the CAM test and on the capillary endothelial cell thymidine incorporation assay (Table I). The high M_r fractions was only positive in the latter assay (Table III). The clinico-pathological features and results of proliferation assay for low M_r fractions are shown in Table IV.

TABLE II

Results of CAM/VIM test on soluble and insoluble fractions of tumour homogenate

Tumour	Residuum	Dialysate
Meningioma - A (5)	—	+
Meningioma - B	—	*
Meningioma - C	—	+
Meningioma - D	—	*

— = no neovascularisation detected
+ = neovascularisation observed
* = probable neovascularisation but obscured by inflammation (possibly caused by strong activity)

N.B.: All samples were applied to the CAM/VIM in 10 mg of lactose containing elvax.

( ) Tumour sample pooled from specimens obtained from several patients. Number of patients in parenthesis.

TABLE III

Patient	MAGS*	Thymidine uptake corrected for controls at 1:100 dilution		
		ME	MEF	MER
1 [68 F]	31	6 166	7 659	1 658
4 [50 M]	50	—	10 112	9 292
9 [34 F]	34	8 207	8 945	4 158
7 [65 F]	37	2 234	2 833	873

MAGS: Microscopic Angiogenesis Grading system
ME: Medium extract whole
MEF: Medium extract filtrate 5,000 M_r
MER: Medium extract retentate 5,000 M_r

TABLE IV

Pt.	Surgeon's assessment	CT	DIVA	MAGS	Low M_r H^3 uptake
1.	v. vascular	+	III	31	7 659
2.	v. vascular	99/48	III	76	
3.	vascular	++	III	34	
4.	vascular	++	II	50	10 112
5.	mod. vascular	++	0	37	
6.	mod. vascular	++	0	36	
7.	not vascular	83/46	I	34	8 945
8.	not vascular	++	III	42	
9.	not vascular	88/47	II	37	2 833
10.	not vascular	+	0	30	

DISCUSSION

This is a preliminary review of data from our study of intracranial tumours and low M_r angiogenic factor. The small numbers limit the conclusions that may be drawn. Nonetheless, our results confirm that there is a low M_r factor extractable from intracranial meningiomas with a potent angiogenic effect, as tested on the CAM model. Gel filtration chromatography further suggest its size to be in the region of 300-600 molecular mass (10). Using thymidine incorporation, fractions with a higher M_r were shown to have an endothelial stimulating effect. The low M_r angiogenic activity described in this paper is probably identical to ESAF (endothelial cell stimulating angiogenic factor) which has a low molecular mass and is able to stimulate capillary endothelial cell proliferation but not aortic endothelial cell proliferation. The high M_r factor may contain carrier bound ESAF but it is probable that some fibroblast growth factor (endothelial cell growth factor) is also present.

Having demonstrated angiogenic activity, the next question is: what does it mean? The clinical and pathological criteria were those available in clinical practice. Of course, their limitations in terms of an objective assessment of tumour vascularity are widely recognised. CT enhancement is not necessarily a reflection of blood flow but may represent altered blood brain barrier — itself a feature of tumour vasculature (11, 12, 13). In addition, the area on CT chosen to quantify enhancement probably does not correspond to the tumour sample used to quantify angiogenic activity. Likewise, angiography does not necessarily equate 'tumour blush' with 'tumour blood flow'. The grading of the angiographic features was subjective but proved consistent when tested with different observers. While the surgeon's assessment of vascularity is notoriously variable, given the difficulties of tumour access, isolation of blood supply and anaesthetic conditions, nonetheless some tumours appear vascular as seen by the high number of capsular vessels when compared with the paucity in 'avascular' tumours in which haemostasis within the tumour is easily achieved.

These features and the histological grading represent the readily available means of albeit empirically and possibly inaccurately assessing tumour vascularity. In our small series, no immediate correlation between the clinicopathological findings was discernible. However, there is a suggestion that age may reduce the amount of factor extracted or produced.

We have not been able to follow up the patients in this study long enough to investigate any correlation between extractable angiogenic activity and prognosis regarding recurrence or speed of regrowth. A larger prospective study of a greater number of cases over a longer time span is under way. In this new study, purified extract will be used.

SUMMARY

Extracts from samples of intracranial meningiomas were tested for angiogen activity. Diafiltration and gel-filtration chromatography were used to separate the extrats into fractions of low and high molecular mass (M_r) and the angiogenic activity of these fractions was assessed by their ability to stimulate capillary endothelial cells to incorporate ^3H thymidine. Angiogenic activity was demonstrated *in all fractions. The high M_r fraction which may contain fibroblast growth factor, did not give a true response on the CAM. Comparison of angiogenic activity was made with the clinicopathological features of each tumour.*

AKNOWLEDGEMENTS

This study was supported by a grant from the North Western Regional Health Authority, UK. Project No. 548.

The authors thank Miss Pam Brown for secretarial assistance in the preparation of this manuscript.

KEY WORDS

Angiogenesis, Angiography, Brain tumour, Computed tomography, Endothelial cell, Meningiomas, Neoplasm.

REFERENCES

1. FOLKMAN (J.), TAYLOR (S.), SPILLBERG (C.): The role of heparin in angiogenesis. *in* Ciba foundation Symposium 100: Development of the vascular system (Pitman 1983), pp. 132-149.
2. FOLKMAN (J.), MERLER (E.), ABERNATHY (C.), WILLIAMS (G.): Isolation of a tumour factor responsible for angiogenesis. J. Exp. Med. 275-278, 1971.
3. AUERBACH (R.): Angiogenesis-inducing factors: a review. Lymphokines 4: 69-88, 1981.
4. SHING (Y.), FOLKMAN (J.), SULLIVAN (R.), BUTTERFIELD (C.), MURRAY (J.), KLAGSBURN (M.): Heparin affinity: purification of a tumor-derived capillary endothelial cell growth factor. Science 223: 1295-1298, 1984.
5. WEISS (J.B.), BROWN (R.A.), KUMAR (S.), PHILLIPS (P.): Angiogenic factor isolated from tumours: a potential low molecular-weight compound. Brit. J. Cancer 40; 493-496, 1979.
6. MCAUSLAN (B.R.), HOFFMAN (H.): Endothelium stimulating factor from Walker carcinoma cells. Relation to tumor angiogenic factor. Expl. Cell Res. 119: 181-190, 1979.
7. FENSELAU (A.), WATT (S.), MELLO (R.J.): Tumour angiogenic factor. Purification from the Walker 256 rat tumour. J. Biol. Chem. 256: 9605-9611, 1981.
8. WARREN (B.A.): Tumor angiogenesis. *in* Peterson H-I (ed.). Tumor Blood Circulation: angiogenesis, vascular morphology and blood flow of experimental and human tumors (CRC Press Inc. 1979), pp. 49-75.
9. BREM (S.), COTRAN (R.), FOLKMAN (J.): Tumor Angiogenesis. A Quantitative Method for Histologic Grading. J. National Cancer Institute 48: 347-354, 1972.
10. LYE (R.H.), ELSTOW (S.F.), WEISS (J.B.): Neovascularisation of intracranial tumours. *in*Walker M.D., Thomas D.G.T. (eds). Biology of Brain Tumour (Martinus Nijhoff Publishers) 1986, pp. 61-66 (in press).
11. GADO (M.H.), PHELPS (M.E.), COLEMAN (R.F.): An extravascular component of contrast enhancement in cranial computed tomography. Part II: Contrast enhancement and the blood-tissue barrier. Radiology 117: 595-597, 1975.
12. DUBOIS (P.J.), DRAYER (B.P.), HEINZ (E.R.), OSBORNE (D.), ROBERTS (L.), SAGE (M.): Rapid serial cranial computed tomography for tumor diagnosis. Neuroradiology 21: 79-86, 1981.
13. VASSILOUTHIS (J.), AMBROSE (J.): Computerized tomography scanning appearances of intracranial meningiomas. J. Neurosurg. 50: 320-327, 1979.

Estrogen and Progesterone Receptors in Central Nervous System Tumors

Roberto BUONAGUIDI, Roberto GIORDANI (°),
Fernando FAGGIONATO, Maria CRISTINA CAGNO, Maria Rita METELLI (°),
Marco FERDEGHINI (°°).

INTRODUCTION

The interest in the study of the influence and the effects of steroid hormones on Central Nervous System (CNS) is increased in recent years, especially to evaluate and explore the possibility of therapeutic hormonal treatment in different neurological diseases (1).

Recently few studies have reported the presence of steroid receptors in meningiomas, other reports have suggested the stimulation of the inhibition of meningioma growth, in vitro, by the steroid hormones or by their pharmacological antagonists (2, 3, 4, 5, 6, 7, 8, 9, 10, 11, 12).

The researchs on hormonal modulation of these CNS solid tumors are based on epidemiological and clinical data : 1) the higher incidence of meningioma in female patients, 2) the rapid progression of clinical symptoms during pregnancy, or luteal phase of the menstrual cycle, 3) the statistically significant association between meningioma and breast carcinoma, 4) the association of meningioma with obesity (13, 14).

From January 1983 to June 1986, 464 patients were treated for CNS tumors at the Institute of Neurosurgery, University of Pisa. 250 patients were males (54 %) and 214 females (46 %). The review of our series (fig. 1) reveals that the meningiomas represent 25 % of all surgically treated CNS tumors. The sex distribution in the different types of tumors is summarized in fig. 2. Of the 82 patients with glioma, 48 (59 %) were males and 34 (41 %) females ; of the 56 patients with glioblastoma, 33 (59 %) were males and 23 (41 %) females; of the 87 patients treated for metastases in CNS, 69 (79 %) were males and 18 (21 %) females.

The male/female ratio in meningioma and in schwannomas is different. Of 115 surgically treated patients with meningioma, 78 (68 %) were females and 37 (32 %) males (ratio 2:1). If we consider the 8 spinal meningiomas, 6 were females and only 2 males (ratio 3:1). Of 37 schwannomas, 23 (62 %) were females and 14 (38 %) males. To explore the sex steroid hormones may play in CNS tumors, we looked for estrogen and progesterone receptors in these tumors.

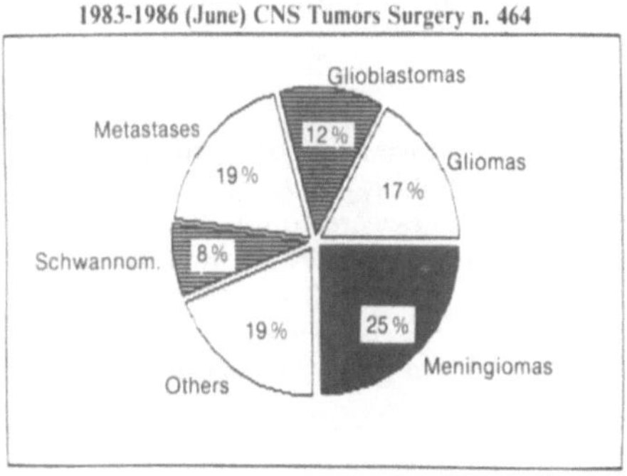

FIGURE 1. The incidence of different CNS tumors in 464 consecutive patients.

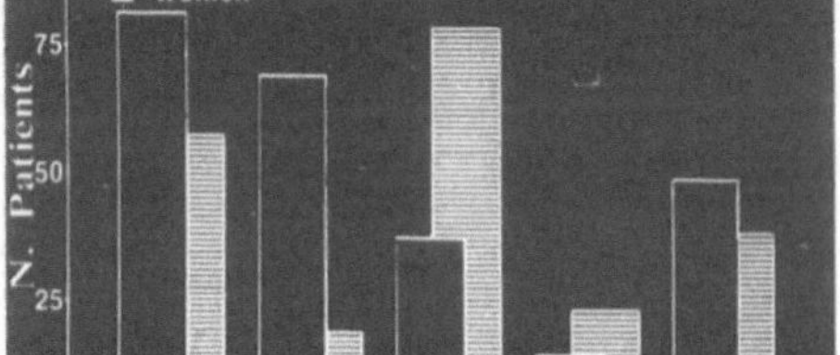

FIGURE 2. Men/women ratio in CNS tumors.

(°) *Institute of Neurosurgery,* (°) *2nd Medical Clinic,* (°°) *Nuclear Medicine, University of Pisa, Pisa, Italy.*

M. Chatel, F. Darcel and J. Pecker (eds.), Brain Oncology. ISBN-13: 978-94-010-8003-3

MATERIALS AND METHODS

Clinical and biopsy data

Estrogen (ER) and progesterone (PgR) cytoplasmic receptors have been examined in 75 CNS tumors (49 meningiomas, 11 schwannomas, 3 astrocytomas, 4 ependymomas, 2 glioblastomas, 2 metastases, 3 pituitary adenomas, 1 cerebellar hemangioblastoma). All the patients received before surgery glucocorticoids. The more consistent group of CNS tumors in our series was that of meningiomas. Tissue samples, randomly selected, were obtained, during the surgery, from 49 patients, 31 females and 18 males. A part of each sample was reserved for histologic examination and the rest was immediately frozen at - 80 °C.

Meningiomas

The mean age of the 115 patients with meningioma was 52 years (range 14 to 72 years). The age distribution of meningioma cases does not demonstrate sex difference (fig. 3). The age of incidence ranged between 30 and 70 years; the peak incidence is around the age of 55.

Of some interest, in our female patients, is the association of meningioma with other previous pathologic conditions, particularly other "endocrine" tumors. 4 patients had been surgically treated for breast carcinoma, 3 for breast cystic hyperplasia, 3 for thyroid cancer, 6 for adenomatous goiter and 2 for GH secreting pituitary adenomas (table 1).

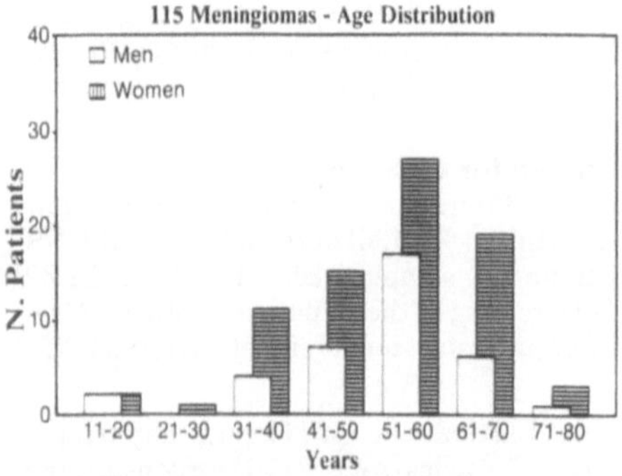

FIGURE 3. Age distribution of meningioma cases.

TABLE 1

Association between meningiomas (78 female patients) and other pathology

	No. Cases	
Breast cancer	4	
Breast cystic hyperplasia	3	
Thyroid cancer	3	
Adenomatous goiter	6	
Pituitary adenomas (Acromegaly)	2	
	18	(23 %)

For histological study all samples were fixed with formalin, embeddded in paraffin and stained with hematoxylin and eosin. The meningiomas were classified as syncitial, fibroblastic, transitional, angioblastic, psammomatous, xanthomatous and atypic (numerous mitotic figures, nuclear pleomorphism and necrosis).

Cytosolic fraction preparation

The frozen tumor samples (1 gm of weight, each) were thawed on ice and homogenized with a Polyton (manufactured by Kinematica instruments) in 10 ml tris buffer, pH 7.4 (EDTA, sodium azide, α-monothioglycerol, sucrose and glycerol). Normally, the tissues were homogenized once, at high speed for 15 sec. If some fragment was seen again, the pulverized tissues were homogenized a second time, allowing a 30 seconds cooling time between each period of homogenization. The homogenates were centrifuged at 100.000 G for 60 minutes, at 2 °C. The supernatant fractions (cytosol) were utilized in the next phases. The protein content of all samples were measured both by the techniques of Waddel and of Lowry.

Estrogen receptor assay

Two doses of cytosol (4 - 5 mg/ml of protein) were incubated for 20 minutes; the first with a 40 μM diethylstilbestrol (DES) and the second with tris buffer.

The unlabeled DES was used to saturate the specific bindings so as to measure the non specific bindings. Then fractions of 200 μl of the two solutions were incubated, for 16 hours at 4 °C, with 50 μl of 2, 4, 6, 7 -^{3}H-oestradiol (7 serial concentrations ranging from 0.7 to 28 nM). At the end of the incubation period, at 4 °C, in all the cytosol preparations 250 μl of dextran-coated charcoal suspension (ratios 10:1) were added to remove free streroid. After 15 minutes the samples were centrifuged at 3000 G for 20 minutes at 4 °C. 200μl of resulting supernatant were used to measure the tritium labeled ligands by a liquid scintillation counter.

Progesterone receptor assay

The progesterone receptor assays were performed according to the guidlines for estrogen receptor assays. Aliquots of cytosol were incubated for 16 hours, at 4 °C, whether with 50 μl of ^{3}H-ORG 2058 (6 serial concentrations ranging from 0.50 to 23 nM) or with 50 μl of 30 μM ORG 2058 to saturate the specific bindings.

Binding determination

Specific binding was determined by substracting non specific binding from total binding. Scatchard plots were constructed from the binding data to determine the dissociation constants (Kd). The cytoplasmic estrogen and progesterone receptors were expressed as fmol/mg of cytosol protein and as fmol/gm of tumor tissue to consider the high vascular component of the CNS tumors. especially of the meningiomas. Samples were considered to be receptor positive if a statistically significant correlation was observed in the Scatchard plot, if the Kd was less than 30 x 10^{-10} mol/l and if the protein content of the cytosol exceeded 2 mg/ml. Threshold values were fixed to 10 fmol/mg of the cytosol protein and to 150 fmol/mg of the tumor tissue for cytoplasmic ER and PgR. Naturally these threshold values, in CNS tumors, are arbitrary levels because we cannot yet correlate the level of hormone receptors with a response to hormonal treatment as it is possible in breast carcinoma (9).

RESULTS

The results are summarized in table II. Of 75 CNS tumors PgR were present in 34 cases (45 %) and ER in 3 cases (4 %). Cytoplasmic PgR, measured in 49 meningiomas, were found in 31 (63 %); in particular in 20 of 31 women (64 %) and in 11 of 18 men (61 %). The level of PgR ranged from 155 to 7850 fmol/gm tumor tissue (fig. 4) of from 11 to 146 fmol/mg cytosol protein (fig. 5).

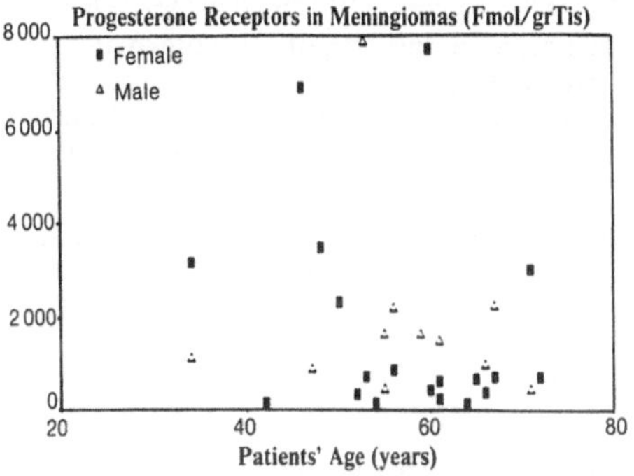

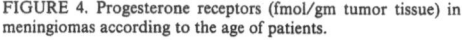

FIGURE 4. Progesterone receptors (fmol/gm tumor tissue) in meningiomas according to the age of patients.

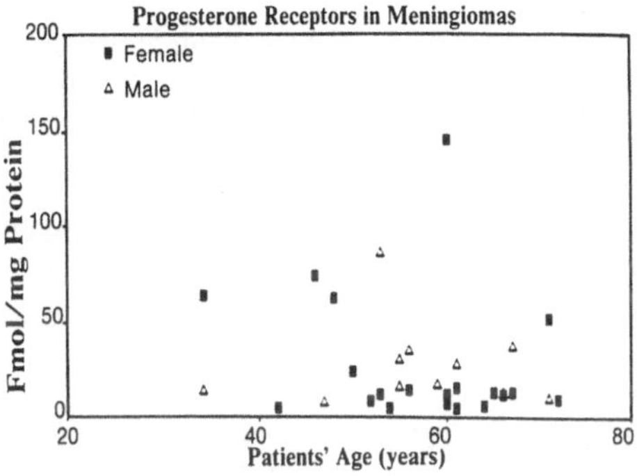

FIGURE 5. Progesterone receptors (fmol/mg cytosol protein) in meningiomas according to the age of patients.

No correlation was found between PgR and the age of the patients (fig. 4, 5), nor was any correlation found between PgR and the histological type (table III). The PgR was not related to the localization of meningiomas. Only two female patients presented ER in the tissue samples (transitional meningiomas); but low bindings of oestradiol were observed: 167 and 437 fmol/gmT respectively. In the other samples of CNS tumors studied only one acoustic schwannoma, one spinal cord mixopapillary ependymoma and the cerebellar hemangioblastoma presented PgR, at level of 259, 2334, 205 fmol/gmT respectively. Only the cerebellar hemangioblastoma had a low level of ER (160 fmol/gmT).

TABLE II

Steroid receptors in central nervous system tumors

Tumors	No. of cases	PgR +	ER +
Meningiomas	49	31	2
Schwannomas	11	1	—
Astrocytomas	3	—	—
Glioblastoma M.	2	—	—
Ependymomas	4	1	—
Pituitary aden.	3	—	—
Metastases	2	—	—
Cerebellar hemangioblastoma	1	1	1
	75	34	3

TABLE III

Histological Type	No. of cases	PgR +	ER +
Syncytial	20	13	—
Transitional	11	6	2
Fibroblastic	5	3	—
Psammomatous	6	4	—
Atypic	4	3	—
Angioblastic	2	1	—
Xanthomatous	1	1	—
	49	31	2

DISCUSSION

A series of 464 patients with CNS tumors were treated during 3 1/2 year period. 75 patients, randomly selected, were studied to evaluate cytoplasmic estrogen and progesterone receptors. We were unable to demonstrate the presence of steroid receptors in astrocytomas, glioblastomas, pituitary adenomas, metastases. Only one of eleven schwannomas presented low PgR level. Only one of four ependymomas presented PgR. The presence of low levels of both steroid receptors was found in the only cerebellar hemangioblastoma examined. If we exclude the case of the female patient with spinal cord mixopapillary ependymoma (PgR: 2234 fmol/gmT or 18.4 fmol/mg cytosol protein), a tumor that can have some hormonal influence, the other CNS tumors, meningiomas excepted, showed only minuscule amounts of steroid receptors.

In contrast to these tumors, our study confirm previous reports that a large portion of human meningiomas is rich in cytoplasm PgR and has low or not detectable levels of ER (2, 3, 14). This fact is not in agreement with the common opinion that the synthesis of PgR is modulated by estrogen through ER. It has been observed that meningioma tissue may resemble T47D human breast cancer cells which lacks free estrogen receptors and in which the synthesis of PgR is not modulated by estrogens (2, 15).

If we consider, in our series of meningiomas, the prevalence, in middle age, of the women and the significant association with other "endocrine" tumors, we can suggest an hormonal control on the growth of meningiomas. However we have not observed relations between the presence or the level of PgR and the age and sex of patients, or between PgR and histological type, or the location of these tumors.

In conclusion we believe that the presence of PgR suggests that meningiomas can be a target tissue for progesterone even if we do not know what role steroid hormones play in the growth of these solid CNS tumors.

SUMMARY

Estrogen and progesterone cytoplasmic receptors have been examined in 75 Central Nervous System tumors (49 meningiomas, 11 schwannomas, 4 ependymomas, 3 astrocytomas, 2 glioblastomas, 2 metastases, 3 pituitary adenomas and 1 cerebellar hemangioblastoma). The sex steroid receptors were determined with a dextran-coated charcoal assay and Scatchard plot analysis.
Progesterone receptors were present, at high levels, in 31 of 49 meningiomas (63 %), but only low and rare amounts of estrogen receptors were detected in the same tissue samples. Of the 26 other CNS tumors only one ependymoma presented a high progesterone receptor level.
Our clinical-epidemiological data of the surgically treated meningiomas (121 cases in 115 patients) and the presence of progesterone receptors suggest that meningioma can be a target tissue for progesterone and so it can be subject to some hormonal influence.

KEY WORDS

Steroid Receptors, CNS Tumors, Meningioma.

REFERENCES

1. POISSON (M.), PERTUISER (B.F.), MOGUILEWSKY (M.), MAGDELENAT (H.), MARTIN (P.M.): Les récepteurs de stéroïdes du système nerveux central. Implications en neurologie. Rev. Neurol. 4: 233-248 (1984).
2. BLANKENSTEIN (M.A.), BLAAUW (G.), LAMBERTS (S.J.), MULDER (E.): Presence of progesterone receptors and absence of oestrogen receptors in human meningioma cytosols. Eur. J. Cancer Clin. Oncol. 19: 365-370 (1983).
3. BLAAUW (G.), BLANKENSTEIN (M.A.), LAMVERTS (S.W.J.): Sex steroid receptors in human meningiomas. Acta Neurochir. 79: 42-47 (1986).
4. CAHILL (D.W.), BASHIRELAHI (N.), SOLOMON (L.W.), DALTON (T.), SALCMAN (M.), DUCKER (T.B.): Estrogen and progesterone receptors in meningiomas. J. Neurosurg. 60: 985-993 (1984).
5. HINTON (D.), MOBBS (E.G.), SIMA (A.A.), HANNA (W.): Steroid receptors in meningiomas. Acta Neuropathol. 62: 134-140 (1983).
6. JAY (J.R.), MACLAUGHLIN (D.T.), RILEY (K.R.), MARTUZA (R.L.): Modulation of meningioma cell growth by sex steroid hormones in vitro. J. Neurosurg. 62: 757-762 (1985).
7. MAGDELENAT (H.), PERTUISET (B.F.), POISSON (M.), MARTIN (P.M.), PHILIPPON (J.), PERTUISER (B.): Progestin and oestrogen receptors in meningiomas. Biochemical characterization, clinical and pathological correlations in 42 cases: Acta Neurochir. 64: 199-213 (1982).
8. MARKWALDER (T.M.), ZAVA (D.T.), GOLDHIRSCH (A.), MARKWALDER (R.V.): Estrogen and progesterone receptors in meningiomas in relation to clinical and pathologic features. Surg. Neurol. 20: 42-47 (1983).
9. MARTUZA (R.L.), MILLER (D.C.), MACLAUGHLIN (D.): Estrogen and progestin binding by cytosolic and nuclear fractions of human meningiomas. J. Neurosurg. 62: 750-756 (1985).
10. SCHOENBERG (B.S.), CHRISTINE (B.W.), WHISNANT (J.P.): Nervous system neoplasms and primary malignancies of other sites: Neurology 25: 705-712 (1975).
11. SCHWARTZ (M.R.), RANDOLPH (R.L.), CECH (D.A.), ROSE (J.E.), PANKO (W.B.): Steroid hormone binding macromolecules in meningiomas: Cancer 53: 922-927 (1984).
12. VAQUERO (J.), MARCOS (M.L.), MARTINEZ (R.), BRAVO (G.): Estrogen and progesterone receptor proteins in intracranial tumors. Surg. Neurol. 19: 11-13 (1983).
13. BELLUR (S.N.), CHANDRA (V.), ANDERSON (R.J.): Association of meningiomas with obesity: Annals of Neurol. 13: 346-347 (1983).
14. TILZER (L.L.), PLAPP (F.V.), EVANS (J.P.), STONE (D.), ALWARD (K.): Steroid receptor proteins in human meningiomas. Cancer 49: 633-636 (1982).
15. HORWITZ (K.B.), MOCKUS (M.B.), LESSEY (B.A.): Variant T47D human breast cancer cells with high progesterone receptor levels despite estrogen and antiestrogen resistence. Cell 28: 633-642 (1982).
16. OLSON (J.J.), BECK (D.W.), SCHLECHTE (J.), LOH (P.M.): Hormonal manipulation of meningiomas in vitro: J. Neurosurg. 65: 99-107 (1986).

Steroid Hormone Receptors and Intracranial Tumors

R. KNERICH (°), M. SCERRATI (°°), G. BUTTI (°), G. SICA (°°°), C. ZIBERA (°°°°), V. NATOLI (°°°), V. SILVANI (°), G. ROBUSTELLI DELLA CUNA (°°°°), G.F. ROSSI (°°) and P. PAOLETTI (°).

INTRODUCTION

Steroid hormone receptors in intracranial tumors have been studied by many authors in recent years. Most of the research has been conducted on the oncotype meningioma while few data are available on gliomas.

In spite of the considerable number of studies on this subject, discrepancies still remain on the results obtained. In meningiomas, for example, there is disagreement on the incidence of estrogen receptors (1), and few data regarding the presence of glucocorticoid receptors are available. On the other hand, series of gliomas are too restricted to allow definite conclusions.

This paper reports the results of the study on the determination of the cytosolic content of glucocorticoid (GR), estrogen (ER), progesterone (PR) and androgen (AR) receptors in meningiomas and gliomas.

MATERIALS AND METHODS

The tissue samples of 35 meningiomas and of 37 gliomas were obtained at the time of surgery from unselected patients. The specimens for the hormone binding assay were immediately frozen in liquid nitrogen and then stored at -80 °C until the time of study. Adjacent samples were taken for histological examination. At the time of assay these frozen tissues were minced with surgical scissors and weighed. They were homogenized in a phosphate buffer (10 mM sodium phosphate, pH 7.4, 1.5 mM EDTA, 10 mM monothioglycerol, 20 mM sodium molybdate, and 10 % v/v glycerol) with three 10-second bursts of an Ultra-Turrax homogenizer. The homogenate was spun at 105.000 g for 1 hour at 0-4 °C in a Beckman Ultracentrifuge. The cytosol was then carefully removed with a Pasteur pipette and its protein content was determined using the method of Lowry et al. (2) in order to obtain a protein dilution of around 2 mg/ml.

Saturation analysis was performed by incubating duplicate samples of cytosol (200 microliters) with increasing concentrations of labelled ligands. 3H-estradiol (0.05-5 nM) was used for ER determination in the presence or absence of an excess of diethylstilbestrol (DES). 3H-ORG 2058 (0.05-5 nM) was used for PR determination in the presence or absence of an excess of the equivalent unlabelled steroid. 3H-dexamethasone (1.0-30 nM) was used for GR determination in the presence or absence of an excess of the equivalent unlabelled steroid. 3H-R1881 (0.1-10 nM) plus a 500 fold excess of triamcinolone acetonide was used for AR determination in the presence or absence of an excess of the equivalent unlabelled steroid.

After incubation overnight at 0-4 °C, the mixtures were treated with 400 microliters of dextran-coated charcoal solution (final concentration: 0.5 % activated charcoal Norit-A; 0.05 % dextran) for 10 minutes at 4 °C. They were then centrifuged at 3.500 g for 10 minutes. An aliquot of the supernatant was added to 10 ml of Insta Gel and the radioactivity was measured. The counting efficiency was approximately 38 %. When the receptors concentrations were sufficient (>10 fmol/mg.prot.), Scatchard plots (3) were constructed for the binding data to determine the dissociation constants (Kd).

(°) Dept. of Surgery, Neurosurgical Sect., University of Pavia, (°°) Inst. of Neurosurgery, "Cattolica" University of Rome, (°°°) Inst. of Histology, "Cattolica" University of Rome, (°°°°) Div. of Oncology, University of Pavia.

M. Chatel, F. Darcel and J. Pecker (eds.), Brain Oncology. ISBN-13: 978-94-010-8003-3

The receptor binding sites are expressed as femtomoles of receptor per milligram of cytosol protein (fmol/mg. prot.). The arbitrary cut-off value of more than 10 fmol/mg. prot. was considered to be indicative of a positive receptor value.
Results were statistically compared using the Student's t-test.

RESULTS

The range of Kd values of the different receptors were as follow: PR: 0.1-0.9 nM; AR: 0.1-0.9 nM; GR: 2-7 nM.

Meningiomas

The mean age of the patients in our study was 58 years (range: 38-78). The male-female ratio was 2/3 (N = 14 vs.21). The histological subtypes were divided as follow: meningotheliomatous N = 15, fibroblastic N = 12, transitional N = 4, psammomatous N = 3, and anaplastic N = 1.

The percentage of receptors positivity and mean concentration are shown in Table I. PR was found to be present in a concentration higher than 10 fmol/mg. prot. in 82.9 % of the cases. The mean concentration was 155.7 fmol/mg. prot. (range: 20.8-570.0). ER was found to be present in 6.1 % of the cases with a mean level of 35.1 fmol/mg. prot. Over 10 fmol/mg. prot. of GR was present in 26 (74.3 %) of the 35 cases with a mean concentration of 79.3 fmol/mg. prot. (range: 16.6-230). In fifty percent of the cases AR had a mean level of 33.9 fmol/mg. prot. (range: 11.8-66.1).

Preoperative dexamethasone therapy was not administered at all to 6 patients (Group 1). Twenty-three patients received therapy with dexamethasone for at least one week before surgery (Group 2). In the remaining 6 cases this therapy was begun only on the day prior to surgery (Group 3). A comparison was made between the receptor concentration and the three dexamethasone depending groups (Table II).

GR were found in all the cases without preoperative therapy (Group 1) with a mean level of 154.5 fmol/mg. prot. (range: 63.6-230); whereas GR were found in 77.3 % of the cases in Group 2 with a mean level of 56.0 fmol/mg (range: 16.6-144.2). In group 3, only fifty percent of cases showed a presence of GR and had a mean concentration of 28.5 fmol/mg. prot. These differences are statistically significant ($p < 0.01$) for Group 1 versus Group 2 and 3. PR were found in 83.3 %, 86.3 %, 83.3 % of the cases for Group 1, 2 and 3 respectively. The mean levels were 207.7, 127.0, and 212.0 fmol/mg.prot. respectively, without any statistical differences (Table II). No differences were noted for either ER or AR based on dexamethasone therapy.

TABLE I

Steroid hormone receptors positivity in meningiomas

Receptor	No. of cases	Percent of positivity	Mean concentration (fmol/mg.pr)
GR	35	74.3	79.3
ER	33	6.1	35.1
PR	35	82.9	155.7
AR	26	50.0	33.9

TABLE II

Preoperative dexamethasone administration and GR and PR positivity in meningiomas

Group	No. of cases	Percent of positivity GR	Mean conc. <(fmol/mg.pr)	Percent of positivity PR	Mean conc. (fmol/mg.pr)
1	6	100	154.5*	83.3	207.7
2	23	77.3	56.0	86.3	127.0
3	6	50	28.5	83.3	212.0

Group 1 = no therapy
Group 2 = therapy one week before surgery (8-16 mg/die)
Group 3 = therapy before surgery (24 mg)
* p 0.01.

Also, no differences in the percentage of presence of the four receptors were noted between males and females (Table III). A statistically significant difference (p. < 0.05) was noted on PR mean levels between male and female. Some relationships were noted between sex hormone receptors and histological subtypes. Only fibroblastic (N = 12) and meningotheliomatous (N = 15) meningiomas are considered in Table IV. PR and AR were higher in the meningotheliomatous rather than in the fibroblastic subtype. However these differences do not reach statistical significance.

TABLE III

Steroid hormone receptors and sex distribution in meningiomas

	MALE			FEMALE		
Receptor	No. of cases	Percent of positivity	Mean conc. (fmol/mg.pr)	No. of cases	Percent of positivity	Mean conc. (fmol/mg.pr)
GR	15	73.3	81.6	20	75	77.6
ER	14	7.1	59.4	20	5	10.7
PR	15	80.0	219.4*	20	85	110.7
AR	11	63.6	33.2	15	40	34.8

* $p < 0.05$

TABLE IV

Steroid hormone receptors and histological subtypes in meningiomas

	FIBROBLASTIC			MENINGOTHELIOMATUS		
Receptor	No. of cases	Percent of positivity	Mean conc. (fmol/mg.pr)	No. of cases	Percent of positivity	Mean conc. (fmol/mg.pr)
GR	12	75.0	75.4	15	80.0	62.9
ER	12	0	—	14	0	—
PR	12	75.0	138.4	15	93.3	199.5
AR	7	42.8	46.0	12	75.0	26.3

Gliomas

The mean age of the 37 cases was 50 years (range: 4-75). There were 20 males and 17 females. Fourteen cases were classified as glioblastomas, 11 as anaplastic astrocytomas, 8 as astrocytomas grade I and II, 2 as ependymomas and 2 as oligodendrogliomas.

TABLE V

Steroid hormone receptors positivity in gliomas

Receptor	No. of cases	Percent of positivity	Mean concentration (fmol/mg.pr)
GR	37	37.8	23.0
ER	37	10.8	17.7
PR	37	5.4	15.9
AR	34	17.6	20.9

Table V shows the general picture of the four sex steroid receptors in gliomas. The percentage of positivity and mean level are generally lower than those observed in meningiomas. GR are the most abundant (mean level: 23 fmol/mg.prot.; range: 10,5-42,4), but they do not seem to be influenced by preoperative dexamethasone therapy. In fact, two of the three cases not treated with dexamethasone do not reveal any detectable level of GR.

It is noted in our series that GR, ER and AR were present more frequently in females than in males but without any great difference in the mean levels (Table VI).

No particular relationship between steroid hormone receptors and histological subtypes (glioblastoma and anaplastic astrocytoma) was found (Table VII).

TABLE VI

Steroid hormone receptors and sex distribution in gliomas

Receptor	MALE No. of cases	MALE Percent of positivity	MALE Mean conc. (fmol/mg.pr)	FEMALE No. of cases	FEMALE Percent of positivity	FEMALE Mean conc. (fmol/mg.pr)
GR	20	25.0	26.3	17	52.9	23.3
ER	20	5.0	22.1	17	17.6	16.2
PR	20	5.0	17.1	17	5.9	14.7
AR	17	5.9	20.3	17	29.4	21.0

TABLE VII

Steroid hormone receptors and histological subtypes in gliomas

Receptor	GLIOBLASTOMA No. of cases	GLIOBLASTOMA Percent of positivity	GLIOBLASTOMA Mean conc. (fmol/mg.pr)	ANAPLASTIC ASTROCYTOMA No. of cases	ANAPLASTIC ASTROCYTOMA Percent of positivity	ANAPLASTIC ASTROCYTOMA Mean conc. (fmol/mg.pr)
GR	14	28.6	29.9	11	27.3	18.5
ER	14	7.1	25.9	11	9.1	11.8
PR	14	0	—	11	9.1	14.7
AR	13	30.7	17.1	9	11.1	13.5

DISCUSSION

The results of the present study demonstrate that meningiomas contain high concentrations of progesterone and glucocorticoid receptors while they contain almost no ER. The problem of the presence of ER has been extensively discussed by some authors (1, 4, 5, 6). We agree that strict criteria must be used in the evaluation of ER positivity (1).

In our study, the effect of preoperative dexamethasone therapy on steroid hormone receptor determination in meningiomas, is clearly demonstrated. GR are significantly reduced both when dexamethasone is chronically administered in variable doses between 8 and 16 mg/daily, and when it is used in preparation for surgery only at the dose of 24 mg in 12 hours. The average quantity of PR is reduced if dexamethasone is chronically administered, but not in a way that is statistically significant. The percentage of PR positivity is not modified by dexamethasone therapy. It is interesting to note that the average quantity of PR is not reduced when dexamethasone treatment begins 12 hours before surgery. This observation requires further studies in order to clarify the role of dexamethasone, and to make eventual interrelations between GR and PR evident (7).

Our study confirms the difference in PR mean levels between fibroblastic and meningotheliomatous subtypes but it is not statistically significant as observed by Poisson et al. (8). No other relationships were found between levels of the receptors and age of patients, location and size of tumors. Only few papers in the literature deal with steroid receptors in gliomas (7-11). In our serie, GR are present in higher percentage of cases and concentration than the other receptors. This observation disagrees with a report (8) in which GR are present only in 1/9 cases, and this fact is not related to dexamethasone therapy.

The limited percentage of positivity of ER and PR suggests a probable limited biological activity of these receptors in gliomas (11).

Differences between male and female were noted in the AR concentration (8); in our study female showed a higher percentage of all receptors except PR than the one observed in male. Even though our serie is not too short, further studies on longer series are necessary to obtain definite conclusions about eventual differences between male and female patients.

SUMMARY

Steroid hormone receptors were evaluated in the cytosol of 72 intracranial tumors (meningiomas and gliomas). The labelled ligands used were: ³H-dexamethasone for glucocorticoid receptor (Gr); ³H-estradiol for estrogen receptor (ER); ³H-ORG2058 for progesterone receptor (PR) and ³H-R1881 plus a 200-fold excess of triamcinolone acetonide for androgen receptor (AR). Bound steroid was measured by the dextran-coated charcoal absorption technique and the number of binding sites and K_D were evaluated from Scatchard plots. Receptors were considered as present above 10 fmoles/mg protein. In meningiomas, GR were found in 74.3 % of the cases, ER in 6.1 %, PR in 82.9 % and AR in 50 %. In gliomas, GR were found in 37.8 % of the cases, ER in 10.8 %, PR in 5.4 % and AR in 17.6 %. Glucocorticoid therapy before surgery affected both the percentage of presence and the level of GR in meningiomas. In facts, tumors from patients treated with dexamethasone showed a lower percentage of GR positivity if compared to the untreated ones. Moreover the mean level of GR decreased.

KEY WORDS

Steroid receptors, Meningiomas, Gliomas, Glucocorticoid.

AKNOWLEDGEMENTS

This research is supported by National Research Council, Rome, Italy, grant no. 85.02059.44, Special Project "Oncologia".

REFERENCES

1. BLANKESTEIN (M.A.), BLAAUW (G.), LAMBERTS (S.W.J.), MULDER (E.): "Presence of progesterone receptors and absence of oestrogen receptors in human intracranial meningiomas cytosol". Eur. J. Cancer Clin. Oncol., 19, 365, 1983.
2. LOWRY (O.H.), ROSENBROUGH (N.J.), FARR (A.L.), RANDALL (R.J.): Protein measurement with the Folin phenol reagent". J. Biol. Chem. 193, 265, 1951.
3. SCATCHARD (G.): "The attractions of proteins for small molecules and ions". Ann. N.Y. Acad. Sci. 51, 600, 1949.
4. SCHNEGG (J.F.), GOMEZ (F.), LEMARCHAND-BERAUD (T.), De TRIBOLET (N.): "Presence of Sex Steroid Hormone Receptors in Meningioma Tissues". Surg. Neurol. 15, 6, 415-1981.
5. TILZER (L.L.), PLAPP (F.V.), EVANS (J.P.), STONE (D.), ALWARD (K.): "Steroid receptor proteins in human meningiomas". Cancer 49, 633, 1982.
6. HAYWARD (E.), WHITWELL (P.K.), BARNES (D.H.): Steroid receptors in human meningioma. Clin. Neuropath. 62, 134, 1983.
7. RENGACHARAY (S.S.), TILZER (L.L.): "A study of dexamethasone receptor protein in human gliomas". J. Surg. Res. 31, 447, 1981.
8. POISSON (M.), PERTUISET (B.), HAUW (J.J.), PHILIPPON (J.), BUGE (A.), MOGUILEWSKY (M.), PHILIBERT (D.): "Steroid hormone receptors in human meningiomas, gliomas and brain metastases". J. Neuro-Oncol. 1, 179, 1983.
9. YU (Z.Y.Y.), WRANGE (O.), GOETHIUS (J.), HATAM (A.), GRANHOEM (L.), GUSTAFSSON (J.A.): "A study of glucocorticoid receptors in intracranial tumors". J. Neurosurg. 55, 757, 1981.
10. PAOLETTI (P.), ASCARI (E.), et al.: "New Aspects on Biochemistry of Brain Tumors". in: Proceedings of 8th International Congress of Neurological Surgery, Toronto (Canada), 1985.
11. MARKWALDER (T.M.), ZAVA (D.T.), MARKWALDER (R.V.): "Sexual Steroid Hormone Receptor Assays in Human Astrocytomas". Surg. Neurol. (Letter to the Editor) 20, 263, 1983.

Steroid Sex Hormones in Non-Pituitary Brain Tumours

C. DAVIS, J. JONES, E. YOSHINO, J. DARLING, G. CARTER,
J. ZAHER, D. THOMAS (°).

INTRODUCTION

It has long been known that meningiomas are commoner in women than men and indeed hormonal manipulation is the second oldest form of treatment in cancer after surgery.

METHODS AND MATERIALS

In the first part of this study we have looked at steroid sex hormone binding in a variety of non-pituitary brain tumours. There are several assay methods available: — The cytosolic method, introduced 20 years ago (1) in the study of breast cancer (2), in which a portion of tumour is analysed using the well established Dextran coated charcoal method with six point Scatchard analysis. The second method is the iso-electric focusing technique, and the third is the nuclear assay which has been open to question. Two further methods have recently been introduced using immunocytostains: The Erica (Abbott Laboratories) oestrogen receptor immunocytostain and more recently the Amersham immunocytostain which is thought to indicate both oestrogen and progesterone receptor activity. Hormone specific binding is thought to be due to the presence of receptors which are polypeptides just beneath the cell membrane and these receptors are also represented in the nucleus. In this study we have used both the Dextran coated charcoal method and more recently the Erica immunocytostain. All assay methods require meticulous tumour collection, storage in liquid nitrogen and careful analysis in a reliable laboratory.

In the second part of this study we have grown ten human meningiomas in monolayer cultures using standard techniques (3). Particular care was used to deprive the calf serum which is the commonly used growing medium, of all hormone and it is possible that many cancer studies using this technique in the past have ignored this vital step. To each of the tumours we added Tamoxifen, Oestradiol and Progesterone in physiological concentrations and the cell proliferation over 32 days have been studied using growth curve and cloning efficiency studies. Meningiomas are slow growing tumours and it is not possible to directly compare this technique with for example gliomas subjected to chemotherapy.

RESULTS

51 oestrogen and progesterone binding analyses using the cytosolic method were undertaken in human brain tumours. Low levels of oestrogen receptor binding were present in five out of eighteen meningiomas, two out of eight gliomas and one germinoma. Two metastases and one acoustic neuroma had no oestrogen receptor binding. Only two of these tumours had anything like markedly raised oestrogen receptor levels as measured by the strictest laboratory criteria (used for breast cancer). One of these was a recurrent cerebellar astrocytoma in a young lady of 21 and the other was a meningioma.

(°) National Hospital for Nervous Diseases. Queen Square, London and Charing Cross Hospital, London.

M. Chatel, F. Darcel and J. Pecker (eds.), Brain Oncology. ISBN-13: 978-94-010-8003-3

Twelves meningiomas analysed for progesterone binding all had markedly raised receptor levels (Table I). Tumour samples taken with a standard cutting diathermy loop had no receptor binding presumably due to the denaturing of the polypeptides while the sample was being collected. There was no histological correlation with progesterone receptor levels in this small series; however it is worth noting that the highest levels were found in menopausal women with sphenoidal tumour which had hyperostosing and extradural elements and of course are likely to recur. Four meningiomas were negative for oestrogen receptor using the Erica immunocytostains.

Half the meningiomas grown in culture were markedly inhibited in a dose dependant manner by the administration of Tamoxifen (table II, fig. 1, fig. 2). This effect was reversed by the concomitant administration of Oestradiol (fig. 1). Progesterone did not seem to affect tumour growth.

TABLE I

Progesterone receptors in meningiomas

	Age	Sex	Site	PR (fm/mg)	Histology
1.	53	F	Sphenoid	308	Angioblastic
2.	46	F	Suprasella	157	Fibrous
3.	58	F	Recurrent sphenoid	156	Fibrous
4.	57	F	Sphenoid	89	Transitional
5.	65	F	Recurrent convexity	76	Meningothelial
6.	60	F	Parasagittal	62	Malignant
7.	56	F	Convexity	51	Transitional
8.	72	M	Dorsal	42	Psammomatous
9a.	35	F	Convexity	42	Transitional
9b.			(Cutting Loop)	0	Transitional
10.	50	M	Parasagittal	40	Transitional
11a.	58	F	Convexity	31	Transitional
11b.			(Cutting Loop)	0	Transitional
12.	55	M	Convexity	17	Transitional

TABLE II

Clinical data and summary of results in 10 patients with meningiomas

Age	Sex	Menopausal status	Location of tumour	Histological type	Tamoxifen		Response to Oestradiol		Progesterone	
					G	C	G	C	G	C
35	F	pre	Convexity	Fibroblastic	+	+	—	—	—	—
31	F	pre	Subfrontal	Transitional	+	+	—	—	ND	ND
64	F	post	Convexity	Syncytial	+	+	—	—	—	—
54	F	post	Convexity	Syncytial	+	+	—	—	ND	ND
53	F	post	Convexity	Transitional	+	NG	—	NG	—	NG
73	F	post	Convexity	Synctial	—	—	—	—	ND	ND
59	F	post	Sphenoid ridge	Transitional	—	—	—	—	ND	—
46	F	post	Suprasellar	Transitional	—	—	—	—	—	—
72	F	post	Parasagittal	Psammomatous	—	NG	—	NG	—	NG
60	F	post	Suprasellar	Synctial	—	—	—	—	—	—

*: Recurrent meningioma; G: Growth curve study; C: Cloning efficiency study; ND: Not done; NG: No growth

DISCUSSION

In discussing these results, one must be aware that the steroid sex hormones are ill understood. Often these hormones seem to have both agonist and antagonist actions at the same time as the blood levels change. Also the relationship between blood levels and receptor status is poorly correlated and the recent NATO breast cancer studies (ref. 4) have suggested that oestrogen receptor status in verified breast cancer does not always correlate well with the administration of Tamoxifen — an anti-oestrogen drug. There has been much recent interest in receptor status and steroid sex hormones particularly in meningiomas and the correlation between prognosis in meningiomas and progesterone receptor levels is clearly important. The mechanism by which Tamoxifen appears to

FIGURE 1

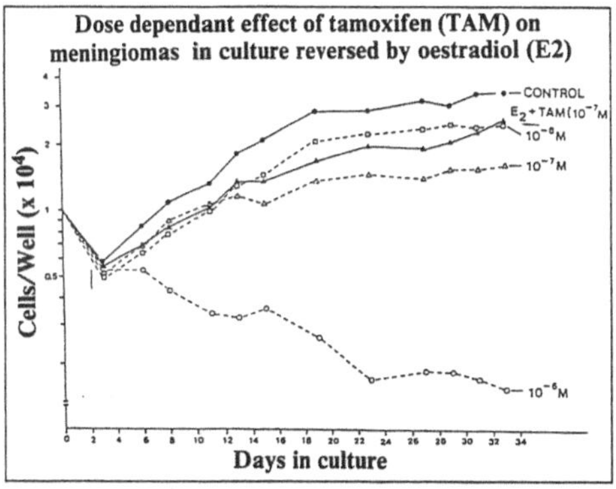

FIGURE 2

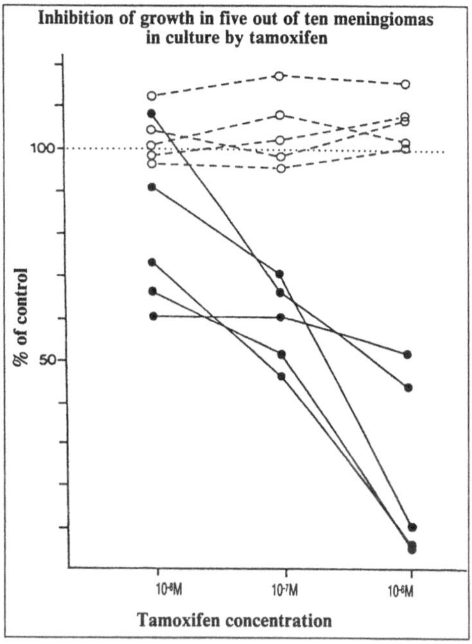

affect these tumours in vitro is ill understood as oestrogen receptor status in these tumours was low. On the clinical side we have used Tamoxifen on two patients and there does appear to be cessation of growth but this takes several months and other workers have not verified these results (5).

It is clear that hormonal manipulation of non-pituitary brain tumours offers exciting prospects (6) and that further work involving a multi-disciplinary approach is required.

SUMMARY

In this study we have investigated the hormone receptor status of non pituitary brain tumours and the effect of hormonal manipulation using Tamoxifen, Progesterone, Oestradiol and combinations of these hormones on in vitro cultures of human meningiomas. It appears that all human meningiomas have progesterone receptors and approximately half the tumours have low levels of oestrogen receptors. The anti-oestrogen drug Tamoxifen appears to inhibit growth in half of cultured meningiomas. The receptor status of other non-pituitary brain tumours is discussed.

KEY WORDS

Brain tumours, Steroid hormone receptors.

REFERENCES

1. SCATCHARD (G.): The Attraction of proteins for small molecules and ions. Ann Ny Acad. Sci. 51, 660-672 (1949).
2. JENSEN (E.V.), SMITH (S.), SOMBRE (E.R. de): Hormone dependency in breast cancer. J. Steroid Biochem. 7, 911-917 (1976).
3. COSTERO (I.), POMERAT (G.M.), JACKSON (I.J.): Tumours of the central nervous system in tissue culture. JNCI. 15, 1319-1339 (1955).
4. BAUM (M.) et al.: Nolvadex Adjuvent Trial Organisation. Lancet. 1, 836 (1985).
5. ZAVA (D.T.), MARKWALDER (T.M.): Biological expression of steroid hormone receptors in primary meningioma cells in monolayer culture. Clin Neuro Pharmacol. 7, 382-388 (1984).
6. OLSON (J.J.), BECK (D.W.), SCHLECTE (J.), LOH (P.): Hormonal manipulation of meningiomas in vitro. J. Neurosurg. 65, 99-107 (1986).

Trials of Hormonal Manipulation of Meningiomas in vivo and in vitro

T.M. MARKWALDER (°) and E. WAELTI (°).

Clinical and epidemiological features (1-4) and the presence of remarkably high titers of a non-estrogen regulated (5-9) high-affinity / limited capacity progesterone receptor (PR) in over 70% of cytosols (10-15, 5-7, 16, 9, 17) are in favour of a sex hormone dependency of tumor growth in meningiomas. We have studied the influence of sexual steroid hormones on growth of primary meningioma cells in monolayer tissue culture and in vivo because adjuvant hormonotherapy would represent, if effective, a desirable therapeutic measure if surgical resection is impossible or only partially practicable because of the tumor location or advanced age.

Antiestrogenic Therapy of Meningiomas

We initially undertook a pilot study which consisted in treating six patients with inoperable, non-operative, or recurrent meningiomas with the antiestrogenic agent tamoxifen (Nolvadex, ICI-Pharma, Luzern, Switzerland) (18, 19) based on the assumption that if meningiomas contain PR, they must also contain estradiol receptors (ER), and thus would respond to hormonotherapy like other hormone-sensitive tumors. Curiously, however, we were not able to detect any specific high-affinity ER in meningiomas (5, 7). Tamoxifen was administered during a 8-12 month period and computer tomographic, scintigraphic, and clinical evidence of an unspecific tumor response was only encountered in one patient after 4 month therapy with tamoxifen. The 2-year results did not indicate a favourable response to antiestrogenic treatment.

Biological Expression of Steroid Hormone Receptors in Primary Meningioma Cells in Monolayer Tissue Culture

Primary meningiomas have been tested for steroid hormone receptors and sensitivity to various steroids and steroid antagonists in monolayer tissue culture (20, 8). We were not able to demonstrate nuclear or cytoplasmic ER in the ten solid tumors or the primary cultures derived from them. PR was present in 50-70% of the solid tumors and some of the primary cultures. Four of four and five of five primary cultures contained, respectively, androgen and glucocorticoid receptors. When one of the cultures was tested for growth sensitivity to estrogen, tamoxifen, progesterone, hydrocortisone, and dihydrotestosterone, the last two had noticeable stimulatory effects on growth by day 5. Interestingly, only androgen and glucocorticoid receptors were present in the primary tumor cells in culture, suggesting that these receptors mediated the effects of their respective hormones on growth. We concluded that much work remains to be done to clarify the role of steroid hormones in the etiology, growth, and function of meningiomas. Some of the most controversial questions that remain unanswered are: 1) What is the biological function of the putative PR expressed in this tumor in the complete absence of ER? 2) Why is PR expressed in the complete absence of ER? 3) Are androgen and glucocorticoid receptors common to all meningiomas? and 4) Will steroid hormone therapy be of benefit in the treatment of this disease? (21)

Effect of Medroxyprogesterone Acetate on the Receptor State of Meningioma Cytosols

Because of the lack of a potent purely antiprogestational agent which can be clinically administered in humans, we have chosen the semisynthetic gestagen medroxyprogesterone acetate (MPA, Depo-Provera 500[R], UPJOHN SA, Zurich, Switzerland) which is thought to display antiestrogenic

(°) Department of Neurosurgery and Institute of Pathology, University of Bern, Bern, Switzerland.

M. Chatel, F. Darcel and J. Pecker (eds.), Brain Oncology. ISBN-13: 978-94-010-8003-3

properties and has a depressive effect on the pituitary-gonadal axis. 15 patients with intracranial or spinal meningiomas have been treated with MPA prior to surgical removal of the tumors with the goal to investigate the influence of MPA on the PR status of meningioma cytosols.

MPA acted as a competitive binder to meningioma-PR: The mean PR values amounted to 15,6 (range 0 - 69) fmol/mg protein and 338,3 (range 0 - 1190) fmol/g tumor, respectively. In comparison, mean PR values of our untreated meningioma series (5, 7) ($n = 58$) amounted to 54,9 (range 0 - 586) fmol/mg protein and 2813 (range 0 - 17168) fmol/g tumor, respectively. The non-normally distributed PR data were compared using the Mann-Whitney test: $0{,}001 < p <= 0{,}01$ at the 5% level of significance.

In cases of two-age resection of meningiomas, MPA significantly decreased PR-activity in the cytoplasm of meningioma cells.

Effect of Medroxyprogesterone Acetate on Growth of Primary Meningioma Cells in Monolayer Tissue Culture

With the exception of one case, we have found that the in-vitro growth rate of MPA-treated meningioma cells was reduced in comparison with untreated meningioma cells in monolayer tissue culture, that MPA impeded the growth rate when administered in the cell cultures, or that in-vitro cultures were not possible with MPA-treated meningioma cells.

The results from the latter two studies (22, 23) lead to the conclusion that medroxyprogesterone acetate binds to meningioma-PR, and, in some cases, MPA reduces the growth rate of primary meningioma cells in monolayer tissue culture. We think that, in patients with inoperable meningiomas, a long-term trial of MPA-therapy might be justified.

SUMMARY

15 patients with intracranial or spinal meningiomas have been treated with the semisynthetic progestational agent medroxyprogesterone acetate (MPA, Depo-Provera[R]) prior to surgical removal of the tumors in order to investigate the influence of MPA on the progesterone receptor (PR) status of meningioma cytosols.

MPA acted as a competitive binder to meningioma-PR: The mean PR-values amounted to 15,6 (range 0-69) fmol/mg protein and 338,3 (range 0-1190) fmol/g tumor, respectively. In comparison mean PR-values of our untreated meningioma series (n = 58) amounted to 54,9 (range 0-586) fmol/mg protein and 2813 (range 0-17168) fmol/g tumor, respectively.

In cases of two-stage resection of meningiomas, MPA significantly decreased PR-activity in the cytoplasm of meningioma cells. With the exception of one case, we have found that the in-vitro growth rate of MPA-treated meningioma cells was reduced in comparison to untreated meningioma cells in monolayer tissue culture, that MPA impeded the growth rate when administered in the cell cultures, or that in-vitro cultures were not possible with MPA-treated meningioma cells.

Conclusions

1. *MPA binds to meningioma-PR.*
2. *In some cases MPA reduces the growth rate of primary meningioma cells in monolayer tissue culture.*

KEY WORDS

Progesterone Receptors, Meningioma, Growth Modulation, Medroxyprogesterone acetate.

REFERENCES

1. CUSHING (H.), EISENHARDT (L.): Meningiomas: Their classification, regional behaviour, life history and surgical end results. Springfied, Illinois: Charles C. Thomas, 1938.
2. WEYAND (R.D.), MacCARTY (C.S.), WILSON (R.B.): The effect of pregnancy on intracranial meningiomas occurring about the optic chiasm. Surg. Clin. North Am 1951, 31: 1225-33.

3. BICKERSTAFF (E.R.), SMALL (J.M.), GUEST (I.A.): The relapsing course of certain meningiomas in relation to pregnancy and menstruation. J. Neurol. Neurosurg. Psychiatry 1958, 21: 89-91.

4. SCHOENBERRG (B.S.), CHRISTINE (B.W.), WHISNANT (J.P.): Nervous system neoplasms and primary malignancies of other sites: the unique association between meningiomas and breast cancer. Neurology 1975, 25: 705-12.

5. MARKWALDER (T.M.), ZAVA (D.T.), GOLDHIRSCH (A.), MARKWALDER (R.V.): Estrogen and progesterone receptors in meningiomas in relation to clinical and pathological features. Surg. Neurol. 1983, 20: 42-7.

6. BLANKENSTEIN (M.A.), BLAAUW (G.), LAMBERTS (W.J.), MULDER (E.): Presence of progesterone receptors and absence of estrogen receptors in human intracranial meningioma cytosols. Eur. J. Cancer Clin. Oncol. 1983, 19: 365-70.

7. MARKWALDER (T.M.), MARKWALDER (R.V.), ZAVA (D.T.): Estrogen and progestin receptors in meningiomas: clinicopathological correlations. Clin. Neuropharmacol. 1984, 7: 368-74.

8. ZAVA (D.T.), MARKWALDER (T.M.), MARKWALDER (R.V.): Biological expression of steroid hormone receptors in primary meningioma cells in monolayer culture. Clin. Neuropharmacol. 1984, 7: 382-8.

9. MARTUZA (R.L.), MILLER (D.C.), MacLAUGHLIN (D.T.): Oestrogen and progestin binding by cytosolic and nuclear fractions of human meningiomas. J. Neurosurg. 1985, 62: 750-6.

10. POISSON (M.), MAGDENELAT (H.), FONCIN (J.F.), BLEIBEL (J.M.), PHILIPPON (J.), PERTUISET (B.), BUGE (A.): Récepteurs d'œstrogènes et de progestérone dans les méningiomes. Rev. Neurol. (Paris) 1980, 136: 193-203.

11. MARTUZA (R.K.), MacLAUGHLIN (D.T.), OJEMAN (R.G.): Specific estradiol binding in schwannomas, meningiomas and neurofibromas. Neurosurgery 1981, 9: 665-71.

12. MAGDENELAT (H.), PERTUISET (B.F.), POISSON (M.), MARTIN (P.M.), PHILIPPON (J.), PERTUISET (B.), BUGE (A.): Progestin and oestrogen receptors in meningiomas. Biochemical characterization, clinical and pathological correlations in 42 cases. Acta Neurochir. 1982, 64: 199-213.

13. SCHNEGG (J.F.), GOMEZ (F.), LE MARCHAND-BERAUD (T.), TRIBOLET (N. de): Presence of sex steroid hormone receptors in meningioma tissue. Surg. Neurol. 1981, 15: 415-8.

14. TILZER (LL.), PLAPP (F.V.), EVANS (J.P.), STONE (D.), ALWARD (K.): Steroid receptor proteins in human meningiomas. Cancer 1982, 49: 633-6.

15. VAQUERO (J.), MARCOS (M.L.), MARTINEZ (R.), BRAVO (G.): Estrogen and progesterone receptor proteins in intracranial tumors. Surg. Neurol. 1983, 19: 11-3.

16. CAHILL (D.W.), BASHIRELAHI (N.), SOLOMON (L.W.), DALTON (T.), SALCMAN (M.), DUCKER (T.B.): Estrogen and progesterone receptors in meningiomas. J. Neurosurg. 1984, 60: 985-93.

17. BLAAUW (G.), BLANKENSTEIN (M.A.), LAMBERTS (W.J.): Sex steroid receptors in human meningiomas. Acta Neurochir. 1986, 79: 42-7.

18. MARKWALDER (T.M.), SEILER (R.W.), ZAVA (D.T.): Endocrine manipulation of inoperable and recurrent meningiomas - a pilot study. In: Spitzy K, Karrer K, eds. Proceedings of the 13th International Congress of Chemotherapy. Vienna: Verlag H. Egermann, 1983.

19. MARKWALDER (T.M.), SEILER (R.W.), ZAVA (D.T.): Antiestrogenic therapy of meningiomas - a pilot study. Surg. Neurol. 1985, 24: 245-9.

20. ZAVA (D.T.), MARKWALDER (T.M.), GOLDHIRSCH (A.): Primary human meningioma cells in monolayer tissue culture: Steroid hormone receptor content and effect of steroid hormones on growth (Abstract 495). J. Steroid Biochem. 1983, Suppl. 19, p. 170.

21. MARKWALDER (T.M.), ZAVA (D.T.): Sex steroid hormones and meningioma cell growth. Letter. J. Neurosurg. 1986, 64: 341-2.

22. MARKWALDER (T.M.), WAELTI (E.), KOENIG (M.P.): Endocrine manipulation of meningiomas with medroxyprogesterone acetate. Part I: Effect of MPA on receptor status of meningioma cytosols. Surg. Neurol. (in press).

23. WAELTI (E.), MARKWALDER (T.M.): Endocrine manipulation of meningiomas with medroxyprogesterone acetate. Part II: Effect of MPA on growth of primary meningioma cells in monolayer tissue culture. In preparation.

PART IV:
BIOLOGICAL AND DIAGNOSTIC IMAGING

Metabolic Studies of Brain Tumours by PET

D.G.T. THOMAS (°), D.J. BROOKS (°°) and T. JONES (°°).

Positron Emission Tomography (PET) provides a relatively non-invasive means of determining the metabolic activity in vivo of normal or abnormal areas of human brain. Suitable positron emitting isotopes include ^{15}O, ^{11}C, ^{18}F, and ^{82}Rb. Many naturally occurring organic molecules can be tagged with these agents and their regional distribution in the brain mapped out in tomographic slices. PET can be used simply as an imaging device, but it has a far greater potential as a means of studying regional cerebral blood flow, oxygen and glucose metabolism, and the transport of substrates across the blood-brain barrier (BBB). The application of PET to study metabolism using tracer kinetic modelling in these areas will be described.

The method which has been employed for measuring regional cerebral blood flow (rCBF), oxygen utilization ($rCMRO_2$) and regional oxygen extraction fraction (rOER) is based on steady-state equations using an extended model to correct for intravascular ^{15}O contributions to the regional cerebral tracer signal (1). Briefly, the method entails sequential inhalation of $C^{15}O_2$ and then $^{15}O_2$ until steady levels of ^{15}O are obtained in the arterial plasma and cerebral tissue. When $^{15}O_2$ is inhaled carbonic anhydrase in red bloods cells rapidly transfers the ^{15}O radionuclide to $H_2{}^{15}O$, and so the cerebral distribution of ^{15}O reflects regional cerebral blood flow. When $^{15}O_2$ is inhaled the regional cerebral ^{15}O uptake reflects both the regional cerebral blood flow and the fraction of oxygen extracted from the arterial blood supplying the region (rOER). The regional oxygen extraction is governed by the metabolic requirements of the cerebral tissue. By comparing the ratio of regional ^{15}O uptake during steady state inhalation of ^{15}O and then $C^{15}O_2$, OER values can be computed. Regional oxygen utilization, $rCMRO_2$, is then derived from the rCBF and rOER taken together with measurement of arterial oxygen content. Regional cerebral blood volume, rCBV, is obtained by labelling red cells with ^{11}CO. There are limitations and errors involved in this approach. However, in practice, blood flow in tumours is found to be highly variable and not coupled to blood volume (2). Low oxygen extraction fractions are a consistent finding. This is a surprising finding as tumour necrosis is often postulated to occur due to tissue ischaemia and infarction. The PET findings suggest that tumours in fact have more than adequate oxygen supply for their metabolic needs. However, the PET method is macroscopic and cannot exclude the presence of microscopic regions of tumour hypoxia below the resolution of the scanner. Regions surrounding the tumour, probably comprising areas of cerebral oedema, characteristically show a coupled reduction in oxygen utilization and blood flow compared to equivalent regions of contralateral brain tissue. However, oxygen extraction fractions in such regions are generally normal. In the contralateral, presumably normal, cortex of brain tumour patients, a significantly depressed oxygen utilization and blood flow, compared to age-matched normal controls, is found (3). This depression in cortical function by tumours is partially reversed following excisional surgery. Administration of dexamethasone, however, has been found acutely to depress both blood flow and blood volume in the contralateral cortex of patients with brain tumours. Radiotherapy has been found to show a progressive fall in oxygen utilization and blood flow in the tumour region, but in the contralateral brain blood flow rises acutely and then subsequently diminishes. However, utilization of oxygen in contralateral brain tissue remains unaltered by radiotherapy.

The analogue of glucose ^{18}F-2-fluoro-2-deoxyglucose (FDG) is transported across the BBB by the same facilitated transport mechanism as normal glucose. Once it has been phosphorylated by hexokinase, FDG-6-phosphate is unable to take part in the reactions of the glycolytic pathway or in glycogen synthesis and is thus essentially trapped in the cells, because dephosphorylation occurs only very slowly. Kinetic models have been developed to relate the ^{18}F tracer distribution following intravenous injection of FDG to regional cerebral glucose utilization. One difficulty with the

(°) Department of Neurological Surgery, The National Hospital, Institute of Neurology, Queen Square, London WC1, (°°) MRC Cyclotron Unit, Hammersmith Hospital, London.

M. Chatel, F. Darcel and J. Pecker (eds.), Brain Oncology. ISBN-13: 978-94-010-8003-3

models is that they rely on a "lumped constant" which relates the relative rates of FDG and glucose transport across the BBB to their relative rates of phosphorylation. The value of this constant in regions of diseased brain is uncertain. A second difficulty is that when the BBB is disrupted, for example in tumours, higher extracellular FDG levels may be achieved leading to artefactual increases in tracer uptake. In spite of these difficulties a number of studies have been carried out on cerebral glucose utilization in tumour patients using this method. In patients studied both for oxygen and glucose utilization it is found that a similar glucose extraction fraction exists for tumours and for cortex. Tumour oxygen extraction is characteristically depressed, indicating that tumours have an increased level of non-oxidative metabolism of glucose compared to normal brain tissue, in the presence of adequate oxygen sypply (4).

Transport of glucose across the BBB in tumours can be studied with ^{11}C-3-0-methyl-glucose, an analogue of glucose that is not metabolised. It has been shown that gliomas have ^{11}C-methyl-glucose extraction fractions up to 30 per cent, compared to 15 per cent extractions observed in normal brain tissue. The BBB is normally highly impermeable to K^+ cations and transport of K^+ is thought to be controlled by ATP-ases situated on the luminal side of endothelial membranes. $^{82}Rb^+$ is a positron emitter, chemically similar to K^+. When infused at a constant rate a steady level of $^{82}Rb^+$ results after four minutes in both arterial plasma and brain tissue. This isotope has been used to measure Rb extraction fractions for cerebral tissue in patients with brain tumour (6). It has been found that Rb extraction is increased in areas of cerebral tumours that also enhance on CT scanning after intravenous injection of iodine compounds. Non-enhancing tumours and normal brain have Rb extractions in the normal range (O-2.5 per cent) (5). In some cases permeability to $^{82}Rb^+$ was shown to be increased following on radiotherapy. Transport of albumin across the BBB can be studied using ^{11}C-methyl-albumin in PET studies. Within the forty minutes period of such PET studies only very slow leakage of albumin into tumour has been found.

PET provided a relatively non-invasive means for studying regional cerebral metabolism in patients with brain tumour and also for studying the effect of treatment on tumour and cerebral function (6). There are some basic scientific problems with several of the quantitative kinetic models and it will be important to perform correlative studies with magnetic resonance spectroscopy and with other biochemical methods. PET relies on an on-line cyclotron for operation and is an expensive technique probably best suited for studies in specialised centres although it may have a limited use as a diagnostic method. However, it does provide unique information about the basic biology of brain tumours in vivo.

SUMMARY

Positron emission tomography (PET) provides a relativly non-invasive method for determining regional concentrations of positron-emitting isotopes in tomographic slices of human brain. PET has been applied to the study of tumour and cerebral metabolism and physiology using tracer kinetic modelling. Results have been obtained for regional blood flow, oxygen utilization, and glucose utilization in cases of brain tumour, as well as for the effects of treatment on these functions. The transport of glucose and other substances into tumour and surrounding brain has also been studied.

KEY WORDS

Metabolism of Brain Tumours, PET, Positron emission tomography.

REFERENCES

1. FRACKOWIAK (R.S.J.), LENZI (G.L.), JONES (T.), HEATHER (J.D.): Quantitative measurement of regional cerebral blood flow and oxygen metabolism in man using ^{15}O and positron emission tomography: theory, procedure and normal values. J. Comput Assist. Tomogr. 1980, 4: 727-736.
2. ITO (M.), LAMMERTSMA (A.A.), WISE (R.J.S.), BERNARDI (S.), FRACKOWIAK (R.S.J.), HEATHER (J.D.), MCKENZIE (C.G.), THOMAS (D.G.T.), JONES (T.): Measurement of regional cerebral blood flow and oxygen utilisation in patients with cerebral tumours using ^{15}O and positron emission tomography: analytical techniques and preliminary results. Neuroradiology 1982, 23: 63-74.

3. BEANEY (R.P.), BROOKS (D.J.), LEENDERS (K.L.), THOMAS (D.G.T.), JONES (T.) and HALNAN (K.E.): Blood flow and oxygen utilisation in the contralateral cerebral cortex of patients with untreated intracranial tumours as studied by positron emission tomography, with observations on the effect of decompressive surgery. Neurol. Neurosurg. Psychiat. 1985, 48: 310-319.

4. RHODES (C.G.), WISE (R.J.S.), GIBBS (J.M.), FRACKOWIAK (R.S.J.), HATAZAWA (J.), PALMER (A.J.), THOMAS (D.G.T.) and JONES (T.): *In vivo* disturbance of the oxidative metabolism of glucose in human cerebral gliomas. Ann. Neurol. 1983, 14: 614-626.

5. BROOKS (D.J.), BEANEY (R.P.), LAMMERTSMA (A.A.), LEENDERS (K.L.), HORLOCK (P.L.), KENSETT (M.J.), MARSHALL (J.), THOMAS (D.G.T.) and JONES (T.): Quantitative measurement of blood-brain barrier permeability using rubidium-82 and positron emission tomography. Cereb. Blood Flow Metab. 1984, 4: 535-545.

6. WISE (R.J.S.), THOMAS (D.G.T.), LAMMERTSMA (A.A.) and RHODES (C.G.): PET scanning of human brain tumours. Prog. exp. Tumor Res., 1984, 27: 154-169.

Study of ^{11}C-L-Methionine Uptake in Brain Gliomas by Positron Emission Tomography: Metabolic Grading, and Effects of Radiotherapy and Intra-Arterial Chemotherapy

J.M. DERLON (°), C. BOURDET (°°), M. CHATEL (°°°), P. BUSTANY (°°)(°°°°), J. THERON (°°°°°), F. DARCEL (°°°), J.P. HOUTTEVILLE (°), A. SYROTA (°°)

The treatment of gliomas remains very disappointing, in spite of a bulk of experimental data and randomized trials over the last years. The inaccuracy of our current methods to investigate the local metabolism of these tumors might partly explain this therapeutic failure. The use of positron emission tomography (PET) provides a promising insight in this field. It allows measuring some physiological and biochemical parameters in the tumorous and peritumoral tissue, and the modification of these parameters after treatment. Many approaches of the tumoral metabolism are possible with PET. We report here our study of intraluminal ^{11}C-L-methionine captation in brain gliomas, in three situations:

— assessment of the histological grade;
— assessment of the radiotherapy effects;
— assessment of the intraarterial chemotherapy effects.

PATIENTS AND METHODS

Twenty-two patients with a histologically confirmed glioma were studied. The detailed protocol of PET exploration has been published along with the first cases of this study (1). Examination has been performed with an ECAT II (R) tomograph (EG&G ORTEC) with the median resolution mode, providing reconstructed images with a 16 mm spatial resolution in both transverse and axial planes. Data were sampled in a plane parallel to the orbito - meatal line, referring to the CT-scan, so as to include a major section of the tumor in this unique slice. There was a two-step exploration:

1. After an IV injection of 560 to 930 MBq of ^{11}C-L-methionine, 12 images were made over a 46 minutes period. The number of events for each image varied from 5.10^5 to 10.10^5 true coincidences. Blood sampling were made via an intravenous catheter during the exploration, in order to measure the ^{11}C-L-methionine activity at the different stages of data sampling.
2. Eighteen hours later the regional cerebral blood volume (rCBV) was measured in the same slice level after a non-saturing IV injection of 2 to 4 mCi of ^{68}Ca G13. The ^{68}GA C13 is bound in plasma with transferrin, a protein which does not cross normally the blood-brain barrier (BBB). This measurement permits one to calculate the intraparenchymatous ^{11}C-methionine activity (after substracting the plasmatic activity), and to localize and assess the areas of BBB disruption inside the tumor.

   Data analysis was performed through the measurement of ^{11}C-methionine activity in the tumor and in the symetric healthy region of interest (ROI) of the opposite hemisphere on the twelfth image. The chosen intratumoral ROI was always the one where the activity was the highest ($\geqslant 90\%$ of the maximum activity of the slice). For each patient, one has computed the ratio R_{MET} between the tumoral activity and the healthy tissue activity:

$$R_{MET} = \frac{\text{(intratumoral activity)}}{\text{(normal tissue activity)}}$$

(°) Department of Neurosurgery, C.H.U., Caen, (°°) S.H.F.J., Orsay, (°°°) Department of Neurology, C.H.U. Rennes, (°°°°) Laboratory of Clinical Pharmacology, C.H.U., Caen, (°°°°°) Department of Neuroradiology, C.H.U. Caen.

M. Chatel, F. Darcel and J. Pecker (eds.), Brain Oncology. ISBN-13: 978-94-010-8003-3

Similarly has the R_{Ga} of ^{68}Ga C13 in the tumor and normal brain been measured. This measurement permitted an assessment of the BBB disruption, which could be correlated with the degree of contrast enhancement on CT-scan.

RESULTS

Metabolic grading (Table I)

In 22 patients, R_{MET} mean values and standard deviations were computed for each histological group. There is a highly significant correlation between the rate of ^{11}C-L-methionine and the histological grade. The difference between grades II and III is significant with $p = 0.045$, and with $p = 0.007$ between grades II and IV. Otherwise, in spite of a higher R mean value for grade IV astrocytomas than for grade III, the difference is not significant ($p = 0.3141$).

The BBB study by CT-scan and ^{68}GA G13 showed, in the vast majority of patients, a good correlation between constrat enhancement on one hand, and R_{Ga} on the other hand: R_{Ga} was > 1 when there was a constrast enhancement, and < 1 in other cases. Nevertheless in three patients (grade III astrocytomas) there was a moderate contrast enhancement with a $R_{Ga} > 1$. R_{MET} in those three patients were respectively 1.5, 1.6 and 1.8.

TABLE I
METABOLIC GRADING

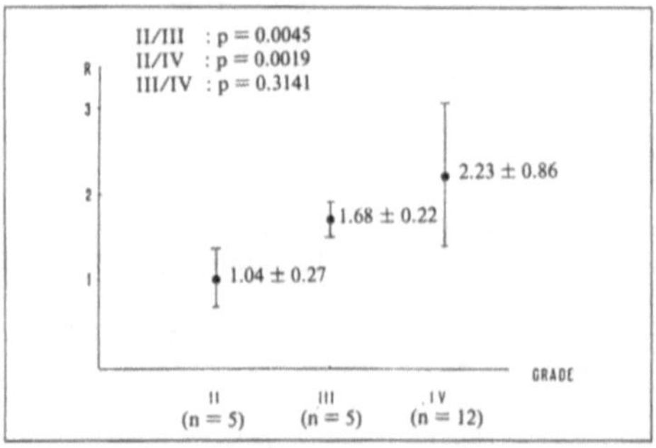

TABLE II
EFFECTS OF RADIOTHERAPY

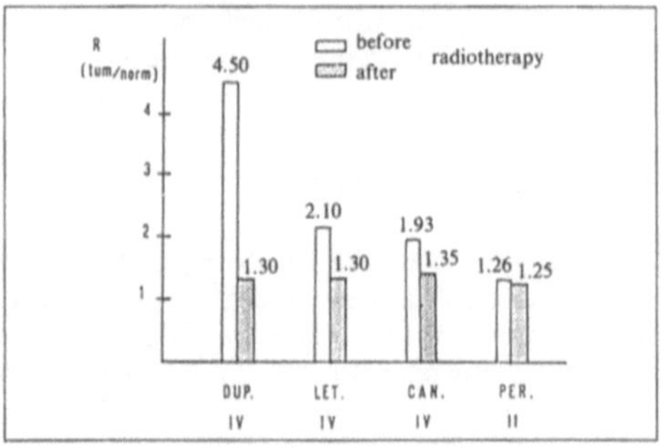

Effects of radiotherapy (Table II)

Four patients were studied before then one month after radiotherapy (60 Gy-eq. on the tumor, in 6 weeks). In three patients with a grade IV astrocytoma, hypermetabolism was noticeably reduced in the area of the tumoral maximum activity. Local analysis of radiation effects can provide more information than this global analysis. Thus, in our third patient (Fig. 1), radiation field was concentrated over a post-surgical residual focus located in the deep insular layers. In this area, PET demonstrated a hypermetabolism with $R_{MET} = 2.5$, which was reduced to 1.2 after radiotherapy. But PET demonstrated also a superficial area in which R_{MET} was 1.5. This focus, not irradiated, exhibited a $R_{MET} = 3.5$ at the end of the radiation course, and the patient died 5 months later from a massive tumoral recurrence growing from the superficial dura.

Early effects of intraarterial chemotherapy

Eight patients were examined before and after a first intra-arterial chemotherapy course, following a protocol further described in this volume by J. THERON et al. (slow infusion of 150 mg BCNU after surpa-ophtalmic internal carotid artery catheterism). In five patients, chemotherapy followed a partial surgical removal of the tumor, before any radiation therapy. In the three other patients, chemotherapy was performed for a tumor recurrence after surgery then radiotherapy. In all patients, the first course of chemotherapy was followed by other courses, each every 6 weeks. In the first five patients, a radiation therapy (60 Gy-tumor in 6 weeks) was performed between the first and the second chemotherapy course. Patients were classified in two groups depending on the clinical outcome:

— group 1 ($n = 3$): improvement (way back to previous activities, complete daily life autonomy) ;

— group 2 ($n = 5$): no improvement (including no complete independance for daily life activities), worsening or death.

The analysis of tumoral activity modifications after chemotherapy ($R = \frac{R_{MET}\text{ post-chemo}}{R_{MET}\text{ pre-chemo}}$) shows (table III) a decrease of the tumor metabolic activity after chemotherapy in group 1 patients ($R = 0.76 \pm 0.17$), but no change in group 2 ($R = 0.98 \pm 0.06$). The difference between both groups (test of Fischer-Peritz) is significant ($p = 0.05$). From this preliminary study, the measurement of ^{11}C-L-methionine uptake therefore seems providing an early assessment of the intraarterial chemotherapy efficiency, with a predictive value for the clinical response along the treatment.

In the same group of eight patients, we studied modifications of R_{Ga} and of blood polyamines levels (spermine and spermidine) before and after the first chemotherapy course. No correlation was disclosed between variations of those parameters and the clinical evolution.

TABLE III
EFFECTS OF INTRA-ARTERIAL CHEMOTHERAPY

Patient	Group. A. Surgery B. Surg + RTH	Grade	M E T - Activ. Ratio tum/norm		^{68}Ga - Activ. Ratio tum/norm		Polyamines Sp Spd		Lenght FW	Clinical Evolution 1. Improvement 2. Stationary 3. Worse 4. Died
			BEFORE	AFTER	BEFORE	AFTER	BEFORE	AFTER		
CHA. D.	A	GBL Left Temporal	1.57	1.37	1.48	1.70	6.04 20.65	9.35 17.5	2 m.	1
HEN. D.	A	III-IV Left Fronto-temporal	1.80	1.51	1.46	1.33	7.21 23.06	10.3 7.1	7 m.	1
LEG. D.	B	GBL Right Frontal	2.00	1.20					17 m.	1
CHE. L.	A	GBL Left Frontal	2.49	2.34	1.40	1.42	8.2 22.6	14.35 51.75	6 m.	2
MOY. F.	B	IV Left Frontal	2.16	1.98	1.20	1.11	9.89 35.25	30.55 106.8	5 m.	2
TRE. J.P.	A	III Left Temporal	1.81	1.99	1.03	1.01	10.3 11.7	11.6 12.3	7 m.	2
DUP. I.	B	GBL Right Frontal	1.30	1.22	1.15	1.01	9.8 11.8	6 11.7	5 m.	3
MAH. G.	A	IV Right Frontal	3.26	3.20	1.50	1.40	9.20 11.43	3.25 5.96	6 m.	4

DISCUSSION

L-methionine is an amino acid uptaken in brain tissue by a facilitated carrying system. In healthy brain tissue, L-methionine is for its greatest part incorporated to protein synthesis, the demethylation route being negligible (2, 3). The injection of L-methionine labeled with ^{11}C on the methyl radical therefore allows brain protein synthesis measurement, which was used in the study of Alzheimer dementias (4). Tumor tissue, in experimental situations or in man, uptakes L-methionine and D-methionine (5) (the latter is not uptaken by normal brain tissue). In tumor cells, the fraction of demethylated methionine (not incorporated to brain protein synthesis) is unknown but probably high. Quantitative assessment of tumor protein synthesis therefore is not available by this method. Nevertheless, it is possible to measure the methionine uptake, and to compare the following activity respectively in tumor and normal brain.

Another study (6) showed a correlation between this uptake level and the degree of tumor anaplasia. Our study confirmed this as concerns the difference between grades II on one hand, III or IV on the other. Some studies using an energy metabolism marker, the ^{18}F-deoxyglucose, disclosed a significant difference between each of the histological grades I to IV (7). But those studies included a greater number of patients than our own series. Another work, using ^{11}C-methyl-glucose, another energy metabolism marker, suggested that ^{11}C-L-methionine uptake allows a more precise delineation of the true tumor spreading.

Assessment of the intraarterial chemotherapy response is of the utmost importance in the present study. It should be very important to have a method for predicting the long term efficiency of a treatment at its very beginning and therefore to change early the chemotherapy protocol. Our eight patients series nevertheless is by far too short, with too much heterogeneity in clinical circumstances and length of follow-up, to allow firm conclusions. But it provides new perspectives in a field where we had until the present time only in vitro antimitograms after tumor cells culturing, this technic being time consuming and not usable in most clinical circumstances.

To conclude, PET is a tool which should provide in the next years a better understanding of glial tumor biology and their response to new therapies. Beside the use of structural (^{11}C-L-methionine) or energy (^{15}O, ^{18}F-FDG, ^{11}C-methyl glucose) metabolism markers, the investigation of other metabolic routes (polyamines) will possibly be of great interest.

SUMMARY

In 22 patients with supratentorial gliomas (grades II to IV), ^{11}C-L-methionine was measured with positron emission tomography (PET). For each case, we computed the ratio R between intra-tumoral activity and activity in the healthy brain tissue of homologous contra lateral area. A significant relationship between R and the histological tumor grade was demonstrated. A significant decrease of R was observed after radiotherapy in grade IV gliomas (3 cases). In 8 patients submitted to intracarotid BCNU chemotherapy, a significant decrease fo R after the first course of treatment was predictive of a good clinical outcome.

KEY WORDS

Positron, Methionine Uptake, Polyamines, Radiotherapy, Chemotherapy,

REFERENCES

1. BUSTANY (P.), CHATEL (M.), DERLON (J.M.), DARCEL (F.), SGOUROPOULOS (P.), SOUSSALINE (F.), SYROTA (A.): Brain tumor protein synthesis and histological grades: A study by positron emission tomography (PET) with C^{11}-L-Methionine. Journal of Neuro-Oncology, **3**, 397-404 (1986).

2. BUSTANY (P.), HENRY (J.F.), DE ROTROU (J.), SIGNORET (P.), CABANIS (E.), ZARIFIAN (E.), ZIEGLER (M.), DERLON (J.M.), CROUZEL (C.), SOUSSALINE (F.), COMAR (D.): Çorrelations between clinical state and positron emission tomography measurement of local brain protein synthesis in Alzeimer's dementia, Parkinson's desease, schizophrenia, and gliomas. (The Metabolism of the Human Brain Studied with Positron Emission Tomography, Greitz T. et al., Raven Press, New-York, 1985).

3. PHELPS (M.E.), BARRIO (J.R.), HUANG (S.C.), KEEN (R.E.), CHUGANI (H.), MAZZIOTTA (J.C.): Measurement of cerebral protein synthesis in Man with positron computerized tomography: model, assumptions, and preliminary results. (The Metabolism of the Human Brain Studied With Positron Emmision Tomography, Greitz T. et al., Raven Press, New York, 1985).

4. BUSTANY (P.), HENRY (J.F.), SOUSSALINE (F.), COMAR (D.): Brain protein systhesis in normal and demented patients: A study by positron emission with ^{11}C-L-Methionine. (Functional Radionuclide Imaging of the Brain, Magistretti Ph. L., Raven Press, New York, 1983).

5. MEYER (G.J.), SCHOBER (O.), HUNDESHAGEN (H.): Uptake of ^{11}C-L-and D-Methionine in brain tumors. Eur. J. Nucl., **10**: 373-376 (1985).

6. LILJA (A.), BERGSTROM (K.), HARTVIG (P.), SPANNARE (B.), HALLDIN (C.), LUNDQVIST (H.), LANGSTROM (B.): Dynamic study of supratentorial gliomas with L-methyl-^{11}C-methionine and positron emission tomography. A. JNR, 6: 505-604 (July/Agust 1985).

7. DI CHIRO (G.), ROBERT (L.), DELAPAZ (L.), RODNEY (A.), BROOKS (Ph. D.), SOKOLOFF (L.), KORNBLITH (P. L.), SMITH (B.H.), PATRONAS (N.J.), KUFTA (C.V.), KESSLER (R.M.), JOHNSTON (G.S.), MANNING (R.G.), WOLF (A.P.): Neurology, **32**, 12: 1323-1329 (1982).

8. BERGSTROM (M.), PETER COLLINS (V.), EHRIN (E.), ERICSON (K.), ERIKSSON (L.), GREITZ (T.), HALLDIN (C.), VON HOLST (H.), LANGSTROM (B.), LILJA (A.), LUNDQVIST (H.), NAGREN (K.): Discrepancies in brain tumor extent as shown by computed tomography and positron emission tomography ysing ^{68}Ga-EDTA, ^{11}C-Glucose, and ^{11}C-Methionine. Journal of computer Assisted Tomography, **7** (6): 1062-1066, (Raven Press, New York, December 1983).

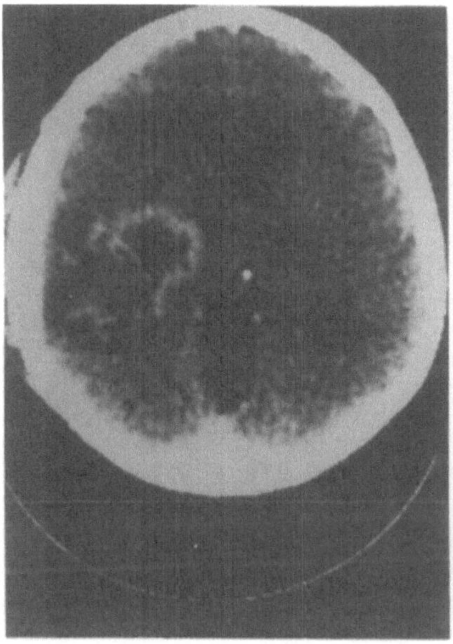

Left
Post-operative CT-scanner showing contrast uptake mainly located in deep structures, in the right hemisphere.

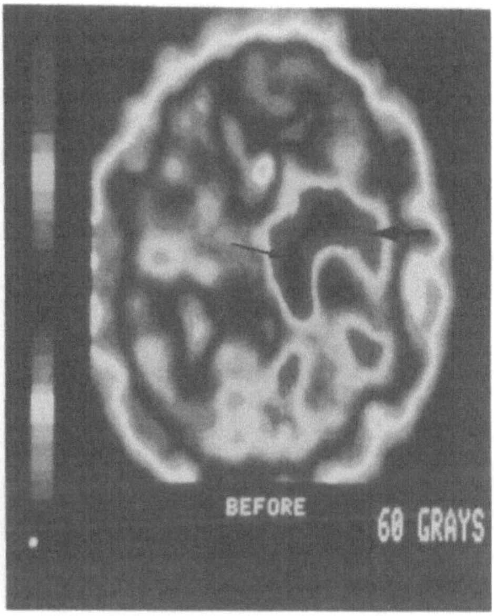

Middle
Pre-radiotherapy PET-scanner showing two loci of increased ^{11}C-MET uptake: deep (thin arrow, $R_{MET} = 2.5$) and superficial (large arrow, $R_{MET} = 1.5$).

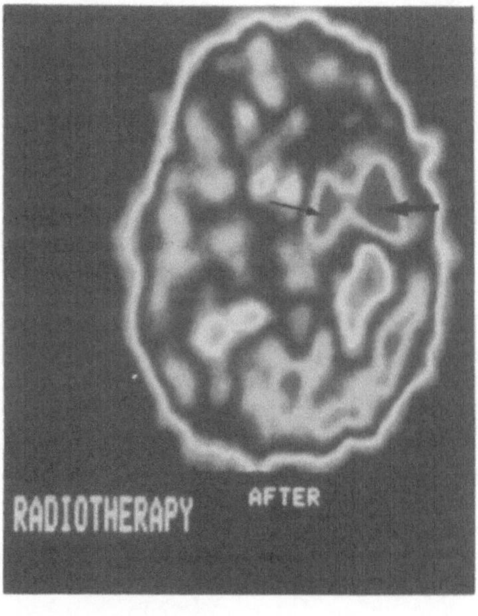

Left
Post-radiotherapy PET-scanner showing a decrease of the methionine uptake in the deep focus ($R_{MET} = 1.2$) but an increase ($R_{MET} = 3.5$) in the superficial one, not included in the radiation field.

FIGURE 1.
REGIONAL EFFECTS OF RADIOTHERAPY — Patient operated of a right temporal grade IV astrocytoma.

Positron Emission Tomography with 11-C-Methionine of Intracranial Tumours compared with Histology of Multiple Biopsies

M. MOSSKIN (°), V.P. COLLINS (°), H. VON HOLST (°), G. NORÉN (°), M. BERGSTRÖM (°).

Patients with clinically suspected intracranial tumours are as a rule examined with computed tomography before and after intravenous injection of contrast medium. This is often sufficient to establish an accurate diagnosis especially in tumours which enhance after contrast injection. Expanding lesions which only lower the attenuation diffusely are much more difficult to delineate.

At the department of neuroradiology of Karolinska Hospital, we have studied intracranial tumours with Positron Emission Tomography using various tracers since 1982. We use 68-Ga-EDTA as a tracer of blood brain barrier disruption and 11-C-glucose to study glucose metabolism. 11-C-methionine was originally introduced with the intention to study protein metabolism. It is quite clear that this tracer shows a cluster of metabolic events. However irrespective of the uptake mechanism, methionine turned out to accumulate in most tumours in an interesting way, hence tumour growth could be better diagnosed.

In order to study the correlation between the extension and histology of supratentorial gliomas and their accumulation of methionine, 38 patients were examined. All examinations were done with the head fixed in an individually made plastic helmet fixed to a baseplate. This fixation allows identical slices to be taken at different occasions. CT was made in all patients before and after contrast medium injection as well as PET using methionine. A stereotactic biopsy using multiple targets was then made guided by the PET examination. A localization box fixed to the baseplate and containing tubes filled with 68-Ga-EDTA supplies reference points for the determination of the stereotaxic coordinates. The baseplate used at CT and PET also serves as a fixation for the stereotactic biopsy instrument.

Histology of the 38 cases was classified according to W.H.O. and grading of Kernohan. Low attenuating lesions without disruption of the blood brain barrier were primarily selected for the study.

32 of 38 cases showed increased accumulation of methionine. Increased accumulation is defined as an uptake higher than that of normal brain. 3 cases showed decreased accumulation and 3 cases accumulation equal to that of normal brain. 4 of these cases were astrocytomas and 2 reactive gliosis.

In 12 cases, there was increased accumulation of methionine combined with a blood brain barrier disruption. All anaplastic astrocytomas and glioblastomas belonged to this group.

In 20 cases, there was increased accumulation of methionine without any trace of blood brain barrier disruption. Histology showed astrocytoma or oligodendroglioma. PET using methionine proved to be of great help to diagnose these tumours correctly.

How reliable is the increased methionine uptake as an indicator of tumour growth? In 22 of the 32 cases with increased uptake, the accumulation of methionine corresponded to the extension of the tumour, as evaluated by stereotactic biopsy.

In 5 cases, tumour growth existed outside the increased accumulation of methionine as determined from one or several biopsies. In 5 of the cases, histology seemed to show a smaller tumour than PET using methionine in that no tumour cells were found in areas with measured uptake. The discrepancies did not seem to be correlated with any particular type of glioma.

(°) *Dept. of Neuroradiology, Tumourpathology and Neurosurgery, Karolinska Hospital, Stockholm, Sweden.*

M. Chatel, F. Darcel and J. Pecker (eds.), Brain Oncology. ISBN-13: 978-94-010-8003-3

The delineation of the tumour was more accurate with PET using methionine than with CT in 24 cases. This is due to the fact that it is often impossible to differentiate a low attenuating tumour from edema, while PET using methionine often shows tumour tissue clearly. In 2 cases PET was less accurate that CT and diffusely growing tumour tissue was found outside the methionine accumulation as in this case of a large frontal astrocytoma.

Histology may be too crude an instrument to differentiate between tumours with different metabolic characteristics. May be PET using metabolic tracers could be more efficient than histology to characterize the biologic nature of tumours.

SUMMARY

1. *Increased accumulation of methionine occured in 32 of 36 gliomas and seems to indicate viable tumour tissue.*
2. *In cases without increased methionine uptake in the entire tumour or in part of it, the delineation of tumour tissue guided by the methionine uptake must be inexact.*
3. *In other cases, a good correlation exists between accumulation of methionine and extension of tumour.*
4. *Delineation of tumour was more accurate with PET using methionine than with CT in 2/3 of the cases.*
5. *Accumulation of methionine lower or equal to ordinary brain tissues indicates astrocytoma or reactive gliosis.*

KEY WORDS

Aminoacid uptake, Methionine, Gliomas, Grading, Positron, PET.

Neuropathology and Regional Imaging of Microcirculation, Tissue pH, Metabolites and Necroses in Cerebral RG2 and F98 Anaplastic Rat Glioma Transplantation Tumors

W. WECHSLER, U. TESKE, G. REIFENBERGER, M. DECKERT, R.J. SEITZ (°), G. MIES (°°), W. PASCHEN (°°) and K.-A. HOSSMANN (°°).

INTRODUCTION

Malignant human gliomas corresponding to grade III and IV are anaplastic ependymomas, anaplastic astrocytomas, anaplastic oligodendrogliomas, anaplastic mixed gliomas and the glioblastoma group (WHO classification, 43). These high-grade gliomas are characterized by an increased rate of cell proliferation and by special regressive changes, such as mucoid and fatty degeneration, cyst formation and in particular by tumor necrobiosis and/or necrosis (33, 46). Size and kind of necroses, however, vary with regard to tumor type and tumor grade. Whereas anaplastic gliomas contain by definition multiple and sometimes abundant necrotic foci, in glioblastomas microscopic necroses of the pseudopalisading type occur as well as macroscopically visible large areas of multicentric necroses.

The pathogenesis of tumor necroses in human malignant gliomas is not well understood. Various factors are discussed to be of importance, e.g. differences in the tumor vascularization detectable by angiography and by morphometric neuropathological analysis with reference to special patterns of the microvasculature of the different tumor types (36), sometimes in combination with BBB, i.e. blood brain barrier disturbances (37). From these data it was assumed that circulatory stasis and regional ischemia should be responsible for tumor necrosis in the first place, perhaps aggravated by stenosis and thrombotic occlusion of tumor blood vessels (46) and by BBB-disturbances. More recently, metabolic peculiarities of both human and experimental brain tumors have been studied (4, 16, 31).

Apart from morphological alterations of tumor tissue in comparison to the histological appearance of normal brain tissue there also exist distinct biochemical and hemodynamic differences between both tissues. Tumor tissue was shown to possess a much lower rate of ATP utilization (18) and to satisfy its energy demand even under normoxic conditions by glycolysis (« aerobic » glycolysis) rather than by oxidative phosphorylation (Warburg, 45). Since aerobic glycolysis is associated with a high lactic acid formation, tumor tissue acidosis was thought to be responsible for the onset of tumor necrosis being amplified during systemic hyperglycemia (1, 5, 19). However, in recent studies on local tumor tissue pH (20, 27, 32) it could be shown that tissue pH of tumor was the same or distinctly higher, i.e. more alkaline, than that of normal brain tissue during normoglycemia and systemic hyperglycemia (MIES et al., International Congress of Neuropathology, September 1986). In autoradiographic studies of local tumor perfusion, focal reductions of flow rates occurred in the central part of the tumor mass where tumor necrosis was seen most frequently (14, 16). Considering the high metabolic rates of tumor tissue, it may be speculated that restriction of glucose delivery to the tumor is more important than tumor tissue acidosis for inducing energy failure and subsequent tumor necrosis. On the other hand, impaired microcirculation of tumor tissue may limit the clearance of acidic equivalents or other toxic waste products thus impairing energy production of tumor tissue (17).

The evaluation of these data is now possible since new methods became available in clinical research (PET). In experimental oncology, VAUPEL (41) studied tumor vascularization, blood flow, oxygen and glucose content *in vivo* in the so called isolated rat transplantation tumor of the kidney

Department of Neuropathology and (°) Department of Neurology, University of Düsseldorf, (°°) Max-Planck-Institut für Neurologische Forschung, Department of Experimental Neurology, Cologne, FRG.

M. Chatel, F. Darcel and J. Pecker (eds.), Brain Oncology. ISBN-13: 978-94-010-8003-3

(DS-carcinosarcoma) and concluded that both oxygen and glucose are essential for tumor metabolism, influencing tumor growth and tumor necrosis. It was postulated that reduced glucose availability is limitating cell proliferation and lack of oxygen is responsible for cell and tissue necrosis. Another *in vivo* technique of a « tissue isolated rat tumor » (MORRIS hepatomas, WALKER carcinosarcoma 256) was developed by SAUER et al. (35) in order to study the utilization of glutamine, ketone bodies, and lactate. Their results suggest that these tumors use oxidation of glucose via aerobic glycolysis depending on substrate availability. Morphological and physiological aspects of the microcirculation in malignant tumors are of increasing importance (42). To measure pathophysiological and metabolic parameters under even more defined conditions, multicellular three dimensional tumor spheroids in culture have become another tool of great significance (8, 24, 25, 26). Tumor spheroids are an intermediate model between tumor monolayer culture and *in vivo* transplantation tumor studies in experimental neuro-oncology.

The objective of our experimental study was twofold, first to determine neuropathologically tumor growth, tumor vascularization and tumor necrosis of syngeneic intracerebral transplantation tumors in rats using two different malignant rat glioma clones, and second to compare the tumor neuropathology with the results of quantitative measurements of regional hemodynamic and metabolic parameters, especially regional blood flow, glucose and lactate content, and tissue pH (17). The two CDF rat glioma clones were established in our laboratory : RG2 is considered as a poorly differentiated anaplastic glioma cell type, while the clone F98 represents an anaplastic cell type with some gliosarcomatous characteristics.

MATERIAL AND METHODS

The primary CNS tumors for the rat glioma clones RG2 and F98 had been induced transplacentally during late fetal gestation by systemic administration of ENU to pregnant inbred CDF rats with the major histocompatibility system H1-1. RG2 and F98 are considered as anaplastic glioma clones ; the morphology in monolayer cultures has been described originally by KO et al. (21) and by KO and KOESTNER (22). According to our experience both clones appear to be rather stable phenotypically. The clones were grown in DMEM supplemented with 5 % fetal calf serum and antibiotics in a humidified atmosphere of an incubator at 37 °C with 5 % CO_2. No mycoplasm contamination could be detected, according to regular examinations by FLOW LABORATORIES.

Cell suspensions of 10^2, 10^3, 10^4, and 10^5 RG2 cells, suspended in 10 μl of DMEM were implanted stereotactically into the right caudate nucleus of adult anesthesized syngeneic rats. For F98 intracerebral transplantation tumors, adult CDF animals received preferentially 10^3 cells by the same stereotactic procedure. Groups of animals were killed in deep ether narcosis after different survival periods, i.e. 5 - 26 days. The brains were immediately removed and either fixed in 4 % buffered formaldehyde or in 70 % ethanol and afterwards routinely processed for neuropathological examination by light microscopy. For immunohistochemistry we used PAP, ABC, and immunofluorescence techniques to determine the immunoreactivity for GFAP, vimentin, neurofilaments, actin, tubulin, cytokeratin, but also for protein S100, NSE, Leu-7, Leu-M1 and fibronectin.

For the morphometric evaluation of the tumor vasculature (vessel volume, diameter, surface and length) and the percentage of tumor necrosis TESKE (40) used for RG2 tumors methods described by CHALKLEY et al. (10) and adapted for tumors by HILMAS and GILETTE (15). These methods could be validated by improved techniques with controlled cardiac perfusion in deep anesthesia and a newly developed technique to visualize vascular endothelia selectively by Ricinus Communis Agglutinin (RCA I) in a ABC procedure (SEITZ, unpublished data). In the latter experiments tumor growth, tumor vascularization and tumor necrosis were evaluated morphometrically by use of an interative image analysing system (IBAS I, Kontron).

Regional blood flow, content of glucose, lactate and ATP, glucose utilization, and local tissue pH were measured quantitatively by autoradiographic, bioluminiscence and fluoroscopic methods in cryostat sections ; for details see HOSSMANN et al. (17).

RESULTS

I. Neuropathology

RG2 and F98 glioma clones can be considered as homogeneous modes for studying anaplastic glioma growth in spite of the fact that both clones present cytologically and histologically some differences in growth behavior. In culture, these clones can be grown as monolayers and as spheroids. The **characteristics of in vitro growth** are summarized in table 1 with respect to doubling time, saturation density, and plating efficiency for monolayer cultures, and with respect to maximal diameter, regressive changes (necrosis, cystic degeneration), adhesiveness, and cell density for spheroids.

TABLE 1: Experimental CDF Rat Glioma Clones in Culture

Culture	RG2	F98
Monolayer		
Plating Efficency (PE)	30 %	50 %
Doubling Time (TD)	18 h	15 h
Saturation Density (SD)	8 x 10^5/cm²	1.8 x 10^6/cm²
Spheroid		
Maximal Diameter	600 um	800 um
Central Necrosis	small	small
Cystic Alterations	?	yes
Doubling Diameter	3 - 12 d	3 - 8 d
Cell Density	medium	high

Early log phases of RG2 monolayers show relatively small fusiform, or stellate cells with fine and long processes and a three dimensional appearance (fig. 1a + b). F98 cells are also of a homogenous bi- and mostly multipolar appearance with a more flattened and larger cell body and shorter processes, but also with a high nuclear-cytoplasmic ratio and irregular cytoplasmic vacuoles (fig. 2a + b). Late log phases and stationary phase cultures demonstrate morphological differences in a better way, especially at higher cellular density for F98 cells with pseudostriated package and a tendency towards multilayered foci when compared with RG2 cultures. Immunocytochemical studies of RG2 monolayer cultures are summarized in table 2; the expression of cytoskeletal proteins indicates similar results for log and stationary phases with prominent vimentin reaction and only minimal and irregular amounts of GFAP in individual cells. S100 protein is variable.

RG2 and F98 spheroids show some differences: while RG2 spheroids are rather fragile with an irregular shape and a loose surface (fig. 1c), F98 spheroids have a higher cell density, a solid and sticky cellular adhesion, a smooth surface and a spherical shape (fig. 2c). Medium and large spheroids of both clones apparently present no large and complete central tissue necrosis with a sharply demarcated zone towards the surrounding peripheral wall of viable and proliferating cells. Regressive changes are of minor importance and follow more an irregular way of cellular necrobiosis with some relation to spheroid size classes (fig. 1d). F98 spheroids present microcystic degeneration in the centre, in the periphery or in the whole spheroid, probably depending on culture conditions (fig. 2d). Multiple mitotic activity occurs in both RG2 and F98 spheroids, especially in the periphery, but also in a reduced way in the centre.

TABLE 2: Studies on the Cytoskeleton of RG2 Glioma Clone in Monolayer Cultures

Immunofluorescence	log phase	stationary phase
Vimentin	+++	+++
GFAP	+	+
Neurofilaments	0	0
Actin	+	+
Tubulin	+	+
Desmin	0	0
Cytokeratin 18	0	0

Tendency of the immunofluorescence reactions: 0 = negative, + = weak and/or rare, ++ = moderate and/or variable, ++ = strong and/or the majority of cells.

In vivo, the neuropathology of spherical **intracerebral RG2 and F98 tumors** is that of a rapidly growing polymitotic anaplastic glioma with many similarities, but also with some differences. All tumors are sharply demarcated against the edematous surrounding brain tissue. Infiltration of the lateral ventricle may occur, while meningeal spreading is rare. RG2 tumors are highly cellular tumors composed of cells with an irregular package and a loose, sometimes serum enriched interstitium; no reticulin fibres are detectable (fig. 3b). F98 tumors are also polymitotic tumors in which the tumor cells are more closely packed and have a marked tendency to grow in a streaming pattern with very fine and delicate reticulin fibres in the intercellular space (fig. 4). The presence of reticulin fibres varies within one tumor and from tumor to tumor. PAS-positive material and collagen are absent. Numerous mitoses appear in all tumors and in nearly all portions of the tumors with no apparent difference between tumor periphery and tumor centre. Quantitative evaluation of mitotic activity has not been obtained so far.

To characterize differentiation properties of RG2 and F98 tumors, **immunohistochemistry** with respect to proteins of the cytoskeleton and other cell markers has been applied to transplantation tumors of different sizes and of different ages (table 3). Negative results were obtained for NSE, neurofilaments, Leu-7 and Leu-M1. RG2 tumors express only small amounts of S100 protein (fig. 3b) and very rarely GFAP in single medium-sized and larger tumor cells and their processes (fig. 3d). Vimentin is present in a large, however, varying amount of the tumor cell population and visible especially in the cytoplasm of the cell bodies (fig. 3c). To our surprise, F98 tumors express small amounts of S100 in individual tumor cells, a higher degree of GFAP in single cells and sometimes in small areas of the tumors, and large amounts of vimentin in numerous, sometimes nearly all tumor cells. Moreover, the tumors were strongly positive for fibronectin (fig. 5a-d).

TABLE 3: Immunohistochemistry of Intracerebral RG2 and F98 Transplantation Tumors in Adult CDF-Rats

	Glioma Clone RG2	Glioma Clone F98
Vimentin	+++	+++
GFAP	+	++
Neurofilaments	—	—
NSE	—	—
S 100	+	+
Leu-7	—	—
Leu-M1	—	—
Fibronectin	—	+++

—: negative, +: less than 10 % of cells positive, ++: 10 % — 50 % of cells positive, +++: 50 % — 90 % of cells positive, ++++: 90 % — 100 % of cells positive.

Tumor growth was studied by TESKE (40) morphometrically in RG2 tumors depending on the initial cell number. The mean survival time of animal groups was 13 days for 10^5 cells, 16 days for 10^4 cells, 22 days for 10^3 cells, and 24 days for all animals receiving 10^2 RG2 cells. As an example, the results of 10^4 RG2 cells induced tumors are summarized with respect to **tumor vascularization** and the percentage of necrotic foci (table 4). After an initial avascular phase, proliferation of small tumor vessels is dependent on the tumor size and the tumor growth in days. Both the relative vessel volume and the mean vessel diameter per tumor reference area increase over time, whereas the ratio of vascular surface area and especially the vessel length decline. At present we are studying RG2 transplantation tumors with more sophisticated techniques, e.g. the selective staining of the vascular endothelia by RCA I, by controlled cardiac perfusion and IBAS I analysis (fig. 6, SEITZ et al., unpublished data). Histopathologically, F98 intracerebral transplantation tumors contain similarly to RG2 tumors in routine paraffin sections only a small amount of narrow or ectatic vessels with very thin walls ; morphometric measurements have not been carried out so far. It is evident that studies concerning tumor vascularization of anaplastic cerebral gliomas must be performed with special techniques.

TABLE 4: Stereotactic Intracerebral Implantation of 10^4 RG2 Cells: Morphometric Evaluation of Tumor Necrosis and Tumor Vascularisation (TESKE 1986)

N° of Animals	Mean Survival days	Volume %	Vascularization (mean values) Surface mm^2/mm^3	Diameter um	Necrosis (%) Length mm/mm^3	Mean	Range
4	17	6	690	18	12	4	0-9
3	16	6	680	18	12	9	2-22
3	14	4	690	13	17	16	11-20
3	12	4	830	10	27	1	0-2

Regressive changes such as **tumor necroses** are irregular from tumor to tumor. Therefore it is difficult to assess exact quantitative data for intracerebral RG2 and F98 transplantation tumors. In this context it should be mentioned that intracerebral transplantation tumors can grow only to a relatively small maximal size determined by neurological deterioration and due to final brain death, in contrast to subcutaneous or renal transplantation tumors. Subcutaneous and renal RG2 transplantation tumors can reach a 10-50 fold size compared to intracerebral tumors, therefore necroses are more pronounced in the non-cerebral transplantation tumors. In the rat brain our studies indicate that microscopic foci of necrosis may disappear during progressive tumor growth due to absorption of the necrotic debris and the proliferation of tumor cells and blood vessels from the neighbourhood, a phenomenon which is illustrated in table 4: tumors 14 days after implantation present the highest percentage of necrosis, i.e. 16 %, while tumors from animals with 16 and 17 days of mean survival show a decline of tumor necroses towards 9 % and 5 %, respectively. All RG2 tumors between 14 and 17 days show a broad range of necrotic volume as an indicator for the irregularity of necrotic events, a phenomenon which is absent in initial and small tumors (table 4). In general, we are inclined to believe that multiple foci of necrosis located irregularly in central or peripheral portions occur more frequently in F98 tumors than in RG2 tumors. Necroses in RG2 tumors appear to be accompanied by protein-rich interstitial fluid and sometimes in combination with cyst formation (fig. 3c), while small and large necroses in F98 tumors are sharply delineated and more of the coagulation-type of necrosis (fig. 4).

II. Pathophysiology and Metabolism

In general, **regional blood flow** is irregular and has a tendency to decrease sometimes markedly from the periphery towards the central portion of the larger tumors. In solid, viable tumor areas the regional blood flow was found to be similar to that of normal grey matter, but hyperemic and hypoemic foci were measured as well. In F98 tumors regional blood flow was absent in tumors with large central or peripheral necroses, whereas in viable portions of the tumors regional blood flow appeared more variable. Blood flow was found to be slightly reduced in the peritumorous edema regions and not in the contralateral hemisphere (fig. 8a).

Regional **content of glucose** was fairly low in both RG2 (fig. 7b) and F98 medium sized and large intracerebral tumors and a declining glucose gradient of concentrations from the tumor periphery to central portions was frequently observed. Tumor glucose content was considerably lower than in the grey matter of ipsi — and contralateral portions of the brain. In contrast, regional **glucose utilization** in tumor tissue was two — to threefold higher in comparison to normal or to edematous brain tissue (fig. 8b). Quantitative assessment of **ATP** in RG2 (fig. 7c) and F98 tumors revealed higher values in tumor tissues when compared with normal brain. Similar results were obtained for the **lactate content** in tumors, which was consistently higher than in normal brain areas (fig. 8d). Quantitative evaluation in F98 tumors demonstrated a fivefold increase of lactate content in the tumor tissue and a twofold increase in the peritumorous edematous zones. Respective metabolite contents of F98 tumors in relation to other brain areas are summarized in table 5.

To measure **regional tissue** pH two methods were used, the *in vitro* umbelliferone method (11) and the autoradiographic ^{14}C-DMO technique (23). As examplified by MIES et al. (27), both techniques offer adequate and similar results in the rat brain under normal and pathological conditions. Most of the intracerebral RG2 and F98 tumors investigated were slightly more alkaline than normal brain tissue (fig. 8c). Quantification of tissue pH in solid regions of F98 gliomas revealed an average value of 7.26 which is about 0.1 units higher than the contralateral grey matter and 0.05 units lower than the value obtained from the peritumoral edematous cortex and grey matter. Similar values were found to be adequate for RG2 tumors. Regions of acidic tissue pH as low as 6.2 were observed only in small areas of the tumors, most frequently related to tumor vessels and their surroundings.

TABLE 5: Quantitative Data of Regional Metabolism and Tissue pH of Intracerebral F98 Transplantation Tumors (HOSSMANN et al. 1986)

Parameter	Region	Ipsilateral	Contralateral
ATP	Tumor	2.58 ± 0.15	——
(μmol/g)	Cortex	2.18 ± 0.27	2.14 ± 0.25
Glucose	Tumor	2.41 ± 0.38	——
(μmol/g)	Cortex	3.55 ± 0.12	2.77 ± 0.10
Lactate	Tumor	6.35 ± 0.46	——
(μmol/g)	Cortex	3.37 ± 0.30	1.32 ± 0.09
pH	Tumor	7.26 ± 0.09	——
	Cortex	7.31 ± 0.05	7.17 ± 0.05

DISCUSSION

The pathogenesis of tumor necroses in malignant human gliomas and in experimental anaplastic gliomas has been a neglected area of research in neuro-oncology for a long time. Tumor tissue necroses in gliomas appear to be dependent on several factors. Especially the hemodynamic and metabolic pathomechanisms of spontaneous tumor tissue necrosis are not yet well understood. For this reason, the relationship between morphological characteristics of tumor tissue, tumor blood flow, tumor glycolysis, the energy - and acid-base status of the tumor tissue was investigated in experimental brain tumors and analysed with recently developed imaging techniques. These allow the local evaluation of the corresponding parameters on intact brain sections thus enabling a precise correlation between hemodynamic and metabolic alterations of tumor tissue and the histological appearance of tumors.

Since the evaluation of these factors and parameters in human malignant gliomas is difficult, we studied tumor growth, tumor vascularization and the development of tumor necrosis in a wel defined experimental system using syngeneic intracerebral transplantation tumors of two different and phenotypically stable malignant glioma clones in adult rat brains. The clones RG2 and F98 represent both rapidly proliferating cells in culture and in vivo. RG2 represents an anaplastic poorly differentiated glioma cell type expressing vimentin and minimal amounts of GFAP and protein S100, while F98 is an even more rapidly growing anaplastic glio-sarcomatous cell type with expression of vimentin, some GFAP and S100, but also large amounts of fibronectin sometimes in association with fine delicate reticulin fibres between the tumor cells. Our immunohistochemical results, especially the GFAP and S100 immunoreactivity (IR) in monolayer cultures, but also the results within intracerebral transplantation tumors underline the glial phenotype of these malignant tumor clones which can be conceived as immature anaplastic astrocytic clones. The strong expression of vimentin, the 57000 molecular weight protein of fibroblast filaments, is the major cytoskeletal component of immature glia (2, 12, 29). The widespread occurence of intermediate filaments of the vimentin type in cultured cells from many vertebrate cell types appears to be a common feature in cultured cells (13). Vimentin has also been observed in various human glioma cells grown in monolayer culture (30, 38, 44). Recently, SAGGU and PILKINGTON (34) demonstrated an inverse relationship between the expression of GFAP and glutamine synthetase (GS) at low and high culture passages, while the distribution of vimentin was constant irrespective of the number of culture passages. It is of interest that the two anaplastic rat glioma clones present only minimal regressive changes as spheroids (maximal diameter below 1 mm), while intracerebral transplantation tumors of medium and large size may have a 0 — 20 % volume of necrosis in the tumor tissue (table 4).

The hypothesis that vascular malnutrition with hypoperfusion and local ischemia may be involved in the development of tumor necrosis is partially supported by our morphometric findings in RG2 tumors. We found a decline in the ratio of the mean values of the vascular surface area and the vessel length with respect to increasing tumor size and tumor age (40). Interestingly, intracerebral spheric transplantation tumors may have low blood flow regions without necrosis and vice versa. Studies of regional blood flow in F98 gliomas dit not correlate exactly with the presence of necrotic areas either. Presumably due to edema and/or compression of adjacent brain tissue blood flow was reduced in the vicinity of tumors as compared to controls. Although oxygen utilization of tumors was not measured in the present study, our hemodynamic and metabolic observations are in accordance with the hypothesis that energy requirements of both anaplastic glioma types are satisfied mainly by glycolysis (17).

The role of glucose on the growth of 9L cells - an MNU induced rat tumor cell line of a gliosarcoma type — in monolayer and tumor spheroid cultures was studied by LI (24, 25). Tumor cells in these studies consume glucose at a rate about four times greater than in normal rodent brain cells. The existence of necrotic zones in multicellular spheroids and in tumors could be attributed to the lack of vital nutrients, although evidence implicating a particular lack of one component over the other remained scanty. The radius of central necrotic zones of 9L spheroids was a function of the spheroid size (diameter) and the calculated critical concentration of glucose for necrosis was below 6×10^{-5} mg/ml. Nevertheless, it would be presumptuous to designate glucose starvation as the only cause of tumor cell and tissue necrosis; other factors, such as oxygen tension, cellular waste products, the lack of other metabolites and pH should have been considered as well. Studying human glioma spheroids (8) with respect to oxygen gradients (6, 7), it was found that glioma spheroids in contrast to carcinoma and sarcoma spheroids have relatively high central pO_2 values, which were considered to be probably due to low oxygen consumption. JÄHDE et al. (19) determined the tissue pH distribution in chemically induced rat transplantation tumors of the CNS and measured pH values by microelectrodes to be between 6.8 and 7.1 in tumors weighing 1.0 — 2.5 g and 6.7 — 7.1 pH values for tumors between 4.0 — 6.0 g weight. These results suggest that extra-cellular tumor pH, in line with our results on tumor tissue pH, appears to be rather independent of the tumor size and the energy state of tumor tissue.

With respect to cerebral transplantation tumors we postulate that tissue pH seems to be a function of the production of acid metabolites, the clearance of these metabolites into the blood or CSF fluid and the buffering capacity of the tumor. Tumor regions with high ATP content were usually alkaline, whereas those with low amounts of ATP, i.e. impaired energy state, tended to be more acid than brain.

Substrate availability of oxygen and/or of glucose is definitively a function of tissue perfusion. Oxygen content of tumor tissue depends on diffusion, whereas delivery of glucose is described by fascilitated transport. Considering the existence of well developed intracellular pH regulation of tumor cells, it is postulated that tumor blood perfusion is more critical for clearance of acid equivalents or other toxic uaste products than for substrate supply, and that spontaneous tumor necrosis may result from both the accumulation of such metabolic products and the lack of nutrients. From our observations we can conclude that local tissue acidosis in anaplastic gliomas seems to be of minor significance for the pathogenesis of tumor necroses.

Whether an influence of chemical mediators, such as tumor necrosis factors, may be involved in tumor necrosis of RG2 and F98 intracerebral transplantation tumors cannot be answered so far. Tumor necrosis factor (TNF), originally discovered by CARSWELL et al. (9) and secreted by macrophages (3), has recently become available as recombinant TNF (28, 39). Both natural and recombinant TNF have been defined as a lymphotoxin, which induces haemorrhagic necrosis in methylcholantren induced sarcomas of BALB/c mice intraneoplastically and systemically.

SUMMARY

Intracerebral stereotactic inoculation of cell suspensions of the CDF anaplastic rat glioma clones RG2 and F98 into the right caudate nucleus of adult syngeneic rats leads to progressive intracerebral tumor growth with survival periods of 2 to 3 weeks dependent on the initial inoculation of 10^2 to 10^5 cells. RG2 represents a poorly differentiated anaplastic glioma cell type expressing vimentin and minimal amounts of GFAP and protein S100, while clone F98 is an even more rapidly growing anaplastic gliosarcomatous cell type with expression of vimentin, some GFAP and S100, but also large amounts of fibronectin in association with fine reticulin fibres. Tumor growth, tumor vascularization and tumor necroses were determined neuropathologically and by morphometric measurement. Cell proliferation and regressive changes were also studied in monolayer and spheroid cultures. Multifocal tumor necroses in RG2 cerebral transplantation tumors varied between 0 to 20% of the tumor volume and appeared to be of a different type in RG2 transplantation tumors compared with F98 tumors. After an initial avascular phase neoproliferation of small tumor vessels is characterized by a decline in the ratio of the mean values of the vascular surface area and the vessel length with respect to increasing tumor size and tumor age, while the relative vessel volume and the mean vessel diameter per tumor reference area increase over time. In general, regional bloodflow decreased from the tumor periphery to the central portions of the tumors, however, low regional bloodflow in F98 gliomas did not correlate exactly with the presence of necrotic areas. Quantitative measurements yield low regional glucose content, an increased rate of glucose utilization, high ATP and lactate content in association with a slightly more alkaline tumor tissue pH suggesting that aerobic glycolysis in the transplantation tumor was sufficient in satisfying tumor energy demand. Local hypoperfusion and/or tumor tissue acidosis appear to be of minor significance for the development of tumor necroses.

KEY WORDS

RG2 and F98 rat glioma clones, monolayer cultures, spheroid cultures, cerebral transplantation tumors, neuropathology, immunohistochemistry, tumor vascularization, microcirculation, metabolism, tissue pH, and tumor necroses.

AKNOWLEGDEMENTS

Supported by the Deutsche Forschungsgemeinschaft, SFB 200.

REFERENCES

1. ARDENNE VON (M.), REITNAUER (P.G.), RHODE (K.), WESTMEYER (H.): In vivo pH-Messungen in Krebs-Mikrometastasen bei optimierter Übersauerung. Z. Naturforsch. **241**: 1610-1619 (1969).
2. BIGNAMI (A.), RAJU (T.), DAHL (D.): Localization of vimentin, the non-specific intermediate filament protein, in embryonal glia and in early differentiating neurons. Developmental Biology **91**: 286-295 (1982).
3. BEUTLER (B.), GREENWALD (D.), HULMES (J.D.), CHANG (M.), PAN (Y.-C.E.), MATHISON (J.), ULEVITCH (R.), CERAMI (A.): Identity of tumour necrosis factor and the macrophage-secreted factor cachectin. Nature **316**: 552-554 (1985).
4. BLASBERG (R.G.), KOBAYASHI (T.), PATLAK (C.S.), SHINOHARA (M.), MIYOAKA (M.), RICE (J.M.), SHAPIRO (W.R.): Regional blood flow, capillary permeability, and glucose utilization in two brain tumor models: prelimminary observations and pharmacokinetic implications. Cancer Treatment Reports **65**: 3-12 (1981).
5. CALDERWOOD (S.K.), DICKSON (J.A.): Effect of hyperglycemia on blood flow, pH, and response to hyperthermia (41 C) of the Yoshida sarcoma in the rat. Cancer Res. **40**: 4728-4733 (1980).
6. CARLSSON (J.), ACKER (H.), NEDERMAN (T.), GLIMELIUS (B.): Glioma spheroids: morphology growth and extra cellular matrix. GBK-Symposium 1985, Cancer Campaign, Gustav Fischer, Stuttgart, New York (1987 in press).
7. CARLSSON (J.), STALNACKE (C.-G.), ACKER (H.), HAJI-KARIM (M.), NILSSON 0(S.), LARSSON (B.): The influence of oxygen on viability and proliferation in cellular spheroids. Int. J. Radiat. Oncol. Biol. Phys. **5**: 2011-2020 (1979).
8. CARLSSON (J.), NILSSON (K.), WESTERMARK (B.), PONTEN (J.), SUNDSTRÖM (C.), LARSSON (E.), BERGH (J.), PAHLMAN (S.), BUSCH (C.), COLLINS (V.P.): Formation and growth of multicellular spheroids of human origin. Int. J. Cancer **31**: 523-533 (1983).
9. CARSWELL (E.A.), OLD (L.J.), KASSEL (R.L.), GREEN (S.), FIORE (N.), WILLIAMSON (B.): An endotoxin-induced serum factor that causes necrosis of tumors. Proc. Nat. Acad. Sci. USA **72**: 3666-3670 (1975).
10. CHALKLEY (H.W.), CORNFIELD (J.), PARK (H.): A method for estimating volume-surface ratios. Science **110**: 295-297 (1949).
11. CSIBA (L.), PASCHEN ((W.), HOSSMANN (K.-A.): A topographic quantitative method for measuring brain tissue pH under physiological and patho-physiological condisions. Brain Res. **289**: 334-337 (1983).
12. DAHL (D.), RUEGER (D.C.), BIGNAMI (A.): Vimentin, the 57000 molecular weight protein of fibroblast filaments, is the major cytoskeletal component in immature glia. Eur. J. Cell Biol. **24**: 191-196 (1981).
13. FRANKE (W.W.), SCHMID (E.), WINTER (S.), OSBORN (M.), WEBER (K.): Widespread occurence of intermediate-sized filaments of the vimentin-type in cultured cells from diverse vertebrates. Exp. Cell Res. **123**: 25-46 (1979).
14. GROOTHUIS (D.R.), MOLNAR (P.), BLASBERG (R.G.): Regional blood flow and blood-to-tissue transport in five brain tumor models. Implications for chemotherapy. Prog. Exp. Tumor Res. **27**: 132-153 (1984).
15. HILMAS (D.E.), GILETTE (E.L.): Morphometric analyses of the microvasculature of tumors during growth and after X-irradiation. Cancer **33**: 103-110 (1974).
16. HOSSMANN (K.-A.), NIEBUHR (I.), TAMURA (M.): Local cerebral blood flow and glucose consumption of rats with experimental gliomas. J. Cereb. Blood Flow Metab. **2**: 25-32 (1982).
17. HOSSMANN (K.-A.), MIES (G.), PASCHEN (W.), SZABO (L.), DOLAN (E.), WECHSLER (W.): Regional metabolism of experimental brain tumors. Acta Neuropath. (Berl.) **69**: 139-147 (1986).
18. KIRSCH (W.M.), SCHULZ (D.), LEITNER (J.W.): The effect of prolonged ischemia upon regional energy reserves in the experimental glioblastoma. Cancer Res. **27**: 2212-2220 (1967).
19. JAHDE (E.), RAJEWSKY (M.K.), BAUMGARTL (H.): pH distributions in transplanted neural tumors and normal tissues of BDIX rats as measured with pH microelectrodes. Cancer Res. **42**: 1498-1504 (1982).
20. JUNCK (L.), BLASBERG (R.), ROTTENBERG (D.A.): Brain and tumor pH in experimental leptomeningeal carcinomatosis. Trans. Am. Neurol. Assoc. **106**: 298-301 (1981).
21. KO (L.), KOESTNER (A.): Morphologic and morphometric analyses of butyrate-induced alterations of rat glioma cells in vitro. J. Natl. Canc. Inst. **65**: 1017-1027 (1980).
22. KO (L.), KOESTNER (A.), WECHSLER (W.): Morphological characterization of nitrosourea-induced glioma cell lines and clones. Acta Neuropathol. (Berl.) **51**: 23-31 (1980).
23. KOBATAKE (K.), SAKO (K.), IZAWA (M.), YAMAMOTO (Y.L.), HAKIM (A.M.): Autoradiographic determination of brain pH following middle cerebral artery occlusion in the rat. Stroke **15**: 540-547 (1984).
24. LI (C.K.N.): The glucose distribution in 9L rat brain multicell tumor spheroids and its effect on cell necrosis. Cancer **50**: 2066-2073 (1982).
25. LI (C.K.N.): The role of glucose in the growth of 9L multicell tumor spheroids. Cancer **50**: 2074- 2078 (1982).

26. MÜLLER-KLIESER (W.): Limitierende Faktoren für die Versorgung von Tumorgeweben. Akademie der Wissenschaften und der Literatur. Funktions-analyse Biologischer Systeme 13, Franz Steiner Verlag Wiesbaden GmbH Stuttgart (1985).

27. MIES (G.), PASCHEN (W.), CSIBA (L.), KRAJEWSKI (S.), WECHSLER (W.), HOSSMANN (K.-A.): Comparison of regional tissue pH measured with the umbelliferone and ^{14}C-DMO technique in rat brain. J. Cereb. Blood Flow Metab. **5**: 247-248 (1985).

28. PENNICA (D.), NEDWIN (G.E.), HAYFLICK (J.S.), SEEBURG (P.H.), DERYNCK (R.), PALLADINO (M.A.), KOHR (W.J.), AGGARWAL (B.B.), GOEDDEL (D.V.): Human tumour necrosis factor: precursor structure, expression and homology to lymphotoxin. Nature **312**: 724-729 (1984).

29. PIXLEY (S.K.R.), DE VELLIS (J.): Transition between immature radia glia and mature astrocytes studied with a monoclonal antibody to vimentin. Developmental Brain Res. **15**: 201- 209 (1984).

30. QUINLAN (R.A.), FRANKE (W.W.): Molecular interactions in intermediate-sized filaments revealed by chemical cross-linking. Eur. J. Biochem. **132**: 477-484 (1983).

31. RHODES (C.G.), WISE (R.J.S.), GIBBS (J.M.), FRACKOWIAK (R.S.J.), HATAZAWA (J.), PALMER (A.J.) THOMAS (D.G.T.), JONES (T.): In vivo disturbance of oxidative metabolism of glucose in human cerebral gliomas. Ann. Neurol. **14**: 614-626 (1983).

32. ROTTENBERG (D.A.), GINOS (J.Z.), KEARFOTT (K.T.), JUNCK (L.), BIGNER (D.D.): In vivo measurement of regional brain tissue pH using positron emission tomography. Ann. Neurol. **15**: 98-102 (1984).

33. RUBINSTEIN (L.J.): Tumors of the central nervous system. Armed Forces Institute of Pathology, Washington (1972).

34. SAGGU (H.), PILKINGTON (G.J.): Immunocytochemical characterization of the A15 A5 transplantable brain tumour model in vivo. Neuropath. and Applied Neurobiol. **12**: 291-303 (1986).

35. SAUER (L.A.), STAYMAN III (J.W.), DAUCHY (R.T.): Amino acids, glucose, and lactic acid utilization in vivo by rat tumors. Canc. Res. **42**: 4090-4097 (1982).

36. SEITZ (R.J.), WECHSLER (W.): Vascularization of human cerebral gliomas: a lectin-cytochemical and morphometric study. Biol. of Brain Tumour, 131-137, eds. M.D. Walker and D.G.T. Thomas, M. Nijhoff. Publ., Boston (1986).

37. SEITZ (R.J.), WECHSLER (W.): Immunohistochemical demonstration of serum proteins in human cerebral gliomas. Acta Neuropath. (Berl.) (1987), in press.

38. SHARP (G.), OSBORN (M.), WEBER (K.): Occurrence of two different intermediate filament proteins in the same filament in situ within a human glioma cell line. Exp. Cell Res. **141**: 385-395 (1982).

39. SHIRAI (T.), YAMAGUCHI (H.), ITO (H.), TODD (C.W.), WALLACE (R.B.): Cloning and expression in Escherichia coli of the gene for human tumour necrosis factor. Nature **313**: 803-806 (1985).

40. TESKE (U.P.): Wachstum und Tumorvaskularisation des maglignen Rattengliomklones RG2 nach syngener intrazerebraler Implantation. Dissert. Neuropath. Inst. der Univ. Düsseldorf (1986).

41. VAUPEL (P.): Atemgaswechsel und Glucosestoffwechsel von Implantations-tumoren (DS-Carcinosarkom) in vivo. Akademie der Wissenschaften und der Literatur. Funktionsanalyse Biologischer Systeme 1, Franz Steiner Verlag Wiesbaden GmbH (1974).

42. VAUPEL (P.), HAMMERSEN (F.): Mikrozirkulation in malignen Tumoren. In: Mikrozirkulation in Forschung und Klinik, Vol. 2. Karger, Basel etc. (1982).

43. WHO: International histological classification of tumours. N° 21: Histological typing of tumours of the central nervous system. ed. K.J. Zülch (1979).

44. WANG (E.), CAIRNCROSS (J.G.), LIEM (R.K.H.): Identification of glial filament protein and vimentin in the same intermediate filament system in human glioma cells. Proc. Natl. Acad. Sci. USA **81**: 2102-2106 (1984).

45. WARBURG (O.): Über den Stoffwechsel der Tumoren. Springer, Berlin (1926).

46. ZÜLCH (K.J.): Brain tumors. Springer, Berlin, Heidelberg, New York, Tokyo (1986).

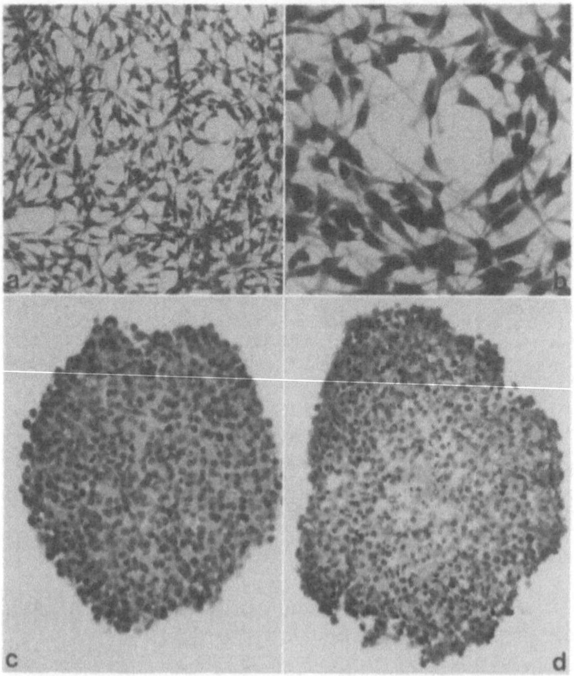

FIGURE 1. Glioma clone RG2 in monolayer and spheroid cultures. a and b early log phases with homogeneous population of stellate and fusiform cells (HE, 150 x and 300 x). RG2 spheroids: c solid vital spheroid with multiple mitoses and no central necrosis, d RG2 spheroid with light central necrobiosis. (HE, c 300 x and d 240 x).

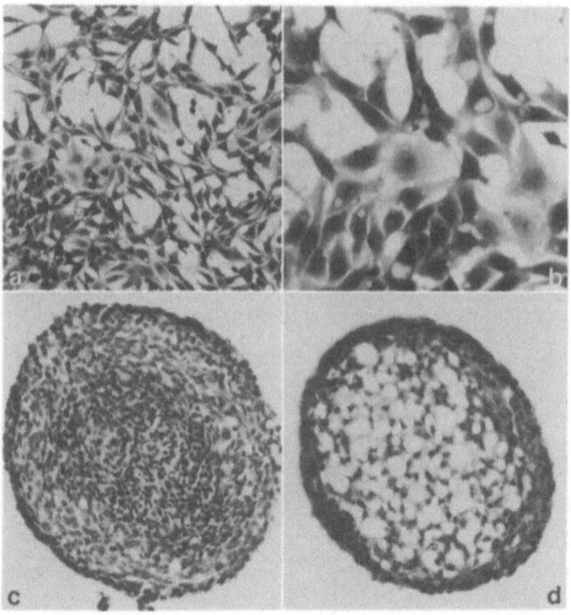

FIGURE 2. Glioma clone F98 in monolayer (a, b) and spheroid cultures (c, d). a and b log phase with semiconfluent areas containing bipolar, multipolar and stellate cells with a tendency for flat cell attachment (HE, 150 x and 300 x). Solid spheroid without necrosis (c) and extensive microcystic changes in d. (HE, c 240 x and d 300 x).

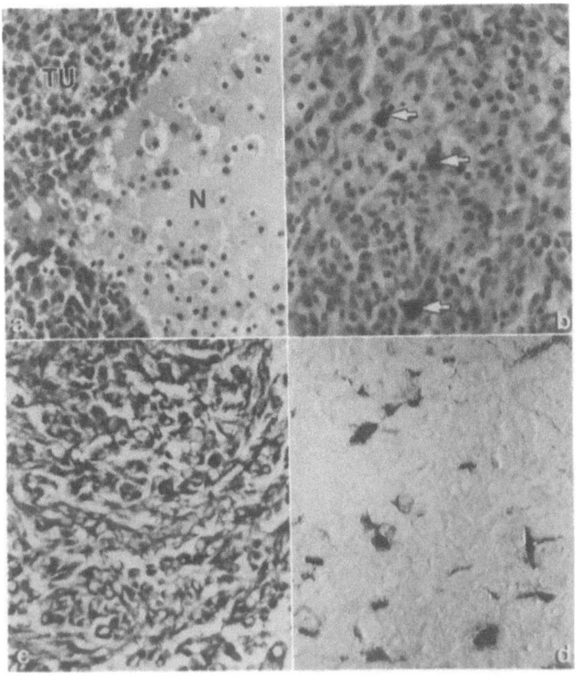

FIGURE 3. Histopathology and immunohistochemistry of intracerebral RG2 tumors. a tumor (TU) with cystic, serum-rich necrosis (N). b vital tumor area with rare S100 positive cells (◄). c High vimentin content in the cell body of the majority of tumor cells, nuclei unstained. d GFAP expression in few larger multipolar cells and their processes, nuclei unstained. (a HE, 300 x, b 380 x, c 300 x, d 350 x).

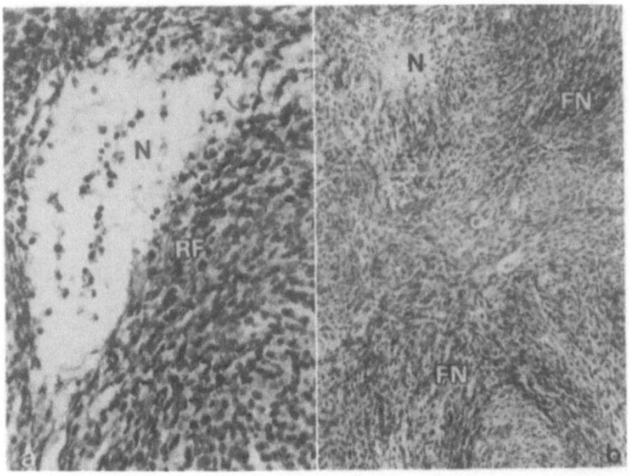

FIGURE 4. Large intracerebral F98 tumor with rhythmic streaming pattern of tumor cell growth. Note foci of necrosis (N) and fine reticulin fibres (RF) in a and in b irregular amounts of fibronectin (FN). (a Tibor-PAP, 300 x, b Fibronectin 100 x).

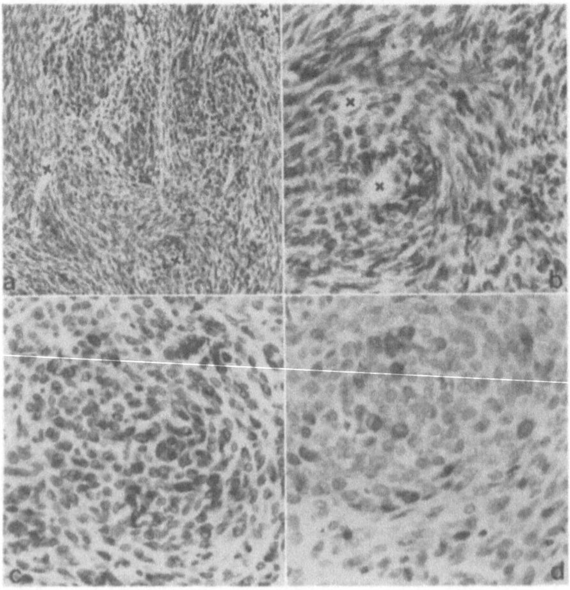

FIGURE 5. Immunohistochemistry of F98 intracerebral tumors. Expression of large amounts of vimentin, x small blood vessels (a and b), of some GFAP (c) and rare protein S100 in single tumor cells (d). (a 150 x, b 380 x, c 380 x, d 380 x).

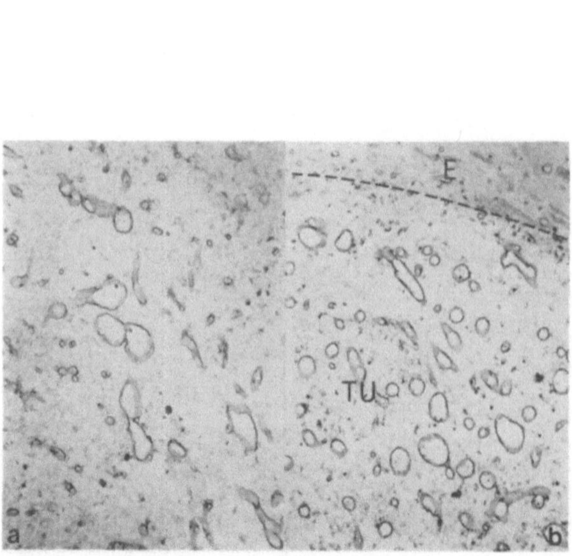

FIGURE 6. Selective staining of vascular endothelia in RG2 tumor with numerous small and ectatic blood vessels by RCA I immunohistochemistry. a central tumor areas after implantation of 10^3 and survival of 18 days. b large tumor after 21 days with more extensive neovascularization in the tumor periphery (TU) as compared to central portions of the tumor (a) and the normal small capillaries in the peritumorous edematous zones (E); dotted line tumor border. (a 120 x, b 120 x).

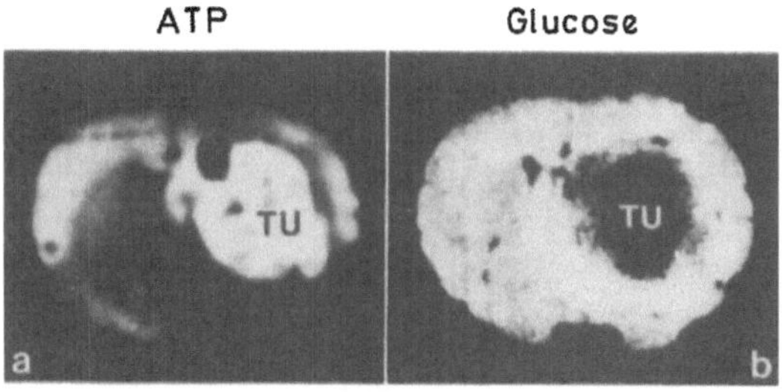

FIGURE 7. Bioluminescent images of regional ATP (a) and glucose (b) in RG2 brain tumor (TU). Note the high tumor ATP content and the very low levels of tumor tissue glucose content, in the same tumor.

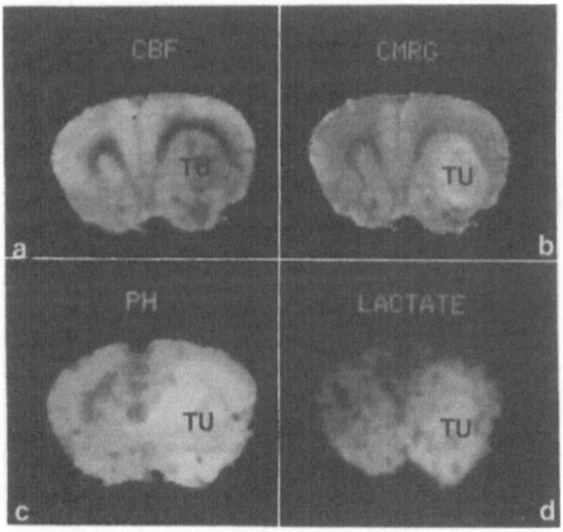

FIGURE 8. a Cerebral blood flow (CBF), b cerebral metabolic rates of glucose (CMRG), c tissue pH (pH) and d lactate content in an experimental F98 brain tumor (TU). Note the decline in tumor blood flow but drastic increase in glucose consumption of the glioma in comparison to the homotopic brain regions. Despite the elevated tumor lactate content, tumor tissue pH is more alkaline than tissue pH of opposite brain structures.

Can Polyamines act as Positron Emitters in Cerebral Oncology? Preliminary results obtained in nude mice bearing human glioblastoma xenografts

V. QUEMENER (°), F. DARCEL (°°), M. CHATEL (°°),
J.-Ph. MOULINOUX (°).

The polyamines, such as putrescine (PUT), spermidine (SPD) and spermine (SPM) are saturated organic compounds which are present in abnormally high concentration in malignant brain tumours (1, 2, 3). In addition, the levels of PUT and SPD in the tumour are, statistically speaking, proportional to the histological grade of the tumour (2, 4). Furthermore, Marton et al. (5, 6) demonstrated that the presence of a brain tumour was associated with a significant increase in the concentration of PUT in the CSF; this type of analysis has been found to be very useful in the management of medulloblastoma (7, 8). In a similar vein, we have observed that the levels of SPD and SPM measured in the red blood cells were significantly elevated in patients afflicted with malignant supratentorial tumours (4). The determination of RBC polyamine levels now appears to have clinical applications, not only for monitoring (9, 10) but also during the post-operative treatment of patients with malignant gliomas (11).

Nowadays, these molecules are considered to be products of metabolic activity closely linked to cell division, and since the mitotic index of normal brain tissue is very low, it is tempting to suggest that polyamines might be used as positron emitters to visualize, *in vivo*, histologically and metabolically different types of human malignant gliomas, by following their proliferative activity.

With this aim in mind, we gave i.p. or i.v. injections of 1-5 μCi of ^{14}C-PUT, ^{14}C-SPD or ^{14}C-SPM (122 mCi/mole) to nude mice bearing sub-cutaneous xenografts of 2 human glioblastomas. One hour after administration of the labelled polyamines, the mice were decapitated and various organs (brain, liver, kidney, muscle, spleen, lung, skin), the tumour and blood samples (red cells and plasma) were taken and solubilised with the aid of Soluene. The radioactivity (dpm/mg tissue or ml blood) of each sample was determined. Three important principles emerged from the results:

a) Whatever the route of administration (i.v. or i.p., Table I) or the choice of labelled polyamine (PUT, SPD or SPM), normal brain tissue contained the lowest level of radioactivity, with about 1/3 of the specific activity observed in the liver, one of the major sites of ^{14}C-polyamine accumulation (Table II).

TABLE I

Tissue and Tumour-Associated Radioactivity (dpm/mg) versus with Brain Labelling (dpm/mg)

Route of administration	Brain	Liver	Spleen	Lung	Kidney	Tumour
I.P. (*)	1	3.9	4.8	3.7	7.2	2.9
I.V. (*)	1	3.4	6.0	3.6	5.2	2.6

(*) 5 μCi of ^{14}C putrescine

b) For each individual animal, again irrespective of the particular labelled polyamine used, the tumour-associated radioactivity was always greater than the radioactivity measured in the brain (Table II).

(°) Groupe de Recherche en Therapeutique Anticancéreuse and (°°) Laboratoire de Neuro-pathologie, CHU de Rennes, Rennes, France.

M. Chatel, F. Darcel and J. Pecker (eds.), Brain Oncology. ISBN-13: 978-94-010-8003-3

TABLE II

Tissue and Tumour-Associated Radioactivity (dpm/mg) compared with Brain Labelling (dpm/mg)

	Brain	Liver	Kidney	Skin	Spleen	Muscle	Tumour
^{14}C Put (1μCi) n = 6	1	5.8 (1.2)	5.4 (1.5)	2.0 (1.0)	8.1 (2)	2.1 (0.5)	5.3 (3.6)
^{14}C Put (5μCi) n = 7	1	9.9 (5.4)	4.7 (2.6)	2.0 (0.5)			5.6 (4.7)
^{14}C Spd (5μCi) n = 7	1	15.3 (20)	9.8 (11)	2.3 (2)			3.3 (1.7)
^{14}C Spm (5μCi) n = 7	1	49 (30)	46 (29)	24 (0.7)			29 (1.5)

I.p. administration of 1-5μCi of ^{14}C-PUT, SPD or SPM to mice bearing gliomas of different volumes.

c) In contrast to our observations with ^{14}C-SPD and ^{14}C-SPM, the tumour uptake of ^{14}C-PUT was significantly correlated with the volume of the tumour, such that the tumour-associated radioactivity (dmp/mg) was inversely proportional to the volume. In other words, the smaller the tumour the greater the uptake of PUT (Figure 1).

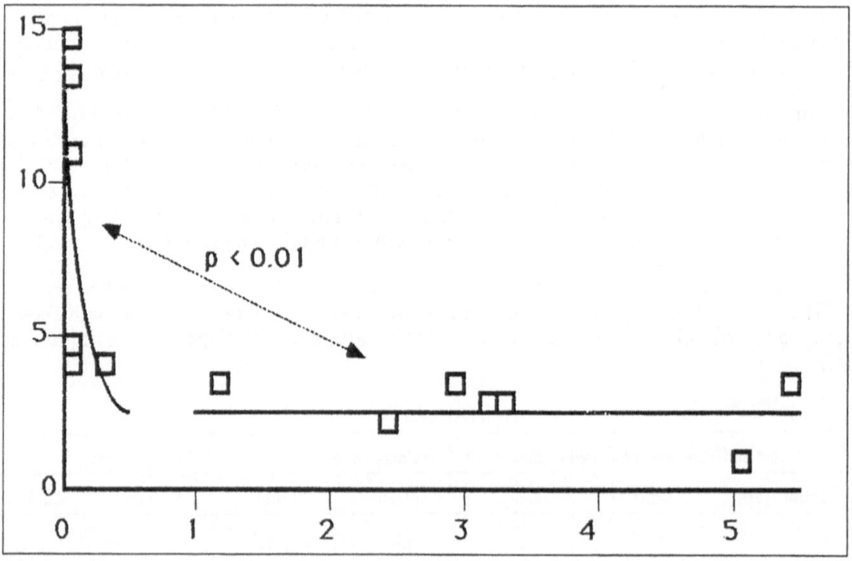

FIGURE 1. Uptake of ^{14}C-Putrescine as a function of tumour volume.
Abscissa: Tumour weight (g)
Ordinate: (dpm/mg tumour) / (dpm/mg brain)

Although this study only involved about thirty animals with xenografts from two different human glioblastomas, these results seem to argue in favour of a role for putrescine in clinical studies by Positron Emission Tomography (PET). Previous results obtained by Volkow et al. (12) using dogs and by Goldman et al. (13) *in vitro*, point in the same direction. Furthermore, the observation that, in this experimental model at least, the incorporation of PUT into the tumour is inversely proportional to the volume is extremely interesting, not just because of the applications in PET, but also in respect to more fundamental studies on the proliferation of malignant glioma *in vivo*.

This work was financed by CNRS (Contract RL 69 n° 866 ONO 315), the Ligue Nationale Française contre le Cancer and the Fondation Langlois. We would like to thank Mme A. Denais, M. C. Martin and M. R. Havouis for their technical assistance.

SUMMARY

Polyamines (Putrescine, Spermidine and Spermine) are aliphatic polycations which have been shown to play major roles in cell proliferation and differentiation This has been shown to be the case in brain tumours.

In such conditions, we planned to explore the polyamine metabolism in patients by means of positron emission tomography (PET).

This leads us to evaluate, as a first step, the polyamine uptake by glioma heterografts in nude mice after intraperitoneal injection of labelled Putrescine, Spermidine and Spermine.

Indaed, polyamine metabolism in a cell is the result of intrinsic synthesis on one hand and extracellular uptake on the other hand. The question to be answered in that protocol was: is this intracellular pathway correlated with the tumour proliferative index and, if this is the case, is the tumour versus normal tissue uptake ratio important enough for being used in a PET study? Series of human glioma grafted nude mice were intraperitoneally injected with ^{14}C Putrescine, ^{14}Spermidine or ^{14}C Spermine.

Injection schedule was planned as to take into account the size of the tumours.

Two conclusions have been gained:
— Only putrescine uptake was significantly increased in the tumour tissue versus normal brain; this ratio being not significant for spermidine and spermine.

— The putrescine uptake by mg of tumour tissue is dependent upon tumour size (decreasing progressivly as the tumour volume increased).

These preliminary findings are in agreement with experimental data obtained in intracerebral grafted rat glioma (Volkow & al.), suggesting that positron emitting putrescine could be a useful probe for exploring human glial tumour proliferation in vivo.

KEY WORDS

Polyamines, Gliomas, Positron, Nude mice, Xenografts.

REFERENCES

1. HARIK (S.J.) et al.: Putrescine as a biochemical marker for malignant brain tumors. Neurology. **28**, 351 (1978).
2. HARIK (S.I.) et al.: Putrescine as biochemical marker of malignant brain tumors, Cancer Res., **39**, 5010-5015 (1979).
3. KREMZNER (L.T.) et al.: Polyamine metabolism in the central and peripheral nervous system. Ann. N.Y. Acad. Sci., **171**, 735-748 (1970).
4. MOULINOUX (J.Ph.) et al.: Polyamines in human brain tumors: a correlative study between tumor, CSF and red blood cell free polyamine levels. J. Neuro-Oncology (JNO), 1984, **2**, 153-158.
5. MARTON (L.J.) et al.: Increased polyamine concentrations in the CSF of patients with brain tumors. Int. J. Cancer, **14**, 731-735 (1974).
6. MARTON (L.J.) et al.: The relationship of the polyamines in the CSF to the presence of central nervous system tumors. Cancer Res., **36**, 973-977 (1976).
7. MARTON (L.J.) et al.: Predictive value of cerebrospinal fluid polyamines in medulloblastoma. Cancer Res., **39**, 993-997 (1979).
8. MARTON (L.J.) et al.: CSF polyamines: a view and important means of monitoring patients with medulloblastoma. Cancer, **47**, 757-760 (1981).
9. MOULINOUX (J.Ph.) et al.: Red blood cell polyamines in malignant glioma patients. Spermidine and spermine blood levels and tumour evolution. J.N. Oncol., in press (1986).
10. CHATEL (M.) et al.: Red blood cell polyamines as biochemical markers of supratentorial malignant gliomas, J. Anticancer Res., in press (1986).

11. THERON (J.) et al.: Intra-arterial chemotherapy with BCNU. Correlations between tumour growing and red blood cells polyamines levels. (Cf. present volume).

12. VOLKOW (N.) et al.: Labelled putrescine as a probe in brain tumors, Sciences, **221**, 673-675 (1983).

13. GOLDMAN (S.S.) et al.: Putrescine metabolism in human brain tumors, J.N. Oncol., **4**, 23-27 (1986).

Conception and Evaluation of a MRI and CT Stereotactic Frame in Neuro-Oncology

F.N. GAGEY, A. BOULIOU, J.M. SCARABIN,
M. CARSIN, J. SIMON, J.D. de CERTAINES.

Stereotactic examinations with CT scan have previously demonstrated their performances but the specific interest of MRI in the neurooncology field requires the transposition of a well established CT scan method into NMR technology (2, 3, 6). Main problems concern the material included in the stereotactic frame (without any ferromagnetic substances), the position of the patient in the imaging system and the visibility of constrast substances in MRI. Regarding these three demands, we have developed a convenient stereotactic frame for both MRI and CT scans. This frame is of very simple use according to the atraumatic fixation on the patient head and allows short time examination compatible with routine use of imaging.

I - STEREOTACTIC FRAME

The stereotactic frame needs an easy pattern of fixation on patient's head (nasion, external auditory meatus) and consists in four triangles (basis 10 cm, height 14 cm) located on the two sides of the skull (two for CT and two for MRI) (figure 1). The coordinates are visualized in both CT and MRI by copper wire (0,4 mm dimameter) and agarose gel with 0,8 g.l^{-1} copper sulfate in polyethylene tube (1,6 mm diameter). An angle of 15° between the CT copper wire of the reference CT triangle and $CuSO_4$ tube of the reference MRI triangle may correct the different positionning of the patient in CT and MRI in order to obtain, in each technique, the bissectris of the reference triangle perpendicular to the slice plane. In MRI apparatus giving oblique slices, this characteristic is not necessary.

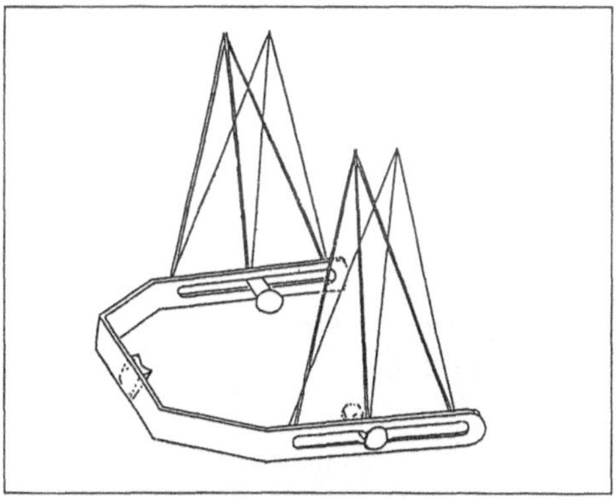

FIGURE 1. CT-MRI stereotactic frame

The frame is adapted to the particular head morphology of each patient by translation of the triangles: the symetry of this adaptation is controled and then the intersection of bissectris and the basis of each triangle must be just in front of the auditory meatus.

II - EXAMINATION MODALITIES

The stereotactic examination includes three different steps:

a) CT scan

The CT scan is performed using iodinated contrast agent on the frame bearing patients. The slice must be perpendicular to the main bissectris of the copper wire triangle.

These copper wires appear as a pair of three points on each lateral side of the skull. Distances between these points allow the calculation of the slice position in referential system.

Groupe SIM, Laboratoire de RMN, Faculté de Médecine, F - 35000 RENNES

M. Chatel, F. Darcel and J. Pecker (eds.), Brain Oncology. ISBN-13: 978-94-010-8003-3

b) MRI

MRI examination is performed in the same conditions as CT but without contrast agents. Agarose gell tubes also appear as three points on each side and allow the same calculation. Two SE pulse sequences are used: TR 500, TE 28 and TR 2000, TE 28 with four echos in order to give informations referring to T1, T2 and spin density. We use a 0,35 T supra-conductive magnet, 2 DFT reconstruction, 9 mm slice thickness and 256^2 matrix size in a field of view of 25,6 cm (pixel size 1 mm).

c) Lateral X-ray examination

The flexibility of the perspex stereotactic frame requires the transfer of localization data on a fixed referential system : we use for that a lateral radiographic view of the frame bearing patient superposing the images of the two lateral triangles under radioscopic control. Conditions of acquisition of this X-ray examination are easily reproducible during cerebral biopsy by superposition of the symetric structures of the skull (external auditory meatus, orbits...). To reduce radiological enlargement, the distance between the X-ray source and the film is 5 meters.

II - DATA ANALYSIS

The used data are the distances between the different points, between the tumor and the nearest triangle and between the anterior and posterior faces of the tumor and the line between the anterior and posterior faces of the tumor and the line between the two triangles bissectris (figure 2). Mathematical analysis gives the slice position coordinates h, ρ and θ (figure 3).

We have the relation :

$$\mathrm{tg}\,\theta : \mathrm{tg}\,\alpha^{-1} . \frac{k-1}{k+1} \quad (1) \text{ with } k = \frac{d_1}{d_2} \text{ (figure 4)}$$

$$h_1 = d_1 \frac{\cos(\alpha+\theta)}{\sin\alpha} \quad (2)$$

$$h_2 = d_2 \frac{\cos(\alpha-\theta)}{\sin\alpha}$$

and ρ is obtained from the two measurements of h in each lateral triangle (figure 5):

$$\sin\rho = \frac{h_1 - h_2}{e} \quad (3)$$

h, ρ and θ calculations starting from a single slice does not give enough precision in slice localization. Then, we use an error minimization by simultaneous analysis of 3 or more adjacent slices. This method requires paralelism and equidistance of the slices.

With : i = the number of the slice

d_{1ij} = the distance d_1 in i slices measured on the right triangle if $j = 1$, and on the left if $j = 2$

d_{2ij} = the distance d_2 in i slices with $j = 1$ or 2.

d_{1ij} and d_{2ij} are related by the following equations :

$$d_{1ij} = k(ai + b_j)$$

$$d_{2ij} = ai + b_j$$

Resolution of this system by the least square method give the value of a and b.

The expression to be minimized is :

$$\sum_{ij} [d_{1ij} - k(ai + b_j)]^2 + [d_{2ij} - (ai + b_j)]^2$$

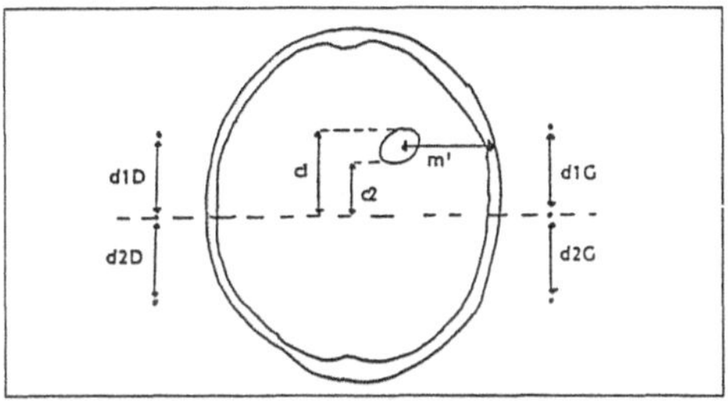

FIGURE 2. Data used : definition of d_1, d_2, c_1, c_2 and m'.

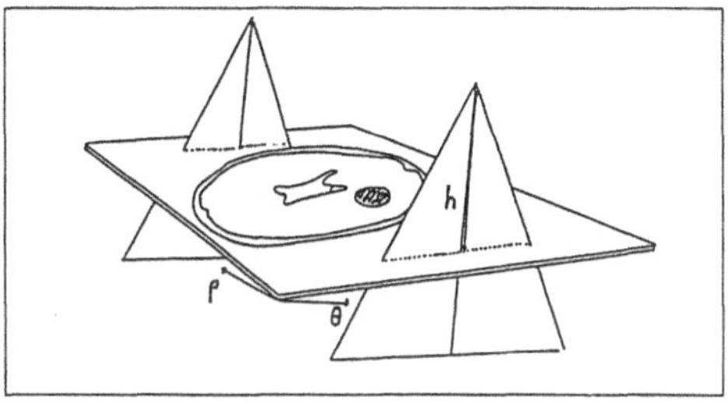

FIGURE 3. coordinates h, ρ and θ of the slice ir the referential system.

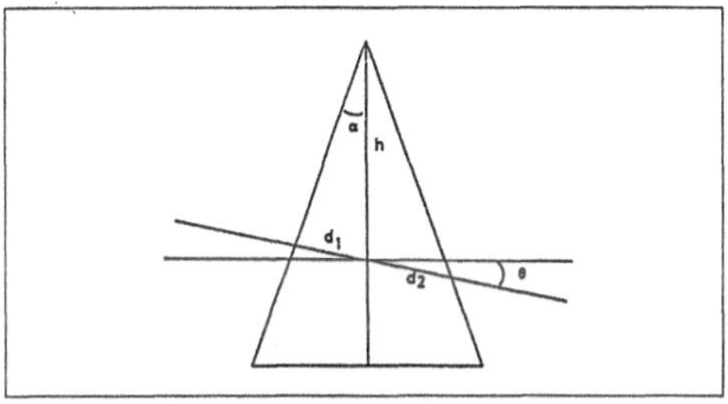

FIGURE 4. h and θ determination.

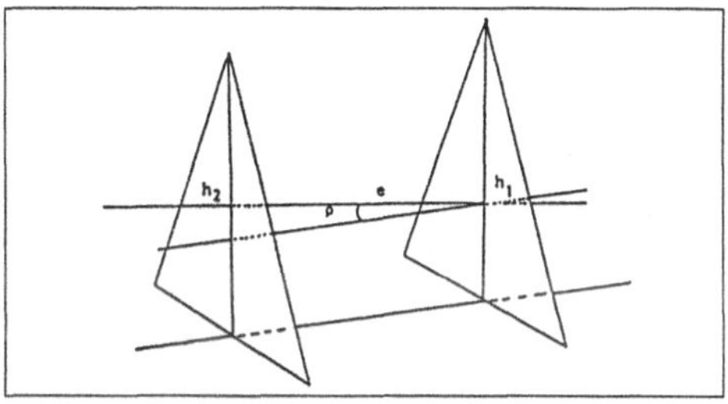

FIGURE 5. ρ determination.

To maintain the linearity of the equations, the calculation include two different steps:

— firstly determination of k :

$$k = \frac{d_{1ij}}{d_{2ij}}$$

The expression to be minimized is :

$$\sum_{ij} (d_{1ij} - kd_{2ij})^2$$

$$\text{and } k = \frac{\sum_{ij} d_{1ij}\, d_{2ij}}{\sum_{ij} (d_{2ij})^2}$$

— secondly, determination of a, b_1 and b_2

$$\sum_{ij} [d_{1ij} - k\,(ai + b_j)]^2 + [d_{2ij} - (ai + b_j)]^2$$

partial derivatives give the following equations :

$$a \sum_i i + b_1 \sum 1 = \frac{1}{k^2 + 1} \sum_i (d_{1i1} + kd_{2i1})$$

$$a \sum_i i + b_2 \sum 1 = \frac{1}{k^2 + 1} \sum_i (d_{1i2} + kd_{2i2})$$

$$2a \sum_i i^2 + (b_1 + b_2) \sum_i i = \frac{1}{k^2 + 1} \sum_i i\, [(d_{1i1} + d_{1i2}) + (d_{2i1} + d_{2i2})]$$

The resolution of this equation system gives a, b_1 and b_2 values, and the determination of d_{1ij} and d_{2ij} minimized values. Then, using equation (1), (2) and (3), we can obtain the coordinate h, ρ and θ of each slice in the referential system. All these operations are computerized using an IBM PC-AT. We may visualize on the screen the detected tumoral lesion in orthogonal projection on the nearest triangle, taking into account the radiological enlargement. By superposing a hard copy of the screen and X-ray image, we have the tumor position.

IV - BRAIN BIOPSY

The patient is maintened on a CGR-Isocentrix chair, under general anesthetics, his head located in exact sagital profile on the Talairach frame. Three angiographic examinations are then performed: the first one in frontal view, the second one in previously described stereotactic conditions, the third one in photogrammetric conditions. The superposition of these two last incidences allows to 3D-visualize the vascular plexus (1, 7). In case of no tumoral hypervascularization, the neurosurgeon may choose the entrance of biopsy needle from which trajectory is always perpendicular to the X-ray film plane. Biopsy samples are selected along this axis and immediatly used for extemporaneous pathologic examination. Haemostasis is carried out by the coagulation of the biopsy axis. In case of failure, a new biopsy will be performed. In these conditions, post-surgical complications are very seldom.

V - EVALUATION OF THE METHOD

Stereotactic examinations have been used for five years and more than 300 patients have undertaken the procedure in our University Hospital. Using proton MRI, problems result from technological consideration, mainly Bo field homogeneity and gradients adjusting. All these technological parameters have been tested using test-objets and protocols for MRI quality control established by a european working group (EEC, project COMAC-BME II.2.3). A specific test-object has been built for our purpose consisting in 8 or 16 mm balls containing a lipidic substance giving contrast with CT, X-ray and MRI. The use of this test-object has shown a geometric error in the position of the ball centres of 2 mm in CT and less than 5 mm in MRI (figure 6 and 7).

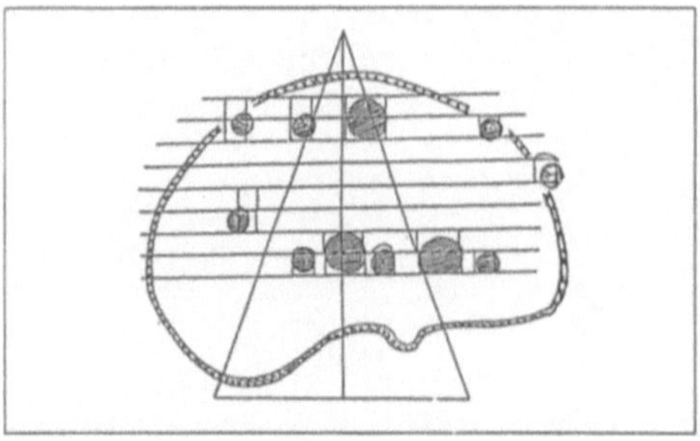

FIGURE 6. CT projection (geometrical error in the position of these ball centres is about 2 mm in CT).

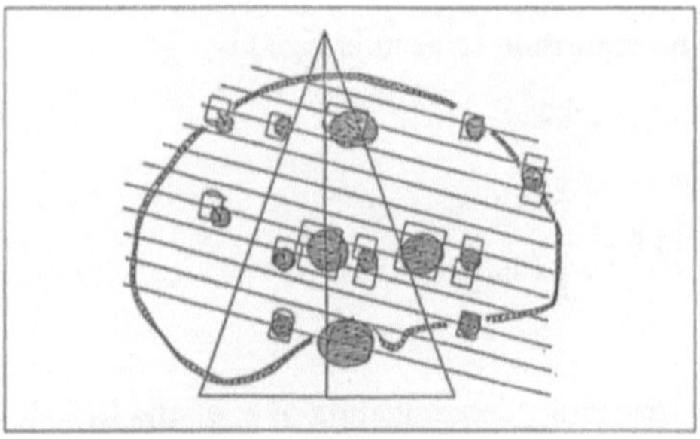

FIGURE 7. MRI projection (geometrical error in the position of these ball centres is about 5 mm in MRI).

VI - FIRST CLINICAL RESULTS

Three cases from our first series will be presented as an example of the method.

— ***Patient G,*** glioblastoma
  - — figure 8 : CT examination
  - — figure 9 : orthogonal projection of tumoral CT image
  - — figure 10 : MRI examination (SE 28/500)
  - — figure 11 : orthogonal projection of tumoral MRI image
  - — figure 12 : comparison of the tumoral volume in CT (thick line) and MRI (narrow line) on the 5 m X-ray examination showing the triangles of the stereotactic frame.

— ***Patient C,*** pineal ependymoma
  — figure 13 : same presentation as in figure 12

— ***Patient S,*** meningioma
  — figure 14 : same presentation as in figure 12

Our first clinical series is in total agreement with the technological evaluation of the method.

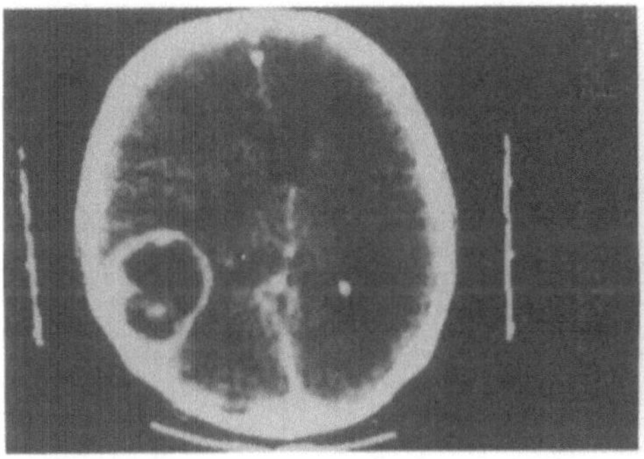

FIGURE 8. Glioblastoma : CT examination.

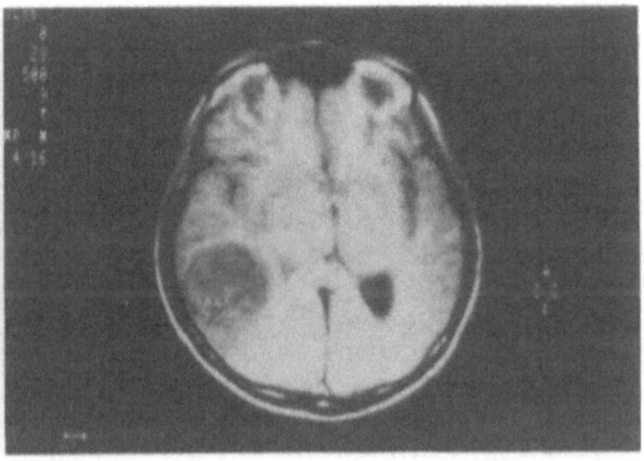

FIGURE 10. Glioblastoma: MRI examination.

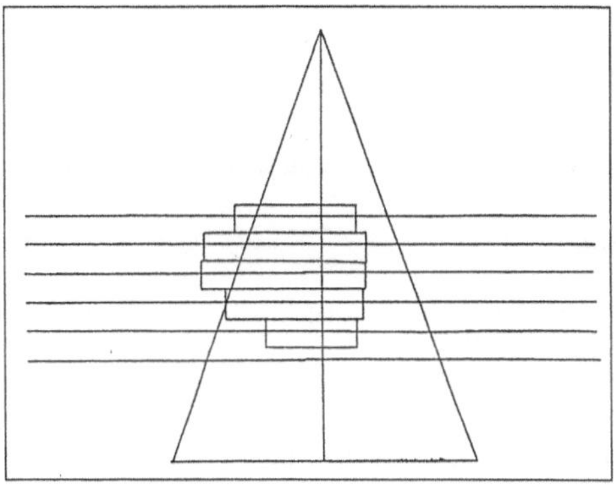

FIGURE 9. Orthogonal projection of tumoral CT images.

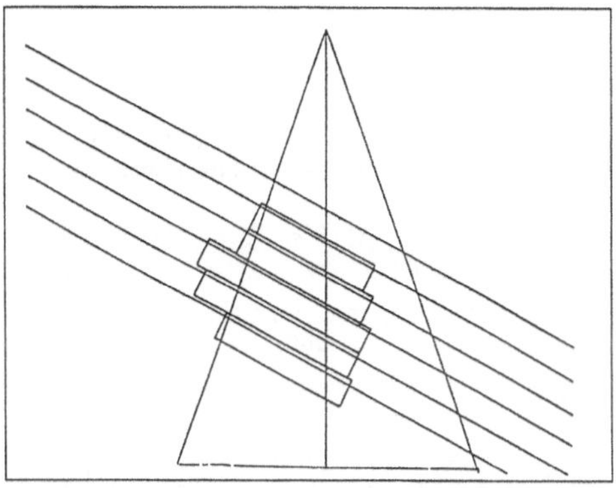

FIGURE 11. Orthogonal projection of MRI images.

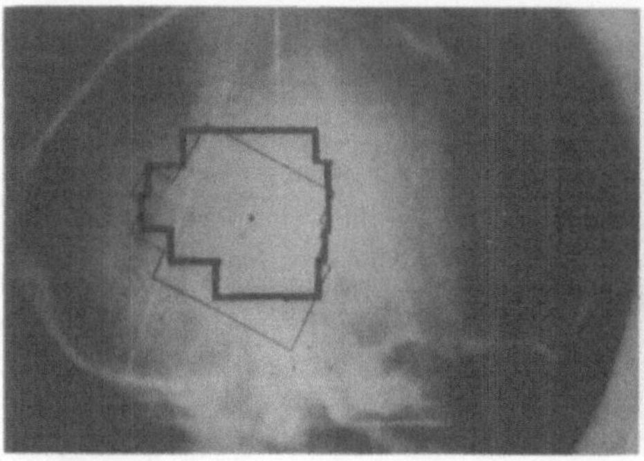

FIGURE 12. Comparison of the tumoral volume in CT and MRI on lateral X-ray.

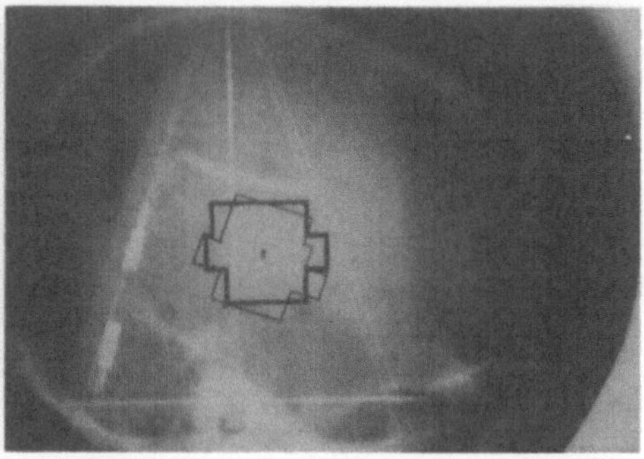

FIGURE 13. Ependymoma: CT projection (thick line) and MRI (narrow line).

CONCLUSION

Stereotactic examinations are already of great interest in all diagnosis strategies. Furthermore, some works are in progress in our University concerning 3D image analysis and synthesis, PACS (Picture Archiving and Communication system), radiotherapy dosimetry (7, 8). They will give new extensions to all the 3D approaches in neurooncology. Then, it seems absolutely necessary to include MRI technology in all methodologies previously developped for CT.

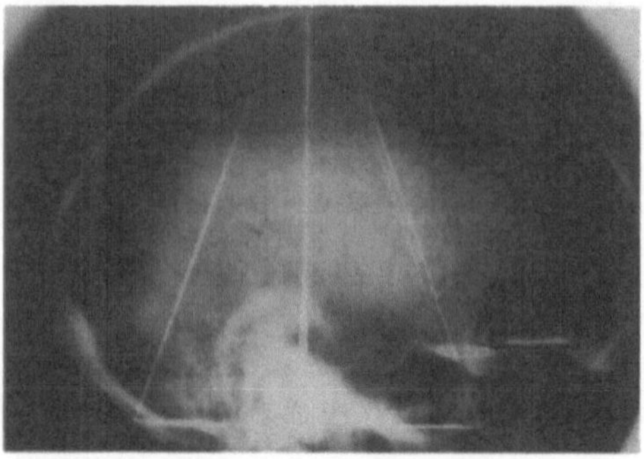

FIGURE 14. Meningioma (same projection).

KEY WORDS

3D Imaging, Brain Tumours Stereotaxy.

REFERENCES

1. GIBAUD (B.), SCARABIN (J.M.), LORIG (B.), CRUETTE (C.): Accurate use of CT scanner stereotaxis and photogrammetry for diagnosis and treatment of cerebral lesions (tumor). Int. Arch. Photogrammetry, 1982, **14** (5) 225-235.

2. KALL (B.A.), KELLY (P.J.), GOERSS (S.J.), EARNEST (F.): Cross registration of points and lesion volumes from MR and CT. IEEE. 1985, 939-41.

3. LEKESSEL (L.), JERNER (T.), LEKESSEL (D.), PERSSON (B.): Visualisation of stereotactic radiolesions by nuclear magnetic resonance. J. Neurol. Neurosurg. Psychiatry, 1985, jan. 48 (1) 19-20.

4. LEKESSEL (L.), LEKESSEL (D.), SCHWEBEL (J.): Streotaxis and nuclear magnetic resonance. J. Neurol. Neurosurg. Psychiatry, 1985, jan. 48 (1) 14-8.

5. PECKER (J.), SCARABIN (J.M.), BRUCHER (J.M.), VALLÉE (B.): Stereotactic aproach to diagnosis and treatment of cerebral tumors. Editions Médicales Pierre Fabre, Paris, 1979.

6. ROSS-DUGGAN (J.W.), PATIL (A.A.), YAMANASHI (W.S.), VALENTINE (J.L.): A stereotaxic system and its application using magnetic resonance imaging. M.R.I. 1986, **4** (2) 138.

7. SCARABIN (J.M.), DUVAUFERRIER (R.), GANDON (Y.), LEGOUT (A.), VELUT (S.), GADAN (R.), MOREAU (J.J.): "Imagerie tridimentionnelle, bilan et perspectives" in *Radiologie et échographie interventionnelles,* tome II, R. Duvauferrier ed., Axone, 1986, p. 743-751.

8. SCARABIN (J.M.), PECKER (J.), LEGOUT (A.), CARSIN (M.), SIMON (J.), GADAN (R.): "Neuroradiologie et neurochirurgie stereotaxiques tumorales" in *Radiologie et échographie interventionnelles,* tome I, R. Duvauferrier ed., Axone, 1986, p. 159-171

MRI and the Surgical Treatment of Low Grade Gliomas

J. BROTCHI (°), D. BALERIAUX (°°), F. DELECLUSE (°°°).

INTRODUCTION

The advent of CT Scan has revolutionized the diagnosis of gliomas, particularly those of low grade. The discovery of such lesions at very early stages, before the appearance of clinical deficits or of radiological signs of compression, has thus allowed surgical treatment that could hopefully be curative in certain cases. However, CT Scan images of « benign » gliomas are often caracterized by a poorly limited hypodensity, making the presurgical evaluation of the limits of the area to be removed very delicate. Furthermore, during the operation itself, we are often made aware of the difficulty in distinguishing the boundaries of these tumors imbedded in the white matter.

Having been able to use Nuclear Magnetic Resonance Imaging (MRI) for tow years now, it has thus been possible for us to compare CT and MRI imaging and to deduce from this comparison a therapeutic strategy.

MATERIEL AND METHODS

Our experience is based on the analysis of 19 patients: all were studied by CT and MRI before surgical treatment. Some underwent an extended tumoral resection, a few even lobectomy, while the others had stereotaxic biopsy performed; we thus have a histological diagnosis in all cases. Were excluded from this study all patients, even if studied by MRI, in whom no definite histological diagnosis could be obtained.

MRI was performed by means of a supra-conductive magnet with a magnectic field of 0.5 tesla (Gyroscan S15). The chosen imaging technic was by spin echo, producing two series of 16 images (E1 and E2), the first at 50 msec, the second at 100 msec with a constant repetition time of 1500 msec. We chose this imaging technic on the basis of a study on contrast analysis: E1 is a reflection of the T1 relaxation time, while E2 ponders T2. These are thus complementary images. Section thickness was of 5 mm. Last, but not least, this study was performed by way of series of semi-axial multisections, which had the advantage of being located in the same planes as that of the CT Scan images, thus making comparison between these two investigational technics much more trustworthy.

Morevover, series of additional multisections in coronal and sagittal incidences were frequently performed, using the same imaging technics.

RESULTS

Of our 19 patients, 17 had a supratentorial low grade glioma (16 astrocytomas, 1 oligodendroglioma), one had a pilocytic thalamo-ventriculo-mesencephalic astrocytoma and one young patient had a pontine astrocytoma vegetating in the fourth ventricle. At CT Scan, tumoural limits were poorly defined in 15 of these cases. In 14 cases could be seen a non contrast enhanced hypodensity, while in 5 cases, a slight modification of the image after contrast injection was noted; there was however no histological incidence.

The study by MRI immediatly showed a greater sensitivity in detection, as well as better contrast between the pathological area and the healthy tissue. However, at this time, MRI is still incapable of distinguishing between tumour and oedema. Sometimes, the E1 images are more eloquent than the E2 images, sometimes the reverse is true; either way, no link with the corresponding histology was found. However, it seemed to us that preponderance of E1 on E2 was more frequently observed in very low grade gliomas such as beginning astrocytomas, but our series is too small to draw any formal conclusion.

(°) Departments of Neurosurgery, (°°) Neuroradiology, (°°°) Neurology. Erasme Hospital, Free University of Brussels, Belgium.

M. Chatel, F. Darcel and J. Pecker (eds.), Brain Oncology. ISBN-13: 978-94-010-8003-3

Comparative analysis of CT Scan and MRI datas showed an equivalent approach in 4 cases out of 19 (fig. 1). Greater sensitivity of MRI in detection of abnormal cerebral tissue, be it tumoural or oedema, was observed in 15 cases out of 19. The lesions appeared much greater in size, as we noticed in many cases, the most spectacular being that of the pilocytic astrocytoma which extended from the thalamus to the pontine area in the brain stem (fig. 2). A few patients underwent MRI analysis after Gadolinium injection. We were able to observe a perfect parallel between contrast enhancement in CT Scan and MRI (4) ; in our study, this last contrast medium was of little benefit. The better definition of abnormal cerebral tissue by MRI, combined with the coronal, sagittal and semi-axial slices which were superimposable with those obtained by CT Scan, allowed us to apply the following strategy:

a. Largest possible excision in surgically accessible areas, with no invalidading sequellae.

b. Stereotaxic biopsy each time the lesion was located in the rolandic or associative zones, the corpus callosum or the basal ganglia.

MRI data allowed us to draw an actual working diagram such as those obtained after stereotaxic biopsy. We knew before surgery what we would remove and we knew the precise limits of our surgical excision. This permitted us to realize a practically total removal in 6 cases, most notably one case of brain stem glioma, with no post-surgical aftermath. In 5 cases, we deliberately practised a subtotal excision, nevertheless as large as possible. The last 8 cases underwent biopsy under stereotaxic conditions.

On the other hand, the anatomical precision of MRI prodded us to greater surgical daring, particularly with the help of the Cavitron in certain delicate areas. There was no post-operative mortality and no aggravation of the prior neurological status.

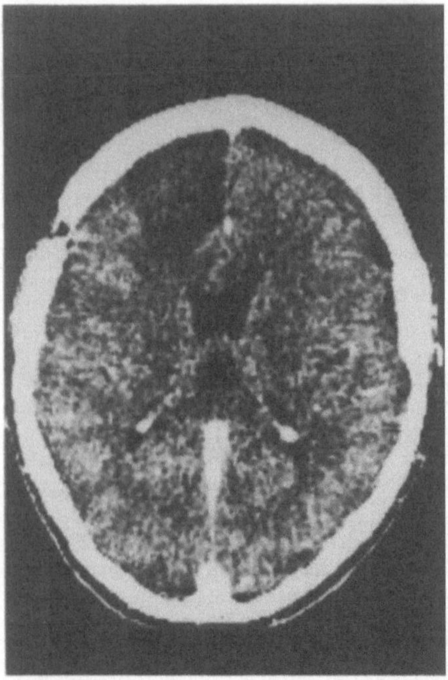

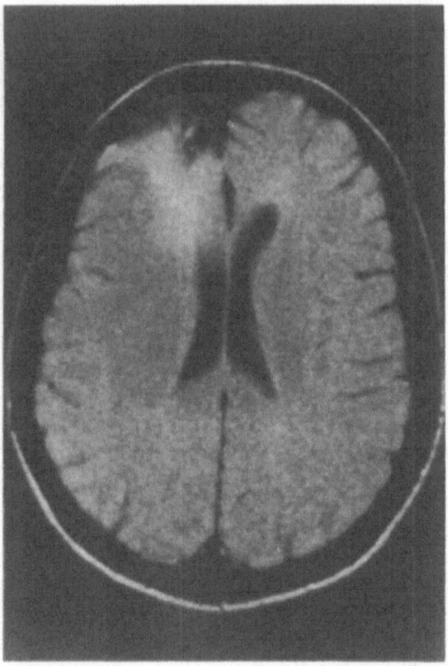

FIGURE 1. Equivalent CT Scan and MRI imaging in a case of right frontal astrocytoma. CT Scan showed a large right frontal hypodensity with no contrast enhancement (1a). MRI showed tumoural infiltration by way of a hypersignal area by first echo (1b).

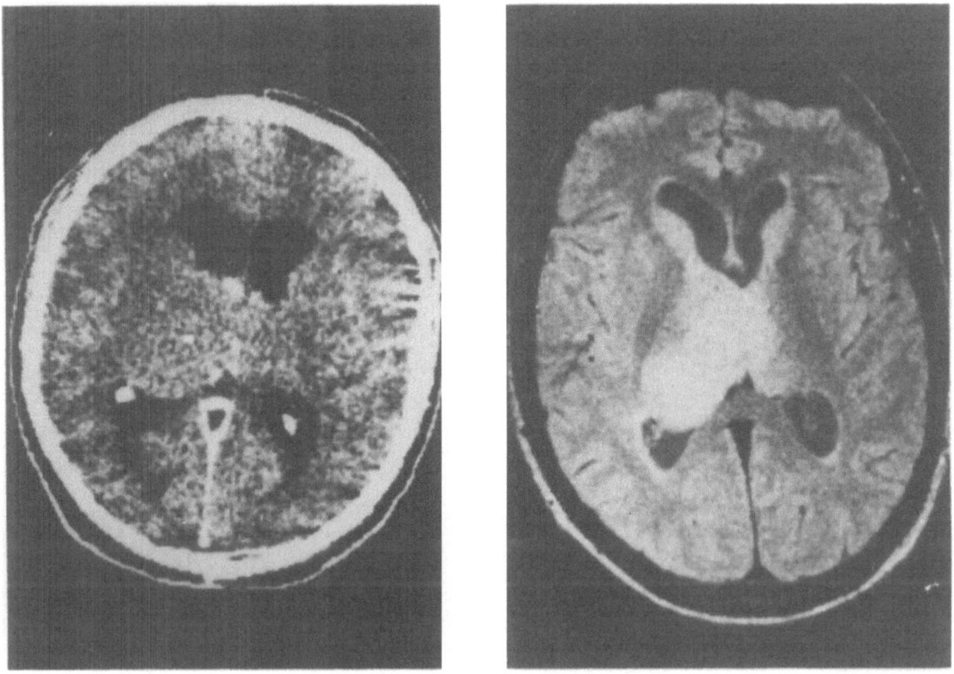

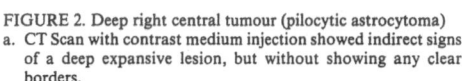

FIGURE 2. Deep right central tumour (pilocytic astrocytoma)
a. CT Scan with contrast medium injection showed indirect signs of a deep expansive lesion, but without showing any clear borders.
b. MRI imaging of the same level allowed a precise workup of the tumoural extension, as shown by the clear hypersignal of the tumoural tissue.

DISCUSSION

Low grade gliomas being by definition infiltrating tumours, their total excision is impossible. However, in view of their slow growth, one can reasonably assume that the length of postsurgical survival is linked with the quantity of tumour removed (8). Classically (8), tumoural resection is limited to the areas whose consistance, texture or colour are clearly pathological. This is true when the surgeon searches for visual references to guide his hand, in order to avoid the risk of operative sequellae but he is then forced to neglect whole areas infiltrated by tumoural cells.

Indeed there may even exist a false plane of separation between what seems to be obviously tumoural tissue and the neighbouring brain, which unfortunately later turns out to be infiltrated.

MRI brings more precise data than CT Scan in the definition of healthy tissue limits (1) but we know that it can not yet make the distinction between tumoural cerebral tissue and oedema (3, 6, 7).

Once we have deliberately decided to define the limits of the surgical act solely on MRI imaging and anatomic contingencies, the operation can be programmed independently of the visual references described above. It is of no consequence if the demarcation between normal and tumoral white substance isn't clear, or if the tumoural borders are uncertain. This way of procedure allows a large ablation in safe conditions.

On the other hand, once the tumour has invaded the contralateral hemisphere, or when it is located in a functionaly dangerous zone, it is more logical to proceed by seried biopsies in stereotaxic conditions (2). As for the brain stem, even if opinions diverge, it is common practice to operate when the tumoural mass bourgeons in the fourth ventricle (5). In our case, MRI showed us such precise anatomical references that, by an intratumoral approach with the Cavitron, we were able to extract pratically all of the tumoural mass, as shown by our postoperative MRI. At this time, with a two years follow-up, the child thus treated is attending school and leading a normal athletic life.

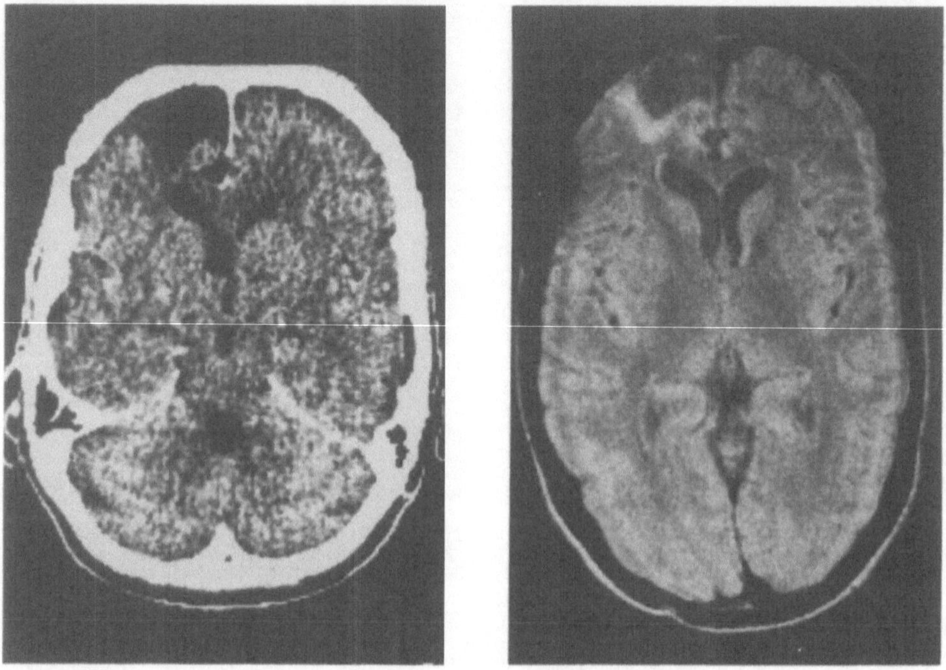

FIGURE 3. Grade II astrocytoma. Postoperative relapse?

a. CT Scan with contrast medium injection. The test showed a hypodense higth frontal sequellae with no clear signs of recurrence.

b. MRI by spin echo TE 50 msec TR 1500 msec. Hypersignal zone on the borders of the previous operative site: tumoural recurrence is strongly suspected (and confirmed on operation).

Furthermore, in the more complex cases of postoperative controls, MRI seemed to us more reliable and more sensitive. For example, while CT Scan showed no clear sign of recurrence in an operated frontal glioma, MRI convincingly showed the apparition of hypersignal areas on the border of the operative site, coinciding with recurrence (fig. 3).

To sum up, it is obviously too early to draw any conclusion as to the prognosis of our patients, our series and our follow-up being much too small. But we can't help but be very enthusiastic about the contribution of MRI in the detection and the operative decision in low grade gliomas.

SUMMARY

The comparative results in a series of 19 intracranial low-grade gliomas allow us to say that Magnetic Resonance Imaging (MRI) is more accurate than Computerized Tomography (CT) scanning in defining the distinct borders of normal brain. However, MRI cannot make the difference between tumour and oedema. But, as the goal of surgery is to remove as much tumor as is safely possible without creating a new neurological deficit, MRI provides a great help in our aggressive policy of resection in low-grade gliomas, the limits of which are based on MRI pictures.

KEY WORDS

MRI, low-grade gliomas.

REFERENCES

1. BREM (H.): Supratentorial astrocytoma. In Long D.M.: **Current therapy in neurological surgery** 1985-1986, (Decker B.C., Philadelphia, 1985), 27-29.

2. COBB (C.A.), YOUMANS (J.R.): Glial and neuronal tumors of the brain in adults. In Youmans J.R.: **Neurological Surgery**, (Saunders, Philadelphia, 1982), 2759-2835.

3. DEBANE (A.), LAVIEILLE (J.), STANOYEVITCH (J.F.), LEGRE (J.): Protocole d'exploration des tumeurs cérébrales en IRM. Intérêt de l'étude des échos multiples. J. Neuroradiology **12**: 290-301 (1985).

4. FELIX (R.), SCHORNER (W.), LANIADO (M.), NIENDORF (H.P.), CLAUSSEN (C.), FIEGLER (W.), SPECK (U.): Brain Tumors: MR Imaging with Gadolinium-DTPA ; Radiology **156**: 681-688 (1985).

5. HOFFMAN (H.J.), BECKER (L.), CRAVEN (M.A.): A clinically and pathologically distinct group of beningn brain stem gliomas. Neurosurgery **7**: 243-247 (1980).

6. LE BAS (J.F.), LEVIEL (J.L.), DECORPS (M.), and BENABID (A.L.): NMR Relaxation Times from Serial Stereotactic Biopsies in Human Brain Tumors. J. of Computer Assisted Tomography **8** : 1048-1057 (1984).

7. RINCK (P.A.), MEINDL (S.), HIGER (H.P.), BIELER (E.U.), PFANNENSTIEL (P.): Brain Tumors: detection and typing by use of CPMG Sequences and in vivo T2 measurements. Radiology **157**: 103-106 (1985).

8. SALCMAN (M.): Supratentorial gliomas: clinical features and surgical therapy. In Wilkins R.H. and Rengachary S.S.: **Neurosurgery**, (McGraw-Hill, New York, 1985), 579-590.

Brain Electrical Activity Mapping in Brain Tumors

S. PRIER (°), C. BENOIT (°).

INTRODUCTION

Brain Electrical Activity Mapping (BEAM) is used in pharmacology (14), psychiatry (10, 11, 12), and neuropsychology (3, 15) as an indicator of the functional state of the brain. Studies of organic brain diseases are of growing number (2, 7, 13), but few are restricted to a specific pathology. In this study, BEAM is applied to brain tumors patients.

MATERIAL AND METHODS

Patients: our study is done on 60 patients (table I), 35 men and 25 wemen, aged from 20 to 74 years (m = 62). The topography of the tumor site is determined by CT-SCAN in all cases. Histology is known by surgery or autopsy. Tumors are dispatched in four groups of progressive depth: I cortical, II cortex and neighbouring white matter, III entirely in the white matter and/or basal ganglia, IV deeper, inferior face of hemispheres and posterior fossa.

Methods: data from 16 standard E.E.G. scalp electrodes are amplified, quantified and stored via a 16 channels polygraph and computer (ALVAR REEGA - 2000 - CARTOVAR). E.E.G. is filtered at 30 Hz using a low-pass 48dB / octave filter. Sampling is made at a rate of 64 c/s, by epochs of 2 seconds, which data are averaged during a sequence of 1 minute. A spectrum of power from 0 to 30 Hz is stored for every electrode and every sequence, on a magnetic disk. Maps of spectral energy are obtained for a frequency band by interpolating the spectral energy between the three nearest electrodes of every point. Classical E.E.G. frequency bands are analysed: Delta (0-3,5 Hz), Theta (4-7,5 Hz), Alpha (8-12,5 Hz), Beta 1 (13-22 Hz) and Beta 2 (22-30 Hz). Display of the power is made using a grey scale: black for the greatest power, white for the least.

RESULTS

BEAM provides a visualisation of the tumoral area in 54 cases out of 60, accurately in 47 cases, with less accuracy in 7 cases of deep seated tumors. These give rise to bilateral slow activity. In 6 patients bilateral theta activity is seen without focus: three deep midline tumors with minimal features and three superficial ones with important bilateral slow activity.

Delta activity is well localized in 25 out of 29 medium depth tumors: groups II and III (Table II, fig 1). 9 out of 20 superficial tumors have bilateral delta activity. 9 out of 25 frontal tumors have

TABLE II

DELTA ACTIVITY

Delta Activity / Tumor Depth		I CORTEX	II CORTICO-SUBC	III SUB-CORTICAL	IV DEEP
Foci	36	7	15	10	4
Widespread	16	9	1	3	3
Few or Lack	8	4	0	0	4
	60	20	16	13	11

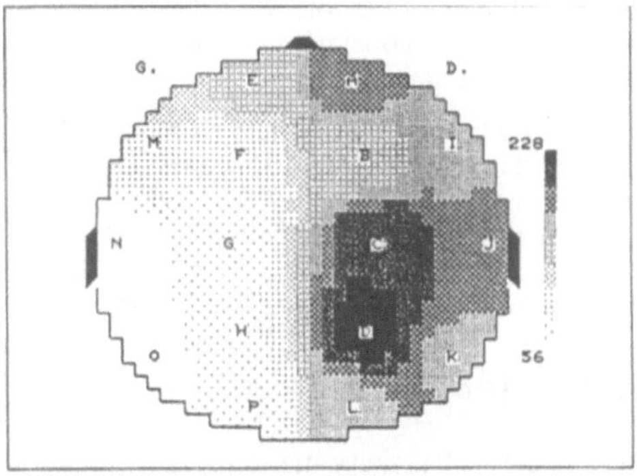

Delta activity. Right Centroparietal Deep Metastatic Carcinoma.

(°) *Service de Neurologie, Hopital Beaujon, 92110 Clichy, France.*

M. Chatel, F. Darcel and J. Pecker (eds.), Brain Oncology. ISBN-13: 978-94-010-8003-3

bilateral delta activity (Table IV). 19 out of 24 Parietal, Temporal and occipital lobes tumors have well focused delta activity. Malignant tumors give more delta activity than tumors with a slower evolution.

TABLE IV

DISTRIBUTION OF DELTA AND THETA ACTIVITY ACCORDING TO THE ANATOMIC LOCATION

		DELTA			THETA		
		FOCI	BILATERAL	LACK	FOCI	BILATERAL	LACK
Fronto-Centrals	25	13	9	3	22	3	0
Others Lobes	24	19	4	1	19	5	0
Deep	11	4	3	4	5	6	0
	60	36	16	8	46	14	0

Theta activity is localized in 16 out of 20 superficial tumors (Table III). Frontocentral lobes have the greatest rate of theta foci, this in 22 of 25 cases (Table IV, fig. 2). Theta activity is more widespread but well lateralized in 41 out of 49 deeper seated hemispheric tumors. Posterior fossa tumors are traduced by bilateral posterior theta activity, prevailing on the tumor side when the lesion is lateralized (fig. 3). Tumors of the parietal, temporal and occipital lobes are traduced by theta as well as delta localized activity.

Alpha activity is decreased on the tumor side in deep-seated lesions. Thus, in cortical tumors of groups I this activity is increased on the tumor side in 13 of 20 cases (Table V). This is more pronouced with malignants tumors but not significant (fig. 4). In some patients Alpha activity is localized near the tumor site. A similar focus has been seen on a post ictal map, but there is not a constant association between such an activity and epilepsy.

Beta 1 activity is decreased on the tumor site in 9 cases, and is symmetrical in 15 cases. Localized beta power is seen in 17 cases, slightly more frequent in gliomas and meningiomas (N.S.) - There is a significant relationship ($P < 0.01$) between localized beta activity and epilepsy.

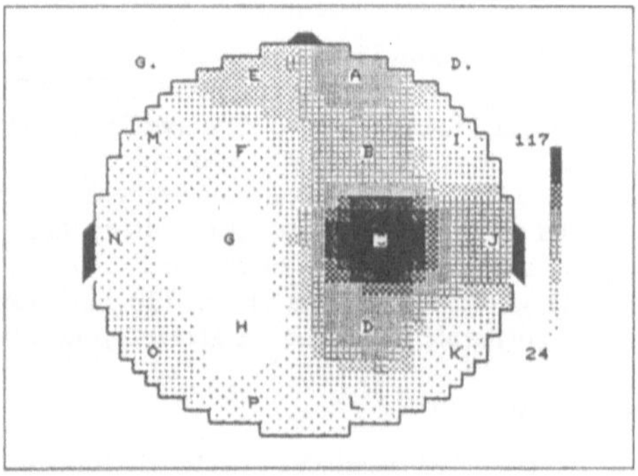

FIGURE 2. Theta activity. Superficial Right Central Metastatic Carcinoma.

TABLE III

THETA ACTIVITY

Tumor Depth / Theta Activity		I CORTEX	II CORTICO-SUBC.	III SUB-CORTICAL	IV DEEP
Foci	46	16	15	10	5
Widespread	14	4	1	3	6
Few or Lack	0	0	0	0	0
	60	20	16	13	11

DISCUSSION

Brain electrical activity mapping is a simple method using quantified E.E.G. by Fast Fourier Transform, non expansive and uninvasive. The patient must be quiet. Moderate drowsiness doesn't prevent the exam (5, 6). We must remind that maps are the display of scalp projected events and not tomographic cuts.

In this study BEAM visualizes tumoral foci in 54 out of 60 cases, accurately in 47. As previously reported (1, 4, 9, 17), localization is more accurate than with conventionnal E.E.G. As all patients explored have an abnormal E.E.G., in no case can this method detect a tumor unnoticeable on the conventionnal E.E.G.

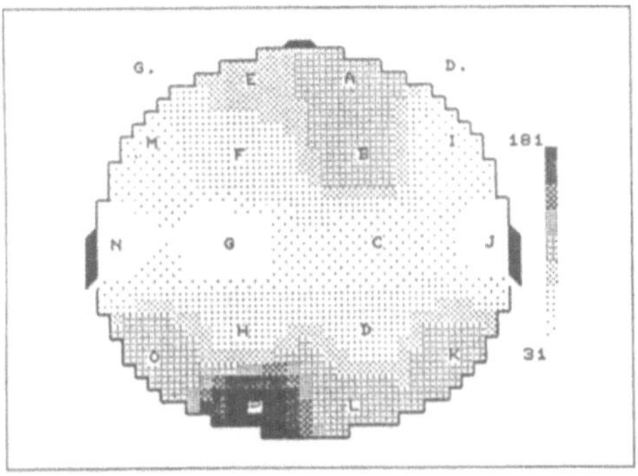

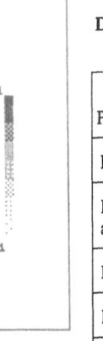

FIGURE 3. Posterior Theta activity lateralized on the left occipital lobe. Left cerebellar hemispheric metastatic carcinoma.

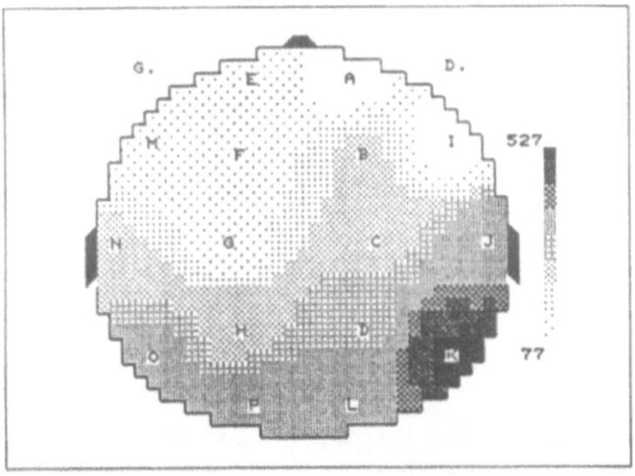

FIGURE 4. Right superficial frontal tumor. Increased ipsilateral alpha activity.

TABLE V
DISTRIBUTION OF ALPHA ACTIVITY ACCORDING TO TUMORS DEPTH

ALPHA PREVALENCE	TUMOR SIDE	OPPOSITE SIDE	SYMMETRICAL
I Cortex	13	3	4
II Cortex and Whitematter	7	6	3
III Subcortical	3	7	3
IV Deep	5	3	3
60	28	19	13

TABLE I
NUMBER OF CASES FOR EACH TUMOR HISTOLOGY, DEPTH AND LOCATION

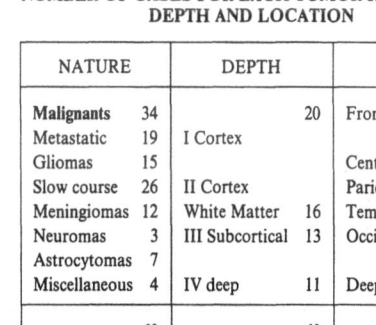

NATURE		DEPTH		LOBE	
Malignants	34		20	Frontal	15
Metastatic	19	I Cortex			
Gliomas	15			Central	10
Slow course	26	II Cortex		Parietal	12
Meningiomas	12	White Matter	16	Temporal	7
Neuromas	3	III Subcortical	13	Occipital	5
Astrocytomas	7				
Miscellaneous	4	IV deep	11	Deep	11
	60		60		60

Theta frequency band is more important than in standard E.E.G. ; when reading an E.E.G. the eyes are attracted by delta waves. On the maps, Theta activity is more frequently localized and contains fewer artifacts than other slow waves.

Delta activity is frequently bilateral and contains eyeball artifacts on the frontal lobes. Delta activity is well localized on the area of groups II and III tumors, of medium depth. This is in agreement with experimental findings of Gloor and al (8) who showed localized polymorphic delta in the cortex overlying a lesion of the white matter.

Changes or asymmetries of alpha and beta activities are more important than in conventionnal E.E.G. in determining lesionnal topography. Decreased alpha activity on the area surrouding the tumor site has been reported (4, 17). Increased localized alpha power has been seen in a case of glioma (18). In our study, changes of alpha activity are dependant of the tumor depth: in superficial lesions (group I), alpha activity is increased on the tumor side. There is no significant correlation between this increase and any history of epilepsy nor polymorphic delta waves on the E.E.G. recording. With deeper tumors, alpha activity is decreased. This could be explained by the interruption of thalamo-cortical fibers in the white matter.

Decreased beta activity on the area overlying the tumor has been described (4, 17). It was so in only 9 cases. Increased localized beta activity is more frequent in our population and there is a significant relationship between it and epilepsy ($p < 0.01$). Part of this fast activity can be due to drugs, but this activity is commonly lateralized, and all our patients received anticonvulsant therapy at the least as a preventive. This fact suggests that localized beta activity could be due to epileptic foci: it has been seen in a case of post ictal period (16).

BEAM does not compete with CT-Scan, it yields a map of the functionnal and not anatomical state of the brain. Nonetheless it provides a visualization of the affected area of the brain more accurate than conventionnal E.E.G. This objective measure from the E.E.G. should be useful to clinicians as an aid in the diagnosis of focal lesions.

SUMMARY

60 patients with histologically confirmed brain tumor have been explored by CT-SCAN, Brain Electrical Activity Mapping (BEAM) and conventionnal E.E.G.

BEAM provides a visualization of the tumoral area in 54 patients out of 60, with accuracy in 47 cases. It never reveals a tumor as none of the conventional E.E.G. is normal. Most of them exhibits significant abnormalities.

Frontal and superficial tumors are detected more reliably by theta than by delta activity. This one has more accuracy for deeper hemispheric, posterior or lateralized tumors. Alpha acitivity is deminished on the area surrounding deep hemispheric lesions and increased on that side in superficial ones.

BEAM provides a more precise location than conventionnal E.E.G. It should be useful to clinicians as an aid in the diagnosis of focal lesions.

KEY WORDS

E.E.G. Mapping, Brain Tumours.

REFERENCES

1. BINNIE (C.D.), BATCHELOR (B.G.), BOWRING (P.A.), BARBY (C.E.), HERBERT (L.), LLOYD (D.S.L.), SMITH (D.M.), SMITH (G.F.) and SMITH (M.): Computer-assited interpretation of clinical E.E.G.s. Electroenceph. Clin. Neurophysiol., **44**: 575-585 (1978).
2. DUFFY (F.H.), ALBERT (M.S.) and Mc ANULTRY (G.): Brain Electrical Activity in Patients with Senile Dementia of the Alzeimer Type. Ann. Neurol. **16**: 439-448 (1984).
3. DUFFY (F.H.), BARTELS (P.H.) and BURCHFIEL (J.): Significance Probability Mapping: an aid in the topographic analysis of Brain Electrical Activity. E.E.G. Clin. Neurophysiol. **51**: 455-462 (1981).
4. DUFFY (F.H.), BURCHFIEL (J.L.) and LOMBROSO (C.T.): Brain Electrical Activity Mapping (BEAM): a method for extending the clinical utility of E.E.G. and evoked potential data. Ann. Neurol., **5**: 309-321 (1979).
5. ETEVENON (P.): Cartographie E.E.G. au cours d'une nuit de sommeil. Communication devant la Société d'E.E.G. et de Neurophysiologie, Tours, 1985.
6. GACHES (J.): Cartographie E.E.G. au cours du sommeil. Communication devant la Société d'E.E.G. et de Neurophysiologie, Tours, 1985.
7. GACHES (J.), ETEVENON (P.): Topographie loco-régionale du spectre E.E.G. chez l'homme: cartographie de deux cas d'accident vasculaire cérébral (dont l'un suivi sous sommeil) Maladies et médicaments **1**: 182-191 (1984).
8. GLOOR (P.), BALL (G.) and SCHAUL (N.): Brain lesions that produce delta waves in the E.E.G. Neurology (Minneap.) **27**: 326-333 (1975).
9. GOTMAN (J.), GLOOR (P.) and RAY (W.F.): A quantitative comparaison of traditional reading of the E.E.G. and interpretation of computer extracted features in patients with supratentorial brain lesion. Electroenceph. Clin. Neurophysiol. **38**: 623-639 (1975).
10. GUENTHER (W.) and BREITLING (D): Predominant Sensorimotor Area Left Hemisphere Dysfunction in Schizophrenia Measured by Brain Electrical Activity Mapping. Biol. Psychiatry **20**: 515-532 (1985).
11. MORIHISA (J.M.), DUFFY (F.H.), WYATT (R.J). Brain Electrical Activity Mapping (BEAM) in Schizophrenic Patients. Arch. Gen. Psychiatry **40**: 719-728 (1983).
12. MORSTYN (R.), DUFFY (F.H.) and Mc CARLEY (R.W.): Altered Topography of E.E.G. Spectral Content in Schizophrenia. E.E.G. Clin. Neurophysiol. **56**: 263-271 (1983).
13. NAGATA (K.), MIZUKAMI (M.), ARAKI (G.), KAWASE (T.) and HIRANO (M.): Topographic Electroencephalographic Study of Cerebral Infarction using Computed Mapping of the E.E.G. J. Cereb. Blood Flow Metabol. **2**: 79-88 (1982).

14. PIDOUX (B.), ETEVENON (P.), CAMPISTRON (D.), PERON-MAGNAN (P.), VERDEAUX (G.) et DENIKER (P.): Aspects topographiques des rythmes rapides médicamenteux en topo-électroencéphalographie quantitative. Rev. E.E.G. Neurophysiol **13**: 35-41 (1983).

15. PRIER (S.), BENOIT (C.) et CAMBIER (J.): Activités verbales, visuospatiales et de calcul mental étudiées par cartographie E.E.G. chez les sujets droitiers normaux. Communication lors de la réunion mixte de la Société d'E.E.G. et de la Société Circulation et Métabolisme du cerveau. Montpellier le 7 juin 1986. A paraître.

16. PRIER (S.), BENOIT (C.) et REDONDO (A.). Résultat de la cartographie E.E.G. au cours des tumeurs cérébrales. Confrontation aux méthodes d'imagerie. Communication devant la Société d'E.E.G. et de Neurophysiologie le 6 décembre 1985. A paraître.

17. SCHNEIDER (J.). Localisation tumorale par l'analyse spectrale et ses données statistiques. Rev. d'E.E.G. Neurophysiol. **6**: 408-414 (1976).

18. SEBBAN (C.L.), RUEL (M.), BAUDRIMONT (M.), BENKEMOUN (G.), DEBOUZY (C.) et MARTEAU (R.): Expression de pathologies cérébrales ischémique, hémorragique, tumorale et dégénératrice sur la cartographie E.E.G. Étude clinique. Br. J. Clin. Pract. Ed. Int. **4**: 22-31 (1984).

An Expert System for the Diagnosis of Brain Tumours in Computer Tomographic Images and Histopathologically

J.R. IGLESIAS, E. KAZNER, J. ESPARZA (°), C. ARUFFO (°°).

INTRODUCTION

For a better understanding and management of the different brain tumours, an equivalent computer tomographic and morphological classification is desirable. An adequate classification leads to a grading of brain tumours and can thus shed some light on their prognosis.

Many variables are dealt with when classifying a given brain tumour, both computer tomographically as well as histopathologically. By using a discriminant analysis it is possible to reduce a great amount of data into few interpretation units. With this method objective criteria are given coefficient values for a linear function and thus ordered in groups (11). It is the purpose of this study to apply a discriminant analysis to classify brain tumours both computer tomographically as well as histopathologically.

TABLE I

Testing of the classification of 177 brain tumours by CT based on a discriminant analysis

Diagnosis by CT	Correct	Incorrect	Total
Astrocytoma	11 (100 %)	0	11
Anaplastic Astrocytoma	15 (88 %)	2 (12 %)	17
Oligodendroglioma	6 (67 %)	3 (33 %)	9
Glioblastoma	25 (93 %)	1 (7 %)	26
Pilocytic Astrocytoma	18 (95 %)	1 (5 %)	19
Ependymoma	13 (100 %)	0	13
Medulloblastoma	14 (88 %)	2 (13 %)	16
Lymphoma	7 (70 %)	3 (30 %)	10
Plexus Papilloma	0	6 (100 %)	6
Meningioma	31 (91 %)	3 (9 %)	34
Metastasis	12 (80 %)	3 (20 %)	15
Total	152 (86 %)	25 (14 %)	177

MATERIALS AND METHODS

A. Computed tomography

A retrospective study of 3 750 computer tomographies (CT) (9) of patients with brain tumours (Table I) was done. The data obtained was used as a data bank or "training field". The presence or absence of the following CT-characteristics was considered in each CT: predominant localization (10 different localizations were taken into account), x-ray absorption, lesion delimitation, multiplicity, calcifications, enhancement after injection of contrast material, post-contrasting enhancement, and perifocal edema. To test our method, we analysed 177 new CT scans. For each case a confirmed histopathological diagnosis based on the World Health Organization's classification of brain tumours (15) existed.

B. Histopathology

In a prospective study, 1684 biopsies of nervous system tumours were analysed using a discriminant analysis and used as a data base. The existence or absence of 50 selected histological items was recorded for the 14 different brain tumours studied (Table II). The same methodology was

TABLE II

Testing of the classification of 532 tumours of the Nervous System based on a discriminant analysis

Neuropathological diagnosis	Number of tumours	1st diagnosis correct	2nd diagnosis correct	False diagnosis
Meningioma	51	50	1	0
Glioblastoma	46	42	2	2
Neurinoma	52	50	2	0
Neurofibroma	61	59	2	0
Astrocytoma	75	67	7	1
Oligodendroglioma	49	45	4	0
Ependymoma	42	38	3	1
Medulloblastoma	26	26	0	0
Metastasis	35	35	0	0
Astroblastoma	5	4	1	0
Angioma	35	35	0	0
Hemangioblastoma	12	12	0	0
Hypophysis Adenoma	35	35	0	0
Neuroblastoma	8	4	1	3
Total	532	502 (94%)	23 (5%)	7 (1%)

(°) Neurosurgical Clinic, Rudolf Virchow Krankenhaus, Augustenburger Platz 1, 1000 Berlin 65.
(°°) Institute of Neurpathology, Klinikum Steglitz der Freien Universität Berlin, Hindenburgdamm 30, 1000 Berlin 45, FRG. On leave from the IIBM-UNAM, Mexico with a DAAD Fellowship.

M. Chatel, F. Darcel and J. Pecker (eds.), Brain Oncology. ISBN-13: 978-94-010-8003-3

applied to obtain a differential diagnosis among meningiomas, glioblastomas, astrocytomas and oligodendrogliomas.

Both for A and B, a personal computer Commodore/8032 (32KB RAM) with a dual-drive floppy disk (8050) was used. The programming language used was Commodore's Microsoft Basic.

Mathematical foundations

Considering that the interpretation of any finding lies equally upon a probability a priori and a conditional probability (3) the values of the probabilities a priori for each diagnosis, both in the CT scans and histopathologically, were calculated (7, 8). The conditional probability was calculated by using a discriminant analysis of the different characteristics or items recorded. Discriminant analyses were calculated separately for CT scans and histological preparations.

RESULTS

In using a discriminant analysis we correctly classified 86 % of the 177 brain tumours in computer tomographies as posteriorly proven with an histological analysis of each of the tumours (Table I).

Histopathologically 94 % of the 532 cases of the testing field were correctly diagnosed. However, if we consider both the 1st and 2nd diagnoses as correct we obtained an accuracy of 99 % (Table II). When calculating the differential diagnoses, we obtained 63 % correctly diagnosed meningiomas (Table III), 85 % glioblastomas (Table IV), 95 % astrocytomas (Table V) and 98 % oligodendrogliomas (Table VI) when considering both the 1st and 2nd diagnoses as correct.

DISCUSSION

From our results, it is evident that a mathematical model such as the one we used provides a structuration of the observed data thus representing an efficient and rapid system for the classification and diagnosis of brain tumours. This system has also been used with success in other central nervous system pathologies (1-2, 4-8, 12-14). However, limitations due to the intrinsic characteristics of each tumour exist. Sometimes the limits between one brain tumour and another are not well defined. In the case of ependymomas and plexus papillomas which have very similar computer tomographic images, our system, which is based on a discriminant analysis, looses accuracy. The same limitations exist when trying

TABLE III

Differential diagnosis of Meningiomas based on a discriminant analysis

Neuropathological diagnosis	Number of tumours	1st diagnosis correct	2nd diagnosis correct	3-5 diagnosis correct
Endotheliomatous	16	10	2	4
Fibroblastic	11	9	2	0
Transitional	5	1	3	1
Psamomatous	8	0	2	6
Angiomatous	4	1	1	2
Angioblastic	2	1	0	1
Malign	4	0	0	4
Meningosarcoma	—	—	—	—
Others	1	0	0	1
Total	51	22 (43%)	10 (20%)	19 (37%)

TABLE IV

Differential diagnosis of Glioblastomas based on a discriminant analysis

Neuro-pathologic diagnosis	Number of tumours	1st diagnosis correct	2nd diagnosis correct	3-5 diagnosis correct
Polymorphic	32	19 (59.4%)	9 (28.1%)	4 (12.5%)
Isomorphic	6	5 (83.3%)	1 (16.7%)	0
Giant Cell	6	4 (66.7%)	0	2 (33.3%)
Gliosarcoma	2	0	1 (50.0%)	1 (50.0%)
Gliomatosis	—	—	—	—
Total	46	28 (60.9%)	11 (23.9%)	7 (15.2%)

TABLE V

Differential diagnosis of Astrocytomas based on a discriminant analysis

Neuropathologic diagnosis	Number of tumours	1st diagnosis correct	2nd diagnosis correct	3-5 diagnosis correct
Fibrillary	33	27	5	1
Protoplasmatic	5	5	0	0
Gemistocytic	—	—	—	—
Pilocytic	14	12	1	1
Subependymal	1	1	0	0
Malign	17	15	1	1
Astroblastoma	5	4	0	1
Total	75	64 (85.3%)	7 (9.3%)	4 (5.3%)

TABLE VI

Differential diagnosis of Oligodendrogliomas based on a discriminant analysis

Neuropathologic diagnosis	Number of tumours	1st diagnosis correct	2nd diagnosis correct	3-5 diagnosis correct
Oligodendroglioma	10	6	4	0
Oligoastrocytoma	23	20	3	0
Malign	16	9	6	1
Total	49	35 (71%)	13 (27%)	1 (2%)

to give a differential diagnosis among glioblastomas since all the subtypes are very similar. In these cases it is necessary to select as items those characteristics which are essentially different in the entities studied.

Due to the fact that we were working with a binary system in which no quantitative data are taken into consideration, our results were not always reliable. Such was the case of psamomatous meningiomas. Psamomatous bodies are seen in all meningiomas, it is only the amount present which makes a tumour psamomatous or not (15). Further refinements to our system in which quantifications are included are now in progress.

In order for an expert system to be successful, the items included must be selected very carefully. Those characteristics which clearly differentiate one tumour from another should be included. Attention should be paid to the fact that items in the data bank should be homogeneous in all entities studied. Only in this manner it is possible to compare and extrapolate results.

Up to now no direct correlation can be made between our computer tomographic diagnoses and the histological ones. Due to the fact that our computer tomographic study was retrospective the type of tumours included differed from those of our histological study. Because we believe it is very important to have a common language among neurologists, neurosurgeons, neuroradiologists and neuropathologists, we are now working on a prospective study of computer tomographies which will hopefully allow us to correlate results to histopathology and thus facilitate the diagnosis and management and which will give insights into the prognosis of each new coming case.

This methodology has been widely used in medicine (1-2, 4-8, 10, 12-14) since it objectivizes the image seen by correlating all the studied items and comparing them to the distribution of each item in the cases with a known diagnosis which are stored in the data bank. It also provides a rapid classification and an excellent archive.

SUMMARY

An expert system for the diagnosis of the most frequently seen brain tumours and their subgroups was designed. This system can be applied to computed tomographies as well as to histopathological sections. We selected 11 items in evaluating computer tomographies and 50 in evaluating histopathological preparations. Subsequently we determined the probabilities of each of these characteristics to appear in each type of brain tumour and determined their coefficients of importance. These coefficients gave us the diagnostic archetype. For all new tumours we determined the likelihood of each characteristic to those of the tumours existing in the data base and transformed our findings to probabilities of similarities by applying Bayes' theorem. Out of 177 computer tomographies with brain tumours 86 % were correctly diagnosed. Whilst 95 % of 532 brain tumours histopathologically examined were accurately diagnosed.

KEY WORDS

Brain Tumours, Computer Tomography, Histopathology, Data Processing, Expert Systems, Discriminant Analysis.

REFERENCES

1. BOULAY (G.H. du), PRICE (V.E.): The diagnosis of intracranial tumours assisted by computer. Br J. Radiol. **41**: 762-781, 1968.
2. BOULAY (G.H. du), TEATHER (D.), HARLING (D.), CLARKE (G.): Improvement in the computer-assisted diagnosis of cerebral tumours. Br. J. Radiol. **50**: 849-854, 1977.
3. ESCUDERO (L.F.): *Reconocimiento de Patrones.* Paraninfo, Madrid, 1977, pp. 1-688.
4. GELERNTER (D.), GELERNTER (J.): Expert systems and diagnostic monitors in psychiatry. Med. Inform. **11**: 23-28, 1986.
5. HIER (D.B.), ATKINSON (G.D.), PERLINES (R.), HILL (H.), EVANS (M.), DESAI (B.), MCCORMICK (W.C.), CAPLAN (L.R.): Can a patient data base help build a stroke diagnostic expert system? Med. Inform. **11**: 75-81, 1986.

6. IGLESIAS (J.R.), SANCHEZ (M.J.), SANDRA (A.), MOHNHAUPT (A.): Computer model of archive and diagnosis of brain tumours based on the WHO classification. EDV für Medizin u. Biologie **14**: 40-44, 1983.

7. IGLESIAS (J.R.), PFANNKUCH (F.), ARUFFO (C.), KAZNER (E.), CERVOS-NAVARRO (J.): Histopathological diagnosis of brain tumours with the help of a computer: Mathematical fundaments and practical application. Acta Neuropath. **71**: 130-135, 1986.

8. IGLESIAS (J.R.), KAZNER (E.), ARUFFO (C.), ESPARZA (J.): A model of semiautomatic type-specific diagnosis of brain tumours by computed tomography: Mathematical fundaments and practical application. Br. J. Radiol. **59**: 895-900, 1986.

9. KAZNER (E.), WENDE (S.), GRUMME (Th.), LAKSCH (W.), STOCHDORPH (O.): *Computertomographie intrakranieller Tumoren aus klinischer Sicht.* Springer, Berlin, 1981, pp. 1-548.

10. ROTTE (K.H.): Zur Anwendung der computergestützten Röntgendiagnostic in der Onkologie. Arch Geschulstforsch. **49**: 347-356, 1979.

11. SPATH (H.): *Cluster-Analyse-Algorithmen zur Objektklassifizierung und Datenreduktion.* R. Oldenburg, Münschen, 1977, pp. 9-217.

12. STEWART (A.), CALA (L.A.): Mathematical method to utilize a computer for diagnosis of site and type of intracerebral mass lesions. Br. J. Radiol. **48**: 97-100, 1975.

13. WILLIS (K.), BOULAY (G.H. du), TEATHER (D.): Initial findings in the computed-aided diagnosis of cerebral tumours using CT scan results. Br. J. Radiol. **54**: 948-952, 1981.

14. WILLIS (K.), TEATHER (D.), BOULAY (G.H. du): An improvement of computer aided diagnosis of meningiomas after CT. Neuroradiology **22**: 255-257, 1982.

15. ZÜLCH (K.J.): Historical development of the classification of brain tumours and the new proposal of the World Health Organization (WHO). Neurosurg. Rev. **4**: 123-127, 1981.

PART V:
CLINICO-PATHOLOGICAL STUDIES

Multi-Centre Epidemiological Study on Primary Cerebral Tumours in the Veneto Region
Preliminary data from June 1st 1985 to December 31 st 1985

P. ZAMPIERI (°), S. MINGRINO (°), D. CERVESATO (°), G.B. SOATTIN (°), E. DI STEFANO (°°), P.L. LONGATTI (°°), M. GEROSA (°°°), C. LICATA (°°°), A. NICOLATO (°°°), L. CASENTINI (°°°°), U. FORNEZZA (°°°°), F. MENEGHINI (°°°°°).

INTRODUCTION

Since June 1st 1985, a multi-centre epidemiological study on primary cerebral tumours has been in progress in the Veneto Region.

The four Neurosurgical Centres of the Region (Padova, Treviso, Verona and Vicenza) are taking part in the research.

Data on anamnesis, clinical findings, neuro-radiology, treatment (surgery, radiotherapy and chemotherapy) and follow-up are collected on each patient.

No pre-set therapeutic protocol is applied, each centre operates independently.

The study is planned to last for two years and we report here the preliminary data regarding the period from June 1st 1985 to December 31 st 1985 (7 months).

GENERAL DATA

A total of 406 patients with intracranial tumour were admitted to the four Neurosurgical Centres; 102 of them had a meningioma, 55 a pituitary adenoma, 51 a metastasis, 18 a dysembryogenetic tumour and 143 a primary cerebral tumour.

Of the 143 gliomas, 125 had a histologically-confirmed diagnosis and 18 had only a clinical-radiological diagnosis (14 were not operated on for surgical contra-indications, 4 for refusal).

A total of 237 patients with intracranial tumours came from the Veneto Region, 207 of them with a primary intracranial tumour and 83 with a primary cerebral tumour,

The estimated average number of residents in the Region for the period in question is 4.367.389.

DATA ON PRIMARY CEREBRAL TUMOURS (125 CASES)

The group of histologically-verified gliomas includes 42 low grade astrocytomas, 57 anaplastic astrocytomas and glioblastomas, 10 oligodendrogliomas, 6 ependymomas, 6 medulloblastomas, 3 lymphomas and 1 pinealoma.

There is a prevalence for the male sex with a ratio M/F of 69 to 56 (55.2 % to 44.8 %).

The age-distribution is shown in the schedule below:

Age	No of cases	%
0-10 ys	8	6.4
10-20	15	12.0
20-30	14	11.2
30-40	8	6.4
40-50	20	16.0
50-60	37	29.6
60-70	18	14.4
> 70	5	4.0

(°) Div. Neurosurgery, Padova, Italy, (°°) Div. Neurosurgery, Treviso, Italy, (°°°) Dep. Neurosurgery, Verona, Italy, (°°°°) Div. Neurosurgery, Vicenza, Italy, (°°°°°) Unit Biostatistics Epidemiology, Fidia labs, Abano Terme, Italy.

M. Chatel, F. Darcel and J. Pecker (eds.), Brain Oncology. ISBN-13: 978-94-010-8003-3

From a general point of view 88.8 % of the patients were in good conditions, 11.2 % were affected by other pathologies, especially heart or lung diseases.

The pre-operative Karnofsky-score ranged between 70 and 100 in as much as 40 % of the cases, between 40 and 70 in 41.9 %, between 0 and 40 in 17.7 %.

The operation consisted in a macroscopically-complete removal of the tumour in 29.5 % of the cases; in 37.7 % a sub-total removal was made; in 13.1 % any incomplete removal was possible and in 19.6 % a biopsy was made.

The overall operative mortality has been 8 %.

There was a percentage of surgical complications of 14.6 %: 6.5 % of haematomas, 5.7 % of oedema, 0.8 % of meningitis and 1.6 % of other complications.

General complications presented in 8.9 % of the cases, more often pulmonary ones (4.8 %).

The post-operative Karnofsky-score ranged between 70 and 100 in as much as 56 % of the cases, between 40 and 70 in 34.2 %, between 0 and 40 in 9.6 %.

PRELIMINARY COMPARISON BETWEEN LOW-GRADE ASTROCYTOMAS AND ANAPLASTIC ASTROCYTOMAS

The data of this study concern only a part of the pre-determinate period and the series of patients is still limited. Therefore it is impossible to draw any conclusion. However it seemed interesting to make a preliminary comparison between the two most numerous classes of gliomas, that is between low-grade astrocytomas (42 cases) on one hand and anaplastic astrocytomas and glioblastomas (57 cases) on the other.

CLINICAL CHARACTERISTICS

		Low-grade astrocytomas %	Anaplastic astrocytomas %
SEX (M/F)		54.7/45.2	59.6/40.3
AGE	0-10 ys	7.1	1.7
	10-20	21.4	0.0
	20-30	11.9	5.2
	30-40	7.1	7.0
	40-50	11.9	22.8
	50-60	28.5	36.8
	60-70	4.7	22.8
	> 70	7.1	3.5
SYMPTOMATOLOGY			
	Progressive course	69.0	84.2
	Sudden onset	9.5	5.2
	Epilepsy	19.0	10.5
	Accidental finding	2.3	0.0
DURATION OF SYMPTOMS			
	0-1 month	38.1	38.6
	1.3 months	16.6	38.6
	3-6 months	14.2	17.5
	6-12 months	9.5	0.0
	>12 months	21.3	5.1
SIGNS ON ADMISSION			
	Intracranial hypertension	40.4	58.9
	Neurological deficit	90.4	89.2
	Mental status abnormalities	31.7	50.0

NEURORADIOLOGICAL INVESTIGATIONS

		Low-grade astrocytomas %	Anaplastic astrocytomas %
CT / DENSITY OF TUMOUR			
	Low density	55.5	30.9
	High density	13.8	9.0
	Mixed	25.0	40.0
	Rim of enhancement	5.5	20.0
CT / CONTRAST ENHANCEMENT		73.5	92.8
CT / CALCIFICATIONS		5.2	1.7
CT / HEMORRHAGE		2.7	10.7
CT / SHIFT OF MIDLINE			
	No	25.6	18.1
	0-5 mm	38.4	38.1
	>5 mm	35.9	43.6
CT / SURROUNDING EDEMA			
	Not significant	51,3	23.6
	< 50 % of tumour size	18.9	32.7
	50-100 % of tumour size	29.7	38.1
	>100 % of tumour size	0.0	5.4
ANGIOGRAPHY			
	Normal	5.2	1.7
	Arterial displacement	31.5	42.8
	Tumour blush	44.7	41.0
	Not performed	18.4	14.2

CHARACTERISTICS OF NEOPLASM

		Low-grade astrocytomas %	Anaplastic astrocytomas %
SITE	Frontal	11.9	14.2
	Temporal	30.9	26.7
	Parietal	28.5	42.8
	Occipital	2.3	8.9
	Corpus callosum	0.0	3.5
	Third ventricle	9.5	0.0
	Brain-stem	4.7	1.7
	Fourth ventricle-vermis	4.7	1.7
	Cerebellar hemisphere	7.1	0.0
DIAMETER	< 2 cm	7.3	7.2
	2-4 cm	48.7	49.0
	>4 cm	43.9	43.6
CONSISTENCY	Firm	14.8	9.6
	Cystic	37.0	28.8
	Soft	48.1	61.5
TYPE OF GROWTH			
	Not infiltrative	13.7	9.6
	Infiltrative	86.2	90.3

KEY WORDS

Brain Tumours, Epidemiology.

(*) This research is supported by the REGIONE VENETO.

Chemically Induced Human Gliomas
Occurrence of Brain Gliomas in three Matchbox Manufacturers
An occupational risk ?

Ph. BRET (°), J. PIALAT (°°),
H. ROBERT, R. DERUTY (°°°), G. FISCHER (°), M. KZAIZ (°).

INTRODUCTION

Very little is known on the aetiology of brain tumours of the glioma group. In most cases encountered in the daily neurosurgical pratice, no particular factor of risk is advocated in view of the past history of patients. The ability of radiotherapy to induce glioblastoma has been established (4). Induction of intra-cranial tumours by inoculation of viruses is supported by several reports (1) and the possibility of a transmission of brain gliomas among a population of non blood relative patients has been recently emphasized (7). Since the pioneering work of Zimmerman using methylcholanthrene (10), many chemicals have been suspected as brain carcinogenic agents. Nitrosourea is routinely used in laboratory to induce brain tumours in rats (5, 6, 8). Acrylonitrile has also experimentally been identified as a brain carcinogen (3). Other substances are regarded as potentially carcinogenic without specificity for the human brain. The role of chemicals is supported by a recent epidemiologic study (9) showing an increased risk for brain tumours in certain occupations. The 3 patients that are the subject of this report were managed at our institution during the 6 past years for brain glioma and had in common the fact that they had been working in a similar workplace in a matchbox factory. This clinical experience suggests an environmental risk factor, possibly occupational.

MATERIAL

Case 1

This patient was aged 57, when she was referred to our department in october 1985. No previous pathological history was notable except for a professionnel bilateral hypoacousia. She experienced sudden visual difficulties. Her examination showed obvious right lateral hemianopsia. She also showed slight speech impairment. Computerized tomography showed a left parietal necrotic mass associated with mass effect and widespread oedema. A craniotomy was undertaken on nov 5, 1985 and a subtotal resection of the tumour was accomplished (P.B.). On histological examination, the diagnosis of isomorphic glioblastoma was stated. The patient died on April 15, 1986. During the post operative course, her relatives had informed us that she had been working for 23 years as a matchbox manufacturer. Furthermore, two of her coworkers who had been employed in the same workplace had been operated on for a brain tumour and subsequently died.

The data seemed to us noteworthy enough to review the clinical course of the mentioned patients and to start a study devoted to the identification of a brain carcinogenic factor in this particular industry. The 2 other patients have been operated on in the same institute by another neurosurgeon (R.D.)

Case 2

P... aged 37 at the time of referral had been employed in the same workplace as patient 1 for 2 non consecutive years (1972-1973 and 1976-1977). Prior to 1972, he had been employed as railwayman. From 1973 to 1976, he had been employed in the marketing department of the same matchbox factory. From 1977 to the initial manifestation of the disease, he had been employed as a printer in the same factory. In 1980, he was treated at several times for a professional dermatosis which was related to exposure to acrylates.

(°) Service de Neurochirurgie C, (°°) Laboratoire d'Anatomie pathologique, (°°°) Service de Neurochirurgie B.
Address : Hôpital Neurologique et Neurochirurgical Pierre WERTHEIMER, 59, boulevard Pinel, 69394 Lyon cedex 3 (France).

M. Chatel, F. Darcel and J. Pecker (eds.), Brain Oncology. ISBN-13: 978-94-010-8003-3

He was admitted to our institution in June 1981. He had showed left progressive hemiparesis associated with ideo motor apraxia. Clinical evaluation showed a left homonymous hemianopsia. CT showed a righ sided parietal necrotic tumour surrounded by brain oedema and slightly enhancing after contrast injection. He was operated on the July 23, 1981 and an subtotal resection of a pleïomorphic glioblastoma was made. Radiotherapy and chemotherapy were given postoperatively. The patient died 12 months after diagnosis was established.

Case 3

C... was aged 42 at the time of referral. He first entered in the matchbox factory in 1967 and he occupied the same workplace as patients 1 and 2 during 9 non consecutive years (1969-1971, 1972-1979). He came to clinical evaluation in June 1979 because he complained of paroxysmal headaches and of visual difficulties. Physical examination disclosed a mild left hemiparesis with bilateral choked disks. CT showed a right frontal heterogenous tumour with mass effect and moderate enhancement following injection. Operation was performed on July 11, 1979. A grade II astrocytoma was found and partially removed. Despite he was given radiotherapy and chimotherapy, the status of the patient progressively deteriorated and he died on April 28, 1981.

RESULTS

The preliminary results of the survey undertaken in collaboration with the occupational medical department of the mentioned factory has led us to consider a brain oncogenic substance as the likely common relationship in this unusual series. Statistically, a brain glioma is expected to occur in 4,3 to 4,9 individuals per 100,000 in the overall population. 440 workers have been employed in the implicated workplace over the period during which our 3 patients are supposed to having been "exposed". The quotient: observed number of gliomas/expected number of gliomas is 139 (681:4,9) would be statistically significant in a larger series. However, a coincidental occurrence of these gliomas seems unlikely and require further investigations. According to the report issued from the medical departement of the factory, a wide range of substances were listed as daily manipulated by matchbox workers. Among those, the followings only were regarded as potential mutagens:

— Formol urea resins and perhaps vinyl cements (scraper components),

— Auramine and other dye components.

As stated in 1985 by IARC (2), auramine only may be potentially carcinogen in man although its ability to cause brain tumours in laboratory animals and in human has not been documented.

Additionaly, one should mention the possible role of hydrocarbon derivates and organic solvents as compounds of lubricating oils used for maintaining mechanical equipment and machines.

DISCUSSION

To our known, no previous report of "professionnal" gliomas occuring under such circumstances is available in the literature. However, many chemical carcinogens have been advocated as possibly responsible for an increased brain tumour risk in several industries (9). Workers usually have multiple exposures and a single chemical risk is difficult to evaluate. The following occupations are thought to carry a potential risk: rubber industry (hexamethylene tetramine, carbon tetrachoride), plastics industry (vinyl choride monomer acrylonitrile), petroleum refining and petrochemical industry (aliphatic and aromatic polycyclic hydrocarbons) and a broad categories of occupations such as those employing or producing formaldedhyde (photograph processors, pathologists, anatomists...), those manipulating phenol compounds (textile industry, weapons industry) and nitrosamines (research laboratories).

Epidemiologic data strongly suggest that a relationship may exist between brain tumours and occupational exposures. Unfortunately, informations on this concern are still controversial and there is a need for a multicentric study including the contribution of neurologists, neurosurgeons, epidemiologists, occupational medicine physicians and laboratory workers. In this view, our experience is of interest because it points out the possible risk of chemically induced glioma in an occupational group in which it had not been mentioned previously. Further developments of this study are directed towards the identification of similar cases and the characterization of the carcinogenic substance. We hope it will prompt other neurosurgeons to report similar cases and to pay a special attention to their patients' present and previous occupation in all cases of brain gliomas.

KEY-WORDS

Glioblastoma, Brain Glioma, Carcinogen, Mutagen, Occupational cancer.

AKNOWLEDGEMENTS

The authors wish to acknowledge for their contribution Professeur Guy PROST, Laboratoire de Médecine du Travail, Faculté Alexis-Carrel, Lyon and Docteur M. FOURNIER, Service de Médecine du Travail de la Manufacture d'allumettes de M...

REFERENCES

1. COPELAND (D.D.), VOGEL (F.S.), BIGNER (D.D.): The induction of intra cranial neoplasms by the inoculation of avian sarcoma virus in perinatal and adult rats. J. Neuropathol. Exp. Neurol., 1975, 34, 340-58.
2. INRS: Produits chimiques carcinogènes pour l'homme. Définitions. Classement. Cahier de notes documentaires n° 123, 1986, 201-03.
3. MALTONI (C.), CILIBERTI (A.), DIMAIO (V.): Carcinogenicity bioassays on rats in acrylonitrile administered by inhalation and ingestion. Med. Sav., 1977, 68, 401-11.
4. PIATT (J.H.), BLUE (J.H.), SCHOLD S.C., BURGER (P.C.): Glioblastoma multiforme after radiotherapy from acromegaly. Neurosurgery 1983, 12, 85-9.
5. PLEVEN (C.): Survenue élective de glioblastomes lors de la manipulation en laboratoire de recherche des dérivés de la nitrosoguanidine. Press Med., 1984, 37, 13.
6. SCHMIDER (H.H.), NIELSEN (S.L.), SCHILLER (A.L.), MESSER (J.): Morphological studies of rat brain tumours induced by N-nitrosomethylurea. J. Neurosurg., 1971, 34, 335-40.
7. SIQUEIRA (E.B.), KRANZLER (L.I.), SCHAFFER (L.): Occurence of glioblastoma multiforme in three closely related patients. Surg. Neurol. 1985, 24, 387-91.
8. SWENBERG (J.A.), KOESTNER (A.), WECHSLER (W.): The induction of tumours of the nervous system with intravenous methylnitrosourea. Lab. Invest., 1972, 26, 74-85.
9. THOMAS (T.L.), WAXWEILER (R.J.): Brain tumors and occupational risk factors. Scand. J. Work Environ. Health 1986, 12, 1-15.
10. ZIMMERMAN (H.M.), ARNOLD (H.): Experimental brain tumors. 1. Tumors produced with methylcholanthrene. Cancer Res., 1941, 1, 919-38.

Prospective Analysis of Grade III and IV Gliomas, With Considerations on Histological Classification. (An E.O.R.T.C. Brain Tumor Group Study)

J.M. BRÜCHER (°), O. DALESIO (°°), G. SOLBU (°°).

The usefulness of a new antineoplastic treatment can be appreciated by comparison to a series of similar cases not receiving this treatment. Treated and untreated tumors have to be histologically classified and the used criteria and nomenclature must be uniform in both arms of the trial.

GRADING SYSTEMS

Using the four-grade system of Broders (1926) for the classification of carcinomas, Kernohan et al (1949) introduced a simplified classification of gliomas in which the grades were estimated histologically by evaluating the numbers of mitotic figures, the percentage of dedifferentiated tumor cells, the extent of necrosis and vascular proliferation, and the degree of pleomorphism. This new classification has been generally well accepted by neurosurgeons and neurologists, who considered the numerous subtypes of the classification of Bailey and Cushing (1926, 1930) as too sophisticated.

The grading system of Kernohan et al (1949) had some biological meaning, but it was based on rather complex and difficult histologic criteria, which were improved later on by Kernohan and Sayre (1952) and Sayre (1956). Nevertheless this classification remained unclear and gliomas were frequently given grade I-II or grade III-IV or even grade II-IV by many pathologists.

In order to avoid the feeling of inaccuracy a three-grade system, as suggested by Ringertz (1950), has been preferred by some pathologists (Schröder et al 1968 a and b, Schröder et al 1970, Nelson et al 1983). The usefulness and accuracy of this three-tiered system have been recently demonstrated by Burger et al (1985) for a large series of gliomas categorized as astrocytoma, anaplastic astrocytoma, or glioblastoma multiforme. The oversimplification of this three-tiered classification can be criticized.

On the other hand a four-grade system has been developed recently by Smith et al (1983) for oligodendrogliomas which were graded A to D, but the survival curves for each tumor grade showed no significant difference between grades B and C. This grading system was based on five histological features amongst which the mitotic rate was not included.

In all these grading systems, the **grades** are understood as histological **stages** in a natural biological evolution of the neoplasm. The astrocytic origin of the glioblastoma has never been demonstrated and so it is not logical to classify this tumor as a highly malignant astrocytic neoplasm.

One of the merits of the « Histological typing of tumors of the central nervous system » proposed by the World Health Organization (WHO) (Zülch 1979) is, above its possible worldwide acceptance, the fact that each tumor entity was simply described and received a biological grade, according to the grading developed by Zülch and Wechsler (1968) and Zülch (1975). This four-grade system, included in the WHO classification of brain tumors, expresses their usual biological behavior in growth and thus the average postoperative survival time of the patients (Zülch 1980, 1986). As emphasized by Smith et al (1983) « the idea of attaching a prognostic estimator to the tumor's name has merit ». Grading of tumors is a response to the daily demand of clinicians. In the WHO classification each tumor entity has a grade which means a clear biological prognostic, and these grades are not to be considered as successive stages in the natural evolution of the tumors.

(°) Neuropathology Department, University of Louvain, avenue Mounier 52, 1200 Brussels (Belgium), (°°) E.O.R.T.C. Data Center, boulevard de Waterloo 125, 1000 Brussels (Belgium).

M. Chatel, F. Darcel and J. Pecker (eds.), Brain Oncology. ISBN-13: 978-94-010-8003-3

WHO CLASSIFICATION

Well differentiated tumors of the nervous tissue are generally characterized by a long history and signs of slow growth, but foci of faster growing activity and lesser differentiation may occur later on. When containing these anaplastic foci, the tumors are called « anaplastic » in the WHO classification. The growth potentiality of these anaplastic tumors is generally lower than that of the actually malignant tumors which show fast growing activity from the beginning and in all the examined areas. In the WHO classification the anaplastic tumors are given the grade 3 and separated from the grade 4 malignant tumors.

The three following examples will facilitate the understanding of the WHO classification, particularly in the controversial field of anaplastic gliomas.

A typical **glioblastoma** is a well circumscribed glioma, often resembling a metastasis (with the CTscan as well as during the neurosurgical approach). Histologically signs of fast growing activity (high cellularity, high mitotic index, poorly differentiated cells) are visible in all the examined areas until the edges of the tumor (fig. 1). Clinical signs of fast growing activity are also noted (short clinical history before and after the surgical excision). Such a glioblastoma is thus a highly malignant tumor from the beginning and in all its parts. Therefore it is considered as a grade 4 glioma.

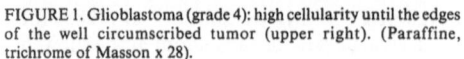

FIGURE 1. Glioblastoma (grade 4): high cellularity until the edges of the well circumscribed tumor (upper right). (Paraffine, trichrome of Masson x 28).

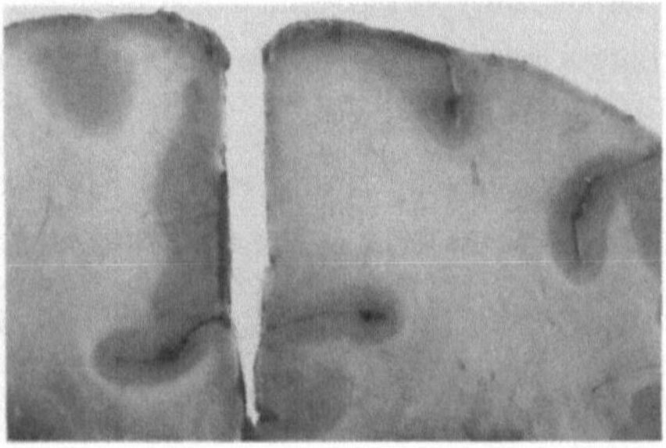

FIGURE 2. Astrocytoma (grade 2) of the right cerebral hemisphere: this ill-defined tumor can only be recognized by a toughened consistency and a pale appearance of the cortex in some gyri.

On the opposite, an **astrocytoma** is a diffuse glioma, appearing on the CTscan as an extended, often bilateral hypodensity. On gross examination by the neuropathologist as well as by the neurosurgeon, the tumor is difficult to recognize because of its ill defined limits (fig. 2). Moderate or poor cellularity, well differentiated astrocytic cells with perivascular feet, and few mitotic figures are typical microscopic features. These signs of slow growing activity correspond to an often long clinical history. **Oligodendrogliomas** also present the same clinical evolution and similar histologic characteristics. These diffuse gliomas cannot be totally excised and a recurrence after several years cannot be excluded by surgical treatment only. Therefore these astrocytomas and oligodendrogliomas are considered as grade 2 gliomas, in opposition to the well circumscribed, benign, intracranial tumors (pilocytic astrocytoma, ependymoma, meningioma, schwannoma, etc.) which are given grade 1 since they can be totally cured by surgical excision.

In some cases of astrocytoma or oligodendroglioma, areas of faster growing activity occur inside the pre-existing, well differentiated neoplasm. The CT scan often shows a diffuse, hypodense tumor containing some denser foci. Histologically these « anaplastic » foci are characterized by higher cellularity (easy to recognize at low magnification) and less differentiated cells with hyperchromatic nuclei and more mitotic figures than in the other parts of the tumor (fig. 3). In some cases these anaplastic foci show such a prominent growing activity (with necrosis and endothelial proliferation) that they offer some resemblance to glioblastoma except the fact that they are surrounded by differentiated, « quiescent » parts of the pre-existing tumor. Such gliomas containing anaplastic foci are called « **anaplastic** » and they are given grade 3. As a matter of fact, the long history and the regional variations of these anaplastic gliomas differ from the characters of the glioblastoma and suggest a moderate growing potentiality of the neoplasm considered as a whole, perhaps due to the nature of the carcinogen agent or to the defense mechanisms of the host or to other unknown factors.

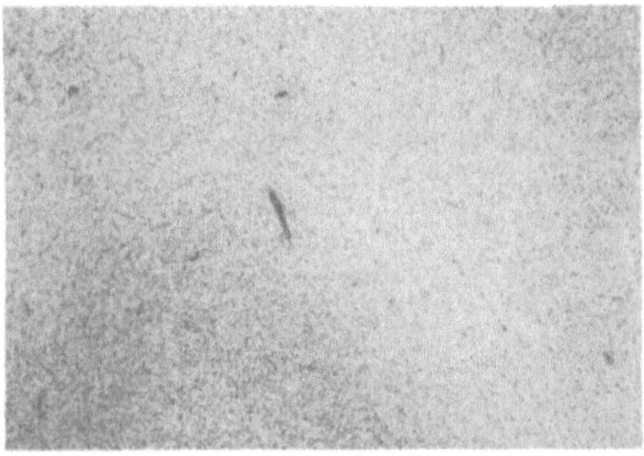

FIGURE 3. Anaplastic astrocytoma (grade 3): diffuse astrocytic tumor of moderate density containing an anaplastic area (bottom left) characterized by higher cellularity, hyperchromatic nuclei, more mitotic figures and less differentiated cells. (Paraffine, haematoxylin and eosin x 28).

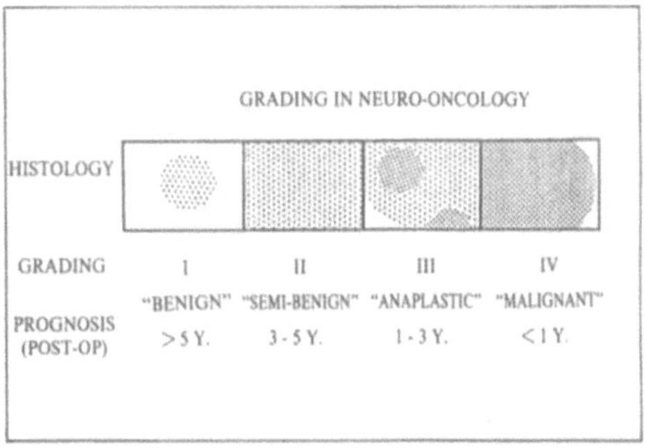

FIGURE 4. Schematic representation of the four-grade grouping of brain tumors according to the biological grading proposed by the WHO classification.

Almost all tumor types of the nervous tissue may present such a focal anaplastic degeneration: for instance, pilocytic astrocytoma, ependymoma, plexus papilloma, schwannoma and meningioma, which are grade 1 neoplasms, may become anaplastic and they are then given grade 3.

On the opposite, tumors with slow growing activity are graded 1 or 2. Grade 1 is given to well circumscribed, benign tumors which can be cured by total excision. Grade 2 tumors are also slow growing neoplasms, but their prognosis is less favourable because of the diffuse character often excluding a total excision.

The four grades of tumors of the nervous system are schematically represented in fig. 4 in which low grades are characterized by low cellularity and sharp limits (grade 1) or diffuse extension (grade 2), and higher grades by high cellularity in some foci (grade 3) or in all parts (grade 4) of the tumor.

PRESENT PROSPECTIVE ANALYSIS

Since the grading system of the WHO classification of brain tumors has a clear biological meaning, it is interesting to verify whether the postoperative evolution is longer for grade 3 than for grade 4 tumors. This opportunity was offered by a series of 202 patients with anaplastic glioma or glioblastoma (trial 26812 of the EORTC Brain Tumor Cooperative Group). After surgical excision these patients underwent classical radiation therapy (6000 rads in a period of 6 weeks: 4000 to the whole brain plus 2000 rads to the tumor). Out of these 202 patients 103 received adjuvant chemotherapy (VM-26 + CCNU: 3 cures in 12 weeks) before the radiation therapy. All these 202 patients have been randomized in the study by 16 institutions from 6 European countries and the neuropathology material has been reviewed by one of us (J.M.B.) without knowledge of the survival. No significant difference was observed between both treatment arms and the detailed results of this study will be published elsewhere.

The survival from surgery of all grade 3 and 4 tumors respectively is presented in fig. 5. These curves show that the grading is a very important prognostic factor. The same is true when we only consider the arm of 99 patients without adjuvant chemotherapy (fig. 6). In this population the survival median was 416 days for the 39 grade 3 patients and 305 days for the 60 grade 4 patients. At 24 months, 9 grade 3 patients (23.1 %) and 1 grade 4 patient (1.7 %) were still alive. Separate analysis of the several types of anaplastic glioma compared to glioblastoma shows a significantly longer survival of patients with anaplastic astrocytoma ($p < 0.001$) and a still longer survival of patients with anaplastic ependymoma or anaplastic oligodendroglioma (fig. 7). Table I shows that the WHO grading is of prognostic value in patients aged less than 50 years as well as in older patients.

COMMENTS

It is the first time that large series of brain tumors diagnosed according to the WHO classification are clinically evaluated in a prospective study performed during a randomized therapeutic trial. It appears clearly that the grading system of the WHO classification is an important prognostic factor, as far as grades 3 and 4 gliomas are concerned.

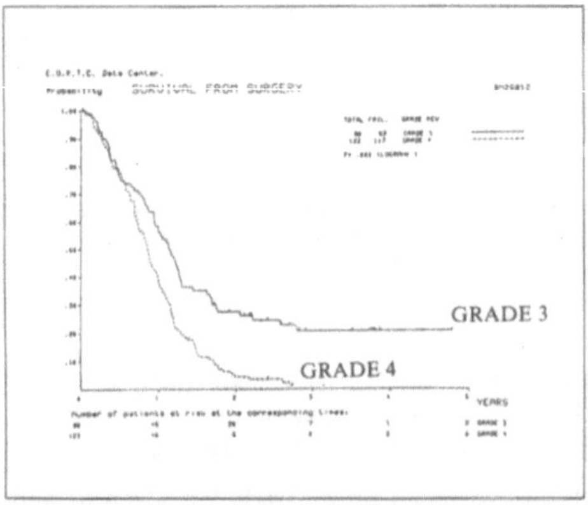

FIGURE 5. Survival curves of 202 operated patients: there is a statistically significant difference between grade 3 and grade 4 when diagnosed by the reviewer according to the WHO classification.

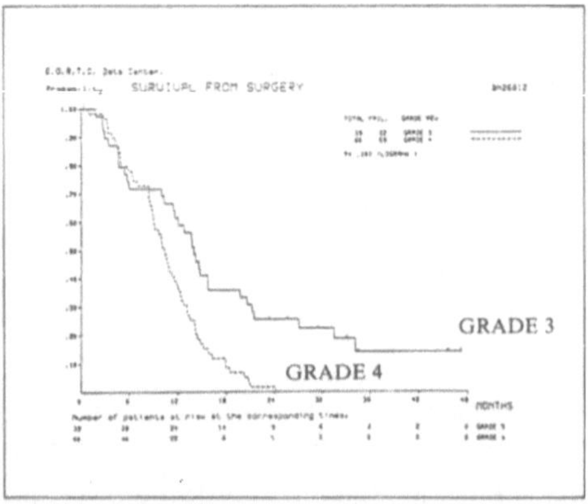

FIGURE 6. When patients with adjuvant chemotherapy are excluded the survival curves from surgery (followed by radiation therapy) show the same difference between grade 3 and grade 4.

Grade 4 tumors show signs of fast growing activity in all their parts and from their beginning. Grade 3 tumors are characterized by the occurrence of anaplastic foci in preexisting, more quiescent neoplasms (grade 1, well delimited, or grade 2, more diffuse).

The diagnosis of grade 3 tumors is based on the recognition of anaplastic foci characterized by higher cellularity, higher mitotic rate and less differentiated cells. By definition these foci of faster growing activity and anaplasia are surrounded with quiescent parts of the preexisting tumor. The latter salient feature makes the main difference between grade 3 gliomas and glioblastoma at least when the neoplastic process is not yet very expanded. At a late stage glioblastomas may gain an infiltrative and diffuse character, and the anaplastic foci of the grade 3 gliomas may invade all the tumor areas which become indistinguishable from the glioblastoma (so-called secondary glioblastoma).

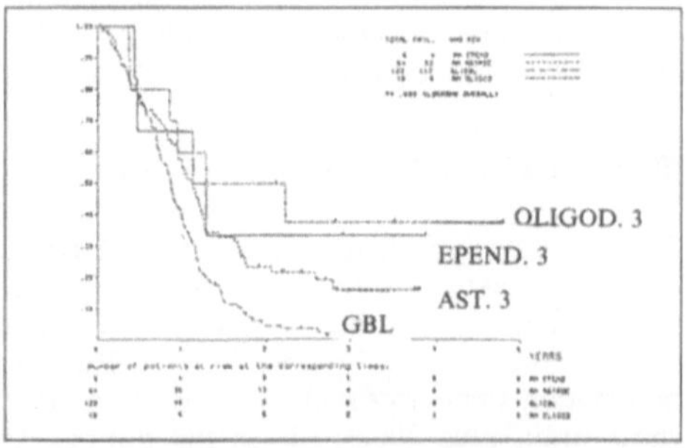

FIGURE 7. The prognosis is definitely less favourable for the glioblastoma (122 cases) than for the anasplastic astrocytoma (64 cases) as well as for the anaplastic ependymoma (6 cases) and anaplastic oligodendroglioma (10 cases).

Thus the main histologic feature of grade 3 gliomas, compared to the grade 4 glioblastoma, is essentially the focal character and not the quality of the anaplasia. For instance, pleomorphous cells, endothelial proliferation and even necroses are not reliable features allowing a distinction between anaplastic gliomas and glioblastomas. This consideration is in accordance with some conclusions of Burger and Vollmer (1980) for whom « the presence of a giant cell neoplasm had a strong positive correlation with survival » and « variables, such as necrosis, endothelial proliferation, and cellularity, dit not have any consistent relationship with prognosis ». Similarly in the recent study of Smith et al (1983) on grading of oligodendrogliomas, the « pleomorphism was the only component of tumor grade which was statistically correlated with survival ».

The present study demonstrates that grade 3 gliomas, as defined by the presence of focal anaplasia, have a definitely better prognosis than grade 4 glioblastoma.

TABLE I

SURVIVAL FROM SURGERY: 201 CASES						
Age at surgery (years)	< 50		⩾ 50		16 - 75	
	Grade 3	Grade 4	Grade 3	Grade 4	Grade 3	Grade 4
Number of patients	34	35	46	86	80	121
Survival: 2 years	15	3	5	2	20	5
	(44.1%)	(8.6%)	(10.9%)	(2.3%)	(25.0%)	(4.1%)
3 years	6	0	1	0	7	0
	(17.6%)	(0.0%)	(2.2%)	(0.0%)	(8.7%)	(0.0%)

KEY WORDS

Gliomas, Grading, Pronostic Factors.

REFERENCES

1. BAILEY (P.), CUSHING (H.): A classification of the tumors of the glioma group on a histogenetic basis with a correlated study of prognosis. J.B. Lippincott (Edit.), Philadelphia (1926).
2. BAILEY (P.), CUSHING (H.): Die Gewebsverschiedenheit der Gliome und ihre Bedeutung für die Prognose. Fischer, Jena (1930).
3. BRODERS (A.C.): Carcinoma: grading and practical application. Arch Path & Lab Med 2: 376-381 (1926).
4. BURGER (P.C.), VOLLMER (R.T.): Histologic factors of prognostic significance in the glioblastoma multiforme. Cancer **46**: 1179-1186 (1980).
5. BURGER (P.C.), VOGEL (F.S.), GREEN (S.B.), STRIKE (T.A.): Glioblastoma multiforme and anaplastic astrocytoma. Pathologic criteria and prognostic implications. Cancer **56**: 1106-1111 (1985).
6. KERNOHAN (J.W.), MABON (R.F.), SVIEN (H.J.), ADSON (A.W.): A simplified classification of gliomas. Proc Staff Meet Mayo Clin **24**: 71-75 (1949).
7. KERNOHAN (J.W.), SAYRE (G.P.): Tumors of the central nervous system. Armed Forces Institute of Pathology, Washington (1952).
8. NELSON (J.S.), TSUKADA (Y.), SCHOENFELD (D.), FULLING (K.), LAMARCHE (J.), PERESS (N.): Necrosis as a prognostic criterion in malignant supratentorial, astrocytic gliomas. Cancer **52**: 550-554 (1983).
9. RINGERTZ (N.): « Grading » of gliomas. Acta Pathol Microbiol Scand **27**: 51-64 (1950).
10. SAYRE (G.P.): The concept of grading gliomas of the central nervous system. J. Intern Coll. Surg. **26**: 440-447 (1956).
11. SCHROEDER (R.), BONIS (G.), MUELLER (W.), VORREITH (M.): Statistische Beiträge zum Grading der Gliome: I. Acta Neurochir (Wien) **18**: 43-56 (1968a).
12. SCHROEDER (R.), BONIS (G.), MUELLER (W.), VORREITH (M.): Statistische Beiträge zum Grading der Gliome: II. Acta Neurochir (Wien) **18**: 186-200.
13. SCHROEDER (R.), MUELLER (W.), BONIS (G.), VORREITH (M.): Statistische Beiträge zum Grading der Gliome: III. Acta Neurochir (Wien) **23**: 1-29 (1970).
14. SMITH (M.T.), LUDWIG (C.L.), GODFREY (A.D.), ARMBRUSTMACHER (V.M.): Grading of oligodendrogliomas. Cancer **52**: 2107-2114 (1983).
15. ZÜLCH (K.J.): Atlas of gross neurosurgical pathology. Springer, Berlin, Heidelberg, New York (1975).

16. ZÜLCH (K.J.) (in collaboration with pathologists from 14 countries): Histological typing of tumours of the central nervous system. International Histological Classification of tumours n° 21. World Health Organization, Geneva (1979).

17. ZÜLCH (K.J.): Principles of the new World Health Organization (WHO) classification of brain tumors. Neuroradiology **19**: 59-66 (1980).

18. ZÜLCH (K.J.): Brain Tumors. Their biology and Pathology. (3d completely revised edition). Springer, Berlin, Heidelberg, New York, Tokyo (1986).

19. ZÜLCH (K.L.), WECHSLER (W.): Pathology and classification of gliomas. Progr. Neurol. Surg. Vol. 2, 1-84, Karger, Basel, New York (1968).

Histological Factors in the Prognosis of Malignant Gliomas

J.N. WILDEN (°), I. MOORE (°), J.S. GARFIELD (°).

INTRODUCTION

The purpose of this study was to explore the hypothesis that duration of survival is related to the degree of de-differentiation or anaplasia in malignant gliomas. Anaplasia was defined as the amount of cellularity, pleomorphism, mitosis, and necrosis. The pathological analysis of these primary brain tumours was aimed at relating the neuropathological findings to biological behavior of the tumour rather than focusing on the neuropathological diagnosis. These two approaches have sometimes been confused in the literature (1), for example, Bailey and Cushing (2) based their histological classification on the resemblance of brain tumours to their embryological counterparts in normal development, whereas as Kernohan and Sayre (3) introduced a system of grading based on the work of Broders (4) relating microscopic appearance to prognosis.

Early neurosurgical series examining the relationship between the pathology of malignant gliomas and prognosis gave a variety of results with respect to the importance of histological features such as amount of cellularity, giant cells, pleomorphism, mitosis, necrosis, and vascularity. For example, Busch and Christensen (5) correlated longer survival with glioblastomas exhibiting a higher degree of cellularity in the tumour, but this result was not corroborated by Davis et al. (6). However, both of these studies showed that a higher proportion of necrosis was an unfavourable prognostic factor and more recently, similar findings were made by the RTOG-ECOG Group (7).

MATERIALS AND METHODS

Data Collection

The following clinical data was obtained for each patient: age at time of surgery, sex, location of tumour, type of treatment, survival time, that is, duration of survival, measured in weeks, from date of surgery to death.

The histological slides of pre-treatment surgical biopsy specimens obtained at craniotomy were reviewed on 53 patients. All patients had been entered into trials co-ordinated by the European Organisation for the Research and Treatment of Cancer (EORTC) between 1976 and 1983 (8 & 9). The criteria for patient's selection into the EORTC trials were as follows: I) diagnosis of a supratentorial malignant astrocytoma based on histology made by two independant, experienced neuropathologists; II) over 16 years of age; III) optimal removal of brain tumour via craniotomy; IV) steroid therapy stopped within 10 days of neurosurgery; V) achievement of post-operative Karnofsky Performance Index (10) of 70 or greater, within 10 days following neurosurgery; VI) expected survival of 8 weeks or more; VII) normal haemopoetic, renal and liver function; VIII) no other serious medical illness.

Post-operatively, all patients received 40 Gy of radiotherapy to the whole brain and 60 Gy to the tumour bed using two opposed parallel beams from a cobalt unit over a period of six weeks. Some patients received further therapy, that is, CCNU, VM 26 or procarbazine whereas others received misonidazole as a radiosensitizer. No significant difference of symptom-free survival or total survival time was found in the different treatment groups, therefore it was considered justified to pool the data from these three trials for the purposes of this study.

(°) Departments of Neurosurgery and Neuropathology, Wessex Neurological Centre, Southampton. UK.

M. Chatel, F. Darcel and J. Pecker (eds.), Brain Oncology. ISBN-13: 978-94-010-8003-3

HISTOLOGICAL ANALYSIS

Haemotoxylin-eosin stained slides sliced approximately 6 microns thick were prepared and viewed under the microscope using a low-power (10 x magnification) and high-power (40 x magnification) field. Each patient's slides were examined without knowledge of survival and the following pathological data recorded by us (JW/IM):

1) Cellularity: was estimated and graded numerically from 1-3 such that, 1+ represented a small increase in cell population, 2+ a moderate increase in cell population, 3+ a large increase in cell population, that is, the whole of the field contained a sheet of cells.
2) Pleomorphism: was estimated as the number of tumour cell populations, as judged by cellular size. 1+ represented uniformity of a tumour cell population, 2+ represented 2 tumour cell populations, and 3+ more than 2 tumour cell populations, that is small, medium and large cells.
3) Mitosis: was estimated as the number of mitotic figures seen in 5 randomly chosen high-power fields (magnification of 40).
4) Necrosis: was estimated as a percentage (increments of 10) of the neoplasm-containing tumour.

In each slide different degrees of anaplasia were assessed according to cellularity, pleomorphism, mitosis and necrosis. The object of this approach was to assess the variability of anaplastic change within the same tumour sections.

STATISTICAL ANALYSIS

For the purposes of analysis patients were divided into those that showed a lower degree of anaplasia defined as cellularities of 1+, or 1 and 2+ compared with those that showed a higher degree of anaplasia defined as cellularities of 2+ or 1+2+3+ or 2 and 3+. Two types of comparison were made, firstly, correlations between histological factors in the patients that had higher degrees of anaplasia and those that had lower degrees of anaplasia. Secondly, comparison was made between histological features and survival similary comparing those patients with higher and lower degrees of anaplasia. The statistical test employed was a non-parametric "T" test, and data was corrected for age.

RESULTS

General Data

53 patients were analysed 33 males and 20 females with an age range of 16 to 64 years, the mean age was 48.03 years.

Correlation between Pathological Variables

21 patients had a lower degree of cellularity, that is, counts between 1 and 2 compared with 32 patients who had higher degree of cellularity, that is, counts of 2 and 3. Patients who exhibited a higher degree of cellularity (Table I) showed a significant correlation between cellularity, pleomorphism and mitosis whereas those with a lower degree of cellularity (Table 2) showed only a significant histological correlation between pleomorphism and mitosis.

TABLE I

Histological Correlations

Higher Degree of Anaplasia	Significant	Not Significant
Cellularity v Pleomorphism	P 0.02	
Cellularity v Mitosis	p 0.01	
Cellularity v Necrosis		p 0.10
Pleomorphism v Mitosis		p 0.50
Mitosis v Necrosis		p 0.10

Correlation between Pathological Variables and Survival Time

Those patients who had a higher degree of cellularity survived significantly longer than those with a lower degree of cellularity and patients exhibiting a higher proportion of necrosis had a significantly shorter survival than those with a lower degree of necrosis (Table III). There was no significant correlations between mean survival and pleomorphism or mitosis.

In summary, Table IV shows the results of correlations between duration of survival and degree of anaplasia. Patients who had a higher amount of cellularity faired significantly better than those that did not, those exhibiting a higher proportion of necrosis faired worse. In those patients who had lower degrees of anaplasia there were no significant histological factors that correlated with survival (Table V).

DISCUSSION

The purpose of this study was to identify histological features of supratentorial malignant astrocytomas which were of prognostic value.

Surprisingly, those patients exhibiting a high degree of cellularity survived longer than those with a lower degree of cellularity. Burger & Vollmer (11) also showed a similar response in a subset of 184 patients with glioblastoma treated with surgery, radiotherapy and BCNU. A further subset treated with surgery and radiotherapy also showed a significant association between giant cell tumours and prolonged survival time. Similar findings had been previously reported by Busch & Christensen (5) when most of their patients also received radiotherapy.

In this study, all patients had an optimal removal of tumour, radiotherapy and some had chemotherapy. This raises the question of whether highly cellular tumours are more radiosensitive which might explain the observations made in this study and the two studies previously noted. Support for this proposition comes from the work of the Duke University Group, who noted that after surgical resection and radiotherapy, glioblastomas frequently enter a "quiescent" stage as shown on CT scan (12).

In a postmortem study of 50 glioblastoma cases (13), eleven patients had glioblastomas resected followed by radiotherapy but died from causes, other than their neoplasm. In these cases the surgical specimens usually contained small anaplastic cells whereas their autopsy specimens contained fibrillated, pleomorphic, gemistocytic astocytes or large bizarre cells. However, patients dying from their disease, following resection and radiotherapy, had brain swelling and proliferation of small anaplastic cells. An interpretation of this result is that radiotherapy is more effective

TABLE II

Histological Correlations

Lower Degree of Anaplasia	Significant	Not Significant
Cellularity v Pleomorphism		p 0.10
Cellularity v Mitosis		p 0.10
Cellularity v Necrosis		p 0.10
Pleomorphism v Mitosis	p 0.02	
Mitosis v Necrosis		p 0.10

TABLE III

Histological Features

	Mean Survival (weeks)		Significance
Amount of Cellularity	Higher	77.20	$p = 0.01$
	Lower	50.60	
Proportion of Necrosis	Higher	42.60	$p = 0.05$
	Lower	61.70	
Degree of Pleomorphism	Higher	66.70	NS.
	Lower	54.10	
Counts of Mitosis	Higher	67.30	N.S.
	Lower	61.70	

TABLE IV

Histological Factors

	Duration of survival	
Higher Degree of Anaplasia	Significant	Not Significant
Cellularity	$p = 0.01$	
Necrosis	$p = 0.05$	
Mitosis		p 0.10
Pleomorphism		p 0.20

TABLE V

Histological Factors

	Duration of survival	
Lower Degree of Anaplasia	Significant	Not Significant
Cellularity		p = 0.20
Necrosis		p = 0.20
Mitosis		p = 0.20
Pleomorphism		p = 0.20

in depopulating the glioblastoma of sensitive small anaplastic elements thereby unmasking less radiosensitive elements such as fibrillary and gemistocytic astocytes. If these preliminary observations are correct then clinical decisions about which patients should receive radiotherapy may partly depend on predominant type of astrocytes rather than the simple criteria of "malignancy".

In this study a high proportion of necrosis was associated with a poor prognosis. In 503 patients with malignant astocytomas in a joint RTOG-ECOG study (7), treated by an optimal removal via craniotomy and adjuvant radiotherapy and chemotherapy, the most decisive histological prognostic factor was one or more foci of coagulation necrosis, resulting in a median survival of eight months compared with twenty-eight months when no foci of necrosis were seen. In earlier studies, Bush and Christensen (5) also found correlation between necrosis and poor survival and most of their patients received radiotherapy, whereas Davis et al. (6) made a similar finding but most of their patients did not receive radiotherapy.

The above studies suggest that when histological features of necrosis are found in malignant astocytomas, prognosis is poor irrespective of subsequent treatment with radiotherapy.

A tentative conclusion from this study and the available literature, is that malignant astocytomas which contain a high preponderance of small anaplastic cells with no areas of necrosis are more likely to be radiosensitive than other types of malignant astrocytomas. These histological factors should be considered when recommending adjuvant therapy.

SUMMARY

A retrospective study has been evaluated of the clinical features of 53 patients from the Wessex Neurological Centre, Southampton, selected for randomization into EORTC Trials.

All patients had a supratentorial malignant glioma, an optimal removal of the tumour, and a post-operative Karnofsky index of greater than 70. A course of post-operative radiotherapy (6000 cGy) was undertaken on all patients and some received adjuvant chemotherapy. Comparison were made between survival and histological data. A summary of results is given.

The results illustrate that prognostic indices can be obtained for patients suffering from malignant gliomas. The implications of the controversial findings that lobectomy and increased cellularity on histological section are related to a better survival will be discussed in relation to other authors.

KEY WORDS

Gliomas, Grading, Pronostic Factors.

AKNOWLEDGEMENTS

The authors are grateful to Professor R. O Weller for his helpful advice and criticism.

REFERENCES

1. McCOMB (R.D.), BURGER (P.C.): Pathologic analysis of primary brain tumours. In Neurologic Clinics, Symposium on Neuro-oncology. Eds. Vick NA, Bigner DD. 1985. 3: 4, 711-728.
2. BAILEY (P.), CUSHING (H.): A classification of the tumours of the glial group on a histogenetic basis with a correlated study of prognosis. Philadelphia, JB Lippincott, 1926.
3. KERNOHAN (J.W.), SAYRE (G.P.): Tumours of the central nervous system. Atlas of tumour pathology. Section X, fasicles 35 and 37. Washington, DC; Armed Forces Institute of Pathology, 1952.
4. BRODERS (A.C.): Carcinoma, grading and practical application. Arch. Pathol. Lab. Med. 1926, 2: 376-381.
5. BUSCH (E.), CHRISTENSEN (E.): The three types of glioblastoma. J. Neurosurg. 1947, 4: 200-220.
6. DAVIS (L.), MARTIN (J.), GOLDSTEIN (S.L.), ASHKENAZY (M.): A study of 211 patients with verified glioblastoma multiforme. J. Neurosurg. 1949, 6: 33-44.
7. NELSON (J.S.), TSUKADA (Y.), SCHOENFELD (D.), FULLING (K.), LAMARCHE (J.), PERESS (N.): Necrosis as a prognostic criterion in malignant supratentorial, astrocytic gliomas. Cancer, 1983, 52: 550-554.

8. EORTC Brain Tumour Group. Evaluation of CNNU, V.M.-26 plus CCNU and procarbazine in supratentorial brain gliomas. J. Neurosurg. 1981, 55: 27-31.

9. EORTC Brain Tumour Group. Misonidazole in radiotherapy of supratentorial malignant brain gliomas in adult patients: a randomized double-blind study. Eur. J. Cancer Clin. Oncol., 1983, 19: 39-42.

10. KARNOFSKY (D.A.), ABELMANN (W.H.), CRAVER (L.F.), BURCHENAL (J.H.): The use of the nitrogen mustards in the palliative treatment of carcinoma. Cancer, 1948, 1: 634-656.

11. BURGER (P.C.), VOLLMER (R.T.): Histologic factors of prognostic significance in the glioblastoma multiforme. Cancer 46: 1980, 1179-1186.

12. BURGER (P.C.), DUBOIS (P.J.), SHOLD (S.C.), SMITH (K.S.), ODOM (G.L.), CRAFTS (D.C.), GIANGASPERO (F.): Computerised tomographic and pathologic studies of the untreated, quiescent, and recurrent glioblastoma multiforme. J. Neurosurg. 1983, 58: 159-169.

13. GIANGASPERO (F.), BURGER (P.C.): Correlations between cytologic composition and biologic behaviour in the glioblastoma multiforme: a postmortem study of 50 cases. Cancer. 1983, 52: 2320-2333.

Supra-Tentorial Gliomas: Multivariate Analysis of Prognostic Factors

A. ROUGIER (°), J.F. DARTIGUES (°°), F. COHADON (°).

INTRODUCTION

Studies of survival time of gliomas are usually correlated to histological grading systems. Therapeutic trials were performed under this reference (14). But actuarial survival curves point out a relative disparity in each well defined histologic group (5,15). This data may be related to exceptions without distinctive feature or may bring out other prognostic factors. A lot of these possible factors have been reported: age, functional status, symptomatology, duration of the pre-therapeutic course, C.T. scan aspects (1, 6, 9, 16, 15). To analyse the liability of each factor for prognosis, the usual method requires a successive stratification of the population: two or more subgroups according, for exemple, to age are broken up into other subgroups according to another factor... This method is quickly restricted by the number of cases in each subgroup and can be considered as valid only if each factor is independant of the others. In fact the prognostic is the result of the interactions between them. So it is most interesting to draw up a multivariate analysis taking into accont simultaneously the whole of these factors. A mathematical modeling strategy is required and founded upon their respective role and their connections.

MATERIALS ANS METHODS

Selection fo patients

A cohort of 192 patients harbouring a supra-tentorial glioma refered to our neurosurgical unit from 1978 to 1983 have been selected. The factors taken-into account for the statistical modeling system and available at the moment of the diagnosis were: age, functional status estimated by a simplified Karnovsky scale (1), epileptic seizures or not as initial symptoms, localisation or not in highly functional area, localisation or not in deep-seated area, tumoral diameter and 4 histological criteria (abnormal cellular density, nuclear polymorphism, neovascularization with endothelial proliferation, necrosis).

Therapeutic policy

When the CT scan disclosed an intracranial lesion likely to be removed without functional hazards, a surgical resection was performed : 96 cases (50 %). 32 tumors (16,6 %) under 35 mm in diameter located in highly functional area or deep-seated zones were treated by stereotaxic implantation of 192 Ir wires (14) after biopsy. When direct surgical approach or interstitial irradiation seemed unreasonable a sterotaxic biopsy was performed : 64 cases (33,4 %). All the patients received 60 GY on the target volume extending 2 cm beyond the outer limit of the tumor. Patients treated by 192 Ir implantation received 35 GY from interstitial irradiation and 35 GY by external radiotherapy. 64 glioblastomas were treated in addition with chemotherapy (teniposide-CCNU).

Statistical analysis

Survival period was chosen as the dependant variable. In a first step Kaplan Meier survival curves were performed according to each histologic pattern and statistical significance was evaluated by the Log-rang test (7). Modeling system was founded on logistic regression: for each factor a predictive coefficient was caculated and tested on the 192 cases with estimation of the mean value and interval of confidence. If the value of the coefficient was zero the factor was redundant with others and considered as without predictive interest. In the other cases the value was corresponding to its predictive significance. Consequently, multivariate analysis with Cox'hazard function gave the estimated survival period for each patient (3).

(°°) Statistics Department, (°) Neuro-Surgery Unit. Hopital Pellegrin, 33076 Bordeaux, France.

M. Chatel, F. Darcel and J. Pecker (eds.), Brain Oncology. ISBN-13: 978-94-010-8003-3

RESULTS

Predictive value of histological criteria

Period of survival is statistically correlated with neovascularisation and necrosis but not with nuclear polymorphism.4 histological groups have been defined: grade 1: abnormal astrocytic proliferation, grade 2: previous data + nuclear polymorphism, grade 3: previous data + neovascularization, grade 4: previous data + necrosis. A significant difference was found only between the junction of grade 1-2 and grade 3-4 providing to select only the operated cases (figure 1).

Multivariate Cox's analysis displayed to select 5 factors with high predictive value: age, pre-therapeutic functional status, epileptic seizures, tumoral diameter. With this procedure only one histologic criteria was selected: neovascularization (figure 2)

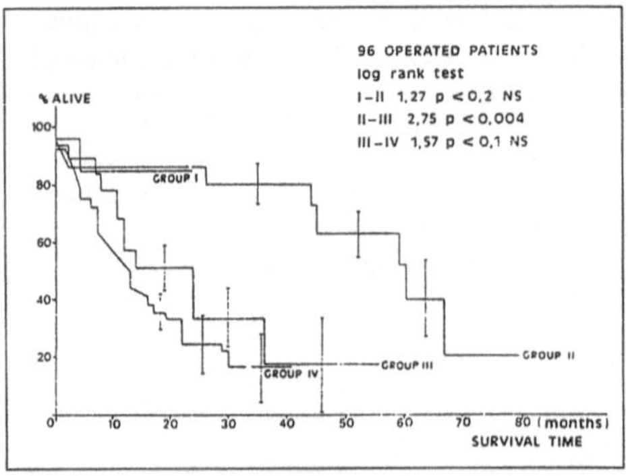

FIGURE 1. Kaplan-Meir survival curves according to histological groups.

FACTORS	COEFFICIENT	INTERVAL OF CONFIDENCE	P
AGE	0.031387	0.006633	0.00001
FUNCTIONAL STATUS	0.635400	0.155019	0.0001
TUMORAL DIAMETER	0.11693	0.004582	0.02
EPILEPTIC SEIZURES	-0.590149	0.239783	0.02
NEOVASCULARIZATION	0.426255	0.208653	0.04

FIGURE 2. Multivariate Analysis using Cox's Model: predictive coefficient of prognostic factors.

In grade 1 and grade 4 surgery seemed to contribute to a longer survival time. But this population is obviously different from the non operated cases. Conséquently it was necessary to differenciate operated and non-operated cases to clarify the predictive value of each factor excluding the surgical part. Multivariate analysis has been performed on three groups: no surgery: 96 cases, « total » surgical resection: 63 cases, sub-total surgical resection: 34 cases. The same association of 5 factors retains its predictive value: age, pre-therapeutic functional status, epileptic seizures, tumoral diameter and neovascularization on the inside of each group.

DISCUSSION

With unifactorial analysis, period of survival is statistically correlated with two histological factors neavascularization and necrosis. With multivariate Cox's model necrosis have not been selected and the predictive value of neovascularization was near the statistical significative limit. The explanation was that histological criteria were highly redundant with a number of other predictive factors (figure 3). Gliomas with necrosis (glioblastomas) arise usually in older patients with defective functional status and epileptic seizures are uncommon. The whole of the worst factors are stored and this phenomenon explains the disappearance of prognostic value of histological patterns. Moreover the prognosis of glioblastomas is said to be better among younger patients and its behaviour comes near to lower grade glioma. Multivariate analysis takes into account the whole clinical aspects. Consequently, histological criteria alone are insufficient to obtain a predictive value of period of survival. Prediction may be improved by injecting supplementary parameters other than histologic : age, functional status, epileptic seizures or not and tumoral diameter. For randomised therapeutic trials, the use of the best predictive model leads to raising the power of the statistical analysis and, possibly, to diminushing the number of cases to point out the therapeutic efficacity.

PROGNOSTIC FACTORS		NUCLEAR POLYMORPHISM yes	NUCLEAR POLYMORPHISM no	NEOVASCULARIZATION yes	NEOVASCULARIZATION no	NECROSIS yes	NECROSIS no
AGE	MEAN	46.9%	39.9%	51.5%	40.5%	53.2%	41.5%
	0-39	15 %	47 %	22 %	49 %	16 %	49 %
FUNCTIONAL STATUS	1	38 %	42 %	20 %	56 %	11 %	54 %
	2	42 %	39 %	59 %	25 %	68 %	26 %
	3-4	20 %	19 %	21 %	19 %	21 %	20 %
EPILEPTIC SEIZURES	YES	15 %	35 %	30 %	56 %	24 %	55 %
TUMORAL DIAMETER	MEAN	52.4%	38.6%	52 %	48.6%	54.2%	47.9%
DEEP-SEATED TUMORS	YES	32 %	25 %	23 %	28 %	29 %	25 %

FIGURE 3. Relationship between histological patterns and non-histological prognostic factors.

SUMMARY

A multivariate analysis using Cox proportional hazards regression model has been performed on a cohort of 192 supra-tentorial astrocytic tumors. The aim of this study was to determine the histologic and non-histologic factors which were strongly correlated with the survival time. 4 histologic patterns had been retained: abnormal cellular density, nuclear polymorphism, neovascularization, necrosis. Non-histologic factors taken into account were: age, functional status, symptomatology, tumoral volume, localisation. The first question was to define the prognostic value of the histological patterns: Kaplan-Meier curves had pointed out the predictive role of neovascularization and necrosis. But, with multivariate analysis, the association of 4 non-histological parameters (age, functional status, epileptic seizures, tumoral diameter) was required to obtain the most valid prediction of survival period. Indeed, histologic criterion was usually redundant with non-histologic factors. This method lead to taking into account cases overlooking to the usual clinical patterns in a same histologic group.

KEY WORDS

Gliomas, Pronostic Factors.

REFERENCES

1. CAUDRY (M.), MAIRE (J.-P.), GUERIN (J.), CELERIER (D.), DEMEAUX (E.), BANAYAN (A.), LEMAN (P.): Gliomes malins sus-tentoriels de l'adulte. Adaptation du traitement aux trois groupes d'une classification clinique : Semaine des hôpitaux. Paris: 59: 453-458 (1983).
2. COHADON (F.), AOUAD (N.), ROUGIER (A.), VITAL (C.), RIVEL (J.), DARTIGUES (J.F.): Histologic and non-histologic factors correlated with survival time in supratentorial astrocytic tumors. J. of neuro-oncology 3: 105-111 (1985).
3. COX (D.R.): Regression models and lifes-tables: Jr Stat. Soc. (séries B) 34: 187-220 (1972).
4. DARA (P.), SLATER (L.M.), TALREJA (D.), ARMENTROUT (S.A.): Long-term survivors of high-grade malignant astrocytomas. Medical and pediatric Oncology: 8: 187-191 (1980).
5. JELSMA (R.), BUCY (P.C.): Glioblastoma multiforme. Its treatment and some factors effecting survival? Arch. neurol. 20: 161-171 (1971).
6. KAPLAN (E.L.), MEIER (P.): Non parametric estimation from incomplete observations. J. Am. Stat. Assoc: 53: 457-481 (1958).
7. KERNOHAN (J.W.), NNABON (R.F.), SVIEN (H.J.), ADSON (A.W.): A simplified classification of the gliomas. Proc. Mayo Clin. 24: 71-75 (1949).
8. LEVIN (V.), HOFFMAN (W.), HEILBRON (D.), NORMAN (D.): Prognostic significance of the pretreatment CT scan on time to progression for patients with malignant gliomas. J. neurosurg. 56, 642-647 (1980).

9. NELSON (J.S.), TSUDAKA (Y.), SCHOENFELD (D.), FULLING (K.), LAMARCHE (J.), PERESS (N.): Necrosis as a prognostic criterion in malignant supratentorial, astrocytic gliomas. Cancer: 52: 550-554 (1983).

10. RINGERTZ (N.): "Grading" of gliomas. Acta, patho. microbiol. Scand 27, 51-64 (1954).

11. ROUGIER (A.), COHADON (F.), PIGNEUX (J.), LOISEAU (H.): La place de l'irradiation interstitielle dans le traitement des gliomes. Neurochirurgie 30: 125-129 (1984).

12. ROUGIER (A.), PIGNEUX (J.), RICHAUD (P.), COHADON (F.): La prise en charge diagnostique et thérapeutique des gliomes malins. Neurochirurgie 27: 315-320 (1981).

13. SALCMAN (M.): Survival in glioblastoma: historical perspective. Neurosurgery: 7: 435-439 (1980).

14. WALKER (M.), GREEN (S.), BYAR (D.), ALEXANDER (E.), BATZDORF (U.), BROOKS (W.), HUNT (W.), MACCARTY (C.), MAHALEY (S.), MEALEY (J.), OWENS (G.), RANSOHOFF (J.), ROBERTSON (J.), SHAPIRO (W.), SMITH (K.), WILSON (C.), STRIKE (T.): Randomized comparisons of radiotherapy and nitroso ureas for the treatment of malignant glioma after surgery. N. Engl. J. Med.: 303: 1323-1329 (1980).

15. WEIR (B.): The relative significance of factors affecting postoperative survival in astrocytomas grades 3 and 4: J. Neurosurg.: 38, 448-452 (1973).

High Graded Astrocytoma: Results of Treatment

A.J. VOETS (°), A. KEYSER (°), M. LENDERS (°),
E. MEIJER (°°).

INTRODUCTION

The outcome in patients with a malignant glioma despite some progress in therapeutic strategies, is still very poor. Numerous reports concerning the results of treatment of high-graded astrocytomas, or more specifically glioblastoma multiforme, have been published in the last three decades (1, 19). Interpretation of results and comparison of these studies is rendered difficult because of use of different pathological classifications, lack of sufficient descriptive data, insufficient statistical analysis or the use of historical or no controls at all, with only few exceptions (1, 8, 18).

As a starting point for further research we performed a retrospective study of our results of treatment of high-graded astrocytomas, on which we like to report here.

METHODS AND MATERIAL

All consecutive patients with a histologically proven astrocytoma grade III and IV, according to the classification of Kernohan (20), who were treated at the Department of Neurosurgery of the Canisius-Wilhelmina Hospital in Nijmegen, The Netherlands, during the period January 1th, 1974, till January 1th, 1983, were included in the study. A subdivision of tumours with histological features of both grade III and grade IV, designated by the pathologist as astrocytoma grade III-IV, was analysed separately. All medical files were reviewed and data were collected concerning age, sex, tumour location, presenting symptom, the interval from first symptom to operation, affection of cranial nerves II, III, IV and VI, operation, the use of radiotherapy, and survival. During the period under study one of the surgeons systematically excluded the use of radiotherapy from treatment in the glioma patients under his care. In this study therefore patients could be stratified according to grade of malignancy and to use of radiotherapy. Statistical analysis was performed by the Statistical-Mathematical Department of our Institute.

RESULTS

Out of 200 patients with a high-grade astrocytoma, who were amenable for study, 71 had to be excluded because of incomplete information concerning survival or the use of radiotherapy. In the immediate post-operative period of fourteen days thirteen patients died, which leaves 116 patients for analysis.

The descriptive data are presented in tables 1 and 2. There are no statistical differences in the characteristics mentioned above between the randomised groups per grade of astrocytoma. Actuarial survival curves are presented in figures 1, 2 and 3.

DISCUSSION

With the exception of a rather high mean age (4, 12, 14, 18); and a high number of affections of cranial nerves II, III, IV and VI (18), our patients are fully comparable with those treated elsewhere. A comparison can be made with the figures in table 3.

(°) Institute of Neurology and (°°) Institute of Neurosurgery, Catholic University, St. Radboudziekenhuis, Nijmegen, The Netherlands.

M. Chatel, F. Darcel and J. Pecker (eds.), Brain Oncology. ISBN-13: 978-94-010-8003-3

TABLE 1

Astrocytoma grade III; descriptive data

	Total	RT	No. RT
Number	38	28	10
Age (in years) mean	47,8	44,2	57,8
median	48,4	45,2	53,7
Male/female	18/20	15/13	3/7
Interval from first symptom to operation (in weeks) mean	36,8	46,2	10,9
median	10 (1-260)	11 (1-260)	8 (3-30)
Presenting symptom			
— headache	13	8	5
— palsies	8	7	1
— fits	14	12	2
— psych. alter	3	1	2
Cranial n. II, III, IV, VI affection			
Operation modality	14/24	11/17	3/7
— biopsy	6	4	2
— partial excision	24	21	3
— total excision	8	3	5
Survival (days) *(4 patients lost for follow-up)	570	664	125

TABLE 2

Astrocytoma grade IV; descriptive data

	Total	RT	No. RT
Number	81	55	26
Age (in years) mean	52,4	50,1	57,4
median	55,8	54,6	60,0
Male/female	56/25	39/16	17/9
Interval from first symptom to operation (in weeks) mean	14,7	18,3	7
Presenting symptom			
— headache	40	24	9
— palsies	25	12	11
— fits	16	11	4
— psych. alter	10	8	2
Cranial n. II, III, IV, VI affection			
Operation modality	32/49	23/32	9/17
— biopsy	10	5	5
— partial excision	59	41	18
— total excision	12	9	3
Survival (days) *(6 patients lost for follow-up)	240	270	68
*Astrocytoma grade III-IV Survival (days)	200	283	63

TABLE 3

Results of treatment from other studies in literature (1, 19). From left to right: authors, year of publication, study period, neurosurgical or radiotherapeutical origin, total number of patients, treatment, number of patients of each treatment modality, percentage of patients surviving

Author		Period		N			Percentage of patients surviving after ... months 3	6	9	12	24	36	60	120
Frankel-German	1958	1924-1952	n.c.	219	r	62	±75	±30	±20	±10	±5	±3	0	
					r+RT	21	±85	±60	±50	±20	±5	±0		
Roth-Elvidge	1960			144	r+RT	144		78		35	18	10	6	
Bouchard-Peirce	1960	1939-1953	r.t.	826	r	23				31,8	6,5			
					r+RT	125				39	20	11,2	7,2	4,0
Bloor et al.	1962	1955-1960	r.t.	95	r	18	±40	±20		±5				
					r+RT	39	±80	±50	±30	±20				
Taveras et al.	1962	1943-1955	n.c.	425	r	36	±40	±15	±5	±5	0			
					r+RT	141	±85	±65	±45	±35	±10	±5	±5	
Hitchcock-Sato	1964	1950-1960	n.c.	225	r	80	±20	±10	±5	0				
					r+RT	63	±80	±70	±50	±30	±10	±5	±5	
Uihlein et al.	1966	1955-1959	n.c.	107	r	59		11,9		5,1				
					r+RT	48		75		29,2	5	3		
Schlienger	1967	1956-1966	r.t.	72	r+RT	72		76		27,5	12,2	6,6	4,3	
Jelsma-Bucy	1967	1945-1964	n.c.	162	r	28	86	46	29	25	11			
					r+RT	42	93	81	50	38	14			
Jelsma-Bucy	1969	1963-1966	n.c.	46	r+RT	46	85	72	54	35	15			
				40	r+RT	40	95	80	60	40	18			
Caldwell-Aristizabal	1971	1964-1971	r.t.	114	r+RT	114	83	64		33	12	4		
Weir	1973	1956-1970	r.t.	248	r	95	1,8 ± 3,6 months							
					r+RT	153	9,6 ± 8,6 months							
Onoyama et al.	1976	1955-1972	r.t.	127	r+RT	127		74		52	29	19	12	
Andersen	1978	1963-1967	r.t.	108	r	57	±55	±20	±15	±0				
					r+RT	51	±65	±45	±25	±20	0			
Jellinger et al.	1979	1970-1979	r.t.	116	r	39		32		5				
					r+RT	31		80		35	3			
Marquardt et al.	1930	1969-1978	r.t.	217	r+RT	61	±63	±40	±20	±15	±10			
Rutten et al.	1931	1957-1978	r.t.	143	r+RT	142	grade III: 24,5 months							
							grade IV: 12,4 months							

— n.c. : originating of a neurosurgical institute
— r.t. : originating of a radiotherapeutic institute
— r. : only surgery
— r+RT : surgery plus radiotherapy
— ± : estimated figures by drooping perpenticulars to absic and ordinates, out of graphics in the original publication.

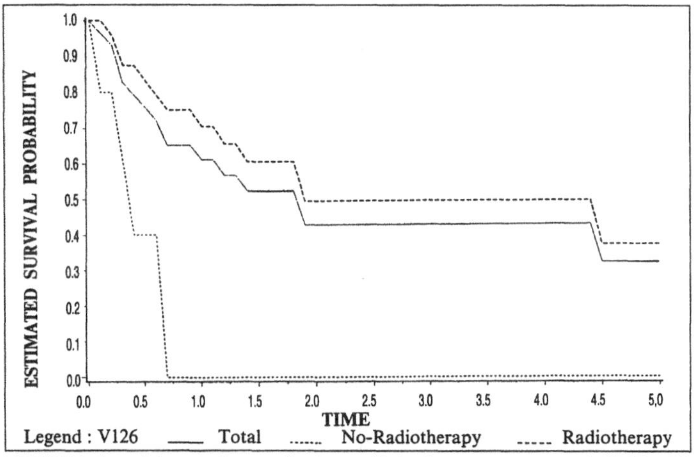

FIGURE 1. Actuarial survival curve of patients suffering from astrocytoma grade III (N = 34)

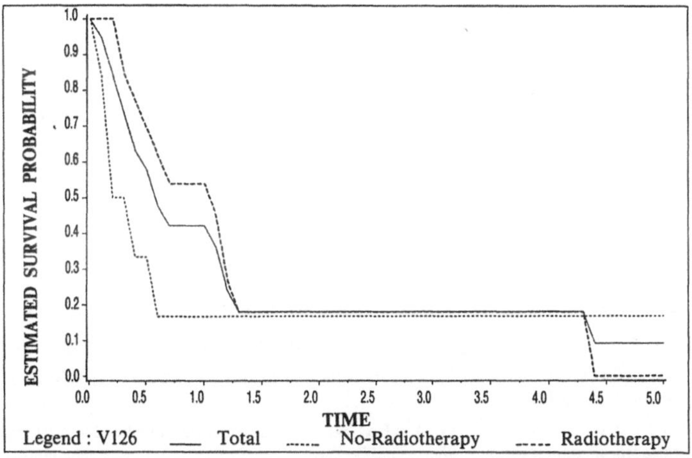

FIGURE 2. Actuarial survival curve of patients suffering from astrocytoma grade III-IV (N = 20)

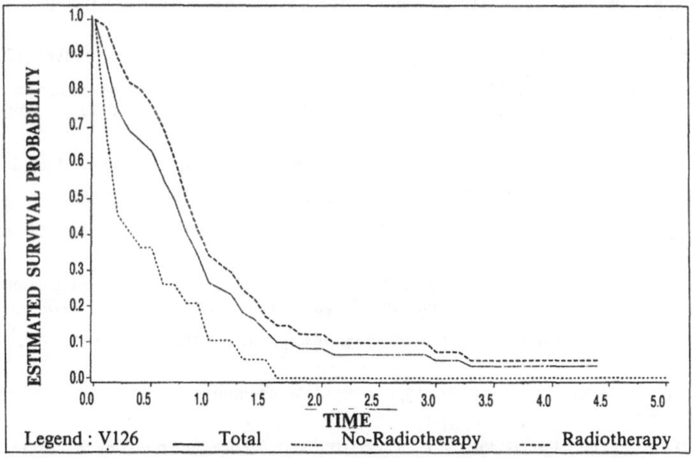

FIGURE 3. Actuarial survival curve of patients suffering from astrocytoma grade IV (N = 75)

Post-operative mortality was low in comparison with that reported from other centers (5, 7, 9, 22). Our results of treatment of patients with a grade III astrocytoma are in the same range as reported by others (15, 21): post-operative radiotherapy prolongs median survival by approximately 18 months. Survival rates in the group III-IV are the same as in grade IV which means that there is no justification that warrants the use of this subdivision. In grade IV post-operative radiotherapy prolongs median survival by approximately 7 months. However, survival curves converge, as shown above, to a line just above zero after two years, which means that the prospects for these patients are really still very poor.

KEY WORDS

Gliomas, Radiotherapy, Surgery.

REFERENCES

1. ANDERSEN (A.P.): Postoperative irradiation of glioblastomas results in a randomised series. Acta Radiol. 1978; 17 (6): 475-484.
2. BLOOR (R.J.), TEMPLETON (A.W.), QUICK (R.S.): Radiation therapy in the treatment of intracranial tumors. A.J.R. 1962; 87: 463-472.
3. BOUCHARD (J.), PEIRCE (C.B.): Radiation therapy in the management of neoplasms of the central nervous system, with a special note in regard to children: Twenty years' experience, 1939-1958. A.J.R. 1960; 84: 610-628.
4. CALDWELL (W.L.), ARISTIZABAL (S.A.): Treatment of glioblastoma. A review. Acta Radiol. 1975; 14: 505-512.
5. FRANKEL (S.A.), GERMAN (W.J.): Glioblastoma multiforme. Review of 219 cases with regard to natural history, pathology, diagnostic methods, and treatment. J. Neurosurg. 1958; 15: 480-503.
6. GLANZMANN (C.), PETERS (T.), HORST (W.), FRIEDE (R.): Indikationen und Ergebnisse der Radiotherapie in der Behandlung von Astrozytomen. Strahlentherapie 1980; 155: 383-387.
7. HITCHCOCK (E.), SATE (F.): Treatment of malignant gliomata. J. Neurosurg. 1964; 21: 497-505.
8. JELLINGER (K.), KOTHBAUER (P.), VOLC (D.), VOLLMER (R.), WEISS (R.): Combination chemotherapy (COMP protocol) and radiotherapy of anaplastic supratentorial gliomas. Acta Neurochir. (Wien) 1979; 51: 1-13.
9. JELSMA (R.), BUCY (P.C.): Treatment of glioblastoma multiforme of the brain. J. Neurosurg. 1967; 27: 388-400.
10. JELSMA (R.), BUCY (P.C.): Glioblastoma multiforme - its treatment and some factors affecting survival. Arch. Neurol. (Chicago) 1969; 20: 161-171.
11. MARQUARD (B.), VOSS (A.C.), MARKEWITZ (A.): Ergebnisse der Strahlentherapie bei 214 primären Hirntumoren und 27 Hirnmetastasen. Strahlentherapie 1980; 156: 371-381.
12. ONOYAMA (Y.), ABE (M.), YABUMOTO (E.), SAKOMOTO (T.), SUYAMA (S.): Radiation therapy in the treatment of glioblastoma. A.J.R. 1976; 126: 481-492.
13. ROTH (J.G.), ELVIDGE (A.R.): Glioblastoma multiforme: A clinical survey. J. Neurosurg. 1965; 17: 736-750.
14. RUTTEN (E.H.J.M.), KAZEM (I.), SLOOF (J.L.), WALDER (H.A.D.): Postoperative radiation therapy in the management of brain astrocytoma-retrospective study of 142 patients. Int. J. Radiat. Oncol. Biol. Phys. 1981; 1: 191-195.
15. SCHLIENGER (M.): Radiothérapie des glioblastomes de l'adulte et de l'enfant. Acta Radiol. 1969; 8: 134-146.
16. STAGE (W.S.), STEIN (J.J.): Treatment of malignant astrocytomes. A.J.R. 1974; 120: 7-18.
17. TAVERAS (J.M.), THOMPSON (H.G.), POOL (J.L.): Should we treat glioblastoma multiforme? A study of survival in 425 cases. A.J.R., 1962; 87: 473-479.
18. UIHLEIN (A.), COLBY (M.Y.), (Jr.), LAYTON (D.D.), PARSONS (W.R.), CARTER (T.L.): Comparison of surgery and surgery plus irradiation in the treatment of supratentorial gliomas. Acta Radiol. 1966; 5: 67-78.
19. WEIR (B.): The relative significance of factors affecting postoperative survival in astrocytoma, grades 3 and 4. J. Neurosurg. 1973; 38: 443-452.
20. KERNOHAN (J.W.), MABON (R.F.), SVIEN (H.J.), ADSON (A.W.): Simplified classification of gliomas. Proc. Mayo Clin. 1949; 24: 71-75.
21. SALAZAR (O.M.), RUBIN (P.), FELDSTEIN (M.L.), PIZZUTIELLO (R.): High dose radiation therapy in the treatment of malignant gliomas: final report. Int. J. Radiat. Oncol. Biol. Phys. 1970; 5: 1733-1740.

Primary Malignant non Hodgkin's Lymphomas of the Central Nervous System Report of two cases with a Predominant Callosal Localization

J. MIKOL (°), M. WASSEF (°), A. GALIAN (°),
F. WOIMANT (°°), C. THUREL (°°°).

INTRODUCTION

Malignant non-Hodgkin's lymphoma (MNHL) of the central nervous system (CNS) has been designated as "microglioma", "malignant lymphoma", "lymphosarcoma", "granulomatous encephalitis", "reticular, perithelial or histiocytic sarcoma". In 1972, Schaumburg, Plank and Adams (28) recognized the histologic similarities between cerebral and extraneural tumors, the existence of primary central nervous system lymphoma, and the importance of appropriate brain biopsy examination. Since then, the increasing frequency of CNS lymphoma has been emphasized. Secondary intracerebral localizations of MNHL were estimated as 8.4% in a multicentric extensive study (14). Primary localizations were considered as 0.7% (9) (1974), 4,5% (16) (1986), 7.6% (18) (1982) of all the MNHL. In 1986 our department observed glial tumors only three times more commonly than primary MNHL. These MNHL were unrelated to acquired or inborn immunodeficiency.

These tumors are solitary or multifocal tumors and have different sizes. They can be nodular or infiltrative (8). Localizations of MNHL are found throughout the CNS; there is a slightly increased incidence of these tumors in the periventricular area. A medial space occupying lesion with bilateral extension is classically diagnosed as a glioma; however such a lesion may indicate a lymphoma. Therefore, the purpose of this study is to report two callosal lymphomas with bilateral extension diagnosed by means of brain biopsy (case 1) or post-mortem examination (case 2).

MATERIALS AND METHODS

Biopsy of right frontal lobe was obtained using a stereotactic method (31) in case 1. Necropsy study was performed for case 2; several fragments of CNS, spinal cord, peripheral nerves and psoas muscle were examined. Serial coronal hemispheric sections (20 microns thick) were obtained between the mammillary bodies and the posterior pulvinar. Sections were stained by means of various histologic methods, including haematoxylin-eosin with or without saffran, Masson Trichrome, periodic acid-Schiff (PAS), Gordon Sweets, May-Grünwald Giemsa, Wölcke, Nissl. Fixed tissues from tumor-involved areas were also studied by means of the peroxydase anti-peroxydase technique for cytoplasmic immunoglobulins (polyclonal antibodies anti-human, alpha, gamma, mu, kappa, lambda, chains, dilution 1/100 DAKO).

Ultrastructural studies were performed on glutaraldehyde-osmic acid (case 1) or formalin fixed tissue (case 2) embedded in epon. Sections were stained with uranyl acetate and lead citrate.

CASE REPORTS

Case 1: The patient was a 59 year old man who worked as an engineer for 18 years at the Atomic Energy Agency. Progressive deterioration with apragmatism, moriatic state and sphincter disturbances were the presenting symptoms. Neurological examination, performed after an epileptic fit, revealed no clinical abnormality. A serum hypergamaglobulinemia was discovered (24%).

(°) Departments of Pathology, (°°) Neurology, and (°°°) Neurosurgery, Lariboisière Hospital, Paris, France, UFR Lariboisière-Saint-Louis.

M. Chatel, F. Darcel and J. Pecker (eds.), Brain Oncology. ISBN-13: 978-94-010-8003-3

Bilateral frontal slow waves were present on EEG. There was a bilateral fronto-callosal hyperdensity more extended on the left side, surrounded by an area of hypodensity on CT Scan (CT) (Pr Merland) (Fig. 1A). By Magnetic Nuclear Resonance (MNR) (Dr Cabanis), there was no sign of compression and the enhancement of the frontal density extended to the splenium of the corpus callosum (fig. 18). Pathologic examination of the frontal cerebral biopsy showed a MNHL.

The abnormal serum monotypic immunoglobulin was of IgM kappa subtype. No antibodies to Human Immunodeficiency Virus (HIV) were detected. Results of clinical examination and other laboratory investigations gave no evidence of extraneural lymphomatous involvement.

A treatment combining corticoids and radiotherapy was initiated (30 grays-12 fractions, 19 days; total irradiation of the brain, C1-C2 and frontal area: Pr Schlienger). Readmission was due to a left hemiparesis with coma; death occurred, after a 5 month survival. Necropsy could not be performed.

Case 2: A 72 year old man, who was employed as dental prosthetist, treated during the last 4 years for non insulin-dependant diabetes mellitus experienced the gradual onset of paresthesias and an acute but regressive visual blurring of the right visual field. A serum gamma 2, lambda 2 monotypic immunoglobulin was subsequently discovered.

Two months later, neurological examination revealed multiple sensory and motor mononeuropathy of the right internal and external popliteal, and ulnar nerves. The deep tendon reflexes were absent in the satellite territories. A Babinski sign was elicited on the right side. Unsteadiness, impairment of cognitive functions, such as constructive apraxia and anterograde amnesia, were present. General examination showed a severely debilitated patient. Subsequently apathy, inconstant spatial and temporal desorientation, occasional instances of confabulation and false recognition were noted. The left hemiparesis observed after an epileptic fit did not regress. Slow delta waves with a left predominance were registered on the EEG. A CT showed a posterior callosal hyperdensity, enhanced after injection, with bilateral extension and hypodensity of the white matter (Fig. 1C-D). Radioisotope examination was evocative of a medial malignant disease. No evidence of extraneural tumoral localization was observed. Studies of HIV antibodies were not done. Electrophysiologic studies showed a distal neurogenic atrophy of the four limbs with a right predominance; conduction velocities were moderately slowed. In account of the deteriorating clinical conditions of the patient, a nerve biopsy could not be performed. Corticoid treatment was initiated. Complications of respiratory disturbances and urinary infection developed. 15 days before death, hyponatremia with hyposmolarity symptomatic of an inappropriate antidiuretic hormone secretion appeared. The patient expired 5 months after clinical presentation.

PATHOLOGIC FINDINGS

Case 1 (Needle brain biopsy examination): The fragment was infiltrated by a highly cellular tumor. The cells were mainly surrounding the vessels and were separated by very thin rings of reticulin fibers extending to the adjoining tissue (Fig. 2A). The large cells, 10 ± 1 microns of diameter, had a basophilic cytoplasm. Nuclei were globular, ovoid or irregular in shape with one or more PAS positive inclusions (Fig. 2B), nuclear diameter ranged from 6 to 9 microns; they contained one or two nucleoli sometimes apposed on the nuclear membrane. There were a few mitotic figures. At the periphery of the tumor, protoplasmic astrocytosis, microglial rod cells and lipid laden phagocytes were present. In a few cells, immunoreactivity patterns for the mu heavy chain included both intranuclear vacuoles and granular or diffuse cytoplasmic staining. The same distribution was shown for the kappa light chain with a more intense staining in more numerous cells (Fig. 2D). No immuno reactivity was detected for the other tested chains.

At the electron microscopic level, the cells were regular. The nuclei (7.2 microns mean diameter), were round, folded or lobulated (Fig. 3A-B) with a dispersed chromatin and several nucleoli. Dilatation of the perinuclear cisternae containing finely granular material and pseudo-inclusions due to cytoplasmic invaginations (cytoplasmic pockets) modified the shape of the nuclei. The cytoplasm of some of the neoplastic cells was poorly differentiated and contained few organelles. Others had a granular reticulum filled with flocculent material similar to the material seen in perinuclear inclusions, and formed a large distended more or less eccentric ergastoplasm (Fig. 3D).

Near the lymphomatous cells, axons were modifed, demyelinated or destroyed. Diagnosis was diffuse B cell MNHL lymphoplasmacytoid type Waldenström like, polymorphic subtype (low grade malignancy in the Kiel Classification (17) and intermediate grade malignancy F for the Working Formulation (35)).

Case 2 (autopsy study): General autopsy examination revealed an acute broncho-pneumonia with several small abcesses. There was no evidence of visceral lymphoma. Bone marrow was rich, without lymphomatous involvement. In the brain, there was a large tumor located in the middle and posterior part of the corpus callosum and the trigones, extending in both sides in the white matter and the posterior cinguli (Fig. 4). It was surrounded by edema and by a colloid material attached to the choroid plexus inside the ventricles. The superior part of the thalami was distorted by the tumoral compression. Microscopic examination of the tumor revealed an extensive diffuse cellular infiltration concentrated around the vessels (Fig. 5A). The cells, 12-15 microns diameter, appeared polymorph with scanty basophilic cytoplasm. Cell nuclei were very large, 9-12 microns diameter; they were irregular, indented or multilobated in shape; their chromatin was fine, ponctuated with 1 to 3 more or less distinct nucleoli (Fig. 5C-D). They were a few mitoses and many pycnotic cells. No immunostaining was obtained with any of the 5 sera tested on formalin fixed material. Electron microscopic studies performed on formalin fixed material showed multilobated nuclei, scanty organelles in the cytoplasm and fragmented membranes. In the areas with dense cellular infiltration, the demyelination was extensive. In other areas, with a less pronounced infiltration, tumor cells were running along the associative pathways. Tumoral cells were mixed with protoplasmic astrocytes, microglial rod cells, and a few lipid laden cells in necrotic areas. In some structures, especially in the grey matter, the microglial rods infiltrated the tissue admixed with diffuse or perithelial tumoral cells and persisting neurons. The tumor had mostly a trigono-callosal posterior location. It extended and lined the ventricles radiating outward in a fan shape. Tumour infiltrated the white matter, with a right predominance, extended into the caudate nuclei, the internal capsule, the thalami, the lenticular nuclei and the subthalamicus areas (Fig. 4D). The midbrain, the pons and the dorsal part of the medulla oblongata were involved. Nodular tumoral foci were also found in cingular, frontal, insular, parietal, and hippocampal gyri. The meninges of the brain stem and the roots of the common motor nerves were infiltrated. The spinal cord, the roots of the peripheral nerves and the cauda equina were normal. The trunks of the peripheral nerves were more or less demyelinated and contained a few lymphomatous cells in the endo and perineurial space, mixed with an abundant lymphoid infiltrate (Fig. 5B). Neurogenic atrophy was present in the muscle. Diagnosis was diffuse MNHL multilobated large cell type which is not actually included in the two classifications (17, 35). It could be classified as high grade malignancy (17, 35), miscellaneous (35) or unclassified (17).

DISCUSSION

In these two cases, the initial symptoms were not specific but their evolution was relatively rapid after the onset of the disease. At a later stage, although the tumor expanded diffusely throughout the CNS the patient 2 exhibited few neurological signs of peripheral or central impairment. Progressively he developped an amnesic syndrome; no precise correlation between the topographical distribution of the brain lesions and the clinical symptoms could be established because all the limbic system was destroyed, although the main, and perhaps initial, infiltration was in the trigones. Few cases of MNHL have been characterized by memory disturbances 9 - 16 - 24 - 33 - 34 and none were quoted in the large series of tumoral disorders of the limbic system (1, 19). An inappropriate antidiuretic hormone secretion developped 15 days before death in patient 2: to our knowledge this finding is very uncommon. It might be due to the infiltration of the hypothalamus. Unfortunately the pituitary gland could not be examined.

The onset of a peripheral neuropathy is very unusual in MNHL (11, 15); only three reports of peripheral neuropathy associated with MNHL of the brain have been published (6, 7, 13) in patients without the Acquired Immunodeficiency Syndrome where the lesions are multifactorial. Peripheral neuropathy might be due to the lymphomatous infiltration of nerves or to a demyelination with secondary axonal degeneration. In case 2, the lesions associated a tumoral infiltration of the roots and an intense inflammatory reaction of peripheral nerves.

The role of CT scan in the diagnosis of lymphoma has been underlined in all large series (3, 5, 10, 23, 30). Various radiographic parameters including density, peri-tumoral modifications, enhancement after contrast medium have been inconstantly interpreted by different authors, due to the absence of specific criteria for the diagnosis of lymphoma. A callosal location has frequently been reported: 67% of cases in multifocal lesions, 25% in localized lesion, i.e., a mean frequency of 43% of all cases (5). But it has to be emphasized that the orbito-meatal CT incidence did not facilitate the distinction between a callosal and a trigonal lesion, as in our case 2. This supports the interest of CT coronal sections and MNR.

All the MNHL are now classified by means of the two pathological classifications used in France (Kiel (17), Working Formulation (35)). Jellinger et al. (12) were the first authors to apply immunocytochemical methods to MNHL of the CNS. In our case 1, the dysglobulinemia isotype was analogous to the one found in the lymphoma and could be interpreted as a tumoral marker (29). In case 2, the monotypic immunoglobulin demonstrated only in the serum was probably in relation with a B cell type lymphoma, but this could not be confirmed by immunocytochemistry. The absence of immunostaining might be due to a long-lasting formalin fixation and/or to the absence of plasma cell differentiation of the tumor cells. This point is important because the multilobated cell lymphoma initially described as a morphologic variant of a T cell type tumor would have a relatively prolonged clinical course. Cases of B cell lymphoma with large multilobated nuclei have been recently recognized (2, 4, 21, 22, 32). No neural involvement was reported, excepted a secondary localization with extension to the CSF (20). Our case 2 is probably the first reported primary multilobated B cell MNHL of the brain.

In conclusion, the incidence of MNHL of the CNS is increasing. These tumors can be difficult to recognize when they are localized in the corpus callosum or the trigone. These data emphasize the value of the biopsy "even in the seemingly hopeless case" (30) performed with stereotactic methods (30) to initiate an early treatment.

SUMMARY

Two cases of malignant non-Hodgkin's lymphoma of the central nervous system are described. Callosal or trigono-callosal involvement, seric monotypic immunoblogulin, and short survival were observed in both cases. In addition, an amnesic syndrome, a multiple mononeuropathy, an inappropriate antidiuretic hormone secretion, and an unusual cellular phenotype were recognized in case 2. The purpose of this study is to emphasize, in these medially located tumours, the advantage of stereotactic biopsy associated with immunocytochemistry and electron microscopy as a diagnostic procedure with therapeutic implications.

KEY WORDS

Malignant non Hodgkin's lymphoma of the central nervous system. Monotypic immunoglobulin. B cell markers. Multilobated nuclei. Lymphoplasmacytoid differentiation. Corpus callosum lymphoma. Trigonal lymphoma. Amnesic syndrome. Mononeuropathy.

ACKNOWLEDGEMENTS

We are indebted to Pr J. Diebold and Dr M.F. d'Agay for advice and to F. Bernard, J. Dellanave, A. Gaste, C. Landolfi, C. Sanchez and M.C. Viot for technical assistance.

Supported by grants of Ligue contre le Cancer (Comité de Paris) and Conseil Scientifique de l'UFR Lariboisière - Saint-Louis).

1. BRION (S.), MIKOL (J.), PLAS (J.): Neuropathologie des syndrômes amnésiques chez l'homme. Rev. Neurol. (Paris), **141**: 627-643 (1985).

2. BURKE (J.S.), WARNKE (R.A.), CONNORS (J.M.), BECKSTEAD (J.H.): Diffuse malignant lymphoma with cerebriform nuclei: a B-cell lymphoma studied with monoclonal antibodies. Am. J. Clin. Pathol., **83**: 753-759 (1985).

3. CELLERIER (P.), CHIRAS (J.), GRAY (F.), METZGER (J.), BORIES (J.): Computed tomography in primary brain lymphoma of the brain. Neuroradiology, **26**: 485-492 (1984).

4. CEREZO (L.): B-cell multilobated lymphoma. Cancer, **52**: 2277-2280 (1983).

5. ENZMANN (D.R.), KRIKORIAN (J.), NORMAN (D.), KRAMER (R.), POLLOCK (J.), FAER (M.): Computed tomography in primary reticulum cell sarcoma of the brain. Radiology, **130**: 165-170 (1979).

6. FINELLI (P.F.): Remote neurological effects of primary malignant lymphoma of brain. Arch. Neurol. (Chic.), **35**: 397-399 (1978).

7. GARAFALO (M.), DANON (M.J.), DONNENFELD (H.), CHUSID (G.J.): Peripheral neuropathy associated with primary malignant lymphoma of the brain. Arch. Neurol. (Chic), **35**: 50-52 (1978).

8. HASSOUN (J.), ANDRAC (L.), GAMBARELLI (D.), TOGA (M.): Lymphomes malins primitifs du système nerveux central. Etude anatomoclinique, ultra-structurale et immunocytochimique. A propos de 23 cas. Ann. Pathol. **1**: 193-203 (1981).

9. HENRY (J.M.), HEFFNER (R.R.), DILLARD (S.H.), EARLE (K.M.), DAVIES (R.L.): Primary malignant lymphoma of the central nervous system. Cancer, **34**: 1293-1302 (1974).

10. HOLTAS (S.), NYMAN (U.), CRONQUIST (S.): Computed tomography of malignant lymphoma of the brain. Neuroradiology, **26**: 33-38 (1984).

11. HUBERT (D.), GEPNER (P.), BAUDRIMONT (M.), KRULIK (M.), BRISSAUD (Ph.), GRAMONT (A. de), SIRINELLI (A.), DEBRAY (J.): Neuropathies périphériques spécifiques au cours des lymphomes non Hodgkiniens. A propos de deux observations. Sem. Hôp. Paris, **60**: 2797-2801 (1984).

12. JELLINGER (K.), RADASZKIEWICZ (Th.), SLOWIK (F.): Primary malignant lymphoma of the central nervous system in man. Acta Neuropathol. (Berl.), 6 (Suppl.): 95-102 (1975).

13. JELLINGER (K.), KOTHBAUER (P.), WEISS (R.), SUNDER (E.): Primary malignant lymphoma of the CNS and polyneuropathy in a patient with necrotizing vasculitis treated with immunosuppression. J. Neurol., **220**: 259-268 (1979).

14. JOHNSON (G.J.), OKEN (M.M.), ANDERSON (J.R.), O'CONNELL (M.J.), GLICK (J.H.): Central nervous system relapse in unfavourable-histology non Hodgkin's lymphoma: is prophylaxis indicated? Lancet, **ii**: 685-687 (1984).

15. KOHUT (H.): Unusual involvement of the nervous system in generalized lymphoblastoma. J. Nerv. Ment. Dis., **103**: 9-20 (1946).

16. KOTASEK (D.), ALBERTYN (L.E.), SAGE (R.E.): A five-year experience with central nervous lymphoma. Med. J. Aust., **144**: 299-303 (1986).

17. LENNERT (K.), MOHRI (N.), STEIN (H.), KAISERLING (E.): The histopathology of malignant lymphoma. Br. J. Hematol. **31** (Suppl.): 193-203 (1975).

18. MACKINTOSH (F.R.), COLBRY (T.V.), PODOLSKY (W.J.), BURKE (J.S.), HOPPE (R.T.), ROSENFELT (F.P.), ROSENBERG (S.A.), KAPLAN (H.S.): Central nervous system involvement in non-Hodgkin's lymphoma: analysis of 105 cases. Cancer, **49**: 586-595 (1982).

19. MIKOL (J.): Désordres du système limbique en rapport avec la pathologie tumorale. Rapport présenté au VIIe Congrès International de Neuropathologie, Budapest: 203-208 (Excerpta Médica 1975).

20. MIKOL (J.): Confrontation Neurologique de la Salpétrière (fév. 1986). Rev. Neurol. (Paris). Sous presse.

21. MIRCHANDANI (I.), PALUTKE (M.), TABACZKA (P.), GOLDFARB (S.), EINSENBERG (L.), PAK (M.S.Y.): B-cell lymphomas morphologically resembling T-cell lymphomas. Cancer, **56**: 1578-1583 (1985).

22. NATHWANI (B.N.), SHEIBANI (K.), WINBERG (C.D.), BURKE (J.S.), RAPPAPORT (H.): Neoplastic B-cells with cerebriform nuclei in follicular lymphomas. Hum. Pathol., **16**, 173-180 (1985).

23. PAGANI (J.J.), LIBSHITZ (H.I.), WALLACE (S.), HAYMAN (L.A.): Central nervous system leukemia and lymphoma: computed tomographic manifestations. A.J.R., **137**: 1195-1201 (1981).

24. PALACIOS (E.), GORELICK (P.B.), GONZALEZ (C.F.), FINE (M.): Malignant lymphoma of the nervous system. J. Comput. Assist. Tomogr., **6**: 689-701 (1982).

25. PILERI (S.)., BRANDI (G.), RIVANO (M.T.), GOVONI (E.), MARTINELLI (G.): Report of a case of non Hodgkin's lymphoma of large multilobated cell type with B-cell origin. Tumori, **68**, 543-548 (1982).

26. PINKUS (G.S.), SAID (J.W.), HARGREAVES (M.D.): Malignant lymphoma T-cell type. A distinct variant with large multilobated cell type with a report of four cases. Am. J. Clin. Pathol., **72**: 540-550 (1979).

27. RUSSEL (D.S.), RUBINSTEIN (L.J.), LUMSDEN (C.E.): Pathology of tumours of the nervous system (E. Arnold 1963).

28. SCHAUMBURG (H.H.), PLANK (C.R.), ADAMS (R.D.): The reticulum cell sarcoma-microglioma group of brain tumors. A consideration of their clinical features and therapy. Brain, **95**: 199-212 (1972).

29. SOTTO (J.J.), RUEFF (A.), BENSA (J.C.), SOTTO (M.F.), GROSLAMBERT (P.), FAVRE (M.), HOLLAND (D.): Lymphomes malins non Hodgkiniens associés à une immunoglobuline monoclonale sérique. Presse Méd., **15**, 569-573 (1986).

30. SPILLANE (J.A.), KENDALL (B.E.), MOSELEY (I.F.): Cerebral lymphoma: Clinical radiological correlation. J. Neurol. Neurosurg. Psych. **45**: 199-208 (1982).

31. THIEBAUT (G.B.), CABANIS (E.A.), LINDEROTH (B.), THUREL (C.), ALFONSO (J.M.), IBA-ZIZEN (M.T.), DESGEORGES (M.). STOFFELS (C.): Intérêt du scanner à rayons X et de l'IRM dans l'approche stéréotaxique. Soc. Neurochir. Langue Française, Déc. 1985, Neurochirurgie, sous presse.

32. WEISS (R.L.), KJELDSBERG (C.R.), COLBY (T.V.), MARTY (J.): Multilobated B-cell lymphomas. A study of 7 cases. Hematol. Oncol.; **3**: 79-86 (1985).

33. WOODMAN (R.), SHIN (K.), PINEO (G.): Primary non-Hodgkin's lymphoma of the brain. A review. Medicine, **64**: 425-430 (1985).

34. ZIMMERMAN (H.M.): Malignant lymphomas of the nervous system. Acta Neuropathol. (Berl.), 6 (Suppl.): 69-74 (1975).

35. National Cancer Institute sponsored study of classifications of non Hodgkin's lymphoma. Summary and description of a Working Formulation for clinical usage. The Non-Hodgkin's lymphoma Pathologic Classification Project. Cancer **49**: 2112-2135 (1982).

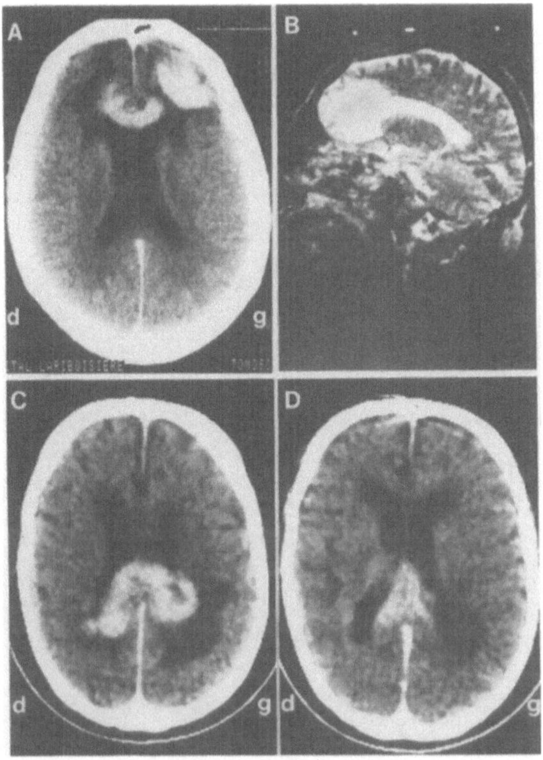

FIGURE 1. A. **(case 1)**: CT scan with contrast medium: fronto-callosal lesion. B. **(case 1)**: MNR: fronto-callosal lesion extending to the splenium. C.-D. **(case 2)**: CT scan with contrast medium: lesion of the callosal splenium.

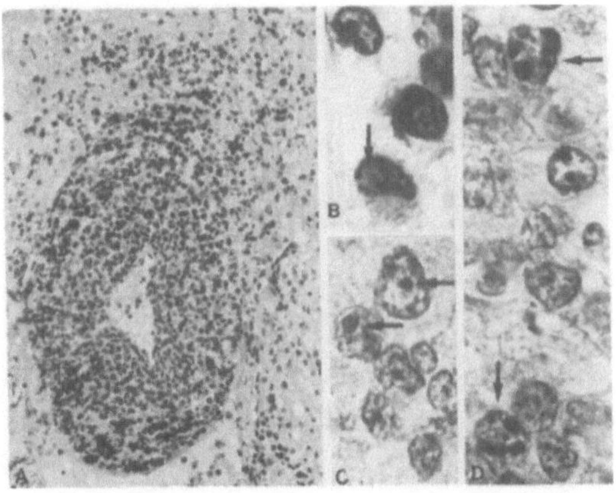

FIGURE 2. **(case 1)** A: Perithelial tumoral cuffing. Haematoxylin-eosin × 192. B.: Intranuclear PAS positive inclusion (arrow) × 1680. C.-D.: Immunostaining of intranuclear inclusions. C.: Mu heavy chain (arrows). D.: Kappa light chain (arrows) PAP method × 1680.

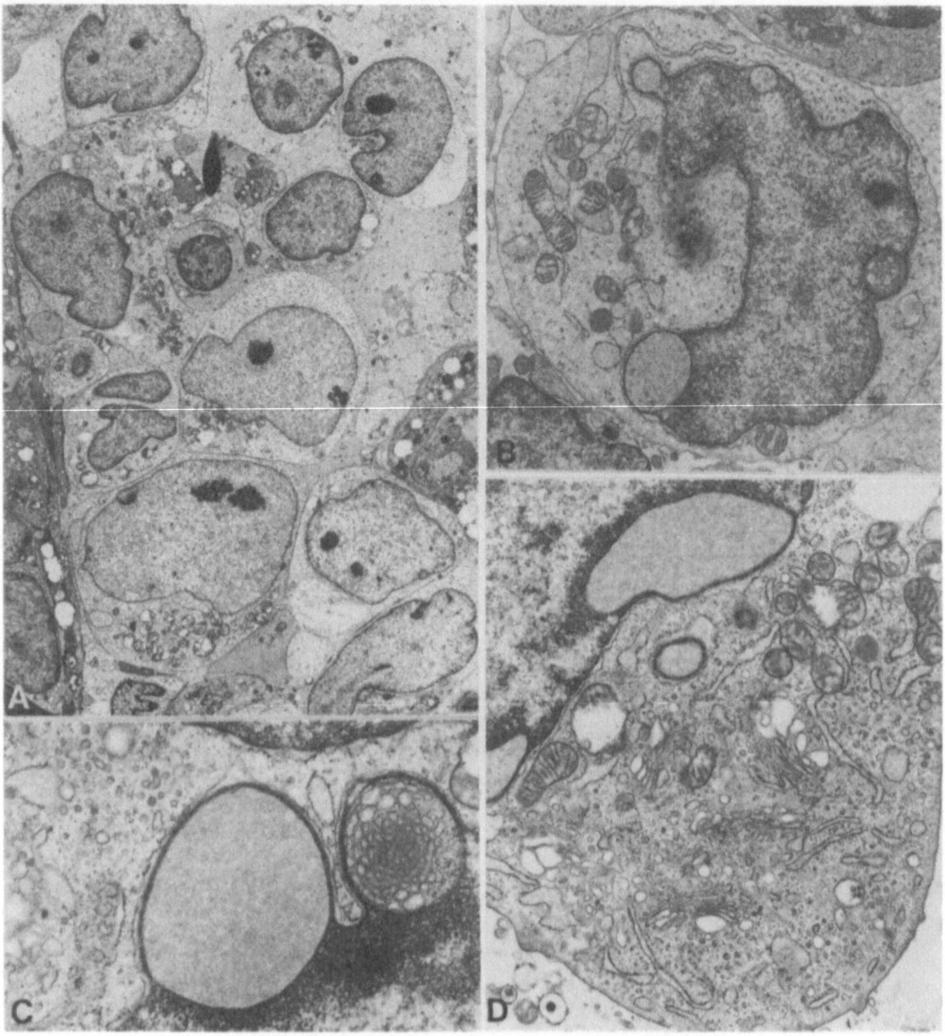

FIGURE 3. **(case 1)**: Electron micrographs: Uranyl acetate-lead citrate. A.: Infiltrating tumoral cells × 2940. B.: Tumoral cell with indented and eccentric nucleus × 12580. D.: Ergastoplasm in a tumoral cell × 7750.

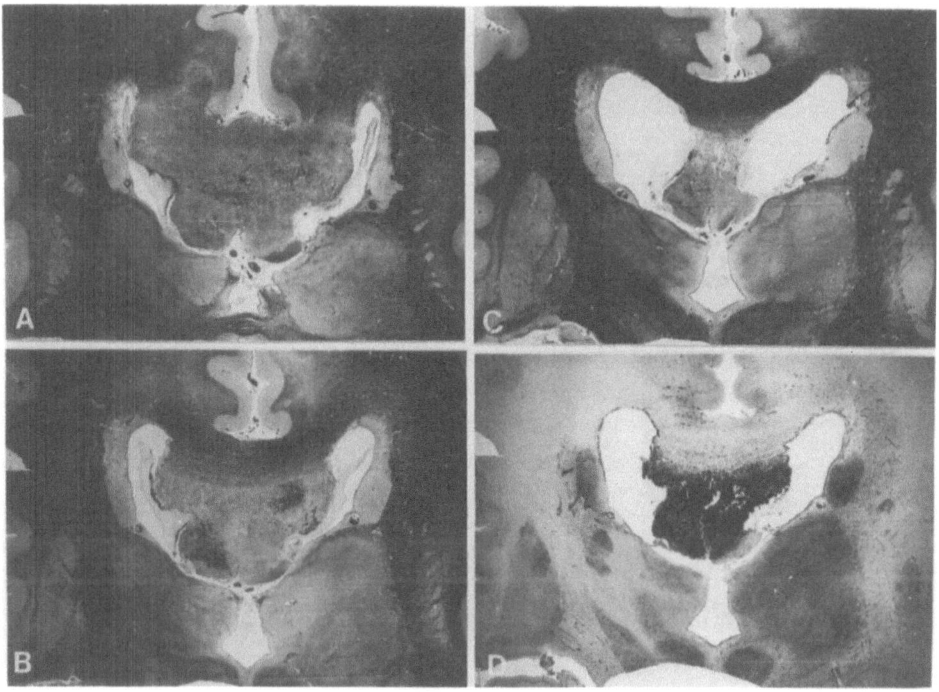

FIGURE 4. (case 2): A.B.C.: Wölcke. D.: Nissl × 1.6. A.-C.: Coronal sections, backwards to forwards, of the tumor: the splenium of the corpus callosum and the trigones were enlarged and demyelinated. D.: Patchy cellular infiltration, lining of the ventricles and radiating tumoral cells in the white matter.

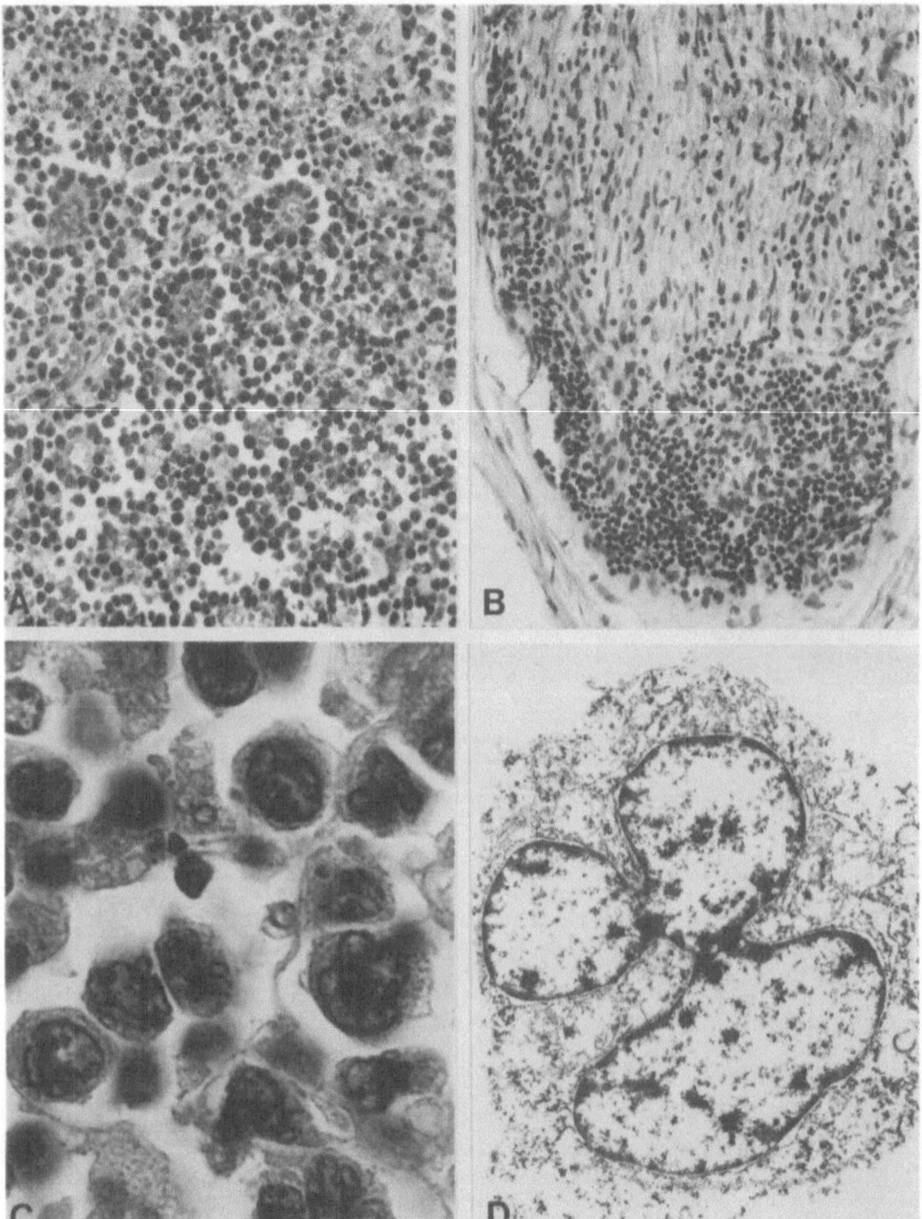

FIGURE 5. **(case 2)**: A. Tumoral cells in the corpus callosum. Haematoxyline-osin × 192. B.: Peripheral nerve: rare tumoral cells mixed with lymphoid infiltrating cells. Haematoxylin-eosin saffron × 192. C.D.: Multilobated cells. C.: Haematoxylin-eosin × 1200. D.: Electron micrograph × 4400.

Tumours of the Pineal Region

C. ALLAIRE (°), A. LEGOUT (°), J. PECKER (°), J.M. SCARABIN (°), B. VALLÉE (°), J.M. BRÜCHER (°°), M. CHATEL (°°°), F. DARCEL (°°°).

During the 1975 Oxford Congress, we proposed the use of stereotactic neuroradiology for the evaluation of pineal tumours and from then, we adopted the following strategy:

— Stereotactic biopsy in all cases, except for highly vascularized tumours.
— Radiotherapy (external or interstitial) for radiosensitive tumours as germinomas, gliomas, pineoblastomas...
— Direct surgical approach for radioresistant tumours as teratomas, pineocytomas, meningiomas...
— Chemotherapy was associated in certain definite histological types (embryonal carcinoma).

Stereotactic procedure was applied to 75 patients with tumours of the pineal region, from 1975 through 1986.

Rationale for the stereotactic procedure:

Many histological types of tumours can develop in the pineal area. Histological determination of the tumours is needed for planning specific management: some are radiosensitive and do not need surgical resection; other ones, benign or malignant, must be removed by surgery.

Although preoperative CT scanners allow to assess many tumoral characteristics, they fail to lead to accurate histological diagnosis. Numerous reports from the litterature confirm this lack of CT criteria to indicate the histological type. Indeed in our experience, several types of tumours had relatively similar CT aspects, and, on the contrary, some histologically proven germinomas mimicked other types of tumours (fig. 1).

Proton Resonance Magnetic Imagery (RMI) improved the diagnosis of anatomical location, especially the tumour extension and its relationships to adjacent structures, but does not either allow the histological determination and not even the grade of malignancy.

Many authors recently pointed out the importance of tumour markers such as human chorionic gonadotrophin, CEA, and alpha-foetoprotein. They are reported to be secreted by certain germ-cell tumours, and their plasma or CSF levels seem to correlate with tumour growth and regression. Such dosages could help to precise the biological characteristics of the lesion, but the need for true histological tumoral tissue study still persists.

Then, the stereotactic procedure seems to be a safe way to assess the histological diagnosis even if resection surgery may be secondarily chosen to reduce the tumour bulk prior to radiotherapy or for tumours which are not likely to respond to radiotherapy.

In our series, prior to biopsy, all patients were submitted to angiographic examination. The number of biopsy samples taken in each case varies from two to four fragments. The obtained tissues were immediately examined by smears, and, later on, by appropriately stained paraffin sections.

Our results are presented according to the W.H.O. Classification of pineal tumours (table 1).

The presence of pineal tumours containing a mixture of malignant elements has been described, but the frequency of such mixed tumours is not known. This data suggests that the adequacy of stereotactic biopsy may be uncertain in rare cases.

RESULTS

Our series include 75 patients with tumours of the pineal region, 52 males (70 %) and 23 females (30 %).

(°) Service de Neurochirurgie C.H.U. Rennes, (°°) Laboratoire de Neuropathologie U.C.L. Bruxelles, (°°°) Laboratoire de Neuropathologie C.H.U. Rennes.

M. Chatel, F. Darcel and J. Pecker (eds.), Brain Oncology. ISBN-13: 978-94-010-8003-3

Their age at the time of diagnosis ranged from 1.5 year to 56 years, with a mean of 23.5 years. The duration of symptoms prior to diagnosis was 7 months (one week to 6 years). A great majority of patients (80 %) presented clinically with increased intracranial pressure. Neuro-Ophtalmological abnormalities were found in 85 % of patients, especially Parinaud's syndrome (50 %).

TABLE 1: Classification of pineal tumours (W.H.O.)

A - Glial cyst

B - Germ-cell tumours
- Germinoma
- Embryonal carcinoma
- Choriocarcinoma
- Teratoma

C - Pineal parenchymal cell tumours:
- Pineoblastoma
- Pineocytoma

D - Para-pineal tumours:
- Glioma
- Gangliocytoma
- Meningioma
- Lipoma
- Dermoïd cyst

E - Vascular lesions

TABLE 2: Pathologic findings in 67 patients with pineal tumours

Glial cyst	1	
Germ cell tumours		35
Germinoma	31	
Teratoma	3	
Embryonal carcinoma	1	
Pineal parenchymal cell tumors		14
Pineocytoma	8	
Pineoblastoma	6	
Gliomas		12
Astrocytoma	6	
Glioblastoma	3	
Spongioblastoma	1	
Oligodendroglioma	1	
Choroid plexus Papilloma	1	
Other tumours		5
Meningioma	2	
Cavernous angioma	1	
Epidermoïd cyst	1	
Medulloblastoma	1	

Histological diagnosis was available in 67 tumours, 60 times by stereotactic biopsy, and seven by direct surgery. No tumoural tissue was found in 3 cases of 63 stereotactic biopsies (table 2). No mortality was related to the procedure. Out of the 63 stereotactic biopsies of pineal region tumours, there were 7 transient incidents, (subarachnoïd hemorrhage, Parinaud's syndrome, hemiparesis), with no sequellae.

Correlations between histology, age and sex ratio are analysed in table 3. Male predominance is important in germinoma. On the contrary, 7 of the 8 pineocytomas are female. Mean age is lower in pineoblastomas, than in pineocytomas.

The results of this procedure are encouraging. Out of 75 patients, 3 cases were unexpected discoveries on CT scanners; 2 additional cases had transient clinical symptoms. These 5 patients had no specific treatment. They have been examined every 6 months and are doing well with a 1 to 3 year follow-up. Other 5 patients were lost to follow-up.

The overall mortality was 25 % (18 patients); no radiotherapy response in 5 cases, and 13 tumour recurrences. 47 patients are still alive, with a median follow-up of 4 years (1 to 10). The five year survival rate was 72 % for germinomas (35 cases). The number of cases is too small and does not allow any conclusion for other types of tumours.

Our data however suggest that:

— Germinomas are highly radiosensitive and have a rather good survival rate.

— Benign Teratomas have an excellent post-operative course.

— Pineocytomas are poorly radiosensitive and may recur after surgery.

— All patients with pineoblastomas died within a year.

In conclusion, stereotactic biopsy procedure allows, in the majority of cases, the histological determination of a pineal lesion. The procedure represents an attractive issue for the choice of an appropriate mode of treatment.

TABLE 3: Age and sex-ratio according to histology

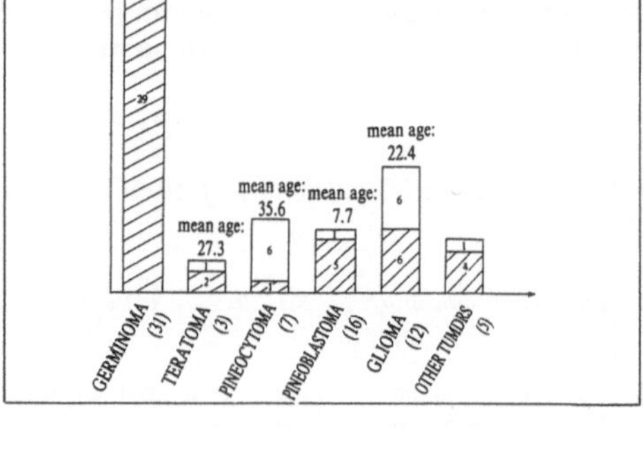

SUMMARY

This study advocates the stereotactic procedure in the management of pineal tumours and in the choice of appropriate mode of treatment.

Stereotactic biopsy allows in the majority of cases the histological diagnosis. Specific management is planned, depending upon the nature of the tumours and its radiosensitivity:
— Radiotherapy for radiosensitive tumours.
— Surgery for poorly and not sensitive tumours.
— Chemotherapy is associated in case of certain definite histological types.

Our series include 75 patients with tumors of the pineal region. Stereotactic biopsy allowed histological diagnosis in 60 cases; in seven other cases, an histological examination was available by surgery.

The tumours were: germ-cell tumors: 35; pineal parenchymal cell tumours: 14; gliomas: 11; glial cyst: 1; other tumours: 6.

The outcome of the patients is analysed: 18 patients (25 %) died, mostly within the first year; 47 patients are alive, with a 4 year median follow-up (1 to 10 years).

KEY WORDS

Stereotaxy, Brain Biopsy, Pineal Tumours.

REFERENCES

1. ALLAIRE (C.): Les tumeurs de la région pinéale: apport de la biopsie stéréotaxique à la décision thérapeutique (A propos de 69 observations). Thèse Médecine, Rennes, 1985.
2. EDNER (G.): Stereotactic biopsy of intracranial space occupying lesions. Acta Neurochir., 1981, **3**: 213-234.
3. FRANK (F.), GAIST (G.), PIAZZA (G.), RICCI (R.F.), STURIALE (C.), and GALASSI (E.): Stereotaxic biopsy and radioactive implantation for interstitial therapy of tumours of the pineal region. Surg. Neurol., 1985, **23**: 275-280.
4. LAPRAS (C.), BRET (P.), and NICOLAS (A.): Experience with direct surgical approach in 52 tumours of the pineal region. Child's Brain, 1981, **8**: 54-55.
5. MOREAU (J.J.), RAVON (R.), CAIX (M.), SALOMON (G.), BRASSIER (G.), and VELUT (S.): Anatomical basis of the microsurgical approch to the pineal gland. Anat. Clin., 1985, **7**: 3-13.
6. NEUWELT (E.A.): The diagnosis and treatment of pineal region tumours (Baltimore, Williams and Wilkivis, 1984).
7. OSTERTAG (G.B.): MENNEL (H.D.), and KIESSLING (M.): Stereotactic biopsy of brain tumours. Surg. Neurol., 1980, **14**: 275-283.
8. PECKER (J.), SCARABIN (J.M.), BRUCHER (J.M.) et VALLEE (B.): Démarche stéréotaxique en neurochirurgie tumorale . Les Éditions Médicales Pierre Fabre, Paris, 1979.
9. SCARABIN (J.M.), PECKER (J.), VALLEE (B.), GUY (G.), LE CLECH (G.), and SIMON (L.): Stereotaxic exploration and biopsy of tumours in the region of tentorial hiatus. J. Neuroradiology, 1978, **5**: 57-68.

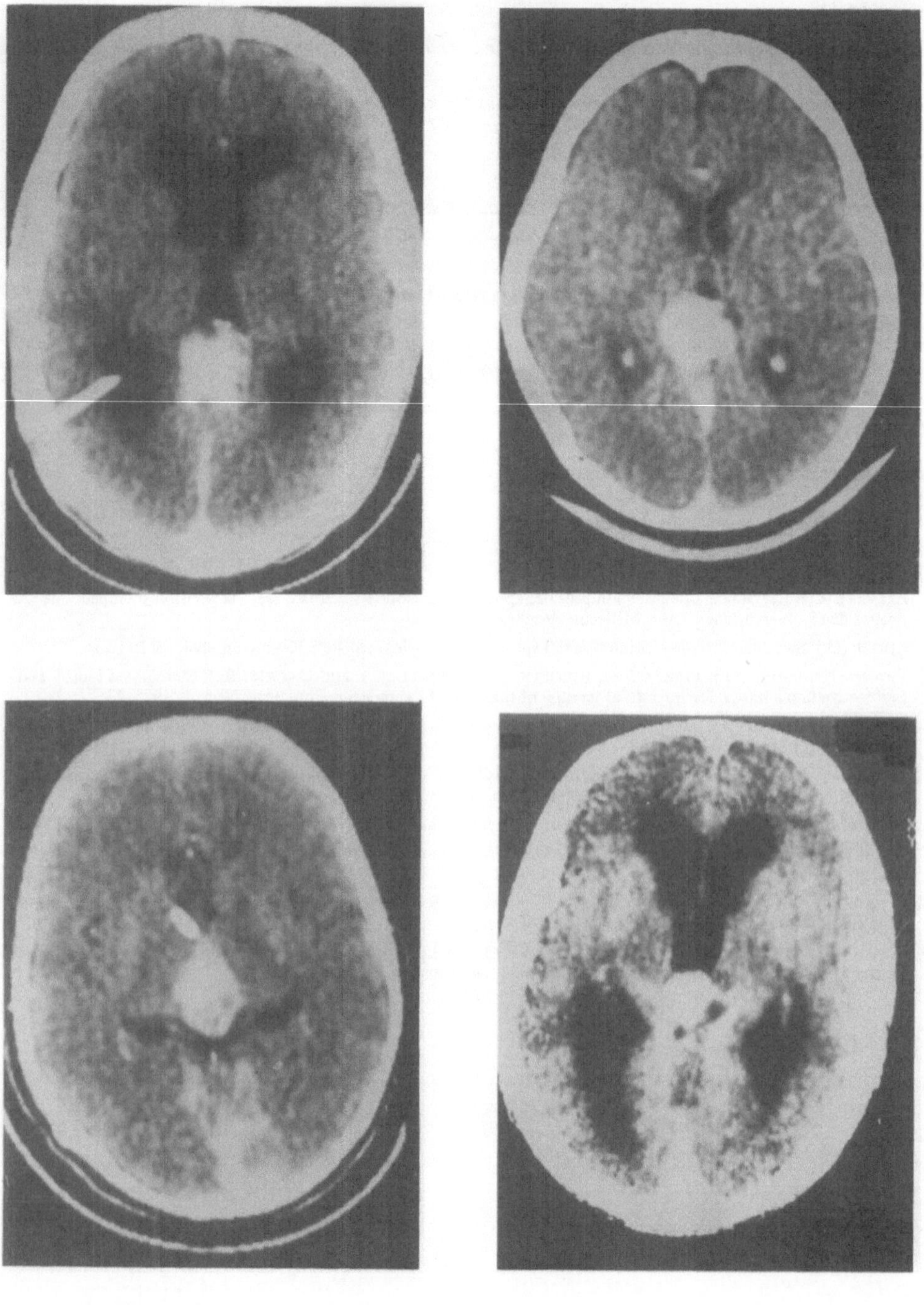

FIGURE 1. Contrast-enhanced tomography showing four cases of similar appearance high-density, iregular midline masses. The histological diagnosis were respectively: a) astrocytoma; b) germinoma; c) pineocytoma; d) glioblastoma.

Meningeal and Intra-cerebral Localizations of Kaposi's Sarcoma in AIDS

F. LABROUSSE (°), C. FONTAINE (°), C. MARCHE (°°), C. FALLET (°), C. VEDRENNE (°).

INTRODUCTION

Kaposi sarcoma (KS) occuring within the central nervous system are rare. We report a case of KS with cerebro-meningeal involvement associated with an Acquired Immune Deficiency Syndrome (AIDS).

This case belong to a series of 63 patients with AIDS who were autopsied at Claude-Bernard Hospital (Paris) between March 1983 and April 1985. This series included 11 additional cases of KS without CNS involvement.

CASE REPORT

A 39 years-old homosexual and heroin-addict french male, was admitted at Claude-Bernard Hospital on March 1985, after experiencing one month of fever, weakness, pain of knees and ankles, headache and cough.

On admission, he was somnolent. A 2-cm diameter purple nodule was noted on the right forearm. Neurological examination disclosed a left homonymous hemianopsia, physical examination was otherwise unremarkable.

The complete blood count disclosed an anemia with a decreased hemoglobin level (7.8 g/100 ml) and a normal number of white blood cells, 7.800/cu mm. The number of lymphocytes was low (746/cu mm) with 209 T4 lymphocytes/cu mm and 234 T8 lymphocytes/cu mm. The T4/T8 ratio was decreased to 0.89. Serum antibodies anti-LAV-HTLV III were positive. No opportunistic infection was biologically detected.

Standard X-rays disclosed a round-shaped opacity in the left inferior pulmonary lobe. On CT-scan, this mass was contrast-enhanced and situated close to the heart and aorta.

CT-head-scan revealed two separate, enhancing, nodular lesions surrounded by edema, one superficially situated close to the dura in the occipital area, the other involved the left parietal lobe.

A biopsy of the cutaneous nodule was performed which demonstrated a typical KS lesion. In addition, the patient underwent a lung lobectomy ; histological examination proved the pulmonary lesion to be a KS localization.

On beginning of April, the patient was more confused and developped right hemiparesia with paresthesia, gastro-intestinal hemorrhage and respiratory failure. He became comatose and died two weeks after the onset of symptoms.

Post-mortem examination disclosed ten 0.5-to-4 cm diameter nodules in the liver, a 7 cm-ulcerated and hemorrhagic tumor in the stomach and numerous hemorrhagic nodules disseminated in both lungs.

In the heart, two 0.5-and-3 cm diameter, grape-like tumor were found in the right auricule.

The lymph nodes were unremarkable.

The occipital tumor (4 cm × 4 cm × 2.5 cm) was attached to the dura and ressembled a meningioma. Necrotic and hemorrhagic changes were found on sections. The 2 cm diameter parietal lesion was located in the white matter. Histologically, all the lesions found at autopsy were KS localization. These tumors and the resected pulmonary mass appeared less differentiated than the cutaneous nodule. These tumors were composed of spindle-shaped cells lining slit-like vascular spaces, and of

(°) Sainte-Anne Hospital Paris, (°°) Claude-Bernard Hospital Paris.

M. Chatel, F. Darcel and J. Pecker (eds.), Brain Oncology. ISBN-13: 978-94-010-8003-3

round anaplasic cells with irregular and enlarged nucleus. Mitosis were frequent. Inflammatory cells infiltrates were found in all locations, iron deposits were present both within the tumors and their periphery. Immunoperoxydase reaction with factor VIII-related-antigen was positive in the cutaneous nodule and pulmonary KS location. A positive but less intense reaction was also found in the CNS locations. This mild reactivity might be related to prolonged formalin fixation time.

DISCUSSION

Review of the litterature indicates that meningeal and cerebral involvements are rare in KS. To our knowledge, only 12 histologically proved cases have been published: 7 cases in classical European or American forms (6 males, 1 female) (1, 4, 6, 10, 11, 12, 15), on African female (13), on American immuno-supressed female (16), one homosexual American male but without study of the patient's immunity (6) and 2 cases in AIDS (8, 9, 18). The dura was involved in 5 patients and the brain parenchyma in 11 cases.

In 9 out of 10 published cases, with general autopsy, cerebro-meningeal locations were associated with heart and/or lung involvement.

This, suggest a metastatic origin for intraparenchymatous cerebral lesions, whereas pure dural location might be related to the multifocal character of KS. The histological type of KS was described only in 6 cases: two were of mixed cellularity and 4 cases were of anaplasic cell type.

Despite the usual extensive involvement of KS in AIDS, LEVY (9) found only 2 cases of KS among 366 patients with AIDS having neurological complications.

KS pathogenesis is complex. Genetic factors may be suspected because of the ethnic predisposition in the European and American forms, and because of the hight ratio of HLA Dr 2 and HLA Dr 5 groups among AIDS patients (14).

According to the presence of CMV-DNA sequences and CMV antigens, within tumoral cells nucleus (5), it seems that viruses are also implicated, mainly cytomegaloviruses (CMV).

Some authors have also demonstrated presence of CMV particles in cytoplasma (3) and herpes-like intranuclear inclusions within KS cells (17). Retrovirus particles have also been observed in KS cells (2, 7).

SUMMARY

The case of a 39 years old homosexual frenchman is reported. The first clinical symptoms noted were: fever, weakness, pains, headache and cough. Physical examination revealed a purplish nodule on the right forearm and a left lateral homonymous hemianopsia. Biologically, the T4/T8 ratio was decreased, antibodies anti-LAV were positive. The cerebral CT scan showed 2 enhancing masses: a right occipital one and a left parietal one. Pulmonary CT scan display a left enhancing mass.

Secondarily appeared an increased mental confusion, a right hemiparesia with paresthesia, a gastrointestinal hemorrage and respiratory failure. The patient died 10 weeks after the onset of the first symptoms.

The autopsy revealed multifocal kaposian lesions involving the liver, the stomach and specially the heart and the lungs. Two intracranial tumours were found: a meningeal one compressing the right occipital lobe and another one in the left parietal lobe.

Histologicaly it was a polymorphous Kaposi's sarcoma (KS) with important anaplastic changes but a vascular component was always found. The immuno-histochemical study with factor VIII related antigen was positive in the cells of the intracranial, cutaneous and pulmonary tumours.

The review of the litterature shows that meningeal and cerebral involvement is rare in the classical forms of KS (10 cases) and also in KS occuring in AIDS (2 cases). Intracerebral localizations are often associated with lung and/or heart involvement suggesting a metastatic mecanism. Histologically anaplastic changes are frequent. The pathogeny of KS is unclear. Some authors mentioned the role of cytomegalovirus, others have found retroviruses particles in KS in AIDS.

KEY WORDS

A.I.D.S., Kaposi, Meninges, Brain Tumours, Lymphomas.

REFERENCES

1. ANTMAN (K.H.), NADLER (L.), MARK (E.J.), MONTELLA (D.L.), KIRKPATRICK (P.) and HALPERN (J.): Primary Kaposi's sarcoma of the lung in an immunocompetent 32 year-old heterosexual white man. Cancer 1984, **54**: 1696-8.
2. DOWNING (R.G.), ELGIN (R.P.) and BAYLEY (A.C.): African Kaposi's sarcoma and AIDS. Lancet 1984, **1**: 470-80.
3. DREW (W.L.), MINER (R.C.), ZIEGLER (J.C.), GULETT (J.H.), ABRAMS (D.I.), GONANT (M.A.), HUANG (E.S.), GROUNDWATER (J.R.), WOLBERDING (P.), MINTZ (L.): Cytomegalovirus and Kaposi's sarcoma in young homosexual men. Lancet 1982, 11: 125-127.
4. EPSTEIN (E.): Extracutaneous manifestations of Kaposi's sarcoma. A systemic lymphoblastoma. Calif. Med. 1957, 87, 98-103.
5. GIRALDO (G.), BETH (E.) and HUANG (E.S.): Kaposi's sarcoma and its relationship to cytomegalovirus (CMV) III -CMV DNA and CMV early antigens in Kaposi's sarcoma. Int. J. Cancer 1980, **26**: 23-9.
6. GORIN (F.A.), BALE (J.F.), HALKS-MILLER (M.), SCHWARTZ (R.A.): Kaposi's sarcoma metastatic to the CNS. Arch. Neurol. 1985, **42**: 162-5.
7. GYORKEY (F.), SINKOVICS (J.G.), MELNICK (J.L.), GYORKEY (P.): Retroviruses in Kaposi-sarcoma cells in AIDS. N. Eng. J. Med. 1984, **311**: 1183-4.
8. KELLY (W.M.), BRANT-ZAWADZKI (M.): Acquired immunodeficiency syndrome: neuroradiologic findings. Radiology 1983, **149**: 485-91.
9. LEVY (R.M.), BREDESEN (D.E.) and ROSENBLUM (M.L.): Neurological manifestations of the acquired immunodeficiency syndrome (AIDS): Experience at UCSF and review of the litterature. J. Neurosurg. 1985, **62**: 475-95.
10. LORING (W.E.) and WOLMAN (S.R.): Idiopathic multiple haemorrhagic sarcoma of lung (Kaposi's sarcome). N.Y. State J. Med. 1965, **64**: 668-76.
11. NESBITT (S.), MARK (P.F.) and ZIMMERMAN (H.M.): Dissemination visceral idiopathic haemorrhagic sarcoma (Kaposi's disease) report of case with necropsy findings. Ann. Intern. Med. 1945, **22**: 601-5.
12. RAMEL (M.E.). Sarcomatose idiopathique hemorragique (Kaposi). Bull. Soc. Franc. Derm. Syph. 1926, **33**: 557-61.
13. RWOMUSHANA (R.J.W.), BAILEY (I.C.), KYALWAZI (S.K.): Kaposi's sarcoma of the brain. A case report with necropsy findings Cancer 1975, **36**: 1127-31.
14. SAFAI (B.): Kaposi's sarcoma: a review of the classical and epidemic forms. Ann. NY. Acad. Sci. 1984, **437**: 373-82.
15. SCHIRREN (C.G.), BURKHARDT (L.): Ein sarcoma idiotaphicum multiplex haemorrhagicum (Kaposi) mit Hirnmetastasen. Arch. Klin. Exp. Dermatol. 1955, **201**: 99-105.
16. SCHNECK (S.A.), PENN (I.): De-novo brain tumors in renal transplant recipients. Lancet 1971, **I**: 983-6.
17. WALTER (P.), PHILIPPE (E.), KHALIL (Th.), NGUEMBY-MBINA (C.), CHAMLIAN (A.): Le sarcome de Kaposi. Un néoplasme vasculaire présumé d'origine virale. Caractères histologiques et ultrastructuraux. Ann. Pathol. 1984, **4**: 19-25.
18. WELCH (K.), FINKBEINER (W.), ALPERS (C.E.), BLUMENFELD (W.), DAVIS (R.L.), SMUCKIER (E.A.), BECKSTEAD (J.H.): Autopsy findings in the Acquired Immune Deficiency Syndrome. JAMA 1984, **252**: 1152-9.

Intracranial Meningiomas with Extracranial Dissemination

Th. WALLENFANG (°), J. BOHL (°°).

Metastases of intracranial meningiomas are very rare, taking into account the frequency of these tumours. A hundred years ago, in 1886, Power (7) published the first account of a woman suffering from a meningioma accompanied by extracranial dissemination to the lungs.

A few years later, in 1889, Klebs (3) reported an example of a meningioma of the cranial arachnoid membrane with histologically identical lung deposits. The tumour was classified as endothelioma of the pia mater. Cushing and Eisenhard (1), in 1938, described a recurrent meningioma which showed malignant degeneration 43 years after the operation. At autopsy, histologically identical tumours were found in the skull and in the lungs.

Later publications, up to 1980, concerning intracranial meningiomas accompanied by metastases have been analysed by Pasquier et al. (6) and Kepes (2).

It is immediately obvious that many authors have observed malignant degeneration and that they noted tumour in the neighbourhood of the major cerebral veins.

From 1956 to 1986, we have operated on 472 instances of intracranial meningiomas. However, we have only observed 3 cases of dissemination outside the skull in the last five years.

Due to the long interval between the first operation and the appearance of metastases on one hand, and on the other to the rarity of this type of outcome, the interpretation of deposits outside the central nervous system remained uncertain until a neuropathological examination could be made.

We would like to describe these three cases, because metastases are probably more common than is generally thought especially when recurrent meningiomas are involved.

First case

In october 1961, a 31 old patient was admitted to the clinic with occipital headaches, accompanied by vomiting, especially in the morning. A clinical examination revealed instability in walking and standing, a tendency to fall forward and cerebellar dysfunction. Papilloedema was seen at the fundus of the eye. An obstructive hydrocephalus caused by a large tumour in the posterior fossa of the skull was diagnosed. Arteriography of the carotid and vertebral arteries confirmed the existence of a meningioma which extended to the tentorium cerebelli.

During the operation the complete extent of the highly vascularised tumour could be seen: it originated in the dura mater at the confluens sinuum and the sinus transversus (this latter was closed) and reached the pontocerebellar junction. The tumour was completely removed, including the affected part of the cerebellar tentorium and of the sinus. Histological examination revealed that it was an angioblastic meningioma of the hemangiopericytic type.

Fifteen years later, in 1978, a second operation was performed. A large recurrent tumour was then discovered with a recent extension between the cerebellum and the right occipital lobe (fig. 1a). The tumour had again arisen in the dura mater next to the resection of the cerebellar tentorium and the remnant of the sinus transversus. Histological examination led to the same result as in 1963, i.e. an hemangiopericytic meningioma (fig. 1c, d).

Three years after the second surgical intervention the patient underwent a successful operation to remove a large tumour in the mediastinum. This was a metastasis of an intracranial meningioma of the hemangiopericytic type. The cellular architecture of the mediastinal tumour was identical to that of the meningioma removed in 1963 (fig. 1b, e).

(°) Department of Neurosurgery and (°°) Institute of Neuropathology, University of Mayence.

M. Chatel, F. Darcel and J. Pecker (eds.), Brain Oncology. ISBN-13: 978-94-010-8003-3

Second case

In spring 1977, a 40 years old patient experienced paresthesia of the right side of the face for the first time; this condition continued to worsen. In addition the patient saw double when looking to the right and suffered from pressure above the right eye. Upon admission to the clinic a right-hand exophthalmia and a malfunction of cranial nerve III leading to partial ophthalmoplegia were noted. The corneal reflex was reduced. By scanning, angiography and tomography of the fossa cranii anterior and media we diagnosed an extended meningioma situated in the medial fossa cranii on the right side. An operation confirmed the clinical result. The tumour stretched from the sphenoid bone and the clinoid apophysis to the pars petrosa ossis temporalis. It had enclosed the internal carotid artery and cranial nerves nerves III, IV, V and VI and had destroyed the summit of the pars petrosa and invaded the cavernous sinus, which was blocked. It had also invaded the sphenoid sinus. The tumour was radically resected including the III rd and VI th cranial nerves and the infraclinoid carotid artery between the pars petrosa and the infraclinoid apophysis. The opening at the base of the skull was covered with the temporal muscle.

Histology showed a hemangiopericytic meningioma (fig. 2b).

For 5 years the patient had no problems except the loss of cranial nerves III and IV on the right side, but later he developed visual disturbances.

In 1983 we diagnosed a large recurrent tumour by scanning and angiography. It extended around the sella turcica and had destroyed the median fossa and the clivus. A second operation seemed impossible (fig. 2a) and X-ray treatment was suggested.

During radiotherapy we noticed osteolytic metastases in the right hip joint and in the ischium (fig. 2d, e). The results of a bone biopsy agreed with the histology of the intracranial meningioma removed in 1978: angioblastic meningioma of the hemangiopericytic type (fig. 2c). The dissemination of meningioma tissue to bone without lung involvement is extremely unusual. For this reason we scanned the lungs and, in fact, discovered multiple metastases.

Third case

In spring 1976, a patient was admitted to the clinic suffering from convulsions. Neurological examination, electroencephalography, radiography of the skull and thorax gave negative results, but brain scintigraphy was positive. Angiography showed a parasagittal and frontocentral meningioma, and an operation was performed. The tumour originated in the falx and had finally blocked the sinus sagittalis superior. On resection of the tumour a plug of meningioma was dislodged from the sinus. The affected part of the sinus was removed together with the body of the tumour. The venous drainage was left intact.

Histology revealed an endothelial meningioma which had penetrated into the dura mater (fig. 4d).

The patient was re-admitted to the clinic in 1981. The scanner showed the presence of three well-defined tumours: a recurrent meningioma in the falx which descended to the corpus callosum, a second fronto-basal meningioma and a third on the right convexity (fig. 3a).

Angiography confirmed these results. In the vicinity of the recurrent meningioma the blood vessels seemed to be pathologically deformed. Only vague contours could be seen of the fronto-basal meningioma. The third tumour received its blood supply exclusively from the external carotid artery.

An x-ray of the lungs showed a single circular deposit of 2-cm diameter in the inferior lobe of the left lung, which was first seen by radiography in 1979. Biopsy of this lung deposit indicated that it was a metastasis of an endothelial meningioma - in accordance with the diagnosis of the brain meningioma resected 3 years earlier.

During a second operation on the skull carried out 5 years after the first, we saw a tumour which had infiltrated the diploe of the skull and the scalp. We removed the meningioma in the right convexity and the recurrent tumour in the falx, which were linked together like the two halves of an hourglass. The recurrent meningioma measured 8 cm in length and 4 cm in width in the cleft between the cerebral hemispheres. Tumour tissue had again invaded the sagittal sinus, making a further resection necessary. Beside the fronto-basal meningioma we discovered two additional tumours in the sinus sagittalis inferior; thus a total of five tumours was removed.

Histological studies indicated a meningioma of mainly endothelial character, thus corresponding exactly with the biopsy of the lung metastasis. The outcome after the operation was complicated by pulmonary embolisms, which sometimes gave only clinical signs; however, some scanner results suggested lung metastases (fig. 3b). The patient died five weeks after the operation as a result of a massive embolism. The autopsy revealed further tumours in the falx (fig. 4c) and confirmed the presence of lung metastases (fig. 4a, b). These had infiltrated the blood vessels and bronchi, and showed regressive changes identical to those seen in the primary tumour (fig. 4d).

DISCUSSION

The relatively small number of publications on the subject leads to the assumption that metastases of meningiomas outside the skull are extremely rare (9,12). The authors seldom describe more than two cases (2, 6, 8, 9, 10, 11).

We can only report on 3 cases of extra-cranial dissemination observed since 1980, although we have operated on 472 meningiomas in the past 30 years, and 98 of these in the last five years. The rate metastases (0.63 %, calculated for 472 meningiomas) is greater than 0.1 % calculated by Strang et al. (11). However, the value of 0.63 % is almost certainly an underestimate. One should remember that only an unusual histological finding will lead to a search through previous clinical notes to arrive at a description of the primary tumour. Tumour deposits outside the skull are often not related to neurosurgical records, especially when the primary tumour has not recurred and a second neurosurgical intervention has therefore not been necessary (6).

Our cases suggest that metastases may result from surgical handling of major veins which have been invaded by tumour, especially when several successive operations are performed. On the other hand, 15 % of the cases of metastases analysed by Kepes (2) originated from meningiomas which were not operated on. According to the observations of Opsahl and Löken (5), and to our own experience, it is possible that the formation of metastases is facilitated when the tumour infiltrates the diploe of the skull and the scalp. Post-operative metastases in the central nervous system carried by cerebro-spinal fluid are even more rare than metastatic deposits outside the nervous system (2, 4, 9, 11). This indicates that release of tumour cells as a result of surgical manipulation cannot be the only factor determining the pathology of metastases. The biological nature of the tumour and the host defence systems play a role which is at least as important, if not more. Among the various types of meningiomas treated in our clinic, angioblastic meningiomas of the hemangiopericytic type are only the third in frequency. Our observations fit into a general pattern emerging from the literature. They indicate that the relatively high incidence of metastases of hemangiopericytic meningioma, 28.9 % in the study of Kepes (2), might reflect the aggressive nature of this tumour, against which neuro-oncologists have so often struggled.

SUMMARY

The authors present three cases of recurrent intracranial meningiomas accompanied by metastases outside the nervous system. Dissemination outside the skull may be seen at the same time as, or several years after, intracranial recurrence. Even years later the histological architecture of the tumours had not changed and was always identical to that of the metastases.

KEY WORDS

Meningioma - Metastases - Histological architecture.

ACKNOWLEDGEMENTS

We are indebted to Professors Wende and Hahn, and Dr. Schweden for permission to use their radiograms.

REFERENCES

1. CUSHING (H.), EISENHARD (L.): The meningiomas: their classification, regional behaviour, live history, and surgical end results. Charles C. Thomas, Springfield, 692-719 (1938).

2. KEPES (J.): Meningiomas: Biology, Pathology, and Differential Diagnosis. Masson Publishing USA, New York, Paris, 190-200 (1982).

3. KLEBS (E.): Die Allgemeine Pathologie. Jena, G. Fischer, Vol. II, p. 628 (1889).

4. LUDWIN (S.K.), CONLEY (F.K.): Malignant meningioma metastasizing through the cerebrospinal pathways. J. Neurol. Neurosurg. Psychiatry **38**: 138-142 (1975).

5. OPSAHL (R.), LÖKEN (A.C.): Meningioma with metastases to cervical lymph nodes. Acta Pathol. Microbiol. Scand. (C) **64**: 294-298 (1967).

6. PASQUIER (B.), COUDERC (P.), PASQUIER (D.), PANH (M.H.), N'GOLET (A.), BARGE (M.), PELLAT (J.): Méningiome récidivant avec métastase pulmonaire. Sem. Hôp. Paris, 55, n° 17-18: 855-862 (1979).

7. POWER (D.): Fibrosarcoma of the dura mater. Trans. Pathol. Soc. Lond. **37**: 12 (1886).

8. RUSSEL (W.O.), SACHS (E.): Fibrosarcoma of arachnoidal origin with metastases. Report of four cases necropsy. Arch. Pathol. **34**: 240-261 (1942).

9. RUSSEL (D.S.), RUBINSTEIN (L.J.): Pathology of tumours of the nervous system, 4 th ed. Baltimore, Williams & Wilkins, p. 91 (1977).

10. SIMPSON (D.): The recurrence of intracranial meningiomas after surgical treatment. J. Neurol. Neurosurg. Psychiatry 20: 22-39 (1957).

11. STRANG (R.R.), TOVI (D.), NORDENSTAM (H.): Meningioma with intra-cerebral, cerebellar and visceral metastases. J. Neurosurg. **21**: 1098-1107 (1964).

12. ZÜLCH (K.L.), POMPEU (F.), PINTO (F.): Über die Metastasierung der Meningiome. Zentralbl. Neurochir. **14**: 253-260 (1954).

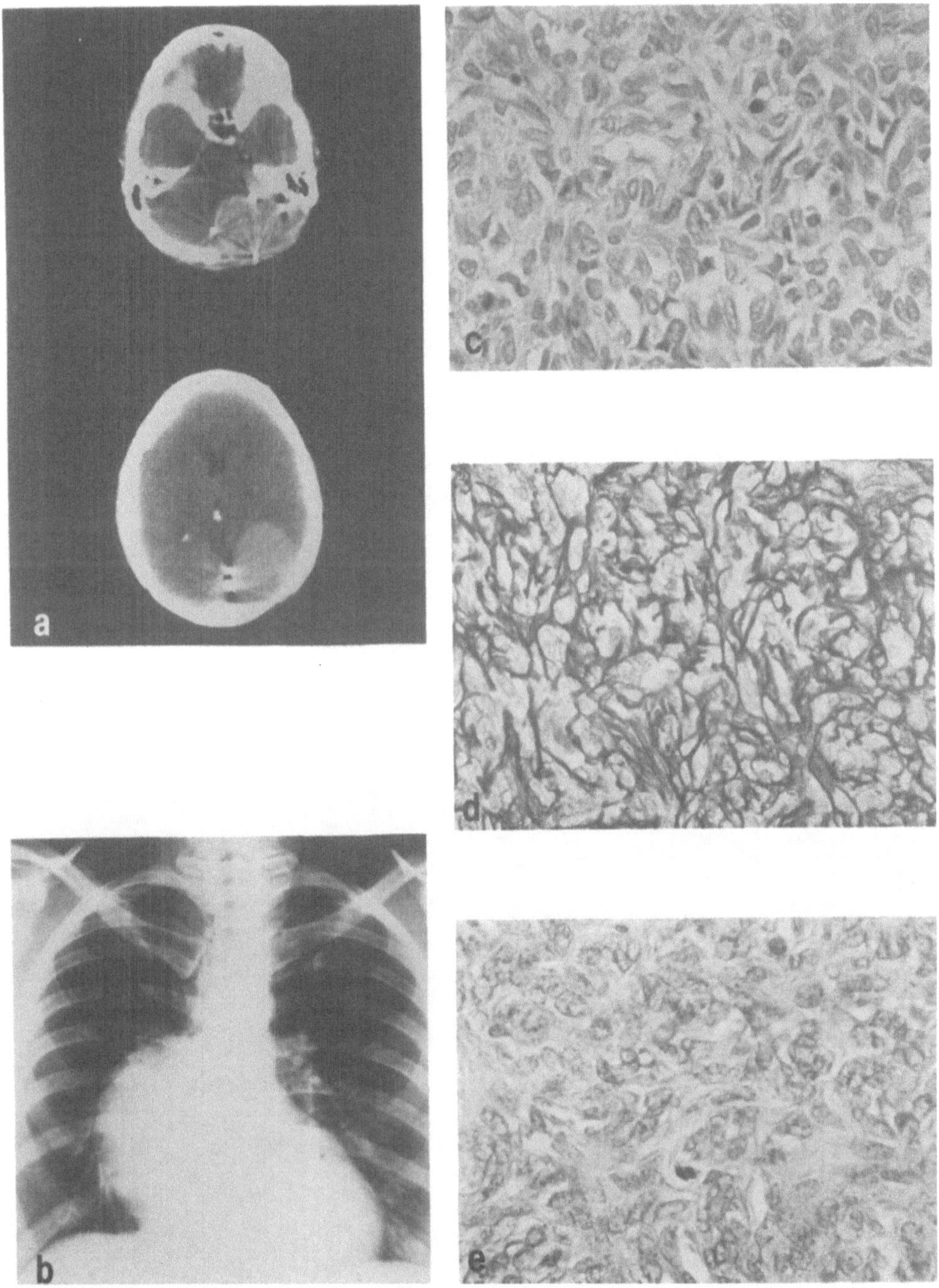

FIGURE 1 a-e.
a) Recurrent meningioma in the tentorium cerebelli diagnosed 15 years after the first operation.
b) Mediastinal metastases 3 years after the second operation.
c) and d) Histological architecture of the recurrent meningioma (x 500), identical to e) that of the metastasis.

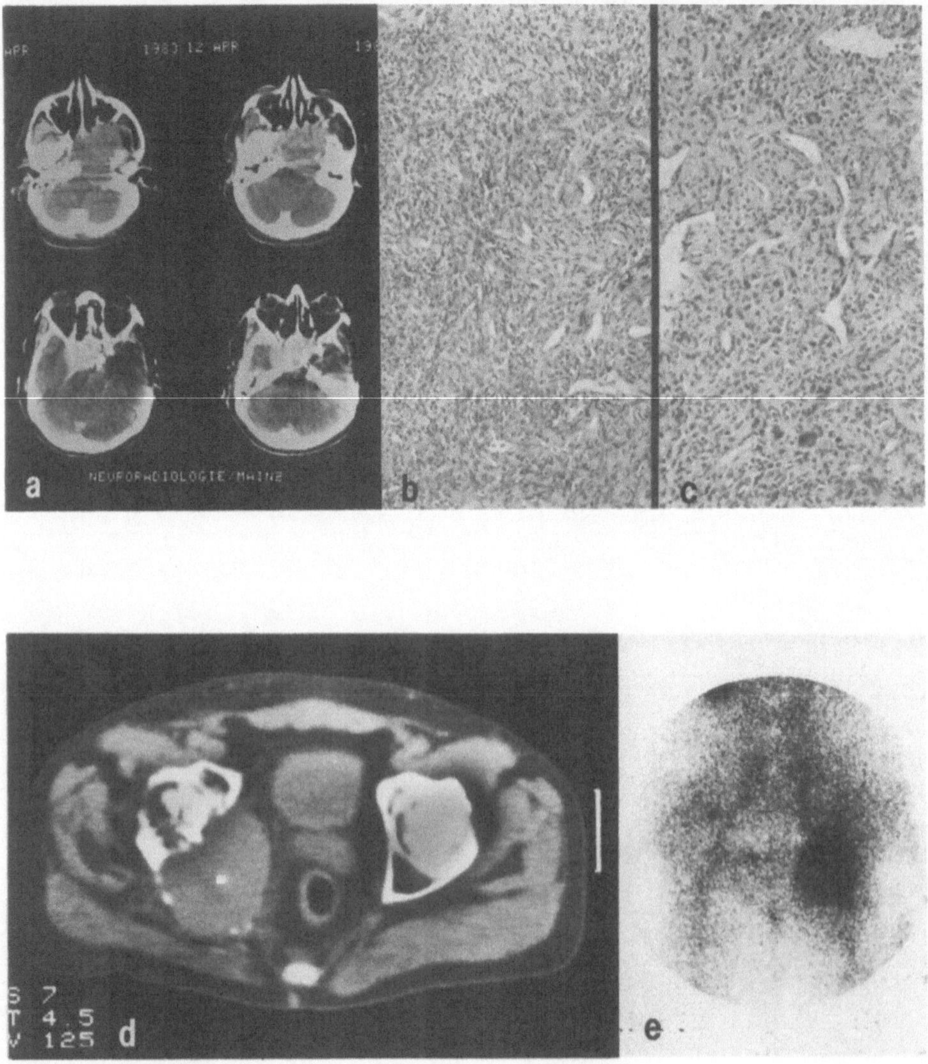

FIGURE 2 a-e.
a) Recurrent meningioma around the sella turcica diagnosed 5 years after the first operation.
b) Histological architecture of the primary tumour (x 150), identical to c) that of the bone biopsy;
d-e) Lytic metastases in the ischium and right hip joint.

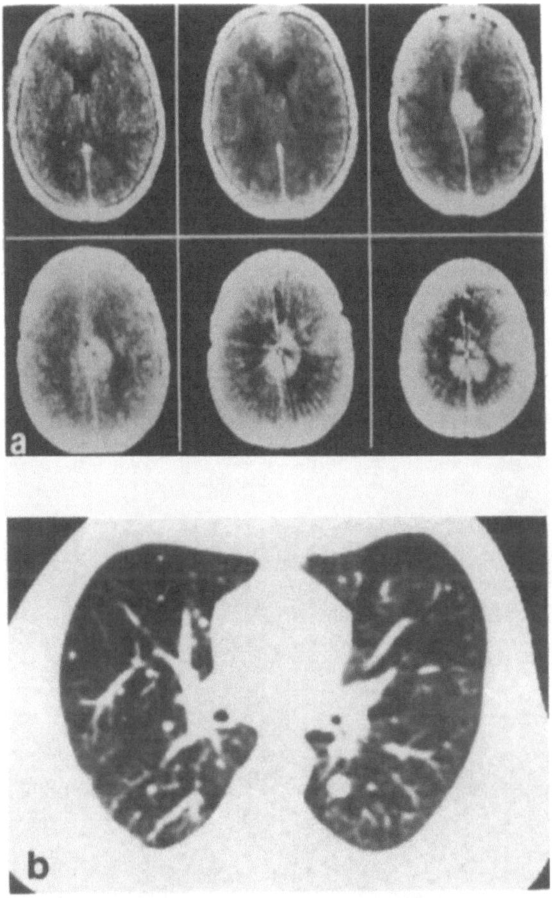

FIGURE 3 a-b.
a) 3 well defined tumours revealed by the scanner: recurrence in the falx, fronto-basal meningioma and tumour in the right convexity.
b) Pulmonary metastases, 5 years after the first operation.

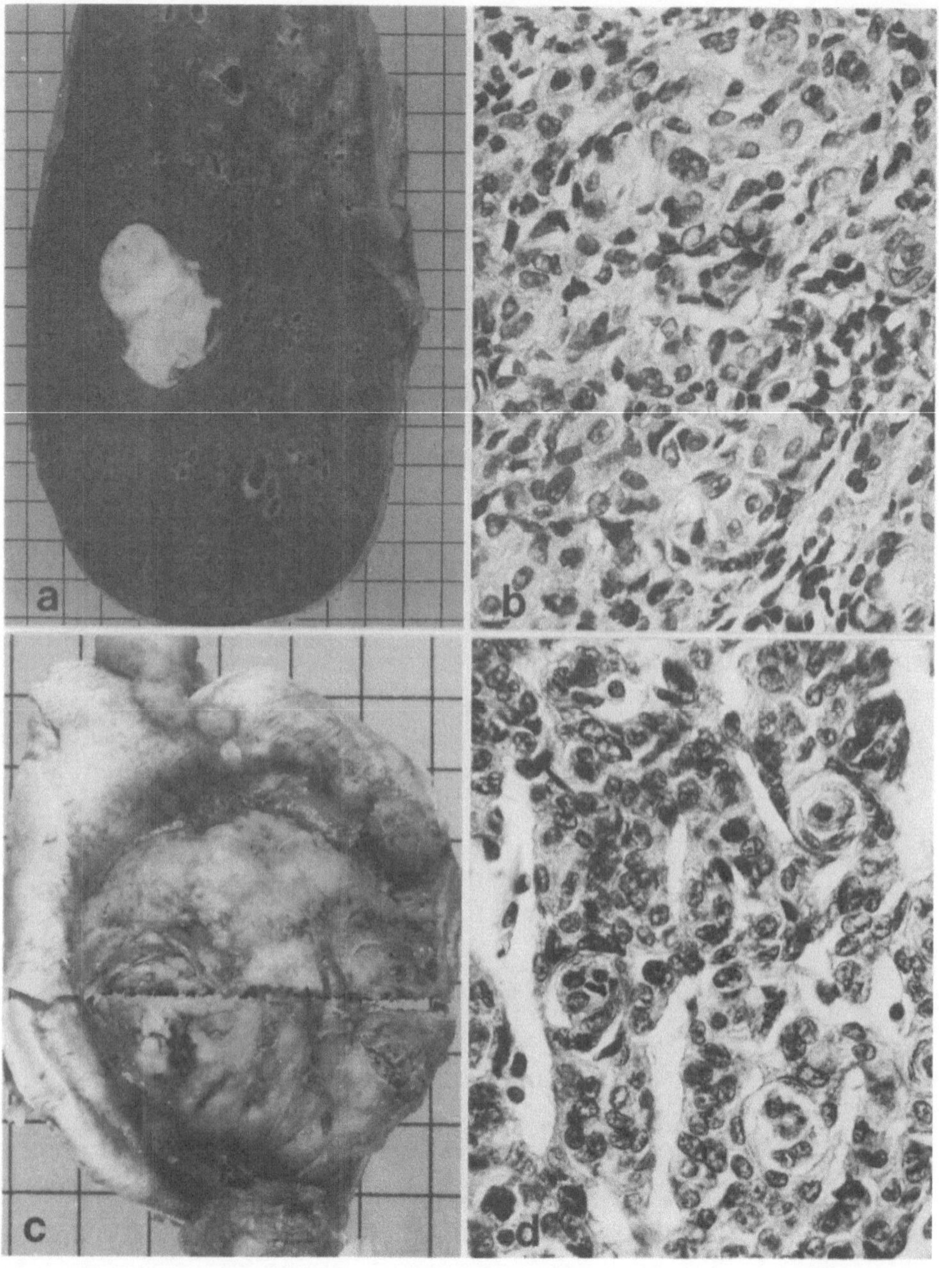

FIGURE 4 a-d.
a) At autopsy, a large pulmonary metastasis.
b) Histological appearance of this metastasis (x 550).
c) Recurrent meningioma in the falx.
d) Histological architecture of the tumour, removed 5 years previously (x 550).

Intracranial Soft Meningiomas:

Diagnostic and Therapeutic Study about 33 Cases

L. VILLETTE (°), I. KRIVOSIC (°°), F. LESOIN (°), A. AUTRICQUE (°), J. CLARISSE (°°°), J.L. CHRISTIAENS (°), M. JOMIN (°).

INTRODUCTION

Among intracranial tumors, meningiomas are the most frequent (10 to 14% of them according to studies).

They usually appear as an extracerebral compact and firm mass repulsing the cortex and highly adhering to dura.

Nevertheless some meningiomas as well as necrotic meningiomas have a very soft consistence, which allows an easy aspiration during their ablation.

Their appearance is similar to fruit jelly or caviar. Their colouris greyish or rosy, sometimes redish when the tumor is haemorrhagic. Their limits are represented by a thin or invisible capsula. Connections with brain are tight: it is a subarachnoid meningioma often inserted in cortex. Moreover the adherence to dura is more important than with usual meningiomas.

MATERIALS AND METHODS

For 24 years, between 1961 and 1985, 33 soft meningiomas have been observed in Lille University Hospital Neurosurgery Department. The patients were 15 males and 18 females; their age varied between 26 and 72 years.

Topography was as follows:
- convexity : 13
- parasagital : 10
- sphenoidal : 6
- intraventricular : 2
- parasellar : 1
- posterior fossa : 1

The lapse of time between the first clinical signs and hospitalization is lower than one year in 25 cases and lower than 6 months in 11 cases. In 4 cases, immediate hospitalization was necessary. The first symptoms are characterized by their sudden occurrence.

In most cases, symptoms are easy to detect, thanks to cerebral signs of irritation or deficit.

Cephalalgias are rare and reveal the occurence of intracranial hypertension.

10 patients exhibited psychological deterioration and 8 suffered from visual deterioration.

DIAGNOSIS

Before intervention diagnosis was usually that of meningioma without any possibility to specify its consistence.

Indeed E.E.G. and radiology are not able to detect features proper to soft meningioma. It seems illusory to expect radiology to be able to precise consistence.

(°) Neurosurgery, C.H.R., 59037 Lille, France, (°°) Neuropathology, C.H.R., 59037 Lille, France, (°°°) Neuroradiology, C.H.R., 59037 Lille, France.

M. Chatel, F. Darcel and J. Pecker (eds.), Brain Oncology. ISBN-13: 978-94-010-8003-3

However, some arteriographic and CT scanographic data can help to put forward a diagnosis of soft meningioma.

In 12 cases, arteriography revealed the same group of signs in favour of soft meningioma:

— Tumoral vascularization by vessels originating from internal carotid artery.
— Vague neovascularization of the circumference of the meningioma whose limits were not well defined.
— Presence of a more or less important net of tumoral veinlets, not early opacified, giving an hairy picture.

It is more interesting to consider the scanographic signs in relation with the diagnosis of consistence.

In 8 cases out of the 10, who beneficited by CT scan, we found:

— a tumor strictly rounded of average and homogeneous density, easily and highly opacified after contrast injection;
— presence of edema around the tumor;
— absence of calcification.

PATHOLOGY

The meningioma considered as soft by surgeons cannot be identified with the « wet meningioma » whose histopathologic form was described by Pierre Masson.

P. Masson's classification is founded upon the similarity between the histologic aspect of arachnoid and the histopathologic aspect of the meningioma.

It distinguishes arachnoidian meningioma and sub-arachnoidian meningioma. The latter may have a dry or wet appearence. The soft consistence made one think that the soft meningioma was a wet meningioma of Masson's classification; in fact, Masson's « wet meningioma » can be very hard; therefore a soft consistence observed during operation was not in favour of wet meningioma as defined in Masson's classification.

In our study, the encountered histologic form was arachnoidian meningioma. No wet meningioma of Masson's classification was found. W.H.O. classification is based upon the cellular aspect without any comparison with arachnoidian histology. This classification, that we usually employ, counts grades of malignancy. In our study, the encountered grades were 5 times grade I, 25 times grade II and 3 times grade III or IV.

The microscopic structure is characterized by the absence or the rareness of collagen, which explains the soft consistence of the tumor.

The aspect may sometimes make one think of an epithelioma metastasis or a glioma.

TREATMENT

In opposition to classical meningioma which are firm, limited by a capsula, out of the cortex and highly vascularized, soft meningiomas are tumors with a gelatinous consistence, with no capsula, situated under arachnoid, and poorly vascularised.

The surgical technique for the ablation of such tumors involves some particularities: incision is not very haemorragic. Usually there is no invasion of bones or dura-mater. The tumor can be removed by aspiration, without important bleeding. This seeming easiness can be opposed to the difficulty of performing cleavage from the cortex. Thus, it may lead to an incomplete albation or to an adjacent decortication. Therefore a post-operative infarction as well as an edema may occur and so one must be very cautious with the surveillance and the therapy following the intervention (anticonvulsants and anti-edema agents).

Prognosis depends upon localization and grading of the tumor and also upon surgical treatment.

Radiotherapy is necessary when grade is high (III or IV), since the risk of recurrence is very important.

CONCLUSION

Soft meningiomas form a particular macroscopic entity whose peroperative diagnosis remains difficult.

Correlation between radiology and pathology must be cautious and does not allow to define its consistence.

Soft meningiomas are young tumors, whose complete and radical treatment requires some precise rules.

SUMMARY

For 24 years, between 1961 and 1985, 33 soft meningiomas have been observed in Lille University Hospital Neurosurgery Department. They are a particular type of meningioma whose consistence allows aspiration during surgical ablation.

Anatomically, they are in connection with arachnoid. Most often they belong to grade II; their evolution potential is important and their growing is rapid.

Diagnosis made before intervention was that of meningioma without any certitude concerning their soft consistence. Indeed there is no specific, electric, radiologic, arteriographic, scanographic signs of this type of meningioma.

Therapy is based on surgery. It is made easier, thanks to the soft consistence of the tumor which allows aspiration. However, cleavage from the cortex is more difficult to perform than with usual meningioma.

Radiotherapy is necessary when grade is high (III or IV) since the risk or recurrence is very important.

KEY WORDS

Intracranial tumors, Soft meningiomas, Surgical treatment.

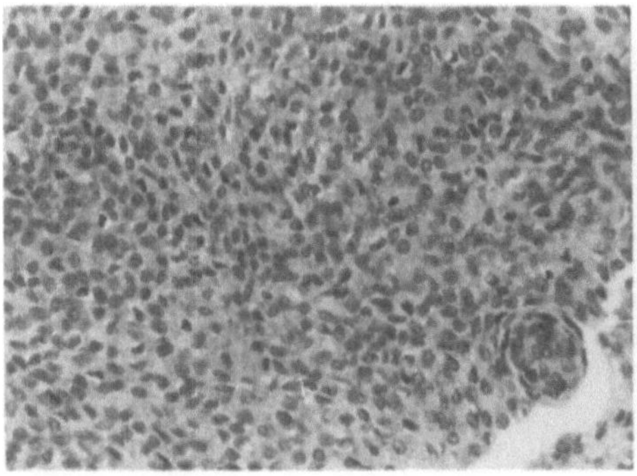

FIGURE 1A. Soft surgeon's meningioma is histologically highly cellular meningothelial type, devoid of fibrosclerosis and calcospherites.

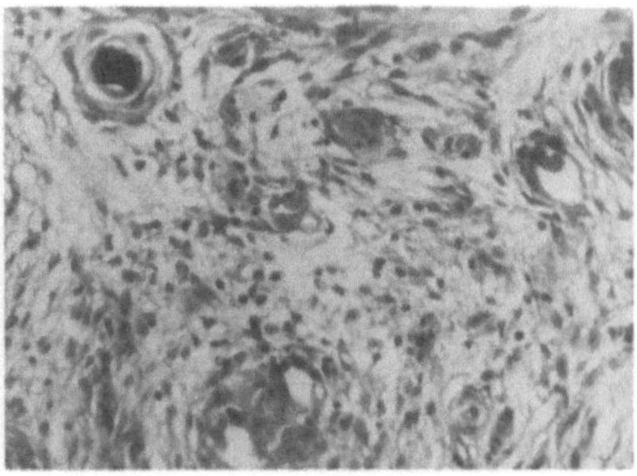

FIGURE 1B. Wet Masson's meningioma has a very loose cellulary, but interstitial « humide » tissue can be fibrosclerous and hard.

Brain Metastases Revealing Lung Cancer.

The Effect of Combined Surgery on Quality and Duration of Survival

F. DUBOIS (°), J.J. LAFITTE (°°), M. ROUSSEAUX (°), F. LESOIN (°°°), F.R. PRUVOT (°°°°).

INTRODUCTION

The initial presentation of a lung cancer by brain metastases is frequent. A single brain metastasis from lung cancer may represent the sole site of metastases (1). Without any treatment, survival is about 4 weeks. Historically, median survival time after brain surgery (2-4), or after whole-brain irradiation (5-7) has ranged between 4 to 6 months. The majority of published studies relevant to this entity, only considers the management of the brain lesion, but does'nt discuss the management of the primary lung tumor, when brain metastasis reveals lung cancer. In this particular situation, the patients who benefitted from bifocal surgery are rare (8-16); so it is rather difficult to evaluate the results of this combined surgical approach, with regard to both the quality and duration of survival. This paper reviews the results of a series of 23 patients with brain metastases revealing a lung cancer, who underwent combined surgical excision of the brain tumor, then of the primary lung lesion.

MATERIALS AND METHODS

Patients and investigations

From 1964 through 1985, 23 consecutive patients who underwent both craniotomy then thoracotomy for brain metastases revealing a lung cancer, were reviewed. There were 20 men and 3 women ranging in age from 41 to 66 years, with a mean age of 52 years. The presenting neurological symptoms were reported in Table I. The pre-treatment functionnal status was graded according to the classification proposed by Winston (4). Two patients were in functional Class I, 7 in Class II, 10 in Class III and 4 in Class IV (Table II).

Neuroradiological investigations demonstrated a single brain lesion in all the patients but 1 (2 lesions in case n° 9). Cerebral angiography was performed in 20 cases, brain scan in 10, and computed tomographic scan in the last 11 patients. The location of the cerebral metastases was sustentorial in 19 patients, and cerebellar in 4 (Table II).

None of the patients had pulmonary symptoms, and the primary lung lesion was demonstrated by chest X-ray films in the 23 cases. Staging of the lung cancer was performed after the pulmonary resection according to the TNM system (17) (Table II)

No other systemic metastases were found on skeletal survey or on liver and spleen scans.

TABLE I
PRE AND POSTOPERATIVE NEUROLOGICAL SYMPTOMS

Preoperative	N° of cases	Postoperative		
		complete regression	improved	stable
Seizures	7	6	1	—
Loss of consciousness	4	4	—	—
Intracranial hypertension	10	10	—	—
Motor deficit	12	7	5	—
Sensitive deficit	6	5	1	—
Aphasia	6	4	2	—
Frontal syndrome	7	5	2	—
Homonymous hemianopsia	5	—	—	5
Cerebellar syndrome	4	1	2	1

(°) Department of Neurology, (°°) Pneumology, (°°°) Neurosurgery and (°°°°) Thoracic Surgery, C.H.U. Lille 59037 France.

M. Chatel, F. Darcel and J. Pecker (eds.), Brain Oncology. ISBN-13: 978-94-010-8003-3

TABLE II
PREOPERATIVE FUNCTIONAL STATUS, SURGICAL TREATMENT, STAGING AND PATHOLOGICAL FINDINGS

Case N°	Age (y)	Preoperative functionnal status *	Site of brain lesion	Thoracic lesion			Histology
				intervention	T	N	
1	53	III	F l	BL	T3-1	NO	Sq
2	47	IV	C l	L	T2-1	NO	Und
3	47	III	FP r	L	T2-1	NO	Ad
4	41	II	P r	L	T2-1	NO	Ad
5	50	III	F l	P	T2-2	NO	Sq
6	45	II	P l	L	T2-1	NO	Sq
7	59	IV	O l	L	T1	N1	Sq
8	59	II	P r	BL	T1	N2	Ad
9	50	III	F l	L	T1	N2	Sq
			O r				
10	64	I	O l	L	T2-1	N1	Und
11	49	II	FP r	P	T2-2	N2	Und
12	51	III	FP r	P	T1	N2	Und
13	61	II	P l	L	T1	N2	Sq
14	43	III	F l	P	T2-3	N2	Sq
15	46	I	FP r	L	T2-3	N2	Sq
16	57	II	C l	L	T2-1	NO	Sq
17	48	II	P l	L	T1	NO	Ad
18	66	II	PO r	L	T3-1	N2	Ad
19	48	I	P l	L	T2-1	N2	Sq
20	50	III	P r	L	T2-2	NO	Sq
21	47	III	C r	L	T2	NO	Sq
22	61	IV	C l	L	T2	N2	Sq
23	53	II	PO r	BL	T2	N2	Sq

* Functional status: I: normal, II: impaired, but able to do the activities of daily living III: impaired, unable to do the activities of daily living, IV: moribund.
Sq = squamous cell ; Ad = adenocarcinoma ; Und = undifferentiated ; L = lobectomy ; BL = bilobectomy ; P = pneumonectomy ; F = frontal, P = parietal, O = occipital ; C = cerebellar, T = tumor, N = node.

Treatment

Gross total excision of the single brain metastasis, and in one case (case n° 9) of two metastases (with an interval of 6 days between the two resections), was followed by excision of the primary lung tumor 18 to 131 days later, with a mean of 43 days. The types of pulmonary resection were pneumonectomy in 4 patients, bilobectomy in 3 and lobectomy in 16 (Table II). In 14 patients histologic studies revealed squamous cell carcinoma, 5 had adenocarcinoma and 4 had undifferentiate carcinoma (Table II).

Postoperatively, 11 patients received chemotherapy, and all the patients treated after 1980 (cases 14-22) received adjuvant whole-brain radiation therapy after surgical resection (60 Gy). Patients with involvement of mediastinal lymph nodes at thoracotomy, were treated by postoperative external radiation therapy to the mediastinum (cases 13, 14, 15, 18, 22).

RESULTS

Short-Term Results

Table I shows the evolution of neurological symptoms after craniotomy. The functionnal status as assessed by the classification of Winston (4) improved in 18 patients (78 %), remained stable in 2 (one Class I, one Class II) and worsened in 1 patient who developed moderate hemiparesis after craniotomy. Two patients (cases 1 and 23) died after thoracotomy, one due to pulmonary embolus, and the other to sepsis, giving a mortality of 8,7 %. After the two operations, 9 patients were in functionnal Class I and 12 in Class II.

Long-Term Results

Survival data, after craniotomy, were calculating using the life-table method. Survival was 87 % at 3 months, 78 % at 6 months, 60 % at 9 months, 39 % at 12 months, 26 % at 18 months. Median survival was 11 months. Three patients were alive at 2 years.

In order to test the quality of survival, the duration of improvement was correlated with longevity. The duration of improvement was evaluated from the time of craniotomy until time of onset of clinical symptoms of brain or thoracic recurrence or systemic dissemination. Then, using actuarial methods, a ratio of duration of improvement to duration of survival was calculated, which determined a palliative index: 89 % of patients surviving at 3 months maintained functional improvement, 67 % at 9 months, 56 % at 18 months.

Recurrent brain metastases occured in 13 patients with 10 at the site of the original brain metastases. 5 of them were treated by a second craniotomy. 4 recurrent lung cancer were observed and 7 diffuse metastases.

DISCUSSION

The data presented here indicated the benefits both in duration and quality of survival of combined surgery in selected patients with single and solitary brain metastases revealing a lung cancer, when both the tumors were surgically accessible.

Metastases from bronchial carcinoma carry a poor prognosis and these patients are usually considered inoperable. However, solitary and single brain metastases from lung cancer are not rare. Single brain metastases are observed in about one third of the cases in large autopsy series (1, 7); solitary brain metastases — without extracranial metastases — are observed in 25 % of the cases; single and solitary brain metastases are observed in 14 % of the cases (1). Several cases of prolonged survival over 18 months, and even possibility of cure with patients alive after 10 years, had been reported after bifocal surgical excision of both the primary and secondary tumors. Table III summarized reported cases from the literature of patients with synchronous presentation of lung carcinoma and metastases to the brain who underwent craniotomy followed by thoracotomy. In our series of 23 cases presented here, the quarter of the patients was alive at 18 months.

Surgical removal of brain metastases rapidly improved neurologicfunction in 78 % of the patients of our series. The 8,7 % 30-day mortality after thoracotomy was that observed in big series of operated lung cancer (18). After the two operations all the surviving patients (91,3 %) were ambulatory and able to carry out activities of daily living. Functional improvement remained until death in at least one half of the patients.

The cause of death was diffuse extracranial metastases in one-third of the patients of our series, and local brain recurrence in two-third of the cases. This rate of neurologically related deaths incited us to complete surgical treatment with adjuvant whole-brain radiation therapy for the last nine patients of our series. However, if Patchell (19) had shown that surgery plus postoperative radiation therapy was superior to radiation therapy alone in the treatment of single brain metastasis from non small cell lung cancer — due to lower recurrence of brain metastases — there is a lack of controlled trials comparing surgery alone versus surgery plus postoperative radiation therapy.

Local control of the bronchial primary carcinoma had been achieved by thoracotomy and maintained until death in 17 patients (74 %). Postoperative radiation therapy to the mediastinum seems to us justified when the mediastinal lymph nodes are involved (20). Sundaresan had demonstrated that agressive surgical treatment of the primary lung tumor was a significant prognostic factor associated with a longer survival time (13). Median survival time was 19 months in a series of 8 patients with synchronous onset of single brain metastasis treated by surgery plus radiation, and lung cancer treated by curative resection. It was 2,5 months in 7 patients who had no resection of the primary tumor (13).

TABLE III
SERIES FROM THE LITERATURE OF PATIENTS WITH BRAIN METASTASES REVEALING LUNG CANCER, TREATED BY BIFOCAL SURGERY

		N° of patients *	Adjuvant Whole-brain RT	Survival **
Flavell	1949	1	+	a 18 months
Mosberg	1976	1	—	a 12 years
Magilligan	1976	4	—	MS 9 months
Salerno	1978	4°	+	d 3 years
				a 10 years
				a 15 years
				a 16 years
Lafitte	1982	17	4/17	MS 10 months
Sundaresan	1983	14	?	MS 8,5 months
		with 8°°	+	MS 19 months
Borelly	1985	4	2/4	MS 4 months
Mussi	1985	10	—	MS 17 months
Dubois	1986	23	9/23	MS 11 months

* Only cases of synchronous onset of brain metastases and lung cancer are reported. ** From time of craniotomy.

a alive
d dead
MS median survival time

° 4 patients/8 with specified adjuvant treatment and survival. °° patients treated in the same center.

A second favorable prognosis factor for the patients who present a single brain metastasis from lung cancer is the absence of systemic disease at time of craniotomy. Recent developments in the field of computerized tomography and echography are helpfull in selecting patients with single and solitary brain metastasis. Echography can identify asymptomatic liver or spleen metastases. CT scanning had increased the diagnostic accuracy of brain metastases: their single or multiple character, their site, and so their possibility to be surgically removed. Only the last 11 patients of our series, treated after 1978, were explored by CT scanning. Improved survival data of patients treated after 1978 (13, 16) illustrates the interest of CT scanning and echography in better selection of patients with the more favorable prognostic factors, to whom bifocal combined excision can reasonnably be proposed.

SUMMARY

From 1964 to 1985, 23 patients with solitary brain metastases as initial presentation of a lung cancer, had both the primary and secondary tumors surgically removed. The interval from craniotomy to thoracotomy ranged from 18 to 131 days, with a mean of 43 days. Results are evaluated with regard to both the quality and duration of survival: the 30-day mortality was 8,7%. Median survival was 11 months. Survival was 26% at 18 months, and 3 patients were alive 2 years after brain surgery. Clinical improvement was achieved in 78% of the patients after craniotomy. After intracranial and thoracic surgery, 21 patients were ambulatory and able to carry out activities of daily living. 50% of this group remained improved all along the duration of survival. Recurrent brain metastases was the cause of death in 2/3 of the patients. So adjuvant whole-brain irradiation seems logic to improve the results. The data of this study indicate that combined surgical treatment in selected cases of primary lung cancer with a solitary and single brain metastases, may indeed improve quality and duration of survival.

KEY WORDS

Metastases, Brain Tumours, Surgery.

REFERENCES

1. GALLUZZI (S.), PAYNE (P.M.): Brain metastases from primary bronchial carcinoma: a stastistical study of 741 necropsis. Br. J. Cancer, **9**: 511-516 (1955).
2. MAC GEE (E.F.): Surgical treatment of cerebral metastases from lung cancer: the effect on quality and duration of survival. J. Neurosurg., **35**: 416-420 (1971).
3. CONSTANS (J.P.), ROUJEAN (J.): Les métastases cérébrales en carcinologie. Neurochirurgie, **20**, suppl. 2, 20-58 (1974).
4. WINSTON (K.R.), WALSH (J.W.), FISCHER (E.G.): Results of operative treatment of intracranial metastatic tumors. Cancer, **45**: 2639-2645 (1980).
5. ORDER (S.E.), HELLMAN (S.), VON ESSEN (C.F.), KLIGERMAN (M.M.): Improvement in quality of survival following whole-brain irradiation for brain metastases. Radiology, **91**: 149-153 (1968).
6. DEELEY (J.J.), EDWARDS (J.M.R.): Radiotherapy in the management of cerebral secondaries from bronchial carcinoma. Lancet, **1**: 1209-1213 (1968).
7. NEWMAN (S.J.), HANSEN (H.H.): Frequency, diagnosis and treatment of brain metastasis in 247 consecutive patients with bronchogenic carcinoma. Cancer, **33**: 492-496 (1974).
8. FLAVELL (G.): Solitary cerebral metastases from primary bronchial carcinoma. Their incidence of cases of successful removal. Br. Med. J., **2**: 736-737 (1949).
9. MOSBERG (W.H.): Twelve year « cure » of lung cancer with metastasis to the brain. JAMA, **235**: 2745-2746 (1976).
10. MAGILLIGAN (D.J.), ROGERS (J.S.), KNIGHTON (R.S.), DAVILA (J.C.): Pulmonary neoplasm with solitary cerebral metastasis. Results of combined excision. J. Thorac. Cardiovasc. Surg, **72**: 690-698 (1976).
11. SALERNO (T.A.), MUNRO (D.D.), LITTLE (J.R.): Surgical treatment of bronchogenic carcinoma with a brain metastasis. J. Neurosurg., **48**: 350-354 (1978).
12. LAFITTE (J.J.) ROUSSEAUX (M.), DUVAL (G.), COMBELLES (G.), LAINE (E.), RIBET (M.), VOISIN (C.), WAROT (P.): Cancer bronchique révélé par métastase cérébrale. Intérêt des exérèses bifocales. Nouv. Presse Med., **11**: 1927-1930 (1982).
13. SUNDARESAN (N.), GALICICH (J.H.), BEATTIE (E.J.): Surgical treatment of brain metastases from lung cancer. J. Neurosurg., **58**: 666-671 (1983).
14. DEVIRI (E.), SCHACHNER (A.), HALERY (A.), SHALIT (M.), LEVY (M.J.): Carcinoma of the lung with a solitary cerebral metastases: surgical management and review of the literature. Cancer, **52**: 1507-1509 (1983).
15. BORRELLY (J.), GROSDIDIER (G.), WACK (B.), MENU (N.), POUSSOT (D.): La chirurgie du cancer bronchique chez les opérés de métastases cérébrales. Med. et Hyg., **43**: 3690-3694 (1985).
16. MUSSI (A.), JANNI (A.), PISTOLESI (M.), RAVELLI (V.), BUONAGUIDI (R.), ANGELETTI (C.A.): Surgical treatment of primary lung cancer and solitary brain metastasis. Thorax, **40**: 191-193 (1985).
17. Codification TNM et cancers broncho-pulmonaires. Rev. Fr. Mal. Resp., **3**: 59-64 (1975).
18. RIBET (M.), VOISIN (C.), LE BERRE (M.), SERGENT (Y.H.), LUGEZ (B.): Le pronostic des cancers bronchiques opérés. Chirurgie, **103**: 199-290 (1977).
19. PATCHELL (R.A.), CIRRINCIONE (C.), THALER (H.T.), GALICICH (J.H.), KIM (J.H.), POSNER (J.B.): Single brain metastases: Surgery plus radiation or radiation alone. Neurology, **36**: 447-453 (1986).
20. MARTINI (N.), FLEHINGER (B.J.), ZAMAN (M.B.): Prospective study of 445 lung carcinomas with mediastinal lymph node metastases J. Thorac. Cardiovasc. Surg., **80**: 390-399 (1980).

PART VI:
NEUROSURGICAL PROCEDURES AND RADIOTHERAPY TRENDS

Therapeutic Modalities in Low-Grade Brain Gliomas

Experience of Neurosurgery Department Sainte-Anne Hospital (J.P. Chodkiewicz, Pr.) (°), Gustave Roussy Institute (*), Tenon Hospital (x).

J.P. CONSTANS (°), A. CASTRESANA (°), C. DAUMAS-DUPORT (°), Ch. HAIE (*), O. MISSIR (°), C. MUNARI (°), A. MUSOLINO (°), M. SCHLIENGER (x), C. VEDRENNE (°).

INTRODUCTION

This retrospective review covers a period during which diagnostic and therapeutic conceptions in cerebral gliomas have made great progress. The development of stereotactic technics and the introduction of computed tomography have permitted a more sophisticated knowledge of the anatomy, the histology and the spatial configuration of these tumors.

METHODS AND MATERIALS

The study is limited to patients seen between 1970 and 1980. It was stopped in 1980 in order to ensure a follow-up period of adequate length.

We have selected 105 cases according to the criterias of degree of malignancy (table 1) after a strict, homogenous and systematic anatomopathological review.

TABLE 1: Low-Grade Gliomas

105	83 Adults		22 Children	
	35 Women	48 Men	10 Girls	12 Boys
%	42.16 %	57.8 %	45.45 %	54.5 %
Mean age	36.5 years	37.8 years	12.6 years	12.9 years

The diagnosis was made from simple biopsy or from serial stereotactic biopsy or from surgical sample (table 2).

TABLE 2: Diagnosis

Serial stereotactic biopsy	82
Simple biopsy	6
Piece surgical	17

The biopsy specimens were studied by neuropathologists in order to determine the histogenic type, the cellular type and the grading of the tumors.

Four criteria were taken into account to define the level of malignancy: nuclear abnormalities, mitosis, necrosis and capillary endothelial proliferation.

Degree A gliomas (Grade I of Kernohan) have none of these parameters. Degree B gliomas (Grade II of Kernohan) have only one of these parameters. The presence of two or more than two parameters characterize the high degree gliomas.

The interest of this group is its histopathological homogeneity. The histogenic types are distributed in: astrocytomas, oligodendrogliomas and mixed oligo-astrocytomas (table 3).

TABLE 3: Histogenic Types

Astrocytoma	82	78.09 %
Oligodendroglioma	7	21.90 %
Mixed oligo-astrocytoma	16	
Pilocytic A.	15	(18.3 %)
Subependymal Giant Cellular A.	3	(3.6 %)
Fibrillary A.	14	(17.07 %)
Protoplasmic A.	7	(8.5 %)
Gemistocytic A.	4	(4.8 %)
Polymorphous A.	39	(47.5 %)
Recklinghausen Disease	3 Pilocytic A. 1 Fibrillary A. 1 Polymorphous A.	
Bourneville disease	1 Subependymal A.	

COMMENTS

The introduction of new techniques, like C.T. Scan renovated the approach to cerebral tumors. The spatial development can be evaluated « in vivo » with the help of C.T. Scan and stereotaxic biopsy exploration.

M. Chatel, F. Darcel and J. Pecker (eds.), Brain Oncology. ISBN-13: 978-94-010-8003-3

Tumor exploration is realized by stereotactic biopsy. Our neuropathologists try to codify the histological information in order to express both histological type and malignancy with the spatial configuration of the tumor (Dr. C. DAUMAS-DUPORT, Laboratory of Pr. C. VEDRENNE). The study of the behaviour of the gliomas within the normal cerebral tissue, shows three distinct types: type I consists of organized tumoral tissue only, Type II consists of tumoral tissue and infiltration of peripheral areas, and Type III consists of isolated tumoral cells. Thirty-three tumors have been explored by stereotactic methods between 1975 and 1979 and 29 in 1979 (with improved techniques of sampling and fixation). The study of the two groups show a prevalence of the A I Type and B II Type; or tumors of degree I (well limited, and of degree II (with peripheral infiltration) (Table 5).

TABLE 5: Spatial Configuration

62 Gliomas	Type I	Type II	Type III	
A	18	1	2	21
B	4	31	6	41

A I = 28.98 %	B I = 6.44 %
A II = 1.61 %	B II = 50 %
A III = 3.22 %	B III = 9.66 %

TABLE 6: Localization

Cerebral Lobes		
Frontal	24	48
Fronto-Basal	1	
Fronto-Parietal	5	
Fronto-Parieto-Temporal	3	
Fronto-Temporal	6	
Fronto-Rolandic	9	
Temporal	9	10
Temporo-Occipital	1	
Parietal	9	17
Parieto-Rolandic	3	
Parieto-Temporal	1	
Parieto-Temporo-Occipital	1	
Parieto-Occipital	3	
Occipital	0	0
Deep		
Lateral Ventricles	1	21
Basal Ganglia	6	
Parietal B.G.	3	
Temporal B.G.	11	
Middle		
Corpus Callosum	2	9
Septum Lucidum	1	
Third Ventricle	5	
Pineal Region	1	

TABLE 7: First Symptom

First Clinic Symptom		%
Partial Epilepsy	72	68.57
Generalized Epileptic Seizures	12	11.42
Intracranial Hypertension	14	13.33
Neurologic Deficit	3	2.85
Psychic Symptoms	2	1.90
Isolated Tremor Hand	1	0.95
Meningeal Hemorrhage	1	0.95

The **topographic site** is more frequently lobar or plurilobar with extension to basal ganglia (table 6). Midline tumors are more frequent in young patients and this represents the preferential location of pilocytic astrocytomas.

The mean age of these patients is below that of patients with higher grade tumors (table 1).

In 80 % of the cases, epilepsy is the initial and for a long time the only symptom (table 7).

TABLE 8: Delay Between First Symptom and Diagnosis

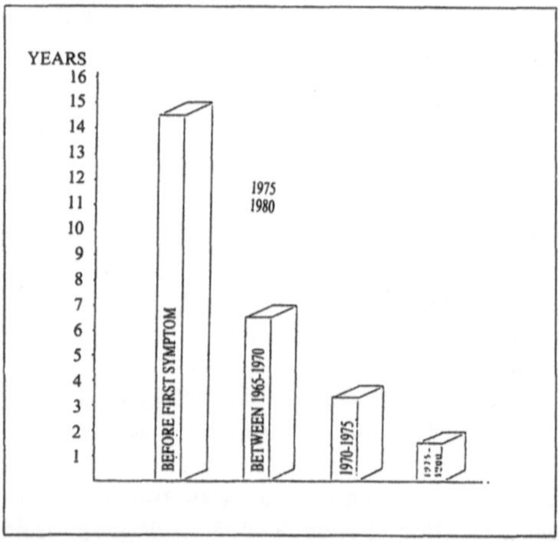

TREATMENT

Since 1975, surgery, radiotherapy or their association were the standard treatments.

The topographic mapping and the histological features (which permit an understanding of the development and the spatial configuration of the tumors in relation to surrounding areas) are the basis of a new **therapeutic approach.**

The stereotactic technique is the basis of interstitial radiotherapy (intratumoral implantation of 192 Ir.) or intra-cavitary-B-irradiation. Brachytherapy can be used alone or in association with external radiotherapy. The stereotactic study of the tumors indicate the target and its volume. The dosimetry is made by computer. The surgical treatment is furthermore directed by the stereotactic findings which specify the anatomic limits of the tumors and their connection with the functional areas.

In our groups, 40 % of the patients were treated by surgery. (table 9).

The inoperable tumors (because of their localization) were treated by radiotherapy in relation to their volume: tumors of less than 3 cm were treated by brachytherapy; between 3 and 5 cm, tumors were treated by brachytherapy and external radiotherapy; tumors of more than 5 cm diameter were treated by external radiotherapy alone.

Most patients were treated by radiotherapy after or before surgery.

TABLE 9: Treatment

Surgery	**41**
Surgery only	13
Surgery before other treatments	19
Surgery after other treatments	9
Radiotherapy	**54**
E.R.T.	19
Interstitial R.T. And/Or Endocavitary B.R.T.	16
Interstitial R.T. + E.R.T.	19
Abstention	10

External radiotherapy

Patients were treated by high energy X-rays (5.5 MV; 18 MV or 25 MV). The advantages of this type of radiation is to spare the skin (thus allowing a second surgical procedure) and to allow hair regrowth.

The irradiated volume consists of the tumoral volume plus a safety margin of 2 to 3 cm in all three dimensions. The C.T. Scan and the stereotactic morphograms help to define the tumoral volume. Dose - fields - fractionation: the standard dose is 55 Gy in 5-6 weeks and 22 sessions. The number of fields depends on the volume and the location of the tumor.

Brachytherapy: the dose administered by brachytherapy only is over 50 - 60 Gy. The I.R.T. is sometimes associated to E.R.T. on « an enveloppe » which correspond to the outer limits of the tumor. The dose is 35 Gy administered in 4 to 10 days. During this time, it is not the radiation dose that has changed but the « volume-target » has been marked out in more detail.

RESULTS

Because the different subgroups of therapeutic combinations are comprised of numerous parameters (anatomic and clinical) that submitted to a multifactor analysis with great difficulty, the evaluation of the data was not easy. Therefore, we have resigned ourselves to conveying them in the form of graphics.

In table X, we compare the survival of patients treated with surgery only (13 patients) with those treated by a combination of surgery and radiotherapy (19 patients). The curves show better results when surgery is associated with radiotherapy. 70 % of patients are still alive 5 years after surgery, and 50 % are alive 6 years after surgery.

We observed also that 50 % of the patients having had other treatment before surgery had a mean, a mean survival of 5 years.

TABLE 10: Survival time after surgery

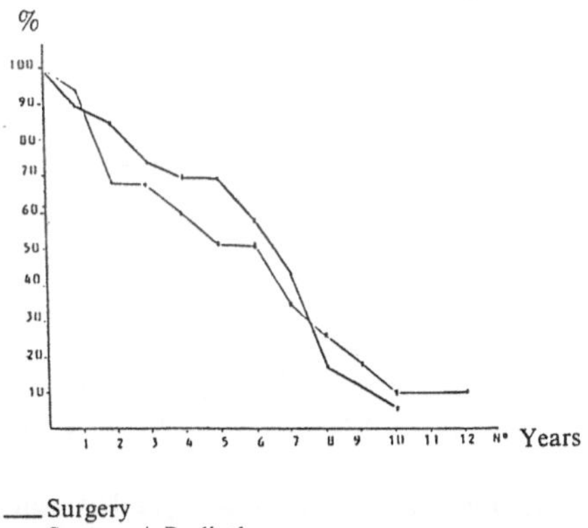

___ Surgery
___ Surgery + Radiotherapy

TABLE 11: Survival time after radiation treatment

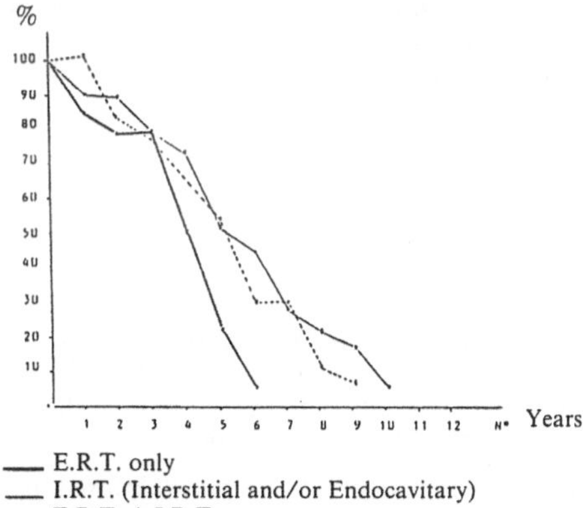

___ E.R.T. only
___ I.R.T. (Interstitial and/or Endocavitary)
\-\-\- E.R.T. + I.R.T.

The patients treated with radiotherapy can be studied in 3 groups: E.R.T. only (19 patients), interstitial radiotherapy or endocavitary-B-irradiation only (16 patients) and combined interstitial and external treatment (19 patients) (table 11).

The overall survival of patients treated for low-grade gliomas is 50 % at 5 years, 20 % at 8 years and 5 % at 10 years (table 12).

In order to gain a better understanding to the results of the different forms of treatment employed and bearing in mind the marked variations in the course of the illness before the initiation of treatment, we have tried to determine the length of survival after the first clinical manifestations in all patients regardless of the treatment (table 13).

TABLE 12: Total survival time with all therapies

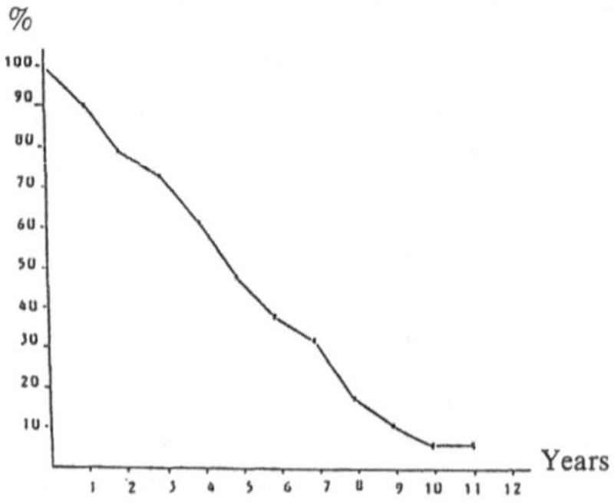

TABLE 13: Total survival time with all therapies

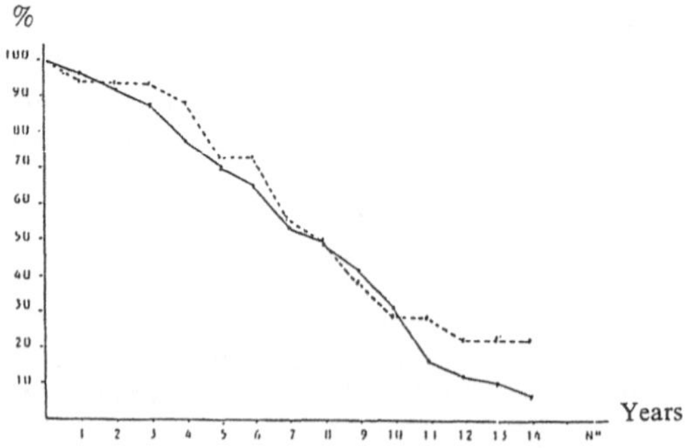

——Degree II after first symptom (66 patients)
- - - Degree I after first symptom (18 patients)

Eighteen patients with tumor of first degree and sixteen patients with tumor of second degree have a superposable survival curve; 85 % at 5 years and 28 % at 10 years. After this time the survival curve reaches a plateau for first degree gliomas.

We have not observed a difference in the group of pilocytic astrocytomas (15 cases) which are reputed to have a better prognosis.

We would have hoped to make a more systematic and exacting analysis of each therapeutic modality. The small number of cases of this series and their extreme variability dit not allow such an analysis.

It certainly is particularly useful to be able to evaluate the length of survival according to tumor position and volume and according to the age, and the general and clinical condition of the patient when the treatment is initiated.

Nevertheless another important and ever basic concept is that of the quality of survival according to the different modes of treatment employed. Thus the criteria for choosing between the various therapeutic procedures must be analysed in detail.

Finally, the place and yet uncertain role of « multifaisceaux » irradiation treatment which may prove to be a new therapeutical solution in a special category of patients, remains to be discussed.

We want to emphasize the importance of corticoid treatment in the development of the disease.

CONCLUSIONS

It seems useful to us to summarize the indications for the different forms of treatment as they evolued out of our experience, in a single table. They arise essentially from two factors the first being topographical: the site (and the volume) of the tumor, and the second histological: the grade of the glioma and its spatial configuration.

By taking these data as a basis, more rational therapeutic solutions may be worked out and we can hope for better results.

TABLE 14: Indications for treatment

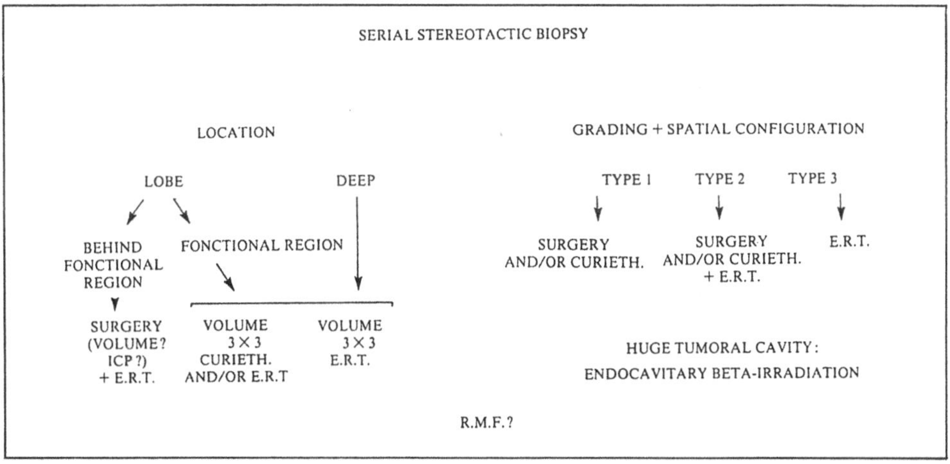

KEY WORDS

« Low-grade » glioma. « Benign » glioma. Grades I and II brain astrocytomas. Oligodendrogliomas. Treatment.

REFERENCES

1. BLOOM (H.J.G.): Intracranial tumors: response and resistance to therapeutic endeavors 1970-1980. Int. J. Radiat. Oncol. Biol. Phys., **8**: 1083-1113 (1982).
2. CONSTANS (J.-P.), SCHLIENGER (M.): Radiothérapie des tumeurs du système nerveux central de l'adulte. Neurochirurgie, **21**: (1975), Suppl. 2, Edit. Masson.
3. DAUMAS-DUPORT (C.), SZIKLA (G.): Délimitation et configuration spatiale des gliomes cérébraux. Données histologiques incidences thérapeutiques. Neurochirurgie, **27**: 273-284 (1981).
4. DAUMAS-DUPORT (C.), MEDER (J.F.), MISSIR (O.), AUBIN (M.L.), SZIKLA (G.): Les gliomes cérébraux: malignité, délimitation et configuration spatiale. Données comparatives, biopsies cérébrales étagées stéréotaxiques, tomodensitométrie (étude préliminaire à propos de 50 cas). J. Neuroradiol., **10**: 51-80 (1983).
5. FAZEKAS (J.T.): Treatment of grade I and II brain astrocytomas. The role of radiotherapy. Int. J. Radiot. Oncol. Biol. Phys., **2**: 661-666 (1977).
6. KELLY (P.J.), OLSON (M.H.), WRIGHT (A.E.): Stereotactic implantation of iridium 192 into CNS neoplasms. Surg. Neurol., **10**: 349-354 (1978).
7. LAWS (E.R.): Neurosurgical management of low grade astrocytoma of the cerebral hemisphere. J. Neurosurgery **61**: 665-673 (1984).
8. PECKER (J.), SCARABIN (J.M.), BRUCHER (J.M.), VALLEE (B.): Démarche stéréotaxique en Neurochirurgie tumorale. Edit. Laboratoires Fabre, 1979, Paris.
9. ROUGIER (A.), COHADON (F.), PIGNEUX (J.), LOISEAU (H.): La place de l'irradiation interstitielle dans le traitement des gliomes. Neurochirurgie **30**: 125-129 (1984).
10. RUBINSTEIN (L.J.): Tumors of the central nervous system in atlas of tumors pathology. Armed Forces Institute of Pathology, 1972, Washington.
11. SALAZAR (O.M.), RUBIN (P.), DONALD (J.), FELDSTEIN (M.L.): Patterns of failure in intracranial astrocytomas after irradiation: analysis of dose and field factors. Am. J. Roentgenol., **126**: 279-292 (1976).
12. SCANLON (P.W.), TAYLOR (W.F.): Radiotherapy of intracranial astrocytomas: analysis of 417 cases treated from 1960 through 1969. Neurosurgery, **5**: 301-308 (1979).
13. SZIKLA (G.): Stereotactic cerebral irradiation. Inserm Symposium N° 12. Elsevier North Holland Biomedical Press, 1979.
14. SZIKLA (G.), BLOND (S.): Bilan stéréotaxique des tumeurs cérébrales. Encycl. Med. Chir., Paris 1980, Radiognostic II/ 31660 E 10-12.
15. SZIKLA (A.), MUSOLINO (A.), MIYAHARA (S.), SCHAUB (C.), ASKIENAZY (S.): Colloidal Rhenium - 186 Endocavitary Beta Irradiation of cystic craniopharyngiomas and active glioma cysts. Long term results. Side effects and clinical dosimetry. Acta Neurochirurgica, 1984, Suppl. **33**: 331-339

Evaluation of Stereotactic Biopsy as an aid to the Management of Supratentorial Tumors:

B. IRTHUM (°), J. CHAZAL (°), M. MOHR (°°), A.M. GEORGET (°°°), P. JANNY (°).

INTRODUCTION

The purpose of this study is to evaluate the advantages brought about by the use of stereotactic biopsies in the treatment of cerebral tumors and especially to appreciate wether the precise knowledge of the nature and grading of these tumors and their exact anatomical situation really permit to define the best therapeutic indication.

This approach, first developped here at the neurosurgical clinic of Rennes by J. Pecker and coworkers, has rapidly convinced us that it was at least a good way for avoiding the poor outcome following some surgical operations.

MATERIAL AND METHODS

Material

One hundred and twenty stereotactic biopsies were performed on 115 patients between January 1982 and April 1986. All of these patients had a CT Scan demonstrating a space occupying lesion in the hemispheres or on the median line (anterior and posterior part of the third ventricle).

A cerebral angiography was performed the day before the biopsy or immediatly before it, and the cases with an abnormal circulation suggesting a malignant tumor were discarded. There were no meningioma nor pituitary adenoma in this series but there were two craniopharyngiomas the diagnosis of which was not clearly established before the biopsy.

Method

A morphogram of the tumor was achieved using a stereotactic neuro-radiological procedure including cerebral angiography, pneumo-encephalography or contrast ventriculography and the data of the CT scan as well.

Our equipment uses the Talairach's frame and is original because only one X ray tube is needed. The patient is seated in the isocentric chair of DIAGNOST N PHILIPS craniographer so that it can undergo a 90° rotation to realize anteroposterior and lateral views with the unique X ray tube. The biopsies are made with a lateral window biopsy cannula designed by Sedan; several fragments of tissue are taken on the trajectory to define the volume of the tumor and the infiltration of the surrounding tissue. Seventy seven patients had one trajectory and 43 patients had two trajectories; 3 to 8 fragments of tissue were obtained for each patient.

RESULTS

Results of the biopsies

Table I shows the results concerning the whole series: the biopsies concluded a diagnosis of certitude in 96 cases, to an undetermined diagnosis although sufficient to give a useful orientation in 8 cases and, in 16 cases it provided no diagnosis.

(°) Neurosurgical Clinic of the University Hospital of Clermont-Ferrand. Hôpital Fontmaure, avenue de Villars, F, 63400 Chamalières. (°°) Institute of Pathology, Hôpital Civil, F, 67000 Strasbourg. (°°°) Department of Neuroradiology, Hôpital Fontmaure, avenue de Villars, F, 63400 Chamalières.

M. Chatel, F. Darcel and J. Pecker (eds.), Brain Oncology. ISBN-13: 978-94-010-8003-3

Five of the diagnoses of certitude were obtained with a single puncture of the lesion (2 abscesses, 2 cystic craniopharyngiomas, one cavernous angioma). In the 91 other cases the histopathological examination provided the diagnosis. Table II shows the wide range, sometimes unexpected, of the lesions.

If we consider that the method failed in the 8 cases of undetermined diagnosis and in the 16 cases where no diagnosis was obtained, we have a total of 24 cases for which we have to search for the reasons of failure.

Table III shows that the target was missed in 12 cases; the fragment of tissue was considered abnormal but no diagnosis could be established in 4 cases; there were 4 undetermined gradings of a glioma and 4 mistakes in the true nature of a malignant tumor.

Complications

They are shown in Table IV: there were 3 deaths (2,5%), 9 persistent neurological impairments and 7 transient neurological impairments.

The origin of these 19 complications were 2 technical failures in the beginning of our practice, 2 intratumoral hematomas and 14 clinical impairments related to an increase of the midline shift without hematoma in the lesion (this mechanism occurred twelve times with malignant gliomas); there was still a case of high intracranial pressure because of acute dysfunction of a shunt. An abnormal circulation in the tumor was seen with Binswanger's about the same frequency in this group of complications (3 out of 19), as in the whole series (30 out of 120).

Accuracy of the pathological examination of stereotactic biopsies

Twenty two patients were operated on with removal of the tumor so that a complete examination of the tumor could be done and the comparison with the first diagnosis after the biopsy was possible.

But only 17 cases could be compared because the tumor was missed by the biopsy in 5 cases.

These comparisons are reported in the Table V. There was one case of discordance on the nature of the tumor: after the biopsy an astrocytoma was diagnosed and after the removal of the tumor the diagnosis was oligodendroglioma. In 3 cases, the grading of the tumor was lower in the biopsy than in the whole tumor.

The remaining 13 cases showed a good correlation on the type and grading of the lesion.

TABLE I

Result of biopsies

	Number of biopsies	Number of patients
Diagnosis of certitude	96	96*
Undetermined diagnosis	8	8
No diagnosis	16	11
TOTAL	120	115

* Five of these patients had 2 biopsies

TABLE II

Pathological results of biopsies

Low grade gliomas		17
— astrocytomas	12	
— oligodendrogliomas	5	
Malignant gliomas		54
— astrocytomas	26	
— oligodendrogliomas	10	
— glioblastomas	18	
Ependymoma (3ᵉ ventricle)		1
Metastasis		2
Malignant lymphomas		9
Germinomas		2
Colloid cyst		1
Hemispheric infarct		1
Hematoma on the way to resorb		1
Viral necrotizing encephalitis		1
Demyelinating encephalopathy		1
Possible Binswanger's encephalopathy		1
TOTAL		91

TABLE III

Analysis of failures

Tumor missed	12
Abnormal tissue, but no diagnosis	4
Undetermined grading of a glioma	4
Mistake in the true nature of a malignant tumor	4
TOTAL	24

TABLE IV

Complications

Deaths	3
Persistent neurological impairments	9
Transient neurological impairments	7
TOTAL	19

Comparison with the clinical diagnosis

We wanted to know what diagnosis would have been established with the clinical, angiographic and CT scan data for these 115 patients. These data were reviewed by two of us and their diagnoses were compared with the final diagnosis based on the clinical, radiological and pathological data. Table VI reports these comparisons and shows that the clinician's diagnosis was correct in 62 cases, but wrong in 53 cases. The diagnosis obtained after the stereotactic biopsy was wrong in 19 cases so that the biopsy corrected the clinician's diagnosis in 34 patients (27%).

TABLE V

Comparisons between pathological results of stereotactic biopsies and tumor removal samples

Discordance on the nature of a tumor	1
Undergrading of a glioma with biopsy in comparison with tumor removal	3
Good correlation on the type and grading of the lesion	13
TOTAL	17

TABLE VI

Comparison between clinician's diagnosis and stereotactic biopsy

Method	Clinician's diagnosis	Stereotactic biopsy (one or two)
Correct diagnosis	62	96
Wrong or undetermined diagnosis	53	19
Number of patients	115	115

DISCUSSION

From the stereotactic biopsy we expected a pathological diagnosis and a better definition of the tumor limits in order to improve the management of these lesions. The first aim was obtained in our opinion because a diagnosis of certitude was established in 83% of the patients.

We think in agreement with Pecker (2) that the pathological data are of most importance for choosing the treatment of pineal tumors because removal of these tumors is not necessary when they are radiosensitive.

Concerning the cortical and infracortical tumors we prefer defining the tumor limits and the pathological diagnosis before discussing the indication of resection of the tumor; finally we decided to remove the tumor only in 22 patients of this series.

We think that the stereotactic biopsy is better for the diagnosis of primary malignant lymphoma of the brain than an operation because these lesions are poorly delimited and often paraventricular.

Our complication rate is similar to the litterature data (1, 2, 3) concerning the intratumoral hematomas, but we observed some cases of impairment with malignant tumors in which occurred an accentuation of the midline shift very likely caused by increment of peritumoral oedema. We wonder about the possible pernicious effect of the sitting position in the mechanism of this oedema. The differences between pathological results obtained by stereotactic biopsy and resection of the tumor are unfrequent especially if the fragments are of good quality and numerous. Certainly an immediate examination of the fragments would have improved the efficiency of the method. The most frequent differences are an undergrading of the tumor with the biopsy. This fact already mentionned, by Pecker (2) is well explained by the frequent heterogeneity of the cerebral gliomas.

The advantages of this method is evident for two reasons; the first is that the clinician's diagnosis is a diagnosis of probability which was wrong in our practice in many cases and was corrected by the biopsy in 27% of cases; the second is difficult to quantify but as such is as important as the first reason because the detailed anatomical information about the tumor location and the knowledge of the pathological data often have convinced us to refuse the operation in order to avoid making some unacceptable sequelae in patients whose prognosis is, with present therapies, evaluated at a few months.

SUMMARY

One hundred and fifteen cases of patients with a CT Scan demonstrating a space occupying lesion of the hemispheres were reviewed in order to confront the clinical, CT Scan and angiographic data on one side and the pathologist's conclusions after stereotactic biopsy on the other side.

The latter were confronted secondly with the complete examination of the tumor in the patients who were operated on.

On the basis of these comparisons the interest of this method of biopsy as an aid for the management of these tumors is discussed.

KEY-WORDS

Brain tumors, Stereotactic biopsy.

REFERENCES

1. BENABID (A.) et Coll.: Les biopsies stéréotaxiques des néoformations intra-crâniennes. Réflexions à propos de 3 052 cas. Neurochirurgie, 31, 295-301, 1985.

2. PECKER (J.), SCARABIN (J.M.), BRUCHER (J.M.), VALLEE (B.): Démarche stéréotaxique en neurochirurgie tumorale (Editions médicales Pierre Fabre, 1979).

3. SEDAN (R.), PERAGUT (J.C.), FARNARIER (Ph.), HASSOUN (J.), TORRES (T.): Place de la biopsie en condition stéréotaxique dans la tactique thérapeutique des gliomes malins. Neurochirurgie, 27, 285-286, 1981.

Intraoperative Ultrasonography in Neurosurgery

V.A. FASANO (°), R. URCIUOLI (°), P. BOLOGNESE (°), G. BROGGI (°).

B-scan real time, Tissutal A-mode and Microvascular Doppler are utilized intraoperatively in the management of brain tumors, vascular malformations, inflammatory lesions and disturbances of liquoral circulation.

The scanhead of the B-scan real time is put on dural surface to explore the operative field in the perspective of the operator, by different scansions and frequencies (3, 5 and 7.5 MHz).

The lesion is localized; its depth, shape, extension are appreciated; the anatomical relations with the median line and with other normal surrounding structures can also be evaluated.

The lesion can be approached through the shortest way with minimal damage of surrounding tissues and radically removed by subsequent echographic controls.

Some surgical manoeuvres (tipping of small-sized ventricles, biopsies, emptying of cysts and abscesses) can be performed more exactly and safely.

The Tissutal A-mode is a technical variation of the traditional A-mode, which selectively increases scattering and diffraction phenomena produced by the interaction between the ultrasound wave and the tissutal cytoarchitecture.

This instrument identifies the pathologic inside the normal tissue, in a small area (5 mm^2) with a spatial resolution of 1 mm.

This was confirmed by histological controls.

Intraoperative Microvascular Doppler (20 MHz) explores vessel's lumen by small shiftable detection gates (0.4 and 1.4 mm ∅).

This instrument can identify the patency of the parent arteries and the definite clipping of the aneurysm.

In AVM's surgery, the nidus, the feeder arteries and their flow can be checked; the radical removal of the AVM can also be verified, by analizing the flow patterns in draining veins.

CONCLUSIONS

The Intraoperative Ultrasonography consents :

— a view of the lesion in the real perspective of the operator;

— to choose the shortest way to approach the lesion;

— to perform a radical removal by means of subsequent echographic controls.

KEY WORDS

Brain Tumours, Surgery, Ultrasonography.

(°) Istituto di Neurochirurgia, Università degli Studi di Torino, Via Cherasco, 15. 10126 Torino.

M. Chatel, F. Darcel and J. Pecker (eds.), Brain Oncology. ISBN-13: 978-94-010-8003-3

REFERENCES

1. ADVANCED INTRAOPERATIVE TECHNOLOGIES IN NEUROSURGERY, Edited by V.A. Fasano, Springer Verlag, Wien, New York, 1986.
2. CHANDLER (W.F.), KNAKE (J.E.), McGILLICUDDY (J.E.), LILLEHEI (K.O.), SILVER (T.M.), 1982: Intraoperative use of real-time ultrasonography in neurosurgery. J. Neurosurg. 57, 157-163.
3. DOHRMANN (G.J.), RUBIN (J.M.): Dynamic intraoperative imaging and instrumentation of brain and spinal cord using ultrasound. Neurol. Clin. 3, 425-437, 1985.
4. DOHRMANN (G.J.), RUBIN (J.M.): Use of ultrasound in neurosurgical operations: a preliminary report. Surg. Neurol. 16, 362-366, 1981.
5. FASANO (V.A.), URCIUOLI (R.), LOMBARD (G.F.), PONZIO (R.M.), LANOTTE (M.M.): The use of laser and CUSA in the treatment of brain stem tumors. International Symposium on Surgery in and around the brain stem and the third ventricle. Hannover, February 18-23, 1985, In press.
6. FRIEDRICH (H.), HANSEL-FRIEDRICH (G.), SEEGER (W.): Intraoperative Dopplersonographie and Hirngefäßen. Neurochirurgia 23, 89-98, 1980.
7. GILSBACH (J.M.): Intraoperative Doppler sonography in neurosurgery. Wien-New York: Springer, 1983.
8. SKALKA (H.W.), CALLAHAN (M.A.), ELSAS (F.J.): Echographic appearance of recurrent orbital retinoblastoma. J. Clin. Ultrastruct. 8, 164-166, 1980.
9. VOORHIES (R.M.), ENGEL (I.), GAMACHE (F.W.), jr., PATTERSON (R.H.), jr., FRASER (R.A.R.), LAVYNE (M.H.), SCHNEIDER (M.): Intraoperative localization of subcortical brain tumors: Further experience with B-mode real-time sector scanning. Neurosurg. 12, 189-194, 1983.

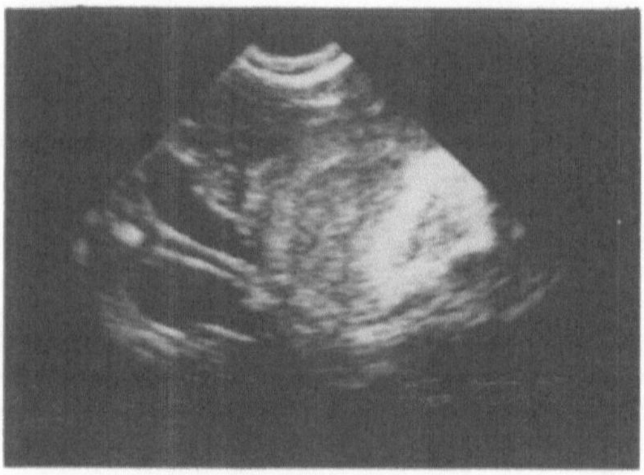

FIGURE 1.

FIGURE 1. **Anaplastic astrocytoma, right hemisphere.**
Frequency 3 MHz, Deepness 8.7 cm, Transversal scansion.
This picture shows:
— the shortest way to approach the lesion through the overlaying tissues,
— the depth of the lesion, its diameter and its shape,
— its anatomical relations with the frontal horns and the falx.

FIGURE 2. **Cerebellar metastasis.**
Frequency 7.5 MHz, Deepness 4.6 cm, Transversal scansion.
B-scan consents to identify the whole tumor: the mean cystic lesion and the smaller solid one. Thus, B-scan consents a radical removal.

FIGURE 3. **Meningioma, right fronto-basal region.**
Frequency 5 MHz, Deepness 6.6 cm, Transversal scansion.
B-scan identifies the borders of the lesion from surrounding edematous (anechogenic) or compressed tissue (slightly hyperechogenic).

FIGURE 4. **Cerebellar hemangioblastoma Tissutal A-mode.**
The instrument distinguishes:
— the normal tissue (flat portion, right side),
— the neoplastic tissue (irregular portion, left side),
— the border between the two tissues.

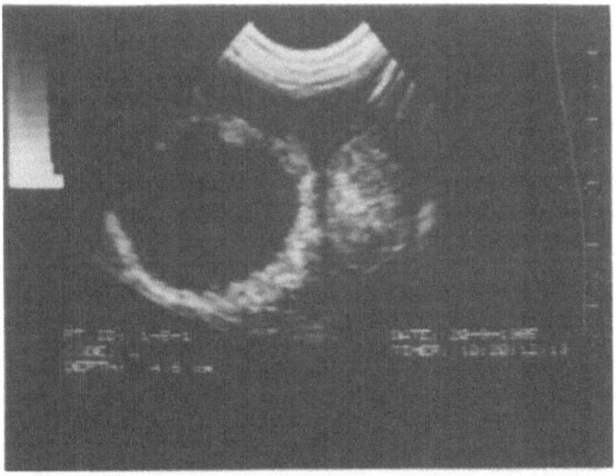

FIGURE 2.

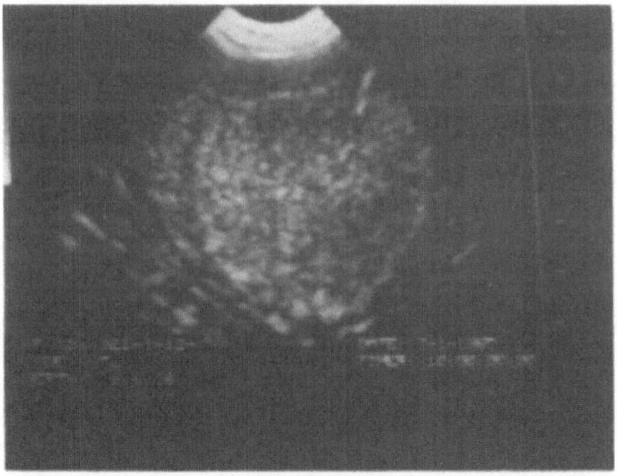

FIGURE 3.

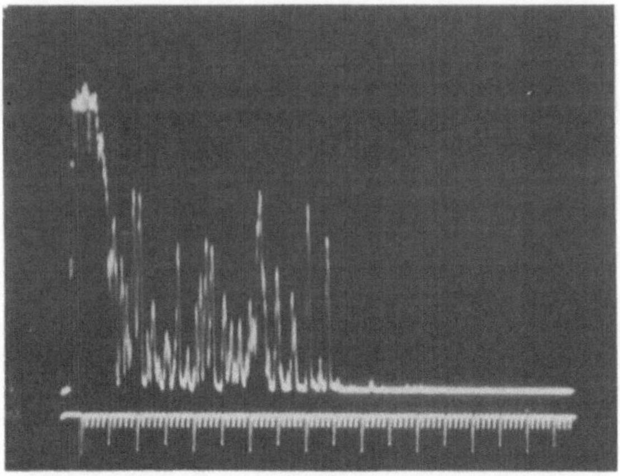

FIGURE 4.

Surgery as Definitive Salvage Therapy for Primary Brain Tumors

R.P. MOSER (°).

INTRODUCTION

The English word "salvage" comes from the Middle French "salver" (to save). In cancer therapy, it refers to the treatment of patients who have failed to respond to or relapsed following front-line therapy. Patients with glial tumors present in all age groups and are generally seen by a neurosurgeon, whose role is both diagnostic and therapeutic (resection or in-situ ablation of the tumor mass). The location of the tumor, its invasive character, and the ability of the surgeon impact on the safety and thoroughness of the operation. The prognosis depends on several factors including the age of the patient, the histology of the tumor, and the patient's performance.

The role of reoperation has been examined in those patients referred to M.D. Anderson Hospital after they had received initial therapy and failed to respond favorably or later developed evidence of tumor relapse. Additional surgery was deemed necessary before other therapeutic modalities could be considered. In the United States, the indications for all types of surgery (including multiple operation for the same tumor) have come under increasing scrutiny by govermental agencies and private-sector health care organizations. When the referred patient has recently undergone craniotomy for the brain tumor, the most obvious questions asked are, "why is a second operation necessary and will it be of benefit?". Three distinct groups of patients have been seen in referral for further treatment and the indications for reoperation examined.

METHODS

Patient Selection

The 33 patients included in this study were referred to M.D. Anderson Hospital and Tumor Institute after having undergone tumor biopsy or subtotal resection as part of their initial treatment. Some patients were referred for radiation therapy whereas others, having already received radiation, were referred for chemotherapy. All pediatric patients were first evaluated in the pediatric neuro-oncology clinic and were seen by the neurosurgical consultant (RPM).

Surgical Criteria

Patients with massive infiltrative tumor, bihemispheral, diffuse subependymal or brainstem involvement were not considered candidates for salvage surgery. Reoperation was performed in an effort to substantially debulk the tumor mass and where possible to achieve complete tumor resection. Conventional operative techniques were employed. Biopsy of the surgical margins for frozen section examination was obtained to help determine the completeness of resection. Postoperative scans were obtained within the first few days after surgery and repeated every 3-6 monts.

RESULTS

Thirty-three patients, who had had a previous craniotomy for tumor, underwent reoperation by one neurosurgeon (RPM) following referral to M.D. Anderson Hospital. There was no perioperative mortality and 1 operative complication (hemiplegia). The average hospital stay was 5 days. Patients

(°) Section of Neurosurgery, Department of Head and Neck Surgery, University of Texas M.D. Anderson Hospital and Tumor Institute at Houston, Texas Medical Center, Houston, TX 77030.

M. Chatel, F. Darcel and J. Pecker (eds.), Brain Oncology. ISBN-13: 978-94-010-8003-3

referred for additional treatment following initial therapy were separated into 3 distinct groups based on the status of their tumor at the time of referral (Table I). Group 1 patients were referred following initial surgery but prior to radiation therapy. In all cases, the first operation failed to adequately deal with the mass effect caused by a large tumor burden. Group 2 patients were referred following initial surgery and radiation therapy or chemotherapy. They all presented with large residual tumors that were not substantially debulked at the first operation. Group 3 patients were also referred after surgery and radiation therapy. They differ from the second group in that they present with clear evidence of new tumor growth rather then symptomatic residual tumor bulk.

TABLE I

Summary of clinical characteristics and present status of 33 salvage surgery patients

	Group 1	Group 2	Group 3
Patients			
No.	10	11	12
Age[1] (range)	6(.9-14)	15(2-34)	38(11-58
Follow-up(months)	24	33	35
Histology[2]			
Astrocytoma	8	6	0
Anaplastic	2	5	7
Glioblastoma	0	0	5
Initial Surgery			
Biopsy only	10	3	2
Resection < 50%	-	8	3
Resection > 50%	0	0	7
Pre-salvage surgery			
XRT	0	10	12
Chemotherapy	0	6	7
Post-salvage surgery			
XRT	2	1	0
Chemotherapy	3	2	5
Present status			
Alive & Well	9	11	6
Progressive disease	1	0	0
Deceased	0	0	6

1 Age in years
2 Nelson et al. (Reference 2)

Group 1 :

Ten patients were included in this first group. All were pediatric patients and the majority had astrocytomas. The remaining 2 patients had anaplastic tumors (1 thalamic, 1 cerebral hemisphere). As of this writing, the average follow-up has been 24 months with a range from 8 to 46 months. Nine patients were well and without evidence of active tumor, whereas 1 patient (thalamic anaplastic astrocytoma) had progressive disease. Only the two patients with anaplastic astrocytomas received radiation therapy. Three patients were placed on a 1 year MOPP chemotherapy program as adjuvant therapy.

Case Report. This 10 month-old infant presented to the local hospital with increasing lethargy, vomiting and inability to stand. At the time of the first operation, a modest resection of an astrocytoma was accomplished (Fig. 1A). The patient failed to improve and was referred to M.D. Anderson Hospital for "emergency" radiation therapy. However, a decompressive surgical resection was felt to be necessary before any additional therapy could be considered. His neurological deterioration was reversed with a near complete removal of tumor (Fig. 1B) and the patient was placed on MOPP chemotherapy. As of this writing, the CT scan showed no evidence of tumor and the child, now 24 months old, was doing quite well.

Group 2 :

The 11 patients examined were older than in the first group and 6 has astrocytomas whereas 5 had anaplastic tumors. Ten of 11 patients had received radiation therapy prior to referral and were now seen for treatment of symptomatic tumor relapse. However, review of their CT scans demonstrated that a large residual tumor burden had remained from the initial operation and that the relapse was more a problem of residual rather then recurrent tumor. As of this writing, the average follow-up time was 33 months, and all 11 patients were well and without evidence of active tumor. Nine patients have received no further therapy beyond the definitive surgical resection.

Case Report. An 11 year-old boy underwent two partial surgical resections, radiation therapy and several courses of chemotherapy over a two-year period for treatment of a left hemisphere astrocytoma (Fig. 2A). Because of increasing mass effect and poor performance status, it was decided to attempt a definitive tumor resection. The intraoperative margins of resection were free of tumor and postoperative scans obtained over the last 33 months showed no evidence of recurrence. The patient has steadily improved and is able to function at an appropriate level for his age (Fig. 2B).

Group 3 :

The 12 patients included in this group were older then those in the first two groups and had either an anaplastic tumor or glioblastoma. All patients had received radiation therapy prior to reoperation and 7 patients had also failed to respond to chemotherapy. Four patients with glioblastoma and 2 with anaplastic astrocytoma have died. The average follow-up time has been 36 months. All patients in this group presented with evidence of new recurrence at the time of referral and underwent an aggressive surgical resection in a attempt to achieve maximum tumor cytoreduction as an adjunct to further therapy. Residual contrast enhancement on the immediate post-operative CT scan was seen in 5 of 6 patients who died despite intensive chemotherapy. As of this writing, the 6 remaining patients were alive and without evidence of tumor. Only 1 of these received additional treatment (chemotherapy) after definitive surgical resection.

Case report. A 29 year-old man was referred for treatment of a recurrent glioblastoma 8 months following subtotal resection, radiation and chemotherapy (Fig. 3A). His only salvage therapy consisted of an en-bloc resection of the tumor along with a wide margin of edematous brain tissue. As of this writing, 12 months later, the patient was engaged in his regular profession, asymptomatic, and with no evident disease on CT scan (Fig. 3B).

DISCUSSION

The 3 groups defined here represent the spectrum of patients being referred to specialized centers for brain tumor treatment. Each patient must be carefully assessed in terms of the quality of their treatment up to the time of referral. The fact that the patient may have recently had a "tumor operation" does not, per se, mean that the surgery was adequate. The Group 1 patients most clearly illustrate this situation. Because of the age of the patients and the relative radioresistence of the tumors, radiation therapy can not be viewed as a substitute for adequate surgical resection. Biopsy alone offers little benefit and, therefore, these patients should be referred to appropriate institutions were definitive surgery can be undertaken as part of the primary therapy.

The Group II patients are similar to the first group in that adequate control of tumor bulk was never achieved with the prior therapy. Most of these patients received radiation therapy without a reduction in the tumor mass. The radiation may have been effective in preventing continued tumor growth and thus afforted the opportunity to reoperate for definitive tumor resection. All of these patients have done very well and, indeed, suggest that apparent symptomatic tumor relapse may be the result of inadequate initial surgery rather than the failure of radiation or chemotherapy.

The essential difference in the Group 3 patients is that new tumor growth rather than residual tumor burden was documented at the time of symptomatic relapse. These patients all had malignant gliomas in which tumor regrowth was, unfortunately, the rule. While reoperation was less likely to be definitive, as of this writing, with a mean follow-up of 43 months, 50% of the patients were well and without evidence of tumor. Despite the fact that many patients with massive infiltrative tumors were not candidates for salvage surgery, a too fatalistic attitude must be avoided (1). In selected patients, referred for further therapy, tumor removal, as a safe, effective, and durable treatment option should not be overlooked (3).

SUMMARY

Certain patients with primary brain tumors, referred to M.D. Anderson Hospital and Tumor Institute for further treatment, have been found to benefit in an immediate and lasting manner from definitive reoperation. Three groups could be identified: 1, patients having inadequate initial surgery and no further therapy; 2, patients with residual tumor burden after radiation and chemotherapy; and 3, patients with recurrent tumor after appropriate therapy. Where adequate control of tumor burden has not been achieve with the first operation, the opportunity to effect a substantive tumor resection and gain a durable remission with a second or even third "dose" of surgery should not be overlooked in our rush to try experimental regimens of uncertain merit.

KEY WORDS

Glioma, Salvage, Surgery, Recurrent Brain Tumors.

REFERENCES

1. FULLING (K.H.), GARCIA (D.M.): Anaplastic astrocytoma of the adult cerebrum. Cancer, 55: 928-931 (1985).

2. NELSON (J.S.), TSUKADA (Y.), SCHOENFELD (D.), FULLING (K.), LAMARCHE (J.), PERESS (N.): Necrosis as a prognostic criterion in malignant supratentorial astrocytic gliomas. Cancer, **52**: 550-554 (1983).

3. SALCMAN (M.), KAPLAN (R.S.), DUCKER (T.B.), ABDO (H.), MONTGOMERY (R.): Effect of age and reoperation on survival in the combined modality treatment of malignant astrocytoma. Neurosurgery, 10: 454-463 (1983).

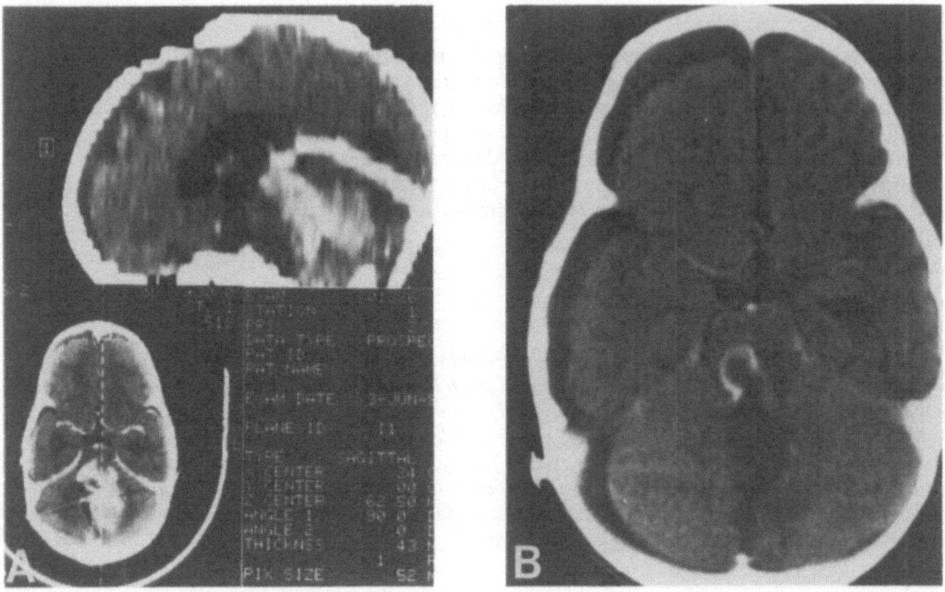

FIGURE 1.
A) Post biopsy CT scan shows minimal tumor resection in symptomatic patient.
B) CT scan after reoperation shows near complete resection of astrocytoma.

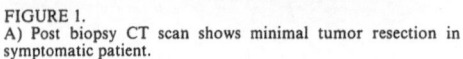

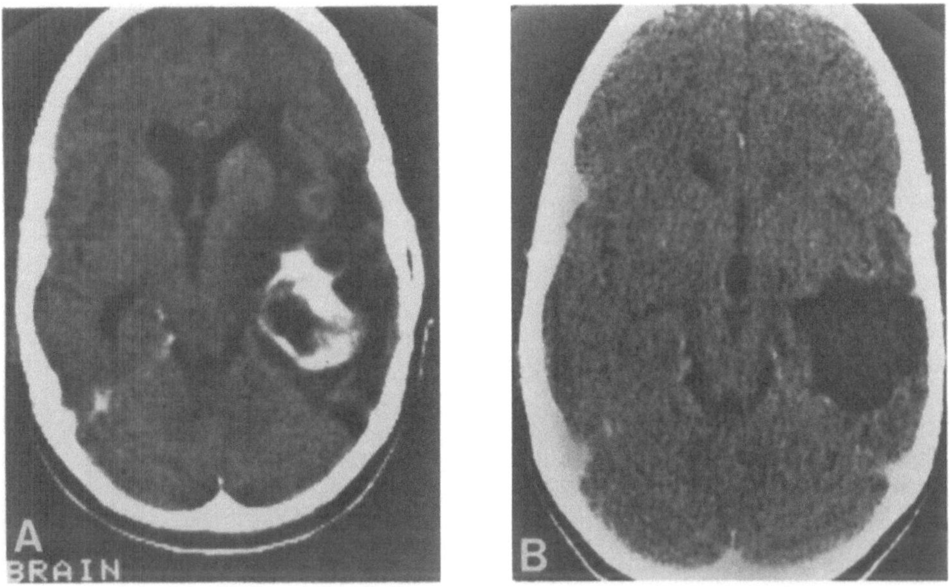

FIGURE 2.
A) Residual astrocytoma following surgery, radiation and chemotherapy over a 2-year period produced increasing symptoms.
B) CT scan, 33 months after tumor resection alone, showed no evidence of recurrence.

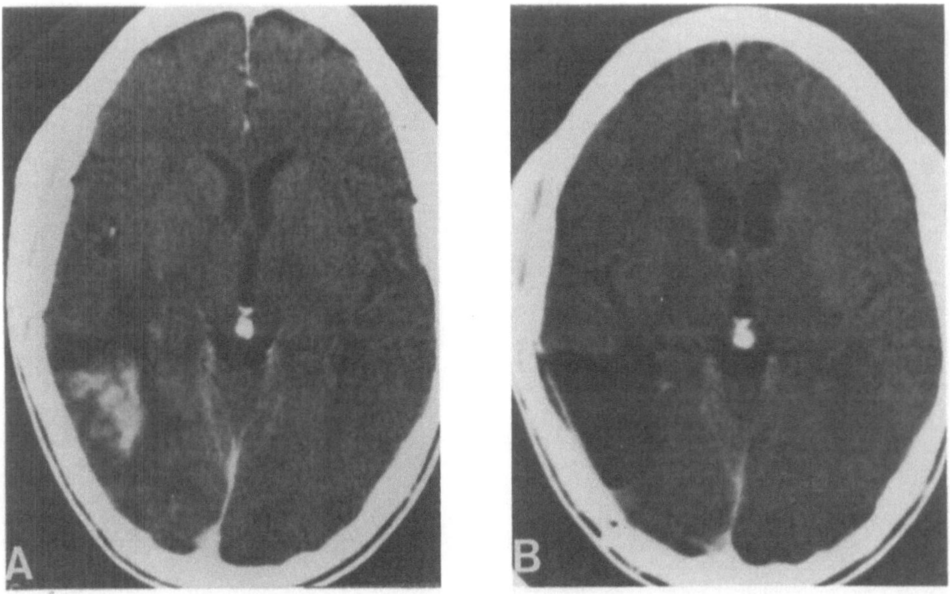

FIGURE 3.
A) Tumor regrowth in patient with glioblastoma was seen on CT scan 8 months after initial surgery, radiation, and chemotherapy.
B) Postoperative scans after en-bloc resection of recurrent tumor continued to demonstrate a durable response to surgical salvage.

Radiation Therapy in the Treatment of Malignant Supratentorial Gliomas: Current Trends and Prospects. A Review.

M. BEN-HASSEL (°), C. CHENAL (°), E. FLEURY - LE PRISE (°).

This International Meeting has given us the opportunity to evaluate the action of ionizing radiations on malignant gliomas.

We shall first consider conventional treatment and then the improvements made in its use: the action of radiosensitizers, high LET radiation, interstitial Curietherapy, multiple beam irradiation.

Conventional Treatment:

Post-operative irradiation of malignant gliomas significantly improves the length of survival without affecting its quality (1, 2). Numerous clinical trials have confirmed these results, which are independent of the extent of tumour removal (3). Toxicity is low, clinically acceptable but certainly underrated (4, 5). Progress in equipment and dosimetry, better target definition due to CT scanning, have not improved on the disappointing results at 18 and 24 months.

The permanent challenge that malignant gliomas represent has motivated many clinical and radiobiological investigations. Much of the work is promising.

Hypoxic Cell Radiosensitizers:

Malignant glioma is a tumour composed of an important number of hypoxic cells. Although local oxygenation is greatly improved by surgical reduction of tumour size and the first sessions of radiotherapy, it remains inadequate. The lack of sufficient, local concentration of oxygen makes the tumour cells resistant to the action of low LET radiations. Three methods are used to combat the radiobiological repercussions of hypoxia:

Hyperbaric Oxygen (6, 7): Oxygen inspired at high pressure (3 to 4 atmospheres) diffuses throughout the brain to a greater distance from the capillaries.

Hypoxic Cell Radiosensitizers: doted with a strong electronic affinity, they reproduce the effect that oxygen has on the hypoxic cells (8).

High LET Radiation: this will be considered later.

Hyperbaric oxygen has not improved results, whether used in conventional or modified fractionation (6). Hypoxic cell radiosensitizers have been found to be toxic (neurotoxicity) at high doses (8). Numerous trials based on different fractions have not proven the superiority of results when Misonidazole, the commonest drug, has been used (9). At the moment, it is impossible to know whether the ineffectiveness is due to the fact that Misonidazole cannot be administered at high doses. The best dose-fractionation relationship has not perhaps been found yet.

High LET Radiations:

Usual radiation (Cobalt 60, linear accelerators) creates few ionizations on its paths. They are known as low LET. High LET radiations (photons, neutrons, heavy atoms, negative pi mesons) have particular effects. Without going into detail (10), let us just note that these radiations are characterized by a great biological effectiveness, even in the absence of oxygen, and/or an extremely accurate spatial distribution (Bragg peak effect). Degenerative lesions of normal brain tissue observed during the first clinical trials using neutrons explain why, for the moment, the bulk of research is aimed at finding an optimum dose-time-fraction relationship (11).

(°) Radiotherapy and Oncology Department, Regional Cancer Institute, 35011 RENNES Cedex.

M. Chatel, F. Darcel and J. Pecker (eds.), Brain Oncology. ISBN-13: 978-94-010-8003-3

Modifications in the Time-Dose Relationship:

Fewer fractions and a higher dose per fraction have led to bad results due to immediate toxicity and serious early and late delayed damage (12). The most encouraging studies are those on hyperfractionation which reduces overall treatment time. By using two series of 30 Gy, we have shown for operated patients a survival rate of 10 % at 2 years after the start of radiotherapy and a median survival of 41 weeks. In the group of biopsied patients, the role played by radiotherapy would seem decisive only in cases of anaplastic astrocytoma (13). The most recent work of the Edmonton Group, Canada, of Douglas and of Fulton in the United States and of the EORTC Radiotherapy Group has confirmed the value of hyperfractionation (14, 15, 16, 17).

Since the publication of these studies and the stagnation in conventional results, Multicentre clinical trials still use conventional radiotherapy as the control arm in randomized trials. No determinant progress has radically altered the quality of our results. Shortening overall treatment time would at least have the merit of generalizing a protocol of which the whole potential has not yet been fully investigated. The case of malignant glioma even warrants comparison with the findings reported in the literature which has now become standard references, and a control by matching historical series. No results, alas, have lent themselves with validity to a controversy which can only be settled by randomization.

Volume Toxicity and Dose-Effect Relationship:

CT scanning allows clinical follow-up of treated patients. It has thus been possible to demonstrate that the vast majority of recurrences occur within the volume of the primary tumour site. But only a few cooperative trials have adopted the principle of an irradiated volume limited to the primary tumour site as defined by the CT scans.

What, however, does a reduction in treated volume mean ? High grade malignant tumours do not benefit from systematic correlation studies between a volume defined by the reference isodose, therapeutic effect and toxicity. We are still a long way from the accuracy with which studies of this type are carried out for other, often less aggressive solid tumours.

Only an exact definition of radiotherapy which is a major factor in treatment can give homogeneous data and avoid important, if not prime, bias in Multicentre trials (a study by the EORTC Radiotherapy Group is in progress). A quality control will determine true toxicity, encourage increased second surgery and post mortems. These procedures have resulted in a radical alteration of therapeutic strategy and in the prognosis of diseases which are now well-controlled (Hodgkin's Disease, ovarian cancer, osteosarcoma).

Interstitial Curietherapy and Per-operative Radiotherapy:

Implant techniques, with or without after-loading, are used in interstitial Curietherapy as for other extra-cerebral solid tumours. Interest should revive given the encouraging results obtained by P.H. Gutin in San Francisco with both 192 Ir and 125 I in after-loading, as well as with the 125 I and the 198 Au as permanent sources (18). More recently, Y. Maruyama associated continuous irradiation techniques and high LET, using the neutron emitter 252 Cf in Curietherapy (19).

Per-operative radiation therapy is another elegant manner of delivering an important dose to the primary tumour site whilst preserving the normal tissue. Finsterer described the technique as long ago as 1915 (20).

Multiple Beam Radiation:

Multiple beam radiation is a highly sophisticated technique which was introduced in Sweden in 1951 (21). It is based on an extremely precise definition of the target volume in stereotactic conditions which have been improved upon by the introduction of the CT scan and NMR (nuclear magnetic resonance imaging). Treatment is delivered to a generally restricted volume by a « cross-fire » technique. Between 100 and 300 beams are used. They come directly from a cobalt 60 unit which has 179 radioactive sources set out in an arc around a virtual centre situated within the tumour. The diameter of the beam ranges from 8 to 14 mm (22). The technique was developed by 0.0. Betti and V.E. Derechinsky at Buenos Aires at the beginning of the 1980s (23).

We would like to emphasize that irradiation is completed in one session and is associated with a very high biological effectiveness. The normal tissue is protected because the doses received are low.

Tumour necrosis occurs during the months which follow irradiation. It is a radiosurgical procedure (24) doted with an effective and specific therapeutic effect, long reserved for the treatment of non-resectable benign tumours and recently extended to malignant gliomas with a diameter of 3 cm.

Boron Neutron Capture Therapy (BNCT):
Boron 10 (10B) is a compound which accumulates in brain tumours and which has been the subject of a number of studies since the first publication by W.H. Sweet in 1952 (25).
Low energy neutron irradiation of Boron causes the Boron to disintegrate [10B (n, d)] by neutron capture resulting in the production of an emission of heavy particles of high energy and of high LET (26). Radiobiological efficacy is high and limited to the volume of Boron distribution.
BNCT is a technique of the future and has already been improved upon by the development of monoclonal antibodies which act as Boron vectors.

Monoclonal Antibodies and Ionizing Radiations:
In radioimmunotherapy, difficulties appear when the approach is discussed. Progress in intra-arterial chemotherapy will certainly make it possible to cross through the blood-brain-barrier, but fluctuations in intra-tumoral vascular permeability represent the limitations in the specificity of such treatment. The dominating problems are linked to the great antigenic variability of malignant glioma cells within the same tumour mass.

An anti-HNTA-Mab pool would provide a response to the needs of radioimmunotherapy by covering several specificities. Progress in the production of new isotopes has led to the concept of an in-vivo generator (27). The elements of radioactive filiation of the chosen isotope in equilibrium with its parents ensure local irradiation. The choice of the mother isotope is determined by its labelling qualities, its half-life and in particular by the high energy beta emissions of the daughter. One of the promising systems is the 66 NI/66 NU. Another method aims at making 10B radioactive. 10B-Mab (28) is subjected to neutron activation and, theoretically, specificities should combine as they are linked to the very nature of Boron and of the monoclonal, its vector.
Ionizing radiations form more than ever an integral part of a pluridisciplinary strategy, where neurosurgeons, neurologists, specialists in nuclear medicine, neuroradialogists, statisticians and radiotherapists all contribute to the treatment of malignant gliomas.
Jean Pecker has always taken part in this collective effort in our Hospital, as well as in numerous national and international scientific organizations. May this communication pay tribute to his brilliant career and bear witness to our collaboration.

KEY WORDS

Gliomas, Radiotherapy.

REFERENCES

1. WALKER (M.D.), GREEN (S.B.), DYAR (D.P.): Randomized comparisons of radiotherapy and nitrosoureas for the treatment9(E.), SATO (F.): Treatment of malignant gliomata. J. Neurosurg. **21**: 497-505 (1964).
2. LE BOLLOC'H (G.): Les tumeurs gliales malignes des hémisphères cérébraux. Thèse de Médecine, Rennes, (1978).
3. HITCHCOCK (E.), SATO (F.): Treatment of malignant gliomata. J. Neurosurg. **21**: 497-505 (1964).
4. KAGAN (A.R.) in: Radiation Damage to the Nervous System, Gilbert H.A. and Kagan A.R., Ed. Raven Press, New York, 183-190 (1980).
5. MIKHAEL (M.A.) in: Radiation Damage to the Nervous System, Gilbert H.A. and Kagan A.R., Ed. Raven Press, New York, 59-91 (1980).
6. LAMPHIER (E.H.): Determinants in oxygenation in clinical applications of hyperbaric oxygen. BOERMA Ed. Elsevier, Amsterdam, 227-283 (1964).
7. CHANG (C.H.) in: Tumours of the Central Nervous System: Modern Radiotherapy in Multidisciplinary Management. Chang C.H. and Housepian E.M. Ed. Masson Publ., New York, 23-30 (1982).
8. GIRINSKY (T.): Radiosensibilisateurs - bases biologiques, les nouvelles voies de recherche. Actualités Carcinologiques, Institut Gustave Roussy.
9. KOGELNIK (H.D.), KARCHER (K.H.), SZEPESI (T.), SCHRATTER-SEHN (A.V.) in: Progress in Radio-oncology II. Raven Press, New York (1982).
10. RAJU (M.R.) Heavy Particle Radiotherapy. Academic Press, New York (1980).

11. CATTERALL (M.), BLOOM (H.J.G.), ASH (D.V.), WALSH (L.), RICHARDSON (A.), UTTLEY (D.), GOWING (N.F.C.), LEWIS (P.), CHAKER (B.): Fast neutrons compared with megavoltage X-rays in the treatment of patients with supratentorial glioblastoma: a controlled pilot study. Int. J. Radiation Onc. Biol. Phys., **6**: 261-266 (1980).

12. KOTALIK (J.F.): Multiple daily fractions in radiotherapy. Cancer Treatment Reviews, **8**: 127-146 (1981).

13. BEN-HASSEL (M. et al.) in: Second International Symposium on the Biology of Brain Tumours. Walker M.D. and Thomas D.G.T. Eds., Martinus Nijhoff (1986).

14. NELSON (D.F.), URTASUN (R.C.), SAUNDERS (W.M.), GUTIN (P.H.), SHELINE (G.E.): Recent and current investigations of radiation therapy of malignant gliomas. Seminars in Oncology, Vol. 13, n° 1 (March), 46-55 (1986).

15. DOUGLAS (B.G.), WORTH (A.J.): Superfractionation in glioblastoma multiforme - results of a phase II study. Int. J. Radiation Onc. Biol. Phys., **8**: 1787-1794 (1982).

16. FULTON (D.S.), URTASUN (R.C.), SHIN (K.J. et al.): Misonidazole combined with hyperfractionation in the management of malignant glioma. Int. J. Radiation Onc. Biol. Phys., **10**: 1709-1712 (1984).

17. EORTC Radiotherapy Group: Communication de résultats préliminaires ; essai irradiation trifractionnée + Misonidazole (1986).

18. GUTIN (P.H.), HOSOBUCHI (Y.), PHILLIPS (T.L.), STUPAR (T.A.): Stereotactic interstitial irradiation for the treatment of brain tumors. Cancer Treatment Reports, 65, (Suppl. 2), 103-106 (1981).

19. MARUYAMA (Y.), CHIN (H.W.), BYRON YOUNG (A.) et al.: Implantation of brain tumors with Cf 252. Radiology, **152**: 177-181 (1984).

20. FINSTERER (H.): Zur Therapie inoperable Magen und Darmkarzinome mit freilegund und nach folgender Röntgenbestrahlung. Strahlentherapie, **6**: 205-213 (1915).

21. LEKSELL (L.) in: Stereotaxis and Radiosurgery-an operative system. Thomas Ch. C., Springfield I11., USA (1971).

22. BACKLUNG (E.O.): Stereotactic Radiosurgery in Intracranial Tumours and Vascular Malformations. In: Advances and Technical Standards in Neurosurgery. Vol. 6, Springer, New York, Berlin (1979).

23. BETTI (O.O.) and DERECHINSKY (V.E.): Irradiation stéréotaxique multifaisceaux. Neurochirurgie, **29**: 295-298 (1983).

24. Stereotactic Cerebral Irradiation, INSERM Symposium N° 12, Szikla G. Ed., Elsevier North Holland Biomedical Press, Amsterdam-Oxford-New York (1979).

25. SWEET (W.H.), JAVID (M.): The possible use of neutron capturing isotopes such as boron 10 in the treatment of neoplasms. J. Neurosurg., **9**: 200-209, 1952.

26. ZAMENHOF (R.G.), MURRAY (B.N.), BROWNELL (G.L.) et al.: Boron neutron capture therapy for the treatment of cerebral gliomas: 1 - Theoretical evaluation of the efficacy of various neutron beams. Med. Phys. **2**: 47-60 (1975).

27. MAUSNER (L.F.): Personal communication in NATO ASI Series, July, 1986: Production and use of prospective radionuclides for radioimmunotherapy.

28. BOURDON (M.A. et al.): Progress in Experimental Brain Tumour Research. Vol. II. Rosenblum M. and Wilson C. Eds., Karger, Basle (1985).

Whole Brain Irradiation is not necessary for the Treatment of Malignant Supra-Tentorial Gliomas

J.Ph. MAIRE (°), M. DAUTHERIBES (°), N. CAUSSE (°), D. CELERIER (°), J. GUERIN (°), M. CAUDRY (°).

INTRODUCTION

Compared with other cancers, supra-tentorial astrocytoma malignancy is not a result of metastatic diffusion but of local recurrence: this suggests that local treatment might be effective. Nevertheless, long term survivors do not exceed 5 to 10% at 3 to 5 years.

Although surgery when feasible is well tolerated, radiation therapy, which is known to prolong survival, is limited by the tolerance-efficacy ratio. Since CT Scans are currently available, radiation damage such as transitory subacute syndrome (1-7), cerebral atrophy (8) and radiation necrosis (9) is often recognized. Furthermore, animal studies have clearly demonstrated that radiation damage is correlated with irradiated volume, total doses and fractionated treatment (2).

The first aim of this retrospective study performed in 1983 was to define the site of tumor recurrence and then to analyse tumor spread within brain parenchyma. The second aim was to reduce irradiated volume.

PATIENTS AND METHODS

Eighty-seven patients with supratentorial malignant gliomas were treated from November 1975 to January 1982. There were 47 men and 40 women whose ages ranged from 14 to 81 (median 52.5 years). Fifty-six glioblastomas multiforme, 22 grade III astrocytomas and 9 non-histologically proved tumors were included in this study. Tumor site was frontal (19 patients), rolandic (7 patients), anterior temporal (10 patients), calloso-frontal (6 patients), posterior hemispherical (parietal, posterior temporal, occipital - 42 patients) or deep-seated (3 patients).

Thirty-six patients underwent a complete surgical resection, and 35 an incomplete one. Eight patients had only biopsy and 9 were not operated. All patients received post-surgical multidrug chemotherapy containing Vincristine, VM 26 and CCNU. Seventy-seven patients were given radiation therapy within 10 to 15 days after surgery. Irradiated volumes did not encompass more than 2/3 of the whole brain during the first part of the treatment corresponding to 2/3 of the total dose. The boost dose was then given to the tumor site plus a 1 to 2 centimeter margin. Total dose and fractionation were not the same for all patients: forty seven patients received 60 Gy in 30 to 33 fractions, and 6 to 6,5 weeks, 23 patients were given 69 Gy in 60 fractions, 2 fractions per day, and for 6 weeks; 9 patients received 17 Gy in 2 fractions and 3 days repeated at a one month interval. Ten patients were not irradiated. All patients received Methylprednisolone during irradiation. Thirteen patients underwent a second craniotomy and one was autopsied.

A pre-operative CT Scan was performed for every patient. The second CT Scan was obtained 4 to 5 months after the first treatment. CT Scan controls were then performed every 2 to 3 months. The total number of reviewed CT Scans was 401, from 2 to 14 per patient (median 4,2). The study of CT Scan 4 to 5 months after the first treatment revealed two principle situations :

— complete remission (CR) was confirmed when CT Scan was normal or in the presence of well defined hypodensity without contrast enhancement or median structure deviation.

— persistant pathological image (PPI) in the presence of hypodensity with contrast enhancement with or without mass syndrome, and which could not be characterized as persistent, recurrent tumor

Services de radiothérapie et de neurochirurgie, Hôpital Saint-André - 1, rue Jean-Burguet, 35070 BORDEAUX CEDEX.

M. Chatel, F. Darcel and J. Pecker (eds.), Brain Oncology. ISBN-13: 978-94-010-8003-3

tumor or radiation necrosis.
Furthermore we studied brain parenchyma near to or at a distance from the initial tumor site.

RESULTS

Table I shows the results of the second CT Scan during the 4th-5th month after the first treatment, and their evolution: thirty one patients presented CR (35%) and 12 of them had tumor recurrence (6 were surgically proved). Among the 56 PPI, 3 progressively disappeared within 10 to 20 months after treatment, while 6 patients were reoperated for a confirmed tumor recurrence. On the whole, 65 patients (74,7%) presented a PPI or a CT Scan recurrence.

TABLE I

Results of the second CT scan performed during the 4th-5th month after the first treatment and their evolutions

SECOND CT SCAN	EVOLUTION DURING FOLLOW UP
31 complete remissions	— 19 complete remissions — 12 tumor recurrences (6 surgically proved)
56 persistent pathological images (PPI)	— 3 complete remissions — 53 PPI of which : - 6 surgically proved recurrences - 1 radiation necrosis (autopsy) - 1 distant radiation necrosis (surgery) - 4 multicentric gliomas - 2 CSF seeding

Sixty-four PPI or CT Scan recurrences were localized within the initial tumor site (98,5%). Tumor recurrence was confirmed for 12 patients after a second craniotomy, and pure radiation necrosis for a thirteenth case at autopsy. One patient died with cerebrospinal fluid seeding confirmed by cytology. Four of the 64 patients presented a second non-contiguous localisation with a concomittent recurrence at the tumor site : there were 2 localizations in the controlateral hemisphere and 2 periventricular subependymal extensions.

The last patient was in CR at the primary tumor site but presented a second localization at five month; craniotomy revealed the presence of radiation necrosis. Nevertheless, this patient died at 7 month from a cerebrospinal fluid extension.

On the whole, only 5 patients presented multifocal CT Scan lesions (5,7%) and in 4 cases, the second localizations was concomittent with a recurrence within the primary tumor site.

During follow up. CT Scan controls showed that tumor progression occurred contiguously to the site of recurrence, according to relatively constant directions (Fig. 1). For example, in frontorolandic localizations, tumor spread towards the controlateral hemisphere was documented for 8/14 relapsing patients, backwards to the parietal lobe for 7/14 patients and downwards to the temporal lobe for 3/14 patients. In posterior hemispherical localizations, tumor spread towards controlateral hemisphere was seen in 15/35 patients, forwards to the anterior temporal lobe for 9/35 patients or to the frontorolandic lobe for 6/35 patients. Lastly in anterior temporal localizations, tumor spread towards the frontal lobe was documented in 2/7 patients, backwards to the temporo-occipital region in 4/7 patients, and to the basal ganglia for 2/7 patients.

DISCUSSION

Our results show that multicentric glioma are uncommon (less than 6% of the cases). We are in agreement with Hochberg et Pruitt (6) who found, after autopsy and/or CT Scans performed on 157 patients, 4% of multicentric gliomas in non treated patients and only 6% in treated ones. On the other hand, 90% of their patients presented a local recurrence within or close to the primary tumor site.

Recently, Green et al. (5) did not find any difference in survival between patients treated with whole brain irradiation and those who received coned-down boost to the tumor volume. Furthermore, it is interesting to note that the best results reported by de Schryver et al. (3) were obtained with small volume irradiation. In addition. Foo et al. (4) have reported on the quality of long term survival in malignant gliomas and conclude that future treatment strategies should investigate less neurotoxic therapies.

Our present results confirm such an approach, as does a recent reevaluation of 173 patients treated from November 1975 to May 1985 in our department. CT Scan survey demonstrates that most recurrence arise within the initial tumor site, and that tumor spread is not random but progresses through contiguous white matter anatomical structures, such as inter and intra-hemispherical fibers (corpus callosum, fasciculus uncinatus, fasciculus longitudinalis superior or inferior). In some cases periventricular sub-ependymal extension was seen. During treatment planning, it is important to include within the target volume, the tumor site and its presumptive extension pathways. CT Scan is at present the best means of defining this volume. Whole brain irradiation is not necessary because with doses given nowadays, it is rarely able to obtain local control; furthermore, whole brain irradiation is given in cerebral parenchyma where tumor extension is rarely possible; it can cause radiation damage which spoils long term survival quality or even shortens it. Reducing the target volume may mean that higher doses of radiation therapy for glioblastoma may be delivered.

SUMMARY

The choice of irradiated volume is one of the most important factor for the treatment of malignant brain tumors. Whole brain irradiation is currently used for patients with glioblastomas, but since CT Scan is now systematically performed, this radiation technique must be reconsidered. In this retrospective study, CT Scan controls performed at 2 to 3 month intervals in 87 consecutive treated patients with supratentorial malignant gliomas showed that: 1) tumor recurrence occurs within the initial tumor site in 98,5% of the cases; 2) tumor invades contiguous anatomical structures through white matter intra-and inter-hemispheric association fibers; 3) multicentric gliomas are uncommon (less than 6% of patients).

Whole brain irradiation with currently given doses seems to be inadequate for three reasons: 1) it is rarely able to obtain local tumor control; 2) it is given in cerebral parenchyma which is not often reached by tumor extension; 3) it can induce radiation damage, which spoils long term survival quality or even shortens it.

Using CT Scan data, it should be possible to restrict the irradiated volume to the tumor site and to presumptive extension pathways. Higher doses may be delivered in this volume.

KEY WORDS

Supra-tentorial malignant gliomas, Radiation therapy, Gliomas.

REFERENCES

1. BOLDREY (E.), SHELINE (G.): Delayed transitory clinical manifestations after radiation treatment of intracranial tumors. Acta. Radiol. Ther. Phys. Biol., 1966, 5, 5-10.

2. CAVENES (W.F.): Experimental observations: delayed necrosis in normal monkey brain. In: Gilbert H.A., Kagan A.R., Radiation Damage to the Nervous system. pp. 1-38, New York, 1980.

3. SCHRYVER (A. de), GREITZ (T.), FORSBY (N.): Localized shaped field radiation therapy of malignant glioblastoma multiforme. Int. J. Radiat. Oncol. Biol. Phys. 1976, 1, 713-716.

4. FOO (S.H.), HIESIGER (E.), WISE (A.) et al.: Quality of long term survival of treated patients with malignant glioma. Proc. ASCO, 1985, 5, 136.

5. GREEN (S.B.), BYAR (D.B.), STRIKE (T.A.) et al.: Randomized comparisons of single or multiple drug chemotherapy combined with either whole brain or whole brain plus coned-down boost radiation therapy for the post operative treatment of malignant gliomas (study 8001). Proc. ASCO, 1986, 5, 135.

6. HOCHBERG (F.H.), PRUITT (A.): Assumptions in the radiotherapy of glioblastoma. Neurology, 1980, 30, 907-911.

7. HOFFMAN (W.F.), LEVIN (V.A.), WILSON (C.B.): Evaluations of malignant gliomas patients during the post-irradiation period. J. Neurosurg, 1979, 50, 624-628.

8. HYMAN (R.A.), LORING (M.P.), LIEBESKING (A.L.) et al.: Computed tomographic evaluations of therapeutically induced changes in primary and secondary brain tumors. Neuroradiology, 1978, 14, 213-218.

9. MIKHAEL (M.A.): Radiation necrosis of the brain: correlation between computed tomography, pathology and dose distribution. J. Comput. Assist. Tomogr. 1978, 2, 71-80.

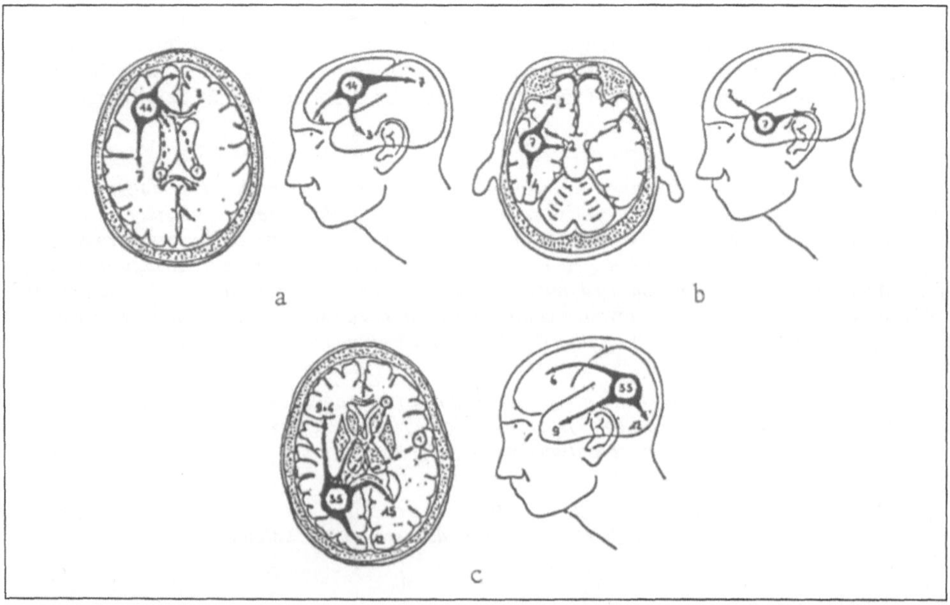

FIGURE 1. CT Scan extension of malignant gliomas - a) frontorolandic localizations
b) anterior temporal localizations
c) posterior hemispheric localizations.

Quality of Treatment Response and Survival in Patients with Supra-Tentorial Malignant Gliomas

J.Ph. MAIRE (°), J. GUERIN (°), M. DAUTHERIBES (°),
H. DEMEAUX (°), F. GUICHARD (°), M. CAUDRY (°).

INTRODUCTION

The outlook for patients with supratentorial malignant gliomas remains poor; until recently, therapeutic results were the same as those reported by Jelsma and Bucy in 1967 (5). Nevertheless, results have been published for heterogeneous patient series, in which treatment is standardized as though it was uniformly efficacious and tolerable. Although host and tumor factors must be analysed in all retrospective studies for comparing therapeutic results, we think as Gilbert et al. (3) that nowadays, treatment could be adjusted to these prognostic factors. Here we present our experience.

PATIENTS AND METHODS

From November 1975 to May 1985, 173 consecutive patients with supratentorial malignant gliomas were treated and followed in our department (96 men and 77 women). Ages ranged from 7 to 81 (median 54,8); 4 patients were less than 15 years old. There were 122 glioblastomas multiforme (GM), 26 grade III astrocytomas (AS III) and 25 non histologically proved tumors (NHP). Seventy-nine complete surgical resections, 48 partial resections and 21 biopsies were performed. In November 1978, we decided to modify our post-operative strategy according to prognostic factors.

This explains the differences between treatments described below. All patients received post-surgical multidrug chemotherapy containing Vincristine, VM 26, CCNU or BCNU. Within 10 to 15 days after the surgical period, all but 31 selected patients were given post-operative radiation-therapy with cobalt 60 and/or 9 MeV photons. Irradiated volumes did not encompass more than 2/3 of the whole brain during the first part of the treatment. The boost dose corresponding to 1/3 of the total dose was then given to the tumor site, plus a 1 to 2 centimeter margin. Total doses and fractionation were not the same for all patients: 91 patients were given 55 to 60 Gy in 30 to 33 fractions over a period of 6 to 7 weeks; 40 patients received 69 Gy in 60 fractions, 2 fractions per day and 6 weeks; 11 patients received 17 Gy in 2 fractions and 3 days, repeated at a one month interval. The 31 remaining patients received only post-surgical chemotherapy.

CT Scan and clinical evaluation were routinely performed. Therapeutic efficacy (Table I) was assessed clinically according to Order and Karnofsky criteria (6-7) and with CT Scan data. A first evaluation was made during the 4th-5th month after the beginning of treatment. Survival curves and statistical analysis were performed according to Peto et al. (8).

(°) Services de radiothérapie et de neurochirurgie, Hôpital Saint-André - 1, rue Jean-Burguet, 35075 BORDEAUX CEDEX.

M. Chatel, F. Darcel and J. Pecker (eds.), Brain Oncology. ISBN-13: 978-94-010-8003-3

TABLE I

Criteria of response to treatment

	CV (Karnofsky)	CT Scan
Complete remission	⩾ 80%	Normal
Partial remission	⩾ 60%	Tumor regression ⩾ 50%
Failure	0-100%	Tumor regression < 50% Progression
Non evaluable	0-100%	Not performed

RESULTS

Median survival (MS) for all patients was 11.5 months; 2 years actuarial survival was 15%.

Tumor factors:

Tumor grade and localisation did not influence either therapeutic response or survival. Nevertheless, NHP gliomas had a significantly worse prognosis ($p < 0.001$).

Host factors:

Age: patients less than 50 years did better than those older than 50. MS was respectively 20 months and 10 months ($p < 0.001$).

Post-surgical neurological status (NS) was the second host factor influencing survival. MS was 14 months for 109 patients with NS 1 or 2, whereas MS was only 7 months for 64 patients with NS 3 or 4 ($p < 0.001$). Six patients with NS 1 or 2 survived beyond 60 months.

Age and NS are two independent factors so that a bifactorial analysis was performed: 3 clinical groups of statistically different prognosis were defined (Table II). Group 1 in which patients were younger than 50 with good post-surgical NS, thus representing 20.2% of the population. The remission rate was 71% (42.5% CR and 28.5% PR) and MS was 25 months. Five patients survived after 60 months without recurrence, 4 of them harboring glioblastoma multiforme. Group 2 represented 37.5% of the patients; only one pejorative factor was present: age ⩽ 50 and NS 3 or 4 (group 2a) or age between 50 and 65 and NS 1 or 2 (group 2b); remission rate was 55% (24.5% CR and 30.5% PR); MS was 13 months. Group 3 was composed of all patients older than 65 and of patients older than 50 with NS 3 or 4; they represented 42.2% of the patients. Remission rate was 17.5% (9.5% CR and 8% PR); MS was 7 months. Differences between the three groups were statistically significant ($p < 0.001$) (Fig. 1).

TABLE II

Clinical classification

Clinical group		Age	Neurological status	Number of patients
Group 1		⩽ 50	1 or 2	35
Group 2	2a	⩽ 50	3 or 4	65
	2b	50 < age ⩽ 65	1 or 2	
Group 3	3a	50 < age ⩽ 65	3 or 4	73
	3b	> 65	1-2-3 or 4	

Therapeutic factors:

Surgical removal was the first therapeutic factor: for non-surgical or only biopsied patients, remission rate was 13%, MS 7,5 months; this is statistically worse than for resected patients ($p < 0.001$), but we did not find any difference between complete and partial resection. For patients with complete resection, remission rate was 59.5% (35.5% CR and 24% PR) and 43.5% for patients with partial resection (16.5% CR and 27% PR) ($p > 0.05$). MS was respectively 14 and 11 months ($p > 0.05$) (Fig. 2).

Fractionated irradiation was the second treatment factor influencing survival. Remission rate was better for 131 patients treated with fractionated irradiation as compared to 11 patients treated with a hypofractionation schedule. All these 11 patients whose median survival was 11 months died during the second year. No complete remission was noted, so we promptly abandonned that irradiation schedule. For patients treated with fractionated or bifractionated irradiation, remission rate was respectively 51.5% and 37.5%, MS 13 and 12 months; 2 year actuarial survival was respectively 23% and 20% ($p > 0.05$).

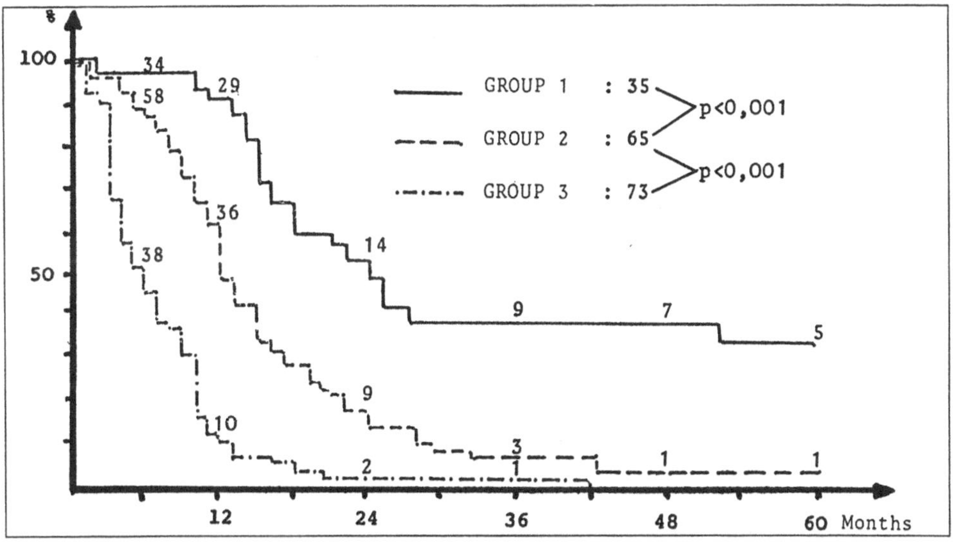

FIGURE 1. Actuarial survival curves according to the three clinical groups.

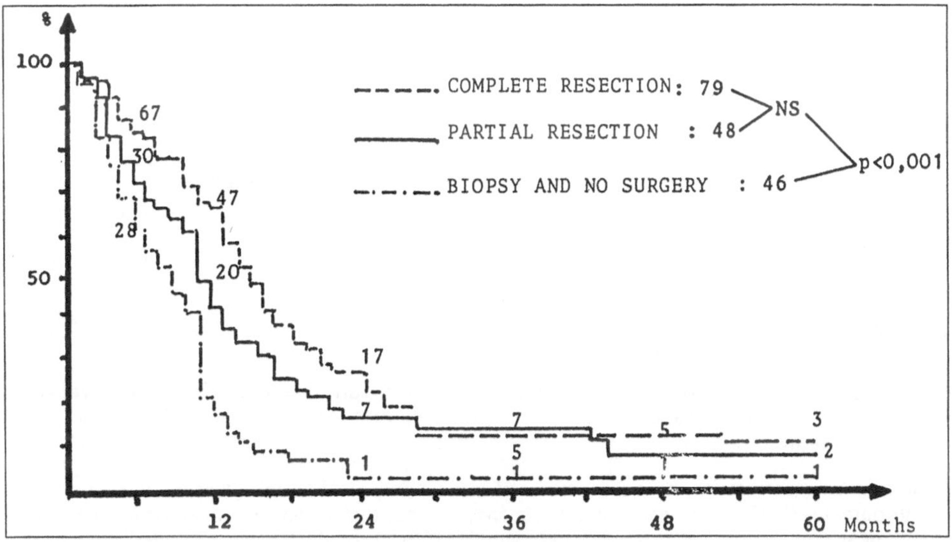

FIGURE 2. Actuarial survival curves according to the extent of tumor removal.

Since November 1978, bifractionnated irradiation has been given essentially to patients belonging to group 2; at that time, we decided to adjust our radiation protocol for this group of patients in order to enhance treatment results. While these patients were retrospectively compared to patients of the same group treated with fractionnated irradiation, no difference either in survival or in remission rate appeared.

Chemotherapy was post-operatively given to all patients of the series; combined with irradiation for 142 patients, its efficacy cannot be assessed. On the other hand, 31 patients included in group 3 only received chemotherapy until remission or death. From November 1978 on, we decided to defer radiation therapy in this patient group because of the poor results obtained with the standard radiation protocol. Thus MS was 5 months after radiation therapy; no CR was obtained. With only post-operative chemotherapy 7 of the 31 patients presented a CR and MS was 8 months. The difference is not statistically significant but the percentage of patients of this group having good familial autonomy rose from 30 to 60% with this therapeutic approach.

Treatment response, assessed during the 4th-5th month after the surgical period, was the last significant factor influencing survival. MS was 17 months for responder patients and only 7 months for non responder and non evaluable patients ($p < 0.001$). For 38 CR patients MS was 19 months and 2 year actuarial survival was 40%; MS was 15 months for 36 PR patients ($p < 0.05$) (Fig. 3).

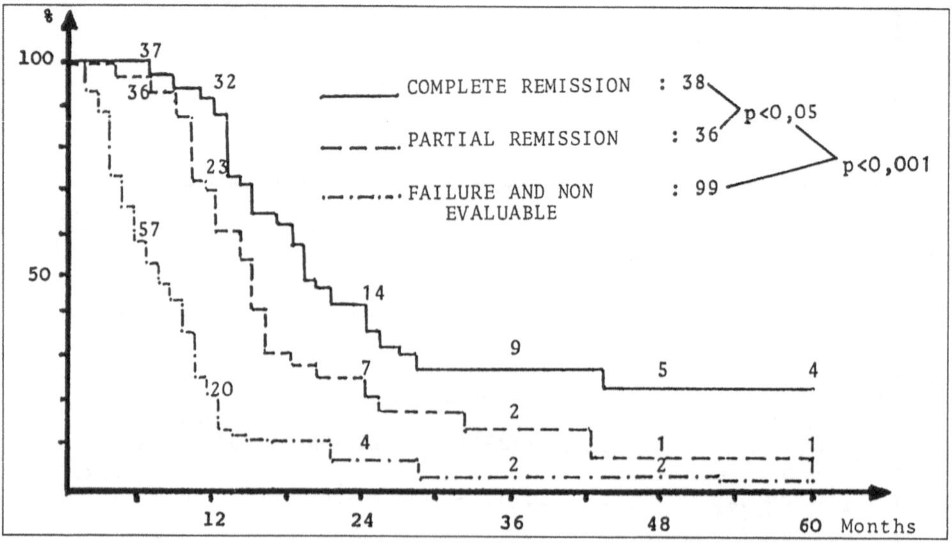

FIGURE 3. Actuarial survival curves according to the treatment response.

DISCUSSION

Our present results confirm our previous work (2-4). Tumor grade does not influence survival and we do not think that grade III and grade IV astrocytomas should be treated differently, whatever the tumor localisation.

As indicated in other series, host factors are of a great importance and of predictive value for patients outcome (3-12-13). It seems that treatment tolerance differs from younger to older patients but it may also be possible that tumor aggressivity differs according to age with identical tumor grades. Post-surgical NS results from cerebral impairment consecutive to the increase of intracranial pressure and to surgery; it also depends on cerebral vascular status. In our series, all patients but one surviving after 2 years had a post-surgical NS 1 or 2; 14 were aged less than 50, 7 between 50 and 65 and none was over 65. Thus age and postsurgical NS are the two most important factors influencing quality of treatment response and survival.

In the light of our current knowledge, surgery is the first treatment to be considered since it may increase survival when combined with other therapies (4-9). The extent of removal does not seem to influence survival; nevertheless, the removal of a larger percentage of tumor mass with the aim of preserving or restoring NS is always the best option. In our experience, patients with poor post-surgical NS do not survive longer than non surgical patients.

Radiation therapy is known to improve survival (1-10-12-13). A dose effect relationship exists (11), and currently given doses are 55 to 60 Gy over 6 to 7 weeks. However, must all patients be submitted to radiation therapy? In our series, patients belonging to group 1 did better after radiation therapy as compared with the other two groups. Forty patients survived 2 years or more. On the other hand, in group 3, MS was only 5 months after irradiation which is hardly different from spontaneous survival. Our policy of deferring irradiation for patients of this group permitted survival quality to be increased without being shortened.

In group 2 which represents more than one third of the patients, we decided to investigate a new radiation protocol. Bifractionated irradiation was tolerated as well as fractionated irradiation but failed to improve survival. New treatment schedules are needed in this group in order to improve the efficacy/tolerance ratio.

Owing to patient heterogeneity, we think that an uniform treatment approach is not a positive one. The total actuarial survival curve has two slopes. There is an initial slope on which median survival can be found; MS is more influenced by prognostic factors than by therapeutic efficacity and could be improved with patient selection. A second slope corresponds to patients who survived thanks to treatment effectivness when the incidence of prognosis factors is reduced, i.e., when uniform patient groups, as defined in our classification, are compared.

The therapeutic goal is also to obtain survival quality in which the patient remains autonomous. In our series, the quality of treatment response was not only evaluated with CT Scan but also with clinical parameters. The first evaluation enables us to predict 4 to 5 months after diagnosis the survival chances for a given patient. When CR is obtained, MS is 20 months and 60 months actuarial survival is 23%. A majority of CR patients previously had the best prognostic factors: group 1 patients (42.8% CR) or NS 1 or 2 patients (34% CR) after complete surgical removal (37.5% CR). Fifteen of the 38 CR patients came from group 1 and 37 had a postsurgical NS 1 or 2. Postsurgical NS was the most important factor influencing treatment response quality and survival.

CONCLUSIONS

We think that:

1 - new studies have to be performed after a post-surgical stratification of patients;

2 - current treatment with surgery and protracted radiation therapy significantly improves survival for patients whose functional status is good;

3 - age is an important factor in tolerance and efficacy of radiation therapy;

4 - at present, when surgery is capable of preserving or restoring NS, it is the first treatment to be indicated, and gives an adequate delay for other therapies to act;

5 - the role of irradiation must be discussed for patients older than 65 and for those older than 50 with poor NS. New chemotherapeutic agents should be tested in this group;

6 - in group 2 we think that new radiation techniques are to be tested in order to improve the efficacy/tolerance ratio;

7 - the place of chemotherapy needs to be reassessed in each group.

Our classification is an excellent guide in the therapeutic approach of supratentorial malignant gliomas, in which treatment should be adapted to the functional status of patients. These three clinical groups are defined by their tolerance to tumor and therapeutic aggressivity.

SUMMARY

Therapeutic goals cannot be the same for every patient with malignant glioma, as the study of 173 cases treated from 1975 to 1985 suggests. In this series, survival is significantly correlated with:

1) host factors: age and post-surgical neurological status;

2) treatment factors: quality of surgical removal which has to be as complete as possible, with the aim of preserving or restoring functional status; quality of adjuvant protracted irradiation given in a limited volume, which is effective only in patients with a good post-surgical neurological status;

3) quality of the initial response to treatment.

From our results, we think that a post-surgical stratification of patients is necessary for defining an adapted and non uniform treatment stragegy.

KEY WORDS

Gliomas, Prognostic factors, Surgery, Radiation therapy.

REFERENCES

1. BLOOM (H.J.G.): Intracranial tumors: response and resistance to therapeutic endeavors. 1970-1980. Int. J. Radiat. Oncol. Biol. Phys. 1982, 8, 1083-1113.
2. CAUDRY (M.), MAIRE (J.P.), GUERIN (J.) et al.: Gliomes malins sustentoriels de l'adulte. Adaptation du traitement aux trois groupes d'une classification clinique. Sem. Hôp. Paris 1983, 59, 453-458.
3. GILBERT (H.), KAGAN (A.R.), CASSIDY (F.) et al.: Glioblastoma multiforme is not a uniform disease ! Am. J. Clin. Oncol. 1981, 4, 87-89.
4. GUERIN (J.), MAIRE (J.P.), CELERIER (D.) et al.: Les facteurs de réponse aux traitements des gliomes malins de l'adulte. Neurochirurgie 1981, 27, 305-314.
5. JELSMA (R.), BUCY (P.C.): The treatment of glioblastoma multiforme of the brain. J. Neurosurg. 1967, 27, 388-400.
6. KARNOFSKY (D.A.), BURCHENAL (J.H.): The clinical evaluation of chemotherapeutic agents in cancer. In: MacLeod C.M. Evaluation of chemotherapeutic agents. Columbia University Press. New York 1949, 191-205.
7. ORDER (S.E.), HELLMAN (S.), VON ESSEN (C.F.) et al.: Improvment in quality of survival following whole brain irradiation for brain metastasis. Radiology 1968, 91, 146-153.
8. PETO (R.), PIKE (M.C.), ARMITAGE (P.) et al.: Design and analysis of randomized clinical trials requiring prolonged observation of each patients. II Analysis and examples. Brit. J. Cancer. 1977, 35, 1-39.
9. ROSSI (G.F.), FEOLI (F.), FERNANDEZ (E.) et al.: The role of surgery in the treatment of supratentorial brain gliomas. In: Multidisciplinary Aspects of Brain Tumor Therapy, Paoletti P., Waker M.D., Butti G., Knerich R. Pub., Elsevier-North Holland Biomedical Press 1979,155-163.
10. SHELINE (G.E.): Radiation therapy of brain tumors. Cancer 1977, 39, 873-881.
11. WALKER (M.D.), STRIKE (T.A.), SHELINE (G.E.): An analysis of dose-effect relationship in the radiotherapy of malignant gliomas. Int. J. Radiat. Oncol. Biol. Physic. 1979, 5, 1725-1731.
12. WALKER (M.D.), GREEN (S.B.), BYAR (D.P.) et al.: Randomized comparisons of radiotherapy and nitrosoureas for the treatment of malignant glioma after surgery. N. Engl. J. Med. 1980, 303, 1323-1329.
13. WEIR (B.): The relative significance of factors affecting postoperative survival in astrocytomas, grades 3 and 4. J. Neurosurg. 1973, 38, 448-452.

Neuropsychologic Impairment in Adults with Brain Tumors after Radiation Therapy

J.Ph. MAIRE (°), B. COUDIN (°), M. CAUDRY (°), J. GUERIN (°).

INTRODUCTION

Radiation therapy given postoperatively to patients with malignant intra-cranial tumors increases survival, compared with surgery alone (1). In the management of certain tumors, a subtential cure rate can be obtained with relatively high doses of radiation given on large brain volumes. Nevertheless, quality of survival must be limited by radiation brain injury classified as acute, early delayed and late delayed. Neuropsychologic impairment is a delayed injury which is well analysed in numerous reports on children. To our knowledge, only one report concerns adults (2), and it would be misleading to extrapolate child results from adult patients, owing to the fact that the child brain is more sensitive to radiation therapy.

In a previous study (3) we found that a significant correlation exists between intellectual impairment and time elapsed from treatment. Since this paper, new patients have been tested and 18 patients have undergone a second, and 5 a third evaluation. This new study confirms the previous one, but we have also found that further intellectual recovery may be observed in some impaired patients during their follow up.

PATIENTS AND TREATMENT METHODS

Fourty-nine adult patients (26 men and 23 women) with primary intracranial tumors were treated and followed in our department. Ages ranged from 15 to 62 (median 37.6) and patients were selected as follows: Karnofsky index was 80% or more and CT Scan did not show any recurrence at the moment of intellectual testing. There were 4 grade I, 9 grade II, 4 grade III astrocytomas, 13 glioblastomas multiform, 8 oligodendrocytomas, 2 ependymomas, 1 pinealoma, 2 meningeal sarcomas, 4 medulloblastomas and 2 non histologically proved tumors.

Thirty-three patients underwent a complete surgical resection, 10 a partial one. Four patients were only biopsied and 7 underwent a ventriculo-cardiac shunt. Immediatly after surgery, 35 patients were given one course of chemotherapy with Vincristine, VM 26 and CCNU or BCNU. When radiation therapy was completed, these patients received from 2 to 12 monthly cycles chemotherapy with the same drugs. Two additional patients with sarcomas received adjuvant Fluorouracile. Ametopterine, Vincristine, Cyclophosphamide and Actinomycine D (12 cycles).

Radiation therapy was usually initiated within 10-15 days after surgery. Total doses and treatment volumes were different according to tumor type and location. Supratentorial gliomas, brain stem gliomas and sarcomas were given 56 to 60 Gy with daily fractions of 1.8 to 2 Gy or 69 Gy in two daily fractions of 1.15 Gy at 8 hours interval, over 6 to 7 weeks, in a tumor bed volume plus a margin. Two only patients with supratentorial glioma and 1 with pinealoma received 40 Gy in a subtotal supratentorial volume, followed by a 20 Gy boost to the tumor bed. The remaining 7 patients with posterior fossa tumors received craniospinal irradiation: 30 to 35 Gy were given at this volume with daily fractions of 1.6 to 1.7 Gy, followed by a 20 Gy boost to the posterior fossa. Irradiation was administered with cobalt and/or 9 MeV photons. All patients received Methyl Prednisolone during irradiation. Antiepileptics (sodium valproate) were systematically given.

FOLLOW UP METHODS

When radiation therapy was completed, patients were examined monthly during chemotherapy or at 2 monthly intervals for non chemotherapy patients. Repeat CT scans were routinely obtained every 3 months during the first two years, and then at 6 to 8 months intervals.

Services de radiothérapie et de neurochirurgie, Hôpital Saint-André - 1, rue Jean-Burguet, 35075 BORDEAUX CEDEX.

M. Chatel, F. Darcel and J. Pecker (eds.), Brain Oncology. ISBN-13: 978-94-010-8003-3

Neuropsychologic testing was performed by one of us (BC). From January 1980 to November 1985, the 49 patients were first assessed between 1.5 and 110 months after the beginning of irradiation (median = 13 months). A second assessment was performed 7 to 37 months after the previous testing for 18 patients. For 5 patients, a third study was performed; the interval between the second and third assessments was 12 to 36 months.

The Weschler Intelligence Scale for Adults (WAIS) was used to evaluate Full Scale Intellectual Quotient (FSIQ) as a result of Verbal and Performance I.Q. (5-6). The method makes it possible to establish a Coefficient of Intellectual Deterioration according to the Babcock method, standardized by Weschler and then brought up to date upon a French population by Pichot (4).

To evaluate Intellectual Deterioration, it would be necessary to know the previous intellectual capacity of each patient which was impossible in our study. The Babcock method avoids this difficulty by using a simultaneous battery of subtests. Some subtests concern only "active" mechanisms (conceptualisation, proximate memory, reasoning, analysis and synthetic processes), and represent non holding subtests. Other subtests concern "passive" mechanisms (previously memorized information), and represent holding subtests. These subtests estimate respectively present and anterior intellectual efficiency.

Their exploitation makes it possible to detect a discriminating impairment of neuropsychologic function by pathological processes, defined by a Deterioration Coefficient (DC). This coefficient cannot be considered as a quantitative approach, but rather represents a deterioration probability. Thus, the probability for a normal adult to have a DC superior to 12% is 0.2 according to Pichot. If, in this study, more than 20% of our patients present a DC > 12%, the tested population is to be considered as significantly deteriorated.

On the other hand, a variation in FSIQ is a quantitative approach for evaluating intelligence changes, because holding and non holding subtests are impaired.

RESULTS

At the moment of this study (November 1985), 37 patients were alive with only one tumor recurrence. Twelve patients are died from the tumor. Median follow up was 54 months (from 9 to 132 months).

A - Initial Evaluation: Vertical study

The results of the 49 initial post-treatment evaluations are given in terms of Deterioration Coefficient and Full Scale IQ.

1 - Deterioration coefficients: Figure 1 shows that 22/49 patients (45%) had a DC > 12%; this was significantly worse than for the normal population defined by Pichot. Nevertheless, DC distribution was heterogenous according to the elapsed time between the beginning of radiation therapy and the psychometric test; it was therefore possible to determine three statistically significant groups of patients (P) :

— the first group (P1) consisted of 11 patients tested from 1.5 month to 4 months;

— the second (P2) was composed of 27 patients tested between 5 and 30 months;

— the third group (P3) included the 11 remaining patients tested beyond 30 months.

In P1, DC did not differ from that of the reference population; on the other hand, for P2 there was a significant positive DC (P = 0.01). Beyond 30 months, there was not more statistical difference of DC in P3.

2 - Full scale intellectual quotients: The median score on each intellectual parameter was assessed by Weschler as Superior (IQ > 110), Normal (90-109), Dull normal (80-89), Borderline (70-79) and

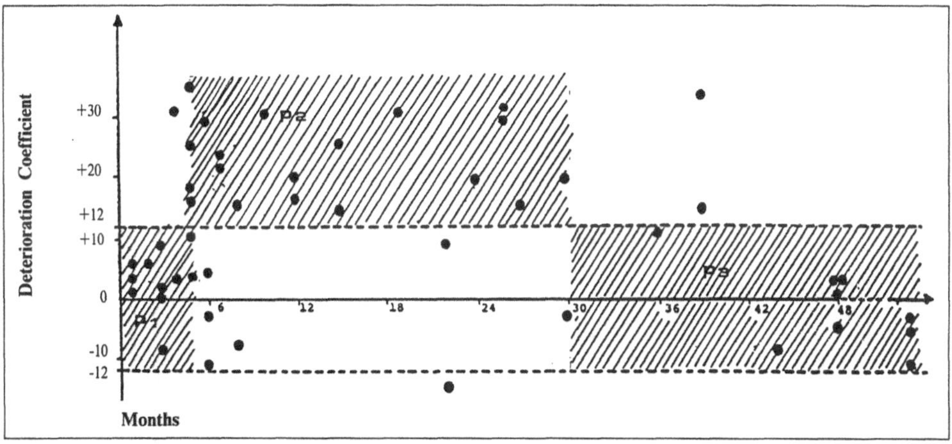

FIGURE 1. Distribution of Deterioration Coefficients of 49 irradiated patients, according to the elapsed time between the beginning of the treatment and the first psychometric test: Vertical Study.

Deficient range (IQ ⩽ 70). This distribution which was too precise for our study, was reduced into two main IQ levels defined as: level 1 (IQ ⩾ 80) and level 2 (IQ < 80).

Analysis of test scores according to the elapsed time from treatment to initial evaluation shows significant correlations within groups P1, P2 and P3. Results are shown in Tabe I: the PI scores do not differ from a normal population, nor do the P2 scores. On the other hand, the percentage of patients in level 2 (IQ < 80) is statistically different in P3 (P = 0.01).

TABLE I

Distribution of FSIQ according to the elapsed time from the beginning of irradiation

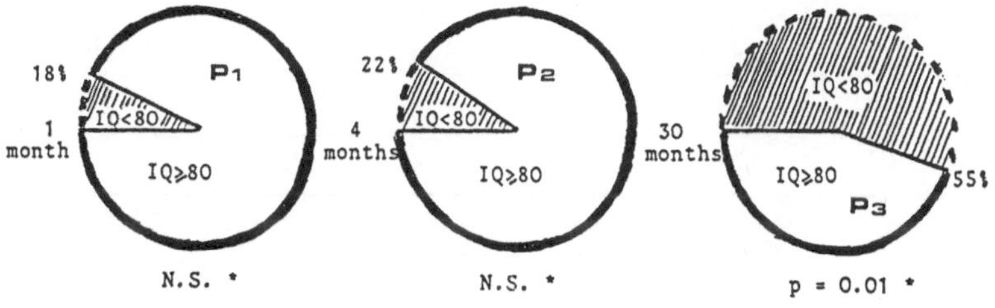

* Compared to a normal population.

B - Second and third evaluations: Horizontal study

1 - Deterioration coefficient: The results of the second test (18 patients) and of the third test (5 patients) are shown in figure 2. They confirm the results of the vertical study for the majority of the patients. During the first year, an increased probability of obtaining a positive DC is evident, whereas beyond two and three years, DC returns to a normal range for most patients. For 5 patients having performed three tests, DC evolution was the same for 4 of them.

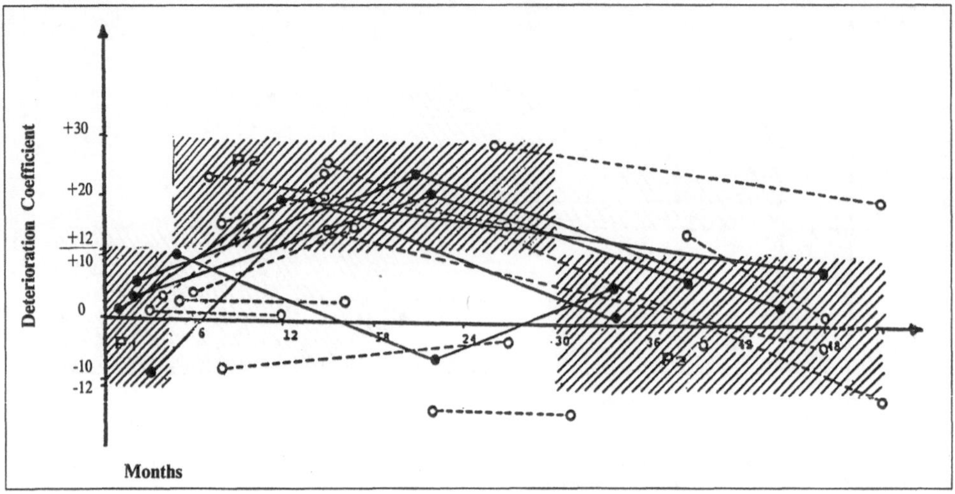

FIGURE 2. Distribution of Deterioration Coefficients of patients that performed two psychometric tests (O - - - O) (18) and three tests (●——●) (5), according to the elapsed time from the beginning of the treatment: Horizontal Study.

2 - ***Intellectual quotients:*** Changes of 5 points or more were necessary for identifying an objective modification of FSIQ. Improvement appeared in 6 patients, deterioration in 4 and stability was seen in 8.

The effect of age at diagnosis seems to be important (Table II). A major improvement was seen in patients less than thirty years old (4/5), whereas a majority of patients between 31 and 50 years remained stable (7/11). Deterioration was noted for the 2 patients over 50 years.

TABLE II

Change in FSIQ according to age at diagnosis (second and third evaluations)

Age (years)	Improvment ⩾ + 5	Stability +/— 4	Deterioration ⩾ — 5
< 30	4	1	0
From 30 to 50	2	7	2
> 50	0	0	2
TOTAL	6	8	4

DISCUSSION

This study was performed on a very selected population. The 49 patients represented about 20% of all adult patients with malignant brain tumors treated by our team during the past 10 years.

The vertical study shows a significant correlation between selective or global neuropsychologic impairment and the time elapsed from treatment. After a 4-5 months delayed period, a significant intellectual deterioration appears, while median FSIQ remains at a normal level. This deterioration only concerns "active" or operational mechanisms (non holding subtests); "passive" mechanisms (holding subtests) are intact.

Furthermore, beyond the second and third years after treatment, DC decreases to a normal level while for a patient majority FSIQ falls. This DC normalisation may be explained by the fact that all mechanisms ("active" and "passive") are affected and virtually prevent the establishment of a mathematical DC. The Deterioration Coefficient and FSIQ are in significant correlation with time elapsed from treatment and could be included in the brain injury classification: early injury (positive DC) and late delayed injury (FSIQ impairment).

Hochberg and Slotnick performed neuropsychologic tests from 12 to 30 months after radiation therapy in 13 selected long term survivor patients without CT Scan recurrence (2). They observed, as in our study, that newly learned tasks requiring attention and immediate solving ability were performed poorly. This fact corresponded to the appearance of a significant selective deterioration, whereas mean Verbal IQ was 98.4 and mean Performance IQ 92. Both scores were in the average range of psychometric intelligence. We agree with their results because median FSIQ was also in the average normal range in our patients tested within 1.5 to 30 months, whereas newly learnt tasks were impaired.

Our horizontal study partially confirms the vertical study. After a second or third evaluation, DC evolution was the same as in our initial study for the majority of patients. However FSIQ was improved in 6/18 patients. Despite a small number of patients limiting statistical signification, the influence of age at diagnosis seems to be important. This later FSIQ improvement was documented in 4/5 patients less than 30 years old and in 2 patients between 30 and 50 years.

Because of patient heterogeneity, we cannot find a significant impact of host defects, tumor location, chemotherapy and radiation doses and volume on intellectual impairement.

CONCLUSIONS

This study confirms and expands our earlier results. Radiation therapy induces neuropsychologic impairment that only fine intellectual evaluation can detect early on; the influence of the post treatment time interval is well documented. After a 4 month latency period, intellectual impairment only affects immediate solving ability (non holding subtests). Beyond a two or three year period, FSIQ deterioration is observed. Nevertheless, if in most instances deterioration remains stable, in some patients younger than 30 years old, later improvement can be seen.

If host, tumor or treatment factors and emotional impact of the disease are to be considered in neuropsychologic deficiency, our first aim is to detect early impairment; this will require more attention and care for such patients. Special psychological and educational assistance and the possibility of returning to work will have a positive impact on FSIQ recovery, especially for younger adult patients. Further studies are needed.

SUMMARY

Neuropsychologic studies were performed in 49 adult patients with primary intracranial tumors, following radiation therapy. In the absence of CT Scan tumor recurrence or neurologic disorders, one (49 patients), two (18 patients) or three (5 patients) intellectual tests were performed with the Weschler Intelligence Scale (WAIS) from 1.5 to 110 months after the beginning of irradiation. Full Scale IQ (FSIQ) and Deterioration Coefficient (DC) were evaluated.

Time elapsed from treatment to initial evaluation (vertical study) revealed 3 statistically different patient groups. During the first 4 months, DC and FSIQ did not differ from a normal population. From 5 to 30 months, there appeared a significant probability of intellectual deterioration ($p = 0.01$), whereas median FSIQ remained at a normal level. Beyond 30 months, deterioration disappeared in terms of DC whereas median FSIQ decreased ($p = 0.01$). Irradiation induces neuropsychologic impairment which may however be transitory especially in younger patients. Age is an important factor in brain tolerance to radiation therapy.

KEY WORDS

Brain tumors, Radiation therapy, Neuropsychologic impairment.

REFERENCES

1. BLOOM (H.J.G.): Intracranial tumors: response and resistance to therapeutic endeavors, 1970-1980. Int. J. Radiat. Oncol. Biol. Phys. 1982, 8, 1083-1113.
2. HOCHBERG (F.H.), and SLOTNICK (B.): Neuropsychologic impairment in astrocytoma survivors. Neurology, 1980, 30, 172-177.
3. MAIRE (J.P.), COUDIN (B.), DEMEAUX (H.) et al.: Incidence probable de l'irradiation cérébrale sur l'efficience intellectuelle. Bull. Cancer 1983, 70, 275-283.
4. PICHOT (P.), and KOUROUSKY (F.): Le quotient de détérioration mentale à l'échelle Wais. Rev. Psychol. Appl. 1969, 19, 273-285.
5. WECHSLER (D.): La mesure de l'intelligence de l'adulte. 2e Ed. Presse Universitaire de France. Paris, 1961.
6. WECHSLER (D.): Echelle d'intelligence de Wechsler pour adultes, Wais. Edition du centre de psychologie appliquée. Paris, 1970.

The Tolerance of Irradiation in Children with Brain Tumour

M. PAMUCKA (°).

INTRODUCTION

Radiotherapy is the principal element in the treatment of brain tumor. Irradiation as well as very kind of treatment is the cause of different unpredictable effects. This is effect of the influence of irradiation on the brain tissues. They were damaged previously by the tumor, intracranial hypertension and surgical procedure. The widespread usage of radiotherapy, in larger and larger doses, and longer survivals of a greater number of patients are the reason for the fact that the problem of damage is one of the principal problems in radiotherapy. This is also a principal in irradiation of children's brain tumor. There are following signs of irradiation damage: dementia, deterioration, mental retardation, hormonal dysfunction (1, 2, 3). There is the atrophy in the region opposite to the tumor in the form of focus of low density in white matter which is observed in computer tomography (CT) (4, 5, 6, 7). These signs are observed in the different span of the time after treatment and in the different intensity (9, 12, 13). The damage is induced by changes and injuries of the blood vessels permeability and the blood-brain-barrier (6, 7, 8, 9, 10). The focus of necrosis in the regions of high doses when the technique of cross-fire was used in white matter in the region opposite to the tumor (5, 11). The injuries imitate the signs of tumor reccurence in the neurological examination and CT (3, 13).

The objective of this work is to describe the cases of postirradiation injuries in children with brain tumor.

MATERIALS AND METHODS

In the years 1974-1984 at the Institute of Oncology in Gliwice and in the Regional Hospital of Oncology in Opole 52 children were irradiated because of brain tumor. In this group there were: 5 cases of astrocytomas I-II, 11-gliomas III/IV, 12-ependymomas, 9-medulloblastomas, 8 cases of brain stem and 7 cases of other kinds of tumor. The age of the children was 2-15 years. Forty four children underwent a surgical procedure before radiotherapy. Twelve children were treated with the help of chemotherapy (CCNU) after radiotherapy. Forty children were irradiated on the whole brain in the doses 38-48 Gy, twelve children on the whole central nervous system (CNS) in the doses 38-42 Gy on the posterior cranial fossa and 28-32 Gy on the spinal cord. Four children did not finish radiotherapy.

The tolerance of radiotherapy was observed in 48 children who received the total planned doses. The tolerance was observed on the basis of some complications. After the end of irradiation the children were examined every 4-6 weeks. The examination consisted of anamnesis and neurological examination with eyeground one and blood morphology.

The complications after irradiation were divided into three groups :

Group 1: The complications which were observed at the time of irradiation and one month after. These were depilation, leukopenia, thrombocytopenia, nausea, vomiting.

Group 2: The complications which were observed at the time of one year after irradiation. There were depilation, anorexia, anaemia, increase of intracranial hypertension.

Group 3: The complications which were observed after the end of the first year. This was only a partial depilation.

(°) Regional Hospital of Oncology, Dep. of Radiotherapy, Opole, Poland.

M. Chatel, F. Darcel and J. Pecker (eds.), Brain Oncology. ISBN-13: 978-94-010-8003-3

RESULTS

Group 1: Leukopenia- was observed in five children. The lowest number of leukocytes was 1800. The leukopenia come back to normal after the break of radiotherapy and administering the typical drugs. Thrombocytopenia was observed in four children. The lowest number of thrombocytes was 60 000/mm^3. The thrombocytopenia came back to normal after the break of irradiation and administering the typical drugs.

Nausea and vomiting were in ten children after the firt days of treatment. These signs disappeared after increasing the dose of Dexamethasone and administering antiemetic drugs.

Depilation was observed in all children in the region of irradiated fields.

Group 2: Anorexia appeared periodically in all children. It started at the time of the second or third month since the end of radiotherapy and administering of Dexamethasone. The typical signs were like in hypoacidity: aversion to eating breakfast, to food with milk and sugar. These signs were decreased after the juice without sugar regular administering. The appetite returned to normal after four to six months after radiotherapy. The children who were treated with adjuvant chemotherapy (CCNU) one year after irradiation had the signs of anorexia from 3-4 to 15-18 months after radiotherapy. These childrens had been administered the appetite drugs.

Anaemia appeared in four children in within 2-3 months time after irradiation. It was in the time of anorexia. These signs disappeared after hematopoetical drugs were administered. Anaemia appeared in eight out of twelve children who received chemotherapy. Anaemia with leukopenia and thrombocytopenia were observed in these children.

These children had been administered hematopoetical drugs and blood. The depilation disappeared at the end of the first year after radiotherapy in all except five children.

Increasing of intracranial pressure was in three children.

A.S. - A two-years-old girl, previously she had surgery and then radiotherapy because of the cerebellar tumor - astrocytoma I/II. She received 38 Gy in 4 weeks on the cerebellum.

Unexpected loss of conscience with convulsions and vomiting followed in twelfth week after radiotherapy. Stasis was on the eyeground. In the neurological examination was found four members paresis to be the strongest on left, without any contact.

In CT of brain there were: cortical atrophy in the frontal regions, a region of low density in the posterior cranial fossa, edema of the whole brain and extension of ventricular system.

This child was subjected to surgery procedure. In the time of craniotomy necrosis was found. Histopathological examination: necrosis. The girl was treated with high doses of Dexamethasone and antiepileptic drugs. She was getting better. Actually, three years after radiotherapy we stated the residual paresis on the left, mental retardation of about two years and on the eyeground atrophy after stasis. Epilepsy was not found.

B.C. - Eight-years-old girl. Tumor of the brain in the right parieto-occipital region. She had surgery procedure. Histopathological examination was glioma malignum. She was irradiated in the dose 40 Gy on the whole brain plus 10 Gy on the tumor bed in five weeks. An unexpected loss of consciousness with vomiting and epilepsy appeared in the twelfth week after radiotherapy. On the eyeground there was stasis. In neurological examination: no contact, without paresis. In CT of brain: area of low density in the left parieto-occipital region, edema of the whole brain. The state of this girl was better after Dexamethasone and antiepileptic drugs administering. This girl is now in a good condition, three and half years after radiotherapy. She has no signs of neurological or mental damage. Her eyeground is right.

J.R. - Two and half-years-old girl. She was treated because of brain tumor in the region of the third ventricle. She has not surgery procedure but received radiotherapy in the doses 40 Gy on the tumor bed during four weeks. Next she had administered chemotherapy : CCNU in the doses 120 mg/m^2 every six weeks for one year.

An unexpected loss of consciousness with vomiting and epilepsy occurred in the time of ten weeks after radiotherapy. She was without contact. On the eyeground there was stasis. CT examination: edema of the whole brain, the area of low density in the midbrain and cortical atrophy in frontal regions. The child received high doses of Dexamethasone and antiepileptic drugs. She was better and chemotherapy was continued. Actually two years after radiotherapy she is well.

The cortical atrophy and areas of low density in white matter were found in CT examination of twenty children. They are without a decline in neurological examination.

Group 3: Partial depilation was observed in five children with distance of retreat.

In this group of forty eight children there was no retardation of growth and hormonal disfunction.

DISCUSSION

The cases presented in this paper can be divided into ones which concern all the patients — depilation and ones which occur in some of them. Depilation, the changes in blood, anorexia, vomiting are complications not dangerous or lasting (12).

The signs dangerous to life are ones which have been described in the three cases as the complications of group 2. These signs had similar courses in all three children: they were observed till 12 weeks after radiotherapy, they began unexpectedly with high intracranial pressure. Edema tissues of brain, cortical atrophy, areas of low density in the part opposite to the tumor were presented in CT examination. Other authors describe similar cases only without cortical atrophy (3, 5, 6, 7, 9, 13).

The treatment was similar in all cases with good effect. It corresponds to other authors (3, 11).

The areas of low density in the region opposite to the tumor or in the tumor bed probably was the effect of brain damage after a long time of high intracranial pressure before surgery procedure. It is possible that the distribution of the expansional forces in the time of tumor growth is similar with the ricochet. The tissues which are damaged by the intracranial hypertension and anaemisation because of pressure on the blood vessels are more sensitive to irradiation (3, 6, 7, 8, 9).

The time of the sign's occurence may be convergent with the moment of retreating Dexamethasone activity. Many authors also describe radioprotectional activity of Dexamethasone (3, 11).

The conclusion drawn from these observations in following: the regions opposite to the tumor should be irradiated with lower doses.

SUMMARY

Fifty two children were irradiated in the years 1974-1984 in our hospital. The tolerance of radiotherapy was observed in 48 children on the basis of developing complications. The complications after irradiation were divided into three groups. In the time of 2-3 months after radiotherapy the increase of intracranial pressure was observed in three children. In CT examination there was a cortical atrophy in the region opposite to the tumor and edema. There was no reccurrence of tumor. The children were treated mainly with high doses of Dexamethasone and antiepileptic drugs. These children are in good health condition after 1-2 years time.

KEY WORDS

Brain tumor in children, Radiotherapy of brain tumor, Tolerance of irradiation, Injuries after radiotherapy.

REFERENCES

1. SHELINE (G.E.): Radiation Therapy of Primary Tumors: Seminars in Oncology, **1**: 29-42 (1975).
2. PAMUCKA (M.): Radioterapia Pierwotnych Nowotorow Mozgu w Materiale Instytutu Onkologii wGliwicach w latach 1960-1976 (Instytut Onkologii-Gliwice, 1981).
3. WARA (W.M.): Radiation Therapy for Brain Tumors: Cancer, **55**: 2291-2295 (1985).

4. HOHWIELER (M.L.), LO (T.C.M.), SILVERMAN (M.L.), FREIDBERG (S.R.): Brain Necrosis after Radiotherapy for Primary Intracerebral Tumor: Neurosurgery: **1**: 67-74, 1986.

5. MARKS (J.E.), BAGLAN (R.J.), PRASSAD (S.C.), BLANK (W.F.): Cerebral Radionecrosis: Incidence and Risk in Relation to Dose, Time, Fractionation and Volume: Int. J. Radiation oncology Biol. Phys.: **7**: 243-252, 1981.

6. CAVENESS (W.F.), KEMPER (T.L.), O'NEILL (R.R.): Delayed Vasogenic Edema Following Irradiation of the Monkey Brain: Dynamic of Brain Edema: Springer Verlag, 1976.

7. ZÜLCH (K.J.): Roentgen Sensitivity of Cerebral Tumours and So-called Late Irradiation Necrosis of the Brain: Acta Radiologica: **8**: 92-109, 1969.

8. CERVOS-NAVARRO (J.), CHRISTMANN (U.), SASAKI (S.): An Ultrastructural Substrate for the Resolution of Post-Irradiation Brain Edema: Dynamics of Brain Edema Springer Verlag-Berlin, 1976.

9. LIEBERMAN (A.), RANSOHOFF (J.): Treatment of Primary Brain Tumors: Medical Clinics of North America: 63/4, 835-848, 1979.

10. REINHOLD (H.S.), HOPEWELL (J.W.): Late Changes in the Architecture of Blood Vessels of the Rat Brain After Irradiation: British Journal of Radiology: **53**: 693-696, 1980.

11. SOFFIETTI (R.), SCIOLLA (R.), GIORDANA (M.T.), VASARIO (E.), SCHIFFER (D.): Delayed Adverse Effects after Irradiation of Gliomas: Clinico-Pathological Analysis: International Symposium of Brain Tumor Therapy-London, 1984.

12. HOFFMAN (W.F.), LEVIN (V.A.), WILSON (C.B.): Evaluation of Malignant Glioma Patients During the Postirradiation Period: J. Neurosurg: **50**: 624-628, 1979.

13. EYSTER (E.F.), NIELSEN (S.L.), SHELINE (G.E.), WILSON (C.B.): Cerebral Radiation Necrosis Simulating a Brain Tumor: **39**: 267-271, 1974.

Human High-Grade Gliomas Grafted into Nude Mice: A Model System to Compare Radiotherapy Schedules

M. BAMBERG (°), M. STUSCHKE (°), V. BUDACH (°), H. SACK (°), S. LUFEN (°).

OVERWIEW OF PREVIOUS WORK

Xenografts in nude mice allow the study of intrinsic sensitivity of tumor cells to cytotoxic therapies in a threedimensional assembly, similar to that in the original tumor. The good correlation between the chemotherapeutic response of xenografts and the tumor in the patient, which validates the model, has been previously outlined (1). The present study was performed in order to evaluate the response of xenografted astrocytomas to different fractionation regimes and to estimate the repair factor a/b.

Between 1980-1985, eight high grade gliomas were successfully xenografted into nude mice. The overall take rate was 5%. All tumors were observed for more than 10 passages (11-36). The xenografts were compared with the original tumors with regard to the DNA content by impulse cytophotometry, histomorphology, karyotype and expression of glial fibrillary acid protein at different passages. An excellent agreement with the original tumor was observed for all tumors from passage 1 to 20.

MATERIALS AND METHODS

Two human astrocytomas Kernohan Grade III-IV, which were established as xenografts in february 1982 (ME) and august 1983 (LI), were used for these experiments. The ME tumor cells are glial fibrillary acid protein (GFAP) — positive (see Fig. 3), while the LI cells do not express this astrocyte specific intermediate filament. ME is a diploid, LI a tetraploid tumor line. Both attributes remained remarkably constant during maintenance of the tumors in nu/nu mice (Fig. 3, 4). The established xenografts were implanted as fragments of 2 mm diameter subcutaneously through an incision at the level of the milk ridge behind the foreleg into 6 weeks old, male nu/nu mice of an outbred NMRI strain. When the tumors reached a volume of 80-240 mm^3, the tumor bearing mice were randomized to the different treatment groups, which consisted of 8-12 animals. The irradiations were performed with a cobalt source at a dose rate of 2.9 Gy/min. Tumors of two mice were irradiated simultaneously in the holding device, shown in Fig. 1. The γ-ray beam was sharply confined by a lead block near the target and a plastic tray near the skin was used to reduce the region of dose build-up in the tumor. To induce hypoxia in the tumor cells, an occlusive plastic clamp was applied to the base of the tumor 10 min. before treatment. Mice were anaesthetized during irradiation by i.p. administration of Ketamine-hydrochloride (150 μg/10 g animal weight) and xylazine-hydrochlorate (100 μg/10 g animal weight) 2 min. before treatment. To construct the growth curve for tumors of a treatment group from the volume versus time data, the median time for reaching a multiple of the initial volume (VO) was estimated by the product-limit method for censored data according to Kaplan and Meier (2). Error bars indicate the region between the 25th and 75th percentile of the distribution of times needed by the tumors in a treatment group for reaching the volume endpoint.

RESULTS

The regrowth curves for the LI and ME xenografts after irradiation are shown in Fig. 5-7, 10, 11 and 12. In the first experiment, the effect of three fractionation schedules on the tumor growth (LI, passage 16) was tested at three dose levels (Fig. 5-9). Endpoint was the growth delay, which can be

(°) Dep. of Radiotherapy, West German Tumour Center, University of Essen, Hufelandstr. 55. D-4300 Essen-1.

M. Chatel, F. Darcel and J. Pecker (eds.), Brain Oncology. ISBN-13: 978-94-010-8003-3

defined as the difference of median times needed by tumors in the treatment and control group, to reach a multiple of the pretreatment volume (VO). For LI, the growth delay at 2 × VO was chosen. Using a recursive procedure, polynomas up to the 2nd degree were fitted to the mean growth delay per fraction versus dose per fraction data. For all fractionation schedules, neither an absolute value nor the b — coefficient became significant. In Fig. 8, the best straight line, passing through the origin was drawn through the cumulated data of all fractionation schedules in this experiment. The slope ($a = 3.74 + 0.22$ d/Gy) was not significantly different from the slopes of lines, fitted to the data of the individual fractionation schedules (1 fraction: $a = 3{,}80 \pm 0.30$ d/Gy; 3 fractions: $A = 3.35 \pm 0.35$ d/Gy; 6 fractions: $a = 3.88 \pm 0.40$ d/Gy). A second experiment was performed with the tumor line LI (passage 21), to confirm the result, that no dose sparing occurs between the fractionation schedules and to determine the oxygen enhancement ratio (Fig. 10-13). Again no curvature was observed in the dose — response relationship. The mean growth delay per fraction agreed within experimental error in the 1 × 2.5 Gy and 2 × 2.5 Gy treatment group for clamped tumors or in the 1 × 1.7 Gy and 2 × 1.7 Gy treatment group for unclamped tumors (Fig. 13). This yields a proof of the hypothesis that different dose fractions in a radiation series are isoeffective, which underlies the a - b model (3). The oxygen enhancement ratio (OER) can be estimated by the quotient of slopes of the oxic ($a = 5.91 \pm 1.0$ d/Gy) and anoxic ($a = 3.15 \pm 0.25$ d/Gy) dose — response relation: $OER = 1.88 + 0.32$. For ME tumors at passage 32, the dose dependence in the 3 fractions schedule is plotted in Fig. 14. Again, a linear dose dependence was found (slope: $a = 0.86 \pm 0.17$ d/Gy). Because less then 50% of the animals reached the endpoint in the 1 fraction and 6 fractions regimes, these data are not recorded here and experiments will be repeated.

DISCUSSION

Two xenografted human tumors of the same histology, astrocytoma Kernohan Grade III-IV, which differ in DNA content and GFAP- expression, showed different absolute radiosensitivities. The LI tumor line was about 4.3 times more radiosensitive than ME, but had a longer volume doubling time (5.4 days) than ME (2.7 days). Comparing the radiosensitivity during maintenance of the xenograft LI, no gross changes were observed (unclamped tumors: $a = 6.8 + 1.0$ d/Gy at passage 8; $a = 5.9 \pm 1.2$ d/Gy at passage 21). The small difference between the slopes in the dose response curves for clamped LI tumors at passage 16 and 21 (see Fig. 8, 13) is probably due to a greater median pretreatment tumor volume in the later experiment (190 vs 100 mm^3). Therefore it can be concluded, that different xenografts exhibit individual responsiveness to radiotherapy, which remains nearly constant during maintenance. In the investigated dose range, which was limited by the median life span of the nu/nu mice after treatment, no curvature was observed in the dose response function. The slopes of the dose response relationship of the different fractionation regimes (Fig. 8) agreed within experimental error. This does not exclude, that the dose response curve may be upward bended for higher doses per fraction but indicates, that the emploied xenografts show no repair of sublethal radiation damage for doses per fraction, clinically used (0.6 - 5 Gy). Lindenberger et al. (4) came to the same result for head and neck carcinoma xenografts and Wheldon et al. (5) for neuroblastoma spheroids. It is concluded that hyperfractionation, which maximize the dose sparing effect for late reacting critical organs with a/b ratios below 7 Gy (6, 7, 8) might increase the therapeutic ratio.

KEY WORDS

Fractionated Radiotherapy, Repair, Human gliomas, Growth delay, Nude mice.

REFERENCES

1. SHORTHOUSE (A.J.), SMYTH (J.F.), STEEL (G.G.), ELLISON (M.), MILLS (J.), PECKHAM (M.J.): The human tumour xenograft, a valid model in experimental chemotherapy? Br. J. Surg. 67, 715-722, 1980.
2. KAPLAN (E.L.), MEIER (P.): Nonparametric estimation of incomplete observations. J. Amer. Statist. Assoc. 53, 457-481, 1958.
3. THAMES (H.D.), WITHERS (H.R.): Test of equal effect per fraction and estimation of initial clonogen number in microcolony assays of survival after fractionated data. Br. J. Radiol. 53, 1071-1077, 1980.

4. LINDENBERGER (J.), HERMEKIND (H.), KUMMERMEHR (J.), DENEKAMP (J.): Response of human tumour xenografts to fractionated X-irradiation. Radiotherapy and Oncology, 6, 15-27, 1986.

5. WHELDON (T.E.), LIVINGSTONE (A.), WILSON (L.), O'DONOGHUE (J.), GREGOR (A.): The radiosensitivity of human neuroblastoma cells estimated from regrowth curves of multicellular tumour spheroids. Br. J. Radiol. 58, 661-664, 1985.

6. FOWLER (D.Sc.): Dose response curves for organ function and cell survival. Br. J. Radiol. 56, 497-500, 1983.

7. BARENDSEN (G.W.): Dose fractionation, dose rate and iso-effect relationships for normal tissue responses. Int. J. Radiat. Oncol. Biol. Phys. 8: 1981-1997, 1981.

8. HORNSEY (S.), MORRIS (C.C.), MYERS (R.): The relationship between fractionation and total dose for X-ray induced brain damage. Int. J. Radiat. Oncol. Biol. Phys. 7: 223-227, 1981.

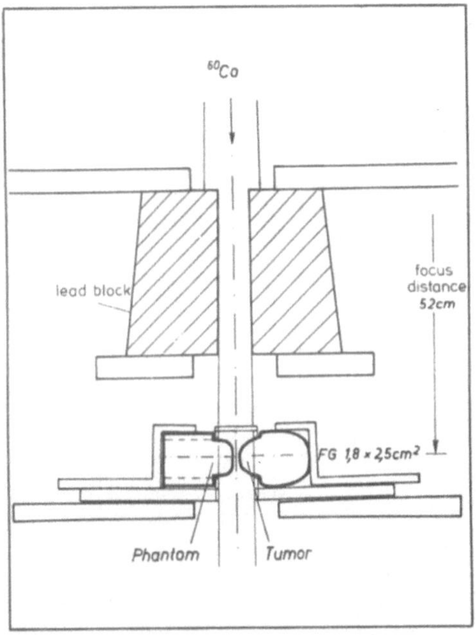

FIGURE 1. Equipment for the irradiation of nude mice at the cobalt unit.

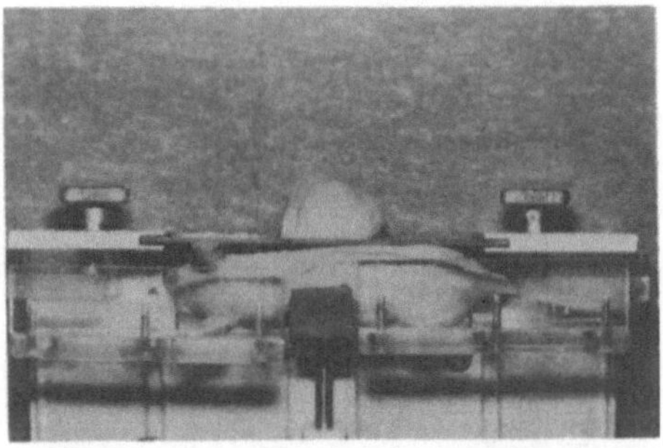

FIGURE 2. Holding device for an anaesthetized mouse during irradiation.

FIGURE 3a. Histology of the astrocytoma Grade III-IV xenograft ME at passage 3 (fig. 3a) and passage 21 (fig. 3b); GFAP - staining; 350x.

FIGURE 3b.

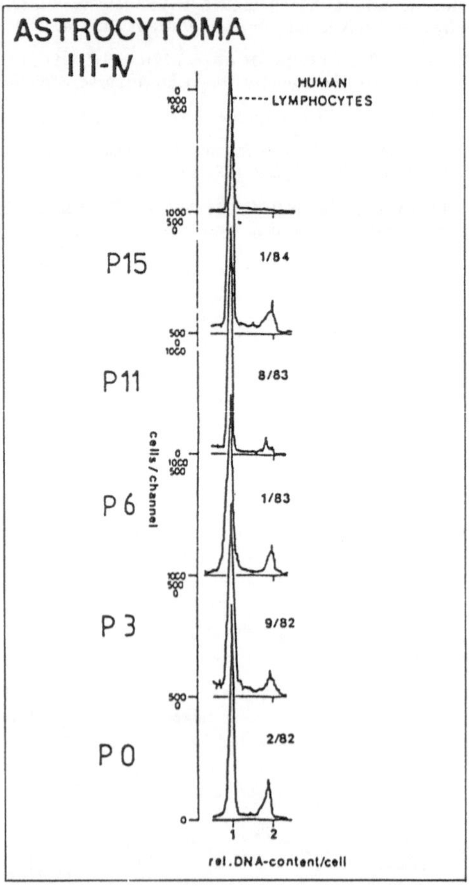

FIGURE 4. Histograms for the DNA content during maintenance of the xenograft ME on nude mice.

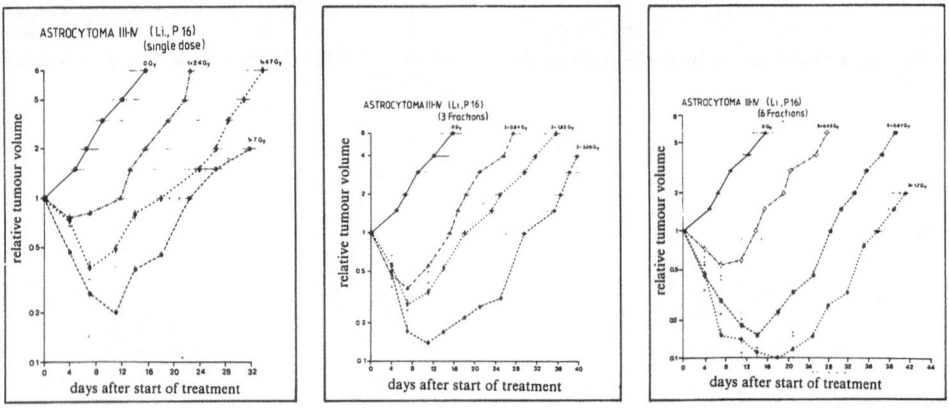

FIGURE 5-6-7. Growth curves of the xenograft LI (human astrocytoma Kernohan Grade III-IV) for different fractionation schedules. Tumors were clamped 10 min. before irradiation. Time between fractions: 5 h.

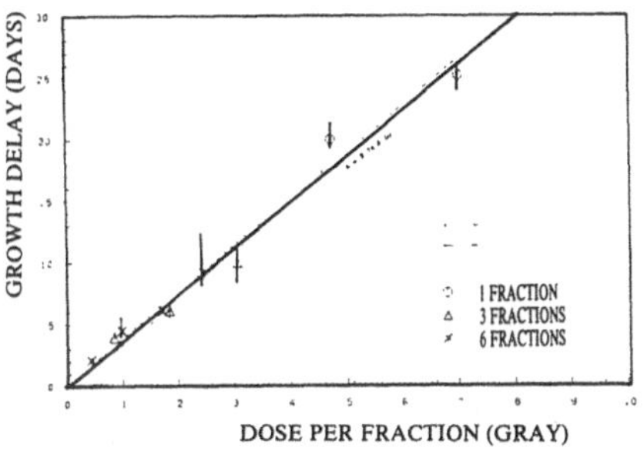

FIGURE 8. Plot of the mean growth delay per fraction versus dose per fraction for the data shown in Fig. 5-7.

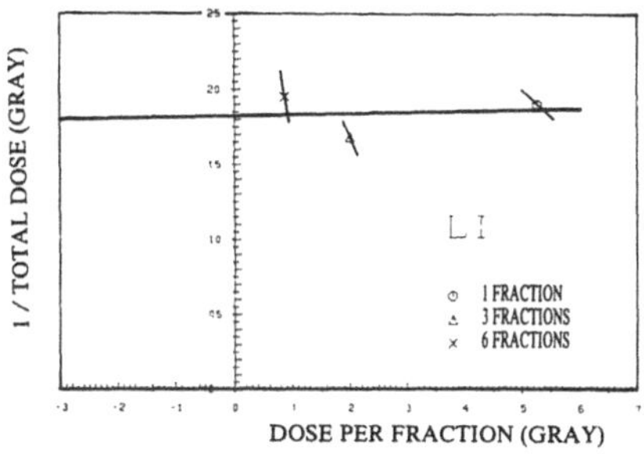

FIGURE 9. Plot of the reciprocal total dose for a growth delay of 20 days against dose per fraction. The slope of the regression line is not significantly different from zero.

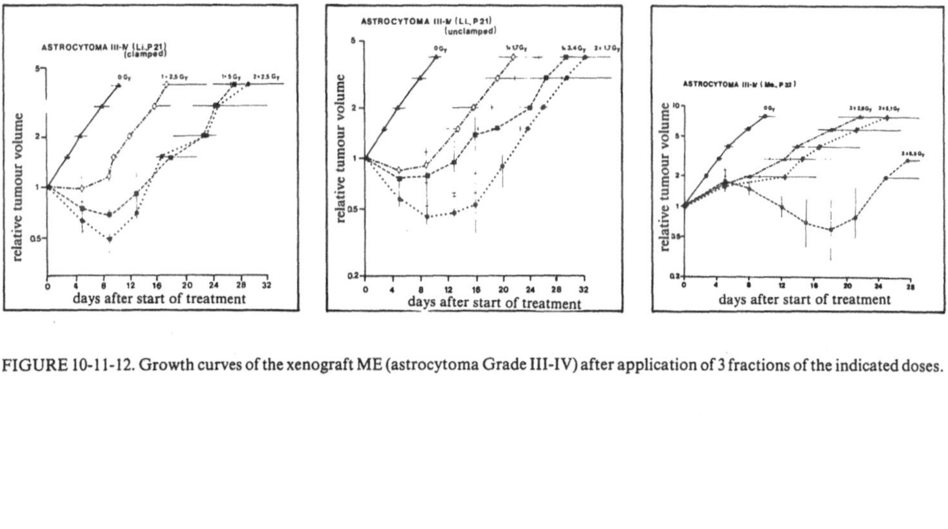

FIGURE 10-11-12. Growth curves of the xenograft ME (astrocytoma Grade III-IV) after application of 3 fractions of the indicated doses.

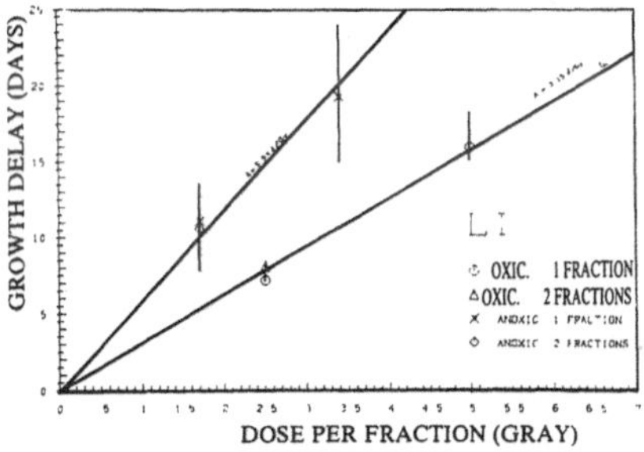

FIGURE 13. Effective dose-response curve for clamped and unclamped LI tumors.

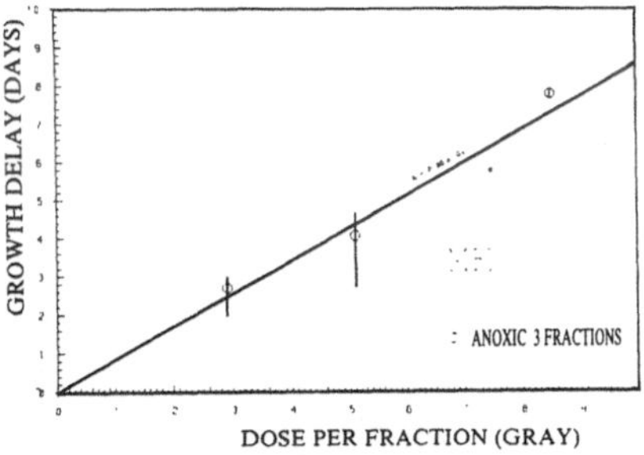

FIGURE 14. Effective dose-response curve for clamped ME tumors.

Pharmacology of the Hypoxic cell Radiosensitizers Ro 03-8799 and SR 2508 in Human Gliomas and Brain Tissue

H.F.V. NEWMAN (°), N.M. BLEEHEN (°), P. WORKMAN (°) and R. WARD (°).

In the treatment of cerebral gliomas, the major problem is that of local tumour control. The role of surbery is inevitably limited by considerations of subsequent neurological deficit. The efficacy of radiotherapy may be limited by a number of factors which include residual tumour bulk and the radiation tolerance of the surrounding brain. A further limiting factor for radiotherapy may be tumour hypoxia; areas of necrosis are often seen in gliomas, suggesting that there may well be adjacent hypoxic and therefore radioresistant cells. Using the 5-nitroimidazole hypoxic cell radiosensitizer metronidazole, it has been shown in a randomised, controlled trial that glioblastoma can be sensitized to radiation in vivo (1). Unfortunately only a few doses could be given because of toxicity. This limitation necessitated using a suboptimal radiation schedule, and the overall results were therefore not improved over those achievable with conventional fractionation. Nevertheless, the principle is established, justifying the investigation of new, less-toxic nitroimidazoles as radiosensitizers for gliomas.

Misonidazole, the first 2-nitroimidazole to be extensively tested, also proved toxic. Peripheral neuropathy limited the total dose to 12 g/m^2, and randomized trials in glioblastoma showed no benefit for its use (2). Two newer agents, Ro 03-8799 and SR 2508, have a much more favourable toxicity spectrum. Furthermore, their toxicities are different from each other, allowing the possibility of combining the agents. It is important however, to attempt to establish the penetration of these drugs into gliomas and adjacent brain, and this paper presents our experience using these two agents.

BACKGROUND: Ro 03-8799 and SR 2508.

Ro 03-8799 is a basic, lipophilic 2-nitroimidazole, with a plasma elimination half-life of around 5 hours. The toxicity consists of an acute syndrome, variously comprising of flushing, sweating, dizziness, drowsiness, mental detachment and nausea. The maximum single dose is 1 g/m^2; fifteen such doses are tolerable, and up to twenty doses of 0.75 g/m^2 may be tolerated. Peripheral neuropathy does not occur. It is more electron-affinic than misonidazole and therefore a more efficient radiosensitizer by a factor of 2-3 in experimental systems (3). In a series of 8 patients given 1 g/m^2 Ro 03-8799 prior to neurosurgery, mean astrocytoma concentration was 18.6 μg/g, and mean brain concentration was 25.1 μg/g. Tissue/plasma ratios were 305% and 372% respectively (4).

SR 2508 is a neutral, hydrophilic 2-nitroimidazole. It is excluded from rodent brain, and would thus be expected to be less neurotoxic. In man it has an elimination half-life of 5 hours. Single doses of 3.7 g/m^2 are tolerable, but peripheral neuropathy limits the total dose of 36-40 g/m^2. Its sensitizing efficacy on a molar basis is equivalent to that of misonidazole, but clearly much higher doses can be given.

When administered together, there appears to be no potentiation of the clinical toxicities of these agents. The acute Ro 03-8799 syndrome is not exacerbated, nor does the peripheral neuropathy of SR 2508 appear earlier than expected. Tolerance has not yet been reached, at twelve doses of 0.75 g/m^2 Ro 03-8799 with 2.5 g/m^2 SR 2508, dosing thrice weekly for one month. Two of three patients at this doses developed a temporary peripheral neuropathy WHO grade 1. There was no adverse pharmacological interaction.

(°) University and Medical Research Council Clinical Oncology Unit, Addenbrooke's Hospital, Cambridge, UK.

M. Chatel, F. Darcel and J. Pecker (eds.), Brain Oncology. ISBN-13: 978-94-010-8003-3

GLIOMA AND BRAIN PHARMACOLOGY: Ro 03-8799 with SR 2508.

The drugs were administered together during neurosurgery for biopsy or resection of suspected gliomas, prior informed consent being obtained from the patients in all cases. The agents were reconstituted in 50 ml of 0.9% saline, and infused intravenously over 10 minutes. Because the availability of the agents was limited, a dose of 0.5 g/m^2 of each drug was used. The time of biopsy was determined by the contraints of the surgery, but every attempt was made to time the infusion so that early (20-30 minute) concentrations could be assessed. All patients had received dexamethasone pre-operatively, and received 100-200 ml of 20% mannitol with the anaesthetic. (The time of administration of the radiosensitizers however was always at least 30 minutes after anaesthesia induction). Blood samples were taken to determine plasma concentrations, and samples of tumour, brain or csf were immediately frozen in solid CO_2 to inhibit any drug metabolism prior to analysis. Nitroimidazole assay was by reversed-phase high performance liquid chromatography.

RESULTS

There was no adverse reactions to the administration of radiosensitizers. Tissue and plasma concentrations from eleven patients are available. The results are shown in Table 1; these have been normalized to a clinically relevant dose of 0.75 g/m^2 Ro 03-8799 with 2 g/m^2 SR 2508.

TABLE I

Concentrations of Ro 03-8799 and SR 2508 (± S.D.) in cerebral lymphoma (1), glioma, brain and CSF normalized to a dose of 0.75 g/m^2 Ro 03-8799 with 2 g/m^2 SR 2508. Tissue/plasma ratios in parentheses.

Tissue	Ro 03-879 μg/g (tissue/ Plasma ratio)	SR 2508 μg/g (tissue/ Plasma ratio)
Glioma : All samples (n = 11)	23.7 ± 18 (275%)	40.6 ± 32 (40%)
Glioma : Clinically viable (n = 7)	33.3 ± 17 (382%)	57 ± 45 (48%)
Glioma : Clinically Frank Necrosis (n = 4)	6.0 ± 3 (63%)	12.3 ± 7.2 (23%)
Normal Brain (n = 2)	29.5, 34.4 (289%)	12.2 50.4 (9%) (33%)
C.S.F. (n = 1)	4.8 (23%)	0.36 (1.1%)

DISCUSSION

It can be seen that in this small series there is a considerable range of results, and this may be due both to patho-physiological processes in the patients, and to experimental artefact. Penetration of the drugs may be affected by such factors and regional tumour vasculature, blood flow and cerebral oedema. There may also be in-vivo drug metabolism in the tumour. Surgical sampling inevitably only assesses a part of any tumour, and surgery may itself interfere with drug access. Furthermore, despite the most rigorous handling of tissue samples, ex-vivo metabolism may occur before the sample is frozen. Nevertheless, taking all eleven tumour samples the mean concentration for Ro 03-8799 is 23.7 μg/g ± 18, (S.D.), with a mean tumour/plasma ratio of 275%. For brain tissue, the ratio is 289%. The concentration of this basic lipophilic agent in tissue over plasma is as expected, and consistent with previous experience. Interestingly, examining those four samples showing gross necrotic liquefaction separately, the concentration of Ro 03-8799 is 6.0 + 3, (S.D.), with a tumour/plasma ratio of 63%, indicating poorer penetration into these areas.

For SR 2508, the mean concentration in eleven tumour samples is 40.6 μg/g ± 32, (S.D.), with a mean tumour/plasma ratio of 40%. For brain tissue, the ratio is 21%. In the four very necrotic samples, the mean concentration of SR 2508 is 12.3 μg/g ± 7.2, (S.D.), for a 23% tumour/plasma ratio. SR 2508 is exhibiting the partial exclusion from the nervous system, as expected for a hydrophilic drug. Indeed, it is evident from Table 1 that whatever the absolute drug levels, the tissue/plasma ratio is always lower for SR 2508 than for Ro 03-8799. Because it is possible to administer a relatively large individual dose of SR 2508 however, significant absolute drug concentrations can still be achieved.

Clearly it will be important to consolidate these early results with more samples, but it is also important to ask what benefit might be expected from the mean radiosensitizer concentrations achieved in this series. Prediction from experimental data is difficult, but assuming that SR 2508 has similar sensitizing efficacy to misonidazole, while Ro 03-8799 is around 2.5 times more efficient, than based on experimental data (3), a single-dose enhancement ratio of 1.5 would seem possible. The limits of tolerability for multiple administrations of the combination have not yet been reached. Based on single-agent data, and the lack of adverse interaction, it is anticipated that at least 18 doses of 0.75 g/m^2 Ro 03-8799 with 2 g/m^2 SR 2508 will be acceptable. It would therefore appear illogical to consider single-agent administration in any further clinical trials of radiosensitizers for malignant cerebral tumours.

SUMMARY

The curability of gliomas may be limited by the presence of hypoxic cells. This hypothesis is supported both by the frequent presence of necrosis in these tumours, and by the fact that metronidazole has been shown to sensitize glioblastoma in vivo. Tumour and brain concentrations achieved using two newer radiosensitizers, Ro 03-8799 and SR 2508, are presented.

Ro 03-8799 is a basic, lipophilic 2-nitroimidazole with a plasma T 1/2 β of 5 hours. The maximum single dose is limited to 1 g/m^2 because of a transient acute central nervous syndrome. Chronic toxicity does not occur. In a series of 8 patients given 1 g/m^2 Ro 03-8799 by intravenous infusion prior to neurosurgery, the mean tumour concentration was 18.6 µg/g, with a tumour/plasma mean ratio of 305%. For "normal" brain the figures were 25.1 µg/g and 372% respectively.

SR 2508 is a neutral, lipophilic 2-nitroimidazole with a T 1/2 β of 5 hours. Single doses of 3.7 g/m^2 are tolerable, but the total dose is limited to 40 g/m^2 by peripheral neuropathy. In combination with 0.75 g/m^2 Ro 03-8799, 12 twice weekly doses of 2.5 g/m^2 SR 2508 do not exceed tolerance. There is no adverse pharmacological interaction. It was therefore decided to administer these agents together during neurosurgery. A total dose of 1 g (0.5-0.75 g/m^2) of each agent was administered intravenously prio to biopsy or lobectomy, the low dose being because of limited drug availability. Eleven patients have been studied. For example, values from a patient with cerebral lymphoma receiving 0.5 g/m^2 of each agent are:

Sample	*Time From*	*Ro 03-8799 (µg/g)*			*SR 2508 (µg/g)*		
	Infusion end	*Plasma*	*Tissue*	*T/P%*	*Plasma*	*Tissue*	*T/P%*
Tumour	*0'*	*15.8*	*19.6*	*123*	*54.9*	*17.4*	*31.7*
Brain	*8'*	*7.7*	*19.7*	*258*	*38.2*	*12.6*	*33.0*

The lower concentrations of SR 2508 in brain is as predicted, while the Ro 03-8799 levels are in accordance with single agent administration. Details for all 11 patients will be presented, and their significance for radiotherapy discussed.

KEY WORDS

Radiosensitizers, Gliomas.

REFERENCES

1. URTASUN (R.C.) et al.: Radiation and high-dose metronidazole in supratentorial glioblastomas. New Engl. J. Med. 244, 1364-7 (1976).
2. BLEEHEN (N.M.): The Cambridge glioma trial of misonidazole and radiation therapy with associated pharmacokinetic studies. Cancer Clin. Trials 3: 267 (1980).
3. WILLIAMS (M.V.) et al.: In vivo assessment of basic 2-nitroimidazole radiosensitizers. Br. J. Cancer. 46, 127 (1982).
4. ROBERTS (J.T.) et al.: A clinical phase 1 toxicity study of Ro 03-8799: plasma, urine, tumour and normal brain pharmacokinetics. Br. J. Radiol. 59, 698, 107-117 (1986).
5. COLEMAN (C.W.) et al.: Initial report of the phase 1 trial of hypoxic cell radiosensitizer SR 2508. Int. J. Radiat. Oncol. Biol. Phys. 10, 1749-54 (1984).
6. NEWMAN (H.F.V.) et al.: A phase 1 study of the combination of two hypoxic cell radiosensitizers, Ro 03-8799 and SR 2508: toxicity and pharmacokinetics. Int. J. Radiat. Oncol. Biol. Phys. **12**: 1113-6 (1986).

Antibody-Guided Irradiation Therapy for Cases of Neoplastic Meningitis

H.B. COAKHAM (°), A.G. DAVIES (°), R.B. RICHARDSON (°), S.P. BOURNE (°),
J.T. KEMSHEAD (°°), J. FABRE (°°°),
J.P. MACH (°°°°), S. CARREL (°°°°),
H. ECKERT (°°°°°) and J.A. BULLIMORE (°°°°°).

INTRODUCTION

Over recent years we have been studying the possibility of targeting radiolabelled monoclonal antibodies to human brain tumours in vivo. This work began with the development of panels of monoclonal antibodies for use in the diagnosis of brain tumour biopsies and cerebrospinal fluid infiltrates (1). Certain of these antibodies were then chosen for use in vivo, labelled with I-131.

When such immunoconjugates are administered intravenously to athymic mice bearing xenografts of human neural tumours, specific antibody targeting can be demonstrated. In these experiments a control antibody labelled differently with I-125 was also employed. Not only were good tumour to normal tissue ratios obtained but true localisation of the specific antibody could be demonstrated (2, 3). Further studies of immunolocalisation in humans with neuroblastoma or glioma showed that tumour could be imaged scintigraphically (4, 5). However, when control antibodies were used, true specificity of uptake was difficult to demonstrate and it was found that a relatively low percentage of the injected dose (per gram) gained access to the tumour following intravenous administration (6). It is likely that this approach can be optimised with the introduction of new antibodies, the use of antibody fragments, modifications of the blood-tumour barrier, and advances in the immunochemistry labelling.

Whilst attempting to solve some of these problems, we are also studying the effects of radiolabelled antibody given directly into the cerebrospinal fluid, and the cases of diffuse neoplasia within the CSF pathways. The direct administration of therapeutic immunoconjugates into body cavities containing tumour has already been attempted with respected to the pleural, pericardial and peritoneal cavities (7). The CSF compartment is ideal for trials of intracavity targeted therapy since it is a less viscous medium and has a natural circulation.

MATERIALS AND METHODS

Clinical Cases

Five patients have been studied, suffering from pineocytoma, CNS teratoma, B-cell non-Hodgkin's lymphoma, medulloblastoma and melanoma. Each case had initial therapy to the primary lesion with good response and later relapsed with evidence of diffuse disease within, or adjacent to CSF pathways. Each case had either failed on conventional therapy or their referring clinicians felt that no further treatment was possible. The cases are described in Table 2 and in the case history below (see Results).

Monoclonal Antibodies

The monoclonal antibodies were highly tumour specific and reacted negatively or minimally with normal tissues. In each case the appropriate target antigen was demonstrated on CSF tumour cells or operative biopsy.

(°) Departments of Neurosurgery and Medical Physics, Frenchay Hospital, Bristol, UK. (°°) ICRF Oncology Laboratory, Institute of Child Health, London, UK. (°°°) Blond-McIndoe Institute, East Grinstead, UK. (°°°°) Ludwig Institute for Cancer Research, Lausanne Branch, 1066 Epalinger, Switzerland. (°°°°°) Radiotherapy and Oncology Centre, Bristol Royal Infirmary, Bristol, UK.

M. Chatel, F. Darcel and J. Pecker (eds.), Brain Oncology. ISBN-13: 978-94-010-8003-3

In each case, an Ommaya reservoir on lumbar CSF infusion chamber was inserted and an initial tracer study carried out using small amounts of specific and control antibody, radiolabelled with I-131 and I-125 respectively in an attempt to demonstrate in vivo specificity and study biodistribution and kinetics (Table 1).

TABLE 1

C.S.F. Radioimmunotherapy Trial - Protocol

1. Case selection: disseminated disease, failure on conventional therapy.
2. Immunostaining of C.S.F. cells or biopsy to show appropriate antigen.
3. Insertion of Ommaya reservoir or lumbar infusion chamber.
4. Thyroid blockade.
5. Tracer study: for assessment of specificity and biodistribution of conjugate
   a) administration of: specific Ab - ^{131}I. 1 mCi
      control Ab - ^{125}I. 1 mCi
   b) scintigraphic imaging
   c) dual channel external gamma counting
   d) regular samples of C.S.F., blood, urine, for gamma counting.
6. Therapy injection: 24-45 mCi ^{131}I-specific Ab (dexamethasone over).
   a) scintigraphic imaging and further biodistribution studies
   b) whole body radiation counting.
7. Follow-up: clinical, radiological and C.S.F. cells / chemistry.

About one week later intrathecal therapy was given using the specific antibody labelled with a high dose of I-131 (Table 2 shows further details).

TABLE 2

Antibody-guided Irradiation: Radiation doses and Results

Case	Diagnosis	Antibody	Radionuclide	Dose mCi	Side effects*	Results
1	Pineocytoma	UJ181.4	^{131}I	24	minimal	Improvement and remission (22 months)**
2	Teratoma	UJ181.4	^{131}I	11	minimal	Died 6 weeks
3	Lymphoma	F8-11-13	^{131}I	43	minimal	Neurological improvement but died 12 months of systemic disease
4	Medulloblastoma	UJ181.4	^{131}I	45	minimal	Improvement and remission (8 months)
5	Melanoma	Mel-14	^{131}I	38	minimal	Improvement with resolution of tumour on CT scan (5 months)

* Mild meningism or perineal paraesthesias ** August 1986

RESULTS

Case Reports

Case 1: A 62 year old man with widespread deposits from a pineocytoma has shown a dramatic and sustained response to intrathecal radio-antibody UJ181.4 (1), remaining in remission at 22 months. Pre-operatively he had been semi-comatose and obtunded prior to therapy but was able to go home three weeks later. At the time of writing he is mentally lucid, having gained 12 Kg in weight and with no evidence of neoplastic cells in the CSF.

Case 2: A child of 3 years and 6 months with an undifferentiated teratoma failed to respond to therapy with UJ181.4 and died of intrathecal disease. There was a complete block in the mid dorsal theca over several segments which meant that antibody could not circulate effectively, or gain access to the centre of this lesion. Target antigen was present on biopsies of the original posterior fossa tumour but there were no CSF cells available for current testing. Also the dose of radiation given was rather low.

Case 3: A 55 year old male presented with a intracerebral B-cell lymphoma which responded to therapy but later recurred in the CSF pathways. This condition did not respond to intrathecal metotrexate. Following treatment with I-131 labelled antibody F8-11-33 (8) he made a sustained neurological recovery over 9 months but then died of systemic recurrence. At autopsy the only evidence of CNS involvement was a small tumour deposit in the septal region of the brain.

Case 4: A 34 year old woman had surgery and radiotherapy for a posterior fossa medulloblastoma, 2 years previously and subsequently developed spinal metastases producing a marked paraparesis. Following intrathecal treatment with radio-antibody UJ181.4 she improved steadily and 6 months later is walking normally and riding a bicycle.

Case 5: A 30 year old woman had an apparently solitary melanoma deposit removed from the Sylvian region of the right hemisphere and was found to have meningeal involvement at craniotomy. Multiple deposits were seen on myelography. She received I-131-Mel 14 antibody (9) and 3 months later is clinically improved with evidence of tumour resolution on CT scan.

Therapeutic results are summarised in Table 2.

The striking feature in all cases was the appearance of the radionuclide scans 7 - 14 days after therapy. At this time any radiolabel that was unbound to tissues should have been eliminated. However, each patient showed a distinctive pattern of uptake which was appropriate to the known sites of tumour. We regard this as supportive evidence for specific binding of the therapeutic conjugates (Fig.). The half-life of gamma emissions from these scintigraphic 'hot spots' were considerably longer than the half-life in CSF and blood (Table 3).

It was not always possible to obtain evidence of specific antibody localisation in the initial tracer studies, probably due to the low amounts of radiolabel (1 mCi) and the differences in attenuation to the tissues of the I-131 and I-125. However, there was a definite trend towards more rapid appearance and higher levels of the non-specific radiolabel in the blood. The most encouraging specificity data was obtained from Case 1 where specific - non-specific antibody ratios were obtained by both external gamma counting and direct counting of CSF cells.

DISCUSSION

Neoplastic meningitis is a serious condition which often carries a survival of a few months. The clinical improvements seen in 4 of 5 cases deemed otherwise untreatable gives cause for encouragement. This is the first known use of antibody-guided irradiation for CSF pathway malignancy and must be regarded as a preliminary study. Dosimetry is complicated and accurate radiation doses have yet to be calculated. No serious side effects have been observed with the doses presently used. We would predict that this therapy would be most suitable for radiosensitive target tumours such as medulloblastomas, neuroblastomas, germinomas and parenchymal tumours of the pineal, and B-cell lymphomas. A number of these cases can relapse after total neuraxis irradiation. It would then be appropriate to use antibodies to target a short track, high energy beta emitter to tumour cells, thus sparing normal nervous tissue from additional excessive radiation.

TABLE 3

The Half-Lives (hours) of ^{131}I labelled Specific Monoclonal Antibody in Patients Following an Intrathecal Therapy Injection

Patient	Tumour (scinti-graphic data)	CSF*	Blood	Whole Body*
JJ	147	42	47	45
JP	NA	15	82	49
BV	146	75**	70	53
ADJ	NA	27	86	59
PS	115	16	92	56

* Where clearance was biphasic, the 2nd half-life has been given.
** Most of the monoclonal antibody left the intrathecal space.

KEY WORDS

Monoclonal Antibody, Intra-thecal Therapy, C.S.F. Neoplastic Meningitis.

AKNOWLEDGEMENTS

We thank Prof. D.D. Bigner for providing antibody 45.6 and Prof. N. de Tribolet for help in obtaining Mel-14.

REFERENCES

1. COAKHAM (H.B.) and BROWNELL (D.B.): Monoclonal antibodies in the diagnosis of intracranial tumours and cerebrospinal fluid neoplasia. In: Recent advances in Neuropathology - 3. Ed. J. Cavanagh. Churchill Livingstone. London, 1986, pp. 25-53.
2. JONES (D.H.), GOLDMAN (A.), GORDON (I.), PRITCHARD (J.), GREGORY (B.J.) and KEMSHEAD (J.T.): Therapeutic application of a radiolabelled monoclonal antibody in nude mice xenografted with human neuroblastoma: tumoricidal effects and distribution studies. *Int. J. Cancer* 35: 715-720, 1985.
3. BOURDON (M.M.), COLEMAN (R.A.), BLASBERG (R.G.), GROOTHIUS (D.R.) and BIGNER (D.D.): Monoclonal antibody localisation in subcutaneous and intracranial human glioma xenografts. *Anticancer Res.* 4: 133-140, 1984.
4. GOLDMAN (A.), VIVIAN (G.), GORDON (I.), PRITCHARD (J.) and KEMSHEAD (J.T.): Immunolocalisation of neuroblastoma using radiolabelled monoclonal antibody UJ13A. *J. Paediatr.* 105: 252-256, 1984.
5. RICHARDSON (R.B.), DAVIES (A.G.), BOURNE (S.P.), STADDON (G.E.), KEMSHEAD (J.T.) and COAKHAM (H.B.): Radioimmunolocalisation of primary cerebral tumours in humans. In: Biology of Brain Tumours. Eds. Walker M., Thomas D.G.T. Dordrecht Martinus Nijhoff, pp. 179-187, 1986.
6. DAVIES (A.G.), RICHARDSON (R.B.), BOURNE (S.P.), KEMSHEAD (J.T.) and COAKHAM (H.B.): Immunolocalisation of human brain tumours. In Bleehen N.M. (ed.). *Tumours of the Brain.* Berlin. Springer-Verlag. p. 83, 1986.
7. COURTENAY-LUCK (N.), EPENETOS (A.A.), HALNAN (K.E.), HOOKER (G.), HUGHES (J.M.B.), KRANSZ (T.), LAMBERT (J.), LAVENDER (P.), MacGREGOR (W.G.), McKENZIE (C.J.), MUNRO (A.), MYERS (J.), ORR (J.S.), PEARSE (E.E.), SNOOK (D.), WEEB (B.), BURCHELL (J.), DURBIN (H.), KEMSHEAD (J.T.) and TAYLOR-PAPADIMITRIOU (J.): Antibody-guided irradiation of malignant lesions: three cases illustrating a new method of treatment. *Lancet,* 1: 1441-1443, 1984.
8. DALCHAU (R.) and FABRE (J.W.): Identification with a monoclonal antibody of a predominantly B lymphocyte - specific determinant of the human leukocyte common antigen. *J. Exp. Med.* 153: 753-765, 1981.
9. CARREL (S.), ACCOLLA (R.S.), CARMAGNOLA (A.L.) and MACH (J.P.): Common Human Melanoma-associated Antigen(s) detected by monoclonal antibodies. *Cancer Res.* 40: 2523-2528, 1980.

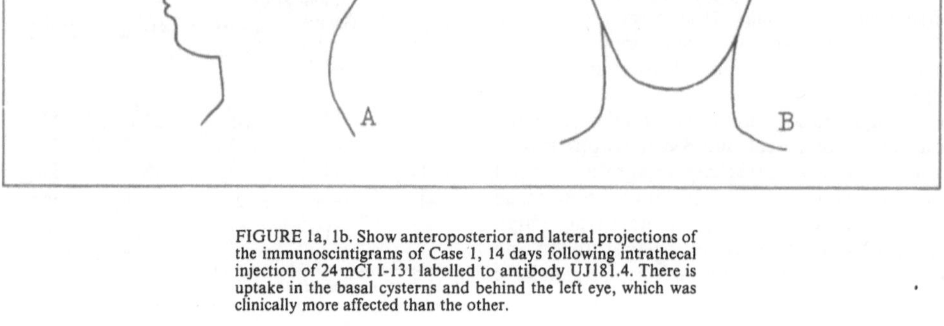

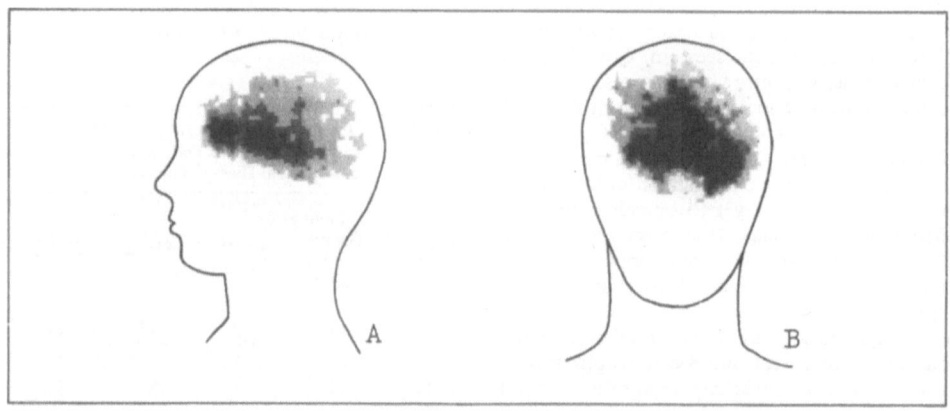

FIGURE 1a, 1b. Show anteroposterior and lateral projections of the immunoscintigrams of Case 1, 14 days following intrathecal injection of 24 mCI I-131 labelled to antibody UJ181.4. There is uptake in the basal cysterns and behind the left eye, which was clinically more affected than the other.

PART VII:
CHEMOTHERAPY AND IMMUNOTHERAPY

An In Vitro Comparative Study of BCNU, VM 26, 5-FU and Ara-A5'P in Treatment of Primary and Secondary CNS-Neoplasms; Potential Clinical Relevance and Clinical Correlations

U. BOGDAHN (°), J. ZAPF (°), H. WEBER (°), G. DÜNISCH (°).

INTRODUCTION

Patients with malignant glial tumours (glioblastoma multiforme, anaplastic astrocytoma) have a poor prognosis with median survival times approaching 50 to 60 months (25, 26); patients with metastatic brain tumours will have even shorter median survival times of approximately 4 months. In vitro assay systems have been one type of approach to improve therapeutic results in these patients, and in some systems good correlations have been demonstrated between predictive test results and clinical courses of brain tumour patients (6, 19, 24). However, discordant predictions (in vitro sensitive/in vivo resistent; in vitro resistent/in vivo sensitive) and insufficient pharmacokinetic data limited the clinical impact of these assays so far. Consequently we have correlated in vitro and in vivo pharmacokinetic data and tried to employ CNS-pharmacokinetic values as far as available in order to improve the predictive capacity of in vitro assays. In correlating sensitivity indices for individual drugs/ tumours with recurrence free intervals of patients, we think there might be another step forward to better in vitro drug sensitivity prediction for individual tumour patients (2).

As most clinical studies on chemotherapy of malignant gliomas have been performed with or compared to BCNU (25, 26), we compared the activities of VM 26, 5-FU and ARA-A5 ' P to that of BCNU. VM 26 and 5-FU currently investigated in an number of clinical studies (12, 21) - therefore we were interested in their in vitro activities. The purine analogue ARA-A5 ' P was originally designed as an antiviral agent and clinical experience is derived mainly from therapy in herpes simplex encephalitis (27). The compound penetrates the BBB (blood brain barrier) very well, resulting in CSF (cerebrospinal fluid) levels of approximately 60% of concurrant plasma levels (14). Its main modes of action are inhibition of DNA-replication and repair-systems, ribonucleotide reductase, adynelate-polymerase, and DNA-and RNA-directed DNA-synthesis; it is also incorporated into DNA (16). The purpose of the preceding paper is mainly to delineate potential activities of ARA-A5 ' P, VM 26 and 5-FU in primary and secondary CNS-neoplasms, and to estimate their possible clinical relevance by relying on clinical correlations for nitrosourea-treated patients.

MATERIAL AND METHODS

Cell cultures: Cell cultures were established from biopsies of 30 patients with primary (N = 21) and metastatic (N = 9) brain tumours (details table 1), as published elsewhere (4, 6). Throughout early passage cells were employed for experimentation (passage No. 2 to 5). Cells were characterized in vitro by cytochemical analysis (HE-stain, PTHA-stain, TRICHROME-stain, NADPH-stain, unspecific esterase and acid phosphatase), detection of glial antigens (Thy-1-20; GE 2-7; GFAP-8; S 100, fibronectin, neurone specific enolase, transferrin receptor, melanoma associated antigen, keratin - DAKOPATS; HLA-A, B, C, and -DR - BECTON-DICKINSON) and by cytogenetic analysis (5). Glial tumours expressed at least 3 of the glial antigens GFAP, S 100, GE 2, melanoma associated antigen or Thy-1. Karyotypes were always pathological, although most glial tumours displayed near diploid karyotypes.

(°) Department of Neurology, University of Würzburg, Joseph-Schneider-Str. 11, D-8700 Würzburg, FRG.

M. Chatel, F. Darcel and J. Pecker (eds.), Brain Oncology. ISBN-13: 978-94-010-8003-3

TABLE 1

Synopsis of clinical data and sensitivity indices for human brain tumour cell lines

No.	Age	Sex	Histology	Location	X-Ray	Chemotherapy	Follow-up	SI_{BCNU}	SI_{VM26}	$SI_{ARA-A5'P}$	SI_{5-FU}
3	72	M	oligodendrogl.	ri fr	—	—	19 (R)	0.439	0.049	0.437	0.114
4	60	F	oligodendrogl.	ri par	—	—	19	0.773	0.027	0.550	0.308
5	5	M	mal.glioma IV	IV ventr	+	PRC, VCR, MTX	11 (S)	0.031	0.026	0.024	0.101
6	63	M	glioblastoma	le par-occ	+	BCNU, VM 26	12 (S)	0.056	0.124	0.105	0.508
7	23	M	ependymoma	L4/L5	+	CCNU	17 (R)	0.063	0.096	0.045	0.131
10	16	F	fibr. astrocyt.	ri fr	—	—	—	0.612	0.696	1.104	0.263
13	13	F	oesteoclastoma	Th 3/4/5	—	—	—	0.116	0.616	1.083	0.493
19	29	M	mal. melanoma	ri temp	—	—	12 (R)	0.776	0.800	0.524	0.370
25	58	F	bronch. carc.	L4/L5	+	—	—	0.842	0.460	0.769	0.961
26	62	F	glioblastoma	bi fr	+	BCNU, VM 26	8 (S)	0.884	0.534	0.613	0.979
27	62	M	glioblastoma	le par-occ	+	BCNU, VM 26	4 (S)	1.116	0.592	0.580	0.275
29	43	M	mal. melanoma	le par	+	—	2 (S)	0.742	1.035	1.073	0.317
31	52	F	meningeoma	le fr-temp	—	—	—	0.888	0.757	0.865	0.191
32	32	M	astrocytoma II	le temp-par	+	—	9	0.993	0.616	0.521	0.181
35	63	M	glioblastoma	le par-occ	+	BCNU, VM 26	6 (S)	0.900	1.080	0.827	0.243
36	65	F	glioblastoma	ri temp	—	—	1 (S)	0.964	0.676	0.639	0.259
37	10	M	hemangiopericyt.	le par	+	—	—	1.483	0.653	0.668	0.291
38	46	F	oligo/astro II	ri temp-par	—	—	—	0.954	0.730	1.009	0.200
43	24	F	Ewing-sarcoma	ri paravert.	+	ADR, CLC, VCR	13 (S)	0.852	0.364	0.449	0.192
46	59	M	bronch. carc.	le par	+	—	—	1.270	1.000	0.644	0.234
47	16	F	ganglioglioma	le par	—	—	—	1.071	0.311	0.250	0.300
48	23	M	fibr. astrocyt.	ri fr-temp	+	—	—	1.436	0.319	0.179	0.239
49	48	M	hypernephr.carc.	ri occ	+	VBL	—	1.270	0.547	0.287	0.220
51	47	M	bronch. carc.	csf	+	MTX	1 (S)	1.071	0.443	1.070	0.262
53	53	F	glioblastoma	ri par-occ	+	BCNU	12 (S)	1.436	0.925	0.717	0.651
54	61	F	thyroid carc.	ri fr-temp	—	—	—	1.873	0.813	0.689	0.637
55	33	M	mal. glioma IV	fr-bas	+	BCNU, VM 26	10 (R)	1.215	0.971	1.116	0.727
56	62	F	astrocytoma IV	le fr	+	BCNU, VM 26	10 (R)	0.771	0.567	0.479	0.311
57	26	M	glioblastoma	le fr-par	+	BCNU, VM 26	8 (R)	0.987	0.692	1.031	0.320
60	19	F	astrocytoma II	le fr-temp	+	—	—	0.845	0.802	0.712	0.247

Assay systems: A microassay was employed to assess drug activity, as published elsewhere (4, 6) single cells are plated in 96-well micro tissue culture plates (flat bottom, COSTAR, 10^3/well) and treated with drugs 24 hrs after plating. After 5 to 8 population doubling times of untreated controls (7 to 14 days) RNA-synthesis is measured by incorporation of (5-6-^{3}H)-uridine (specific activity 27Ci/mmol, AMERSHAM BUCHLER) employing a liquid scintillation counting protocol. Dose response curves for individual tumours and drugs were derived from inbition of RNA-synthesis of treated cells relative to untreated controls.

Pharmacology: For each drug in vitro and in vivo pharmacological data had to be obtained. **BCNU:** in vivo data have been obtained from LEVIN (15), in vitro data from GIANNINI (9). Calculations were made for 1 hr exposure. **VM 26:** in vivo data were mainly derived from STEWART (23-CNS-parenchyme values) and ALLEN (1). In vitro pharmacokinetic parameters were derived from own experiments employing an in vitro bioassay. **5-FU:** in vivo CNS-parameters were calculated based on data from KERR (10), ALMERSJÖ (3) and OBRECHT (17), in vitro data were taken from SOMADOSSI (22). **ARA-A5 ' P:** in vivo parameters were taken from LEPAGE (4) and PREIKSAITIS (18), in vitro data were determined by a HPLC-protocol, performed kindly by H.G. LÖBERING at THILO-research laboratories (Table 2). Calculations for the latter 3 compounds were made for continuous exposure.

Correlation of in vitro and in vivo pharmacokinetics: For the drugs a correlation curve of c $\times$ t (concentration time product = μmol $\times$ hrs/l)-values and in vitro drug concentrations was established, employing in vitro pharmacokinetic data. In vivo achievable maximal (CNS) concentration time products were then correlated to a corresponding in vitro drug concentration, resulting in a maximum in vitro exposure dose equivalent to the maximum in vivo exposure dose ("cutoff"-concentration).

Evaluation of in vitro dose response curves: Dose response curves for each drug were evaluated from the lowest to the "cutoff"-concentration, the drug effect then being expressed as SI-value: Si = Auc_x/Auc_{cut} (Auc_x = area under theoretical 100% survival curve to "cutoff"-concentration; Auc_{cut} = area under survival curve of tumour cell line).

Clinical correlation: SI-values for 22 patients treated with nitrosoureas (BCNU, CCNU) and radiation have now been accumulated to be compared with respective recurrence free intervals; a preliminary correlation analysis has been performed for this purpose.

RESULTS

Pharmacology: Pharmacokinetic parameters including results of own in vivo pharmacokinetic experiments are summarized in table 2.

Drug effects: Sensitivity indices calculated for each drug and cell line are depicted in table 1. Mean sensitivity indices for different drugs and primary/metastatic brain tumours as well as number of tumours with SI-values below 0.8, 0.5, and 0.2 are given in table 3. SI-indices related to high grade malignant gliomas and infratentorial/other gliomas are shown in table 4.

Clinical correlations: Correlations of SI-values and time to tumour progression for 22 patients (most of these patients are not included in this study - Table 1) treated with nitrosoureas is depicted in fig. 1; predictive time to tumour progression may be either given as a minimal prognosis (r = -0.91), when tumours with worst prognosis have been taken for correlation only, or as regular prognosis, when all tumours have been taken for correlation (r = - 0.84). A KAPLAN-MAIER plot of the identical correlation with a given (arbitrary) discriminatory SI $\leqslant$ 0.5 or SI $>$ 0.5 is shown in fig. 2.

TABLE 2

	peak C (§)	$T_{1/2}$ (hrs)	c x t (&)	« cutoff » (§)
BCNU: in-vivo:	9.2	1.13	4.77	—
in vitro:	—	0.35	—	9.0 (ihr)
VM_{26}: in-vivo *:	21.5	8.88	107,7	—
in vivo :	0.39	—	5.25	—
in vitro :	—	43.2	—	0.15 (ctd)
ARA-A5 ' P: in-vivo:	30.0	0.14-4.5	287,1	—
in vitro:		2.6	—	75 (ctd)
5-FU: in vivo:	100	0.25	51.9	—
in vitro:	—	0.1	—	410 (ctd)

*: plasma; :tumor tissue; (ihr/etd): exposure ihr or continous; § = μmol/l; & = μmol x hrs/l.

TABLE 3

Mean sensitivity indices of primary and metastatic brain tumour cells / drug effectivity

	SI_{BCNU}	$SI_{5\text{-}FU}$	$SI_{ARA\text{-}A5'P}$	SI_{VM26}
prim. CNS-Tumours	0.819	0.329	0.594	0.535 (N = 21)
metastatic Npl.	1.052	0.410	0.732	0.675 (N = 9)
all tumours	0.890	0.351	0.635	0.577 (N = 30)
	BCNU	5-FU	ARA-A5'P	VM26
prim. CNS-Tumours	(N)	(N)	(N)	(N)
SI < 0.8	7	20	15	18
SI < 0.5	4	17	7	7
SI < 0.2	3	6	4	5
CNS-Metastases				
SI < 0.8	2	8	6	6
SI < 0.5	—	7	2	3
SI < 0.2	—	—	—	—

TABLE 4

Correlation of sensitivity index with tumour histology

	Astrocytomas GR.IV Glioblastomas / N = 10		Low-GR. gliomas / N = 9 Infratentor: tumours	
BCNU	SI = 0.836	$\sigma = 0.434$	SI = 0.765	$\sigma = 0.382$
VM26	SI = 0.619	$\sigma = 0.323$	SI = 0.421	$\sigma = 0.282$
ARA-A5 ' P	SI = 0.68	$\sigma = 0.284$	SI = 0.569	$\sigma = 0.345$

SI in this table = mean SI.

Table 1: Synopsis of clinical data and neuropathology, as well as sensitivity indices for brain tumour cell lines. Abbreviations: Follow-up (months); SI = sensitivity index; PRC = procarbazine; VCR = vincristin; CCNU = lomustine; ADR = adriamycin; CLC = cyclophosphamide; R = recurrence; S = survival.

Table 2: Synopsis of pharmacokinetic data for BCNU, VM 26, ARA-A5 ' P and 5-FU. The in vivo plasma-pharmacokinetics for VM 26 is listed for completeness only.

Table 3: Upper part: synopsis of mean sensitivity indices for different drugs; lower part: the number of tumours is given, which has a sensitivity index below 0.8, 0.5 or 0.2 for a given drug.

Table 4: Differences in mean sensitivity indices for astrocytomas IV/glioblastomas and astrocytomas III, other gliomas and infratentorial CNS-neoplasms are given.

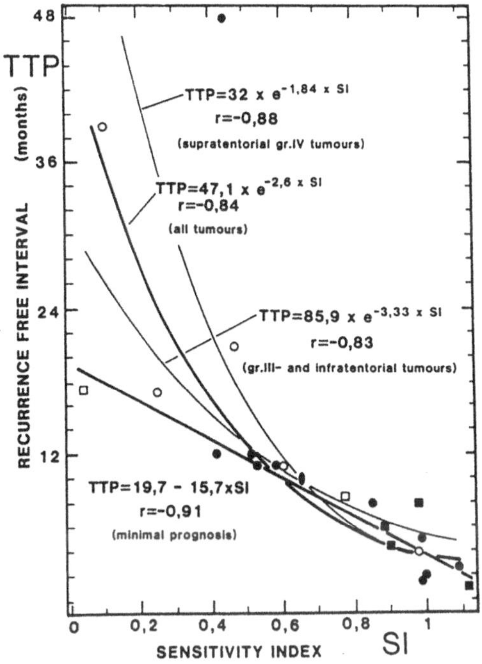

FIGURE 1

FIGURE 1.

Correlation of sensitivity index SI and relapse free interval for 22 patients with primary malignant brain tumours, who have been operated, treated with radiotherapy and nitrosoureas only; most patients are not included in table 1. Minimal prognosis: this correlation has been found by combining a given SI-value with the corresponding shortest relapse free interval. TTP = time to tumour progression. For a given patient's SI — determined by drug screening on his/her tumour — a probable TTP for an individual drug (in this graph BCNU) may be predicted. A minimal prognosis will be also available.

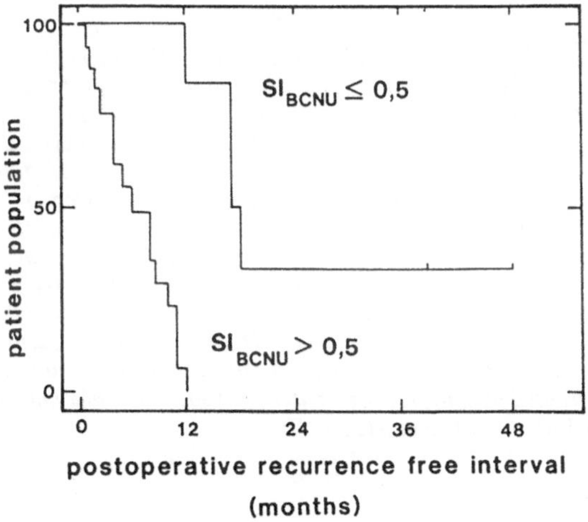

FIGURE 2

FIGURE 2.

KAPLAN-MAIER plot of relapse free intervals for the same 22 patients (as in fig. 1), discriminated by SI-values below and above 0.5. Mean relapse free intervals for patients with SI $\leqslant$ 0.5 were 25.6 months, for those with SI $>$ 0.5 ($p < 0.001$).

DISCUSSION

In this present study 3 out of 21 primary CNS neoplasms (14.3%) were highly sensitive to BCNU ($SI < 0.2$) - this proportion corresponds very well to the number of longterm survivors among patients with anaplastic gliomas who were treated with BCNU (25, 26). In our clinical correlation of SI-values with recurrence free intervals (fig. 1) an SI of < 0.2 is also associated with a prognosis for long time to tumour progression of more than 2 years; interestingly, this may be even longer, if analysis is made for high grade supratentorial astrocytomas alone. Unfortunately, the proportion of tumours with such a small SI is quite limited with nitrosourea-therapy. Although we do not have clinical correlations for the other drugs investigated, and we do not know whether these correlations will resemble that for BCNU. Considerably more tumours had SI-values below 0.5 and even below 0.2 for 5-FU, but also for VM 26 and ARA-A5'P. On a statistical basis (WILCOXON test), 5-FU, VM 26 and ARA-A5'P were all significantly ($p < 0.001$) more active than BCNU. There are no clinical data available for ARA-A5'P to validate these findings; but clinical results for VM 26 (12) and 5-FU (21) so far did not show any spectacular effects. Clinical application is performed, however, as a bolus infusion, although VM 26 is strictly and 5-FU may be a cell cycle phase specific agent, requiring almost continuous exposure of cells to be effective. As dose modifying effects of the BBB have been respected in our investigations and VM 26 and 5-FU are active agents under in vitro conditions, a proposal is made for a modified clinical application as a continuous rather than a bolus infusion.

Preliminary observations indicate an anti-tumour activity of ARA-A5'P in vitro systems (6, 11) and in some animal tumours (13). Because of its excellent BBB-penetration and its rather low and reversible toxicity (18, 28) this compound seemed to be an attractive candidate in brain tumour chemotherapy. In this in vitro study, it was more active than BCNU in primary and secondary brain tumours. There was no cross-resistance to the other drugs tested. However, in some patients there may be extremely high serum deaminase levels leading to more rapid drug inactivation; although ARA-A5'P seems to be more resistant to serum deaminase than ARA-A, this is still a limiting factor for clinical administration.

Metastatic brain tumours displayed relatively high resistance to the four agents investigated — as would have been expected from the clinical experience. However, we could show that some of these metastatic tumours seemed to be at least accessible to 5-FU with an $SI < 0.5$ - and to VM 26 and ARA-A5'P in a smaller proportion. Therefore we propose that individual chemotherapy screening might be especially helpful in patients with brain metastases to delineate those patients, who might benefit from drug therapy, and to save the remainders from drug toxicity.

SUMMARY

BCNU (carmustine), VM 26 (teniposide), 5-FU (5-fluorouracil) and ARA-A5'P (vidarabin-monophosphate) were compared in their activities against 30 cell lines of primary ($N = 21$) and secondary ($N = 9$) brain tumours, which were characterized in tissue culture by cytochemical, immunological and cytogenetic analysis. Drug sensitivity was determined by an in vitro microcytotoxicity assay based on in vivo and in vitro pharmacokinetics (AUC) of respective drugs. Cells were exposed to the drugs in vitro; after 5-8 population doubling times of untreated cells RNA-synthesis was determined employing a liquid scintillation counting protocol: Inhibition of RNA-synthesis relative to untreated controls was calculated for dose-response curves. Drug effects were expressed in terms of a sensitivity index SI ($SI = 1$ complete resistance). Mean SI-values for primary CNS-neoplasms were 0.82 (BCNU), 0.54 (VM 26), 0.33 (5-FU), and 0.59 (ARA-A5'P). Metastatic brain tumours were less sensitive to all four agents; high grade gliomas were less sensitive to all drugs than grade III gliomas and infratentorial tumours. Clearcut crossresistance was not observed for any drug. A correlation of SI-values and recurrence free intervals for nitrosourea treated patients is presented ($r = -0.91/-0.84$) and may allow some extrapolation of in vitro results for VM 26, 5-FU and ARA-A5'P.

KEY WORDS

BCNU, Vidarabin-Monophosphate, 5-Fluorouracil, Teniposide, Brain Neoplasms, Gliomas, in vitro assay, clinical correlations.

REFERENCES

1. ALLEN (J.M.), CREAVEN (P.J.): Comparison of human pharmacokinetics of VM 26 and VP 16, two antineoplastic epipodophyllotoxinglucopyranoside derivatives. Europ. J. Cancer 11: 697-707, 1975.
2. ALI-OSMAN (F.S.), MAURER (R.): In vitro cytostatic drug testing in the human stem cell assay: a modified method for the determination of the sensitivity index. Tum. Diag. Ther. 4: 1-5, 1983.
3. ALMERSJÖ (O.E.), GUSTAVSON (B.G.), REGATH (C.G.), WALEN (I.): Pharmacokinetic studies of 5-Fluorouracil after oral and intravenous administration in men. Acta Pharm. Toxicol. 46: 329-336, 1980.
4. BOGDAHN (U.), RUPNIAK (H.T.R.), ALI-OSMAN (F.), ROSENBLUM (M.L.): Characterisation of human malignant brain tumour cells in vitro and comparison of three different in vitro assays to determine their sensitivity to BCNU. In: Voth D, Krauseneck P. Chemotherapy of gliomas. Walter de Gruyter, Berlin, New York, 1985, p. 321-328.
5. BOGDAHN (U.), DÜNISCH (G.), SCHMIDT (G.), WEBER (H.), ZAPF (J.): Characterization of human primary and metastatic brain tumours in vitro. J. Neurol., manuscript in preparation, 1986.
6. BOGDAHN (U.): Chemosensitivity of human malignant brain tumours. J. Neurooncol. 1: 149-166, 1983.
7. TRIBOLET (N. de), CARREL (S.), MACH (J.P.): Brain tumour associated antigens. Progr. Exp. Tum. Res. 27: 118-131, 1984.
8. ENG (L.F.), VANDERHAEGEN (J.J.), BIGNAMI (A.), GERSTL (B.): An acidic protein isolated from fibrous astrocytes. Brain Res. 28: 351-354, 1971.
9. GIANNINI (B.), LEVIN (V.A.): Determination of in vitro pharmacokinetics of different nitrosoureas. Unpublished results; BTRC, UCSF, San Francisco, Ca USA.
10. KERR (I.G.), ZIMM (S.), COLLINS (J.M.) et al.: Effects of intravenous dose and schedule on cerebrospinal fluid pharmacokinetics of 5-fluorouracil in monkeys. Cancer Res. 44: 4929-4932, 1984.
11. KUFE (D.W.), MAJOR (P.B.), MUNROE (D.), EGAN (M.), HARRICK (D.): Relationship between incorporation of 9β-D-arabinofuranosyl-adenine and cytotoxicity. Cancer Res. 43. 2000-04, 1983.
12. KRAUSENECK (P et al.): Current project of the German Brain Tumour Study Group. Unpublished results.
13. LEE (F.H.), CARON (N.), KIMBALL (A.P.): Therapeutic effects of 9β-D-Arabinofuranosyl-adenine and 2-Deoxycoformycin combinations on intracerebral leukemia L1210. Cancer Res. 37: 1953-55, 1977.
14. LEPAGE (G.A.), NAIK (S.A.), KATAKKAR (S.B.), KALIK (A.): 9β-D-arabinofuranosyl-adenine-5-phosphate metabolism and excretion in humans. Cancer Res. 35: 3036-3040, 1975.
15. LEVIN (V.A.): A pharmacologic basis for brain tumour chemotherapy. Sem. Oncol. 2: 57-61, 1975.
16. MULLER (W.E.G.), ZAHN (R.K.), BITTLINGMEIER (K.), FALKE (D.): Inhibition of herpes virus DNA-synthesis by 9β-D-arabinofuranosyl-adenin in cellular and cell-free systems. Ann N Y Acad. Sci. 184: 34-48, 1977.
17. OBRECHT (J.P.), WEBER (W.), CANO (J.P. et al.): 5-Fluorouracil. A comparative pharmacokinetic study and preliminary results of a clinical phase I study. In: Recent Res. Cancer Res. Vol. 29: 101-107, Springer Verlag, Berlin, New York, 1979.
18. PREIKSAITIS (J.K.), LANK (B.), NG DK, et al.: Effect of liver disease on pharmacokinetics and toxicity of 9β-D-arabinofuranosyl-adenine-5-phosphate. J. Inf. Dis. 144: 358-364, 1981.
19. ROSENBLUM (M.L.), GEROSA (M.), WILSON (C.B.), BARGER (G.R.), PERTUISET (G.S. et al.): Stem cell studies of human malignant brain tumours. J. Neurosurg. 58: 170-176, 1983.
20. SEEGER (R.C.), DANON (Y.L.), RAINER (S.A.): Definition of a Thy-1 determinant on human neuroblastoma, glioma, sarcoma and teratoma cells with a monoclonal antibody. J. Neurol. 128: 983-989, 1982.
21. SHAPIRO (J.R.) et al.: Current project of the American Brain Tumour Study Group. Unpublished results.
22. SOMADOSSI (J.P.), GEWIRTZ (G.A.), DIASIO (R.B.) et al.: Rapid catabolism of 5-fluorouracil in freshly isolated rat hepatocytes as analysed by HPLC. J. Biol. Chem. 257: 8171-8176, 1982.
23. STEWART (D.J.), RICHARD (M.T.), HOGENHOLZ (H.) et al.: Penetration of Teniposide (VM 26) into human intracerebral tumours. J. Neurooncol. 2: 315-324, 1984.
24. THOMAS (D.G.T.), DARLING (J.L.), PAUL (E.A.): Assay of anticancer drugs in tissue culture: relationship of relapse free interval and in vitro chemosensitivity in patients with malignant glioma. Br. J. Cancer 51: 525-532, 1985.
25. WALKER (M.D.), ALEXANDER (E.J.), HUNT (W.E.), MCCARTY (C.S.) et al.: Evaluation of BCNU and / or radiotherapy in treatment of anaplastic gliomas. J. Neurosurg. 49: 333-356, 1978.
26. WALKER (M.D.), GREEN (S.B.), BYAR (D.P.): Randomized comparison of radiotherapy and nitrosoureas for the treatment of glioma after surgery. NEJM 303: 1323-1329, 1980.
27. W6HITLEY (R.J.), SOONG (S.J.), DOLIN (R.) et al.: The collaborative study group: Adenine-arabinoside therapy of biopsy-proved herpes simplex encephalitis. NEJM 297: 289-294, 1977.
28. WITLEY (R.J.), TUCKER (B.C.), KINKEL (A.W.) et al.: Pharmacology, tolerance, and antiviral activity of vidarabine-monophosphate in humans. Antimicrob Agents Chemother. 18: 409-415, 1980.

Heterogeneity in Chemosensitivity and Acquisition of Drug Resistance in a Murine Model of Glioma

R. BRADFORD (°), J.L. DARLING (°), and D.G.T. THOMAS (°).

INTRODUCTION

Brain tumours are amongst the most devastating and difficult forms of cancer to control. Although some human gliomas respond to adjuvant therapy with cytotoxic agents, they invariably recur. These failures may be the result of inadequate drug delivery but may also occur because of the development of drug resistance within the tumour. Apparent drug resistance may occur because cells are able to effectively repair drug-induced damage (1) or because of the presence of a number of different drug resistant clones within the tumour (2, 3, 4, 5). The presence of such heterogeneity should be considered in the development of in vitro and in vivo models for the study of tumour cell drug sensitivity.

Cell line VMDk P497 derived from the VM spontaneous murine astrocytoma (SMA) (6) retains astrocytic features in vitro (7) and can be transplanted intracerebrally into syngeneic animals to produce tumours with a pleomorphic cell population and the features of a malignant glioma (8). Moreover, six clonal cell lines have been obtained from P497 which express dissimilar morphological, antigenic, kinetic and chromosomal properties (9). We have used this model system to investigate changes in chemosensitivity in vitro after drug treatment of VM mice bearing P497 intracerebral tumours.

MATERIALS AND METHODS

Cell Lines: The cell line VMDk P497 was originally the gift of Dr D. Bigner, Duke University Medical Center, USA. The cloned cell lines, designated A8, B2, B6, C12, D2 and F1, were the gift of Dr H. Koppel, Institute of Psychiatry, London.

Maintenance of Cells in Culture: The methods for the maintenance of cell cultures have previously been described (7).

Chemosensitivity Assay: The chemosensitivity assay used was the ^{35}S-methionine assay which has been described in detail elsewhere (9, 10, 11). The spectrum of in vitro chemosensitivity of parental P497 and the six cloned cell lines was established against a panel of nine cytotoxic agents (see Table 1 for drugs and abbreviations used). Quadruplicate determinations for each drug were performed on two separate occasions and a mean value of the ID_{50} (dose of drug which inhibited protein synthesis by 50%) was calculated.

Treatment of Tumour-bearing Animals: Intracerebral tumours were established by inoculating 10^6 P497 cells, harvested from a monolayer culture, into the right cerebral hemisphere of anaesthetised VM mice. Sixteen days following inoculation, groups of mice were treated with either PCB 100 mg/kg, VCR 270 μg/kg or CCNU 6 mg/kg daily for five days. One group of mice were untreated and served as controls. When animals became moribund, as a result of their tumour, they were sacrificed and the tumour-bearing hemisphere removed aseptically. Single cell suspensions prepared from these tumours were used to initiate monolayer cultures. The spectrum of in vitro chemosensitivity of the derived cell lines was then determined.

(°) *Gough-Cooper Department of Neurological Surgery, Institute of Neurology, Queen Square, London WC1, UK.*

M. Chatel, F. Darcel and J. Pecker (eds.), Brain Oncology. ISBN-13: 978-94-010-8003-3

TABLE 1

Chemosensitivity of Clonal Cell Lines Derived from the VMDk P497 Cell Line

	Mean ID_{50} µg/ml							
DRUG	P497	A8	B2	B6	C12	D2	F1	Fold Difference[1]
PCB	543.0	471.0	673.0	573.0	419.0	448.0	160.0	4.2
VCR	0.00018	0.016	0.054	0.070	0.061	0.0 53	0.005	14.0
CCNU	3.68	7.78	14.30	13.38	7.83	7.71	3.36	4.3
BCNU	3.56	3.10	10.43	5.41	9.33	11.21	3.30	3.6
VDS	0.0033	0.014	0.058	0.042	0.085	0.0044	0.042	20.2
ADM	0.02	0.15	0.13	0.25	0.23	0.068	0.19	3.4
C-PLAT	0.17	0.25	0.33	0.35	0.98	0.53	0.31	3.9
BLM	0.16	0.12	0.38	0.35	036	0.41	0.27	3.4
5-Fu	1.68	0.41	0.35	0.37	0.14	0.25	0.28	2.9

1. Fold difference in ID_{50} between least and most sensitive clone.

PCB - procarbazine, VCR - vincristine, VDS - vindesine, ADM - adriamycin, C-PLAT - cis-platinum, BLM - bleomycin, 5-Fu - 5-fluorouracil.

RESULTS

Table 1 shows the calculated mean ID_{50} for parental P497 and the six clones against the panel of drugs used in this study. It is clear that differences in chemosensitivity exist amongst the clones for all nine drugs tested. The widest variation in sensitivity between the clones was observed for the vinca alkaloids VCR and VDS, where the ID_{50}'s varied between 14.0 and 20.2 fold respectively. For three of the clones B2, B6 and C12 the ID_{50} for VCR was more than 300 times greater than that for the parental cell line P497.

Four derivative cell lines were established from the parent VMDk P497. These were designated 497-C (1), 497-P(1), 497-V(2) and 497-CC(1). They were derived from a single control animal and from single animals treated with PCB, VCR and CCNU respectively. Table 2 shows the increase or decrease in chemosensitivity of these derived cell lines. The cell line derived from an untreated tumour, 497-C(1) exhibited small changes in sensitivity to CCNU, BCNU, VDS, C-PLAT and 5-FU.

TABLE 2

Changes in Chemosensitivity of Cell Lines Derived from VMDk P497

	Mean ID_{50} ($\mu g/ml$)	Fold Change in ID_{50} of derived lines			
DRUG	P497	497-C(1)	497-P(1)	497-V(2)	497-CC(1)
PCB	534	NC*	↑ x 2	R**	NC
VRC	0.00018	NC	NC	↑ x 105	NC
CCNU	3.7	↑ x 2.7	NC	↑ x 4.7	NC
BCNU	3.6	↓ x 4.6	NC	↑ x 5.4	NC
VDS	0.0033	↓ x 2	NC	↑ x 71	↓ x 8.4
ADM	0.02	NC	↑ x 3	↑ x 8	↑ x 3.5
C-PLAT	0.17	↓ x 3.5	NC	NC	↓ x 13
BLM	0.16	NC	NC	NC	↓ x 11
5-FU	1.68	↓ x 9.3	↓ x 8.8	↓ x 54	↓ x 22

* - No change in sensitivity (less than 2 fold change in ID_{50})
** - Resistant (ID_{50} greater than 1000 $\mu g/ml$)

In vivo treatment with CCNU induced no change in the sensitivity to the nitrosoureas of cell line 497-CC (1). Changes in sensitivity of this cell line followed a similar pattern to 497-C (1). 497-P (1) exhibited a two fold increase in the ID_{50} of PCB. The greatest changes in sensitivity were observed with cell line 497-V (2). There was a 105 fold increase in the ID_{50} of VCR and a 71 fold increase for the related vinca alkaloid VDS. 497-V (2) also exhibited decreased sensitivity to PCB, CCNU, BCNU and ADM but the ID_{50} of 5-Fu decreased by 54 fold.

DISCUSSION

Tumour heterogeneity has been well documented for many tumours including gliomas (12). Differential chemosensitivity has also been demonstrated in clonal subpopulations of human glioma (13, 14). Heterogeneity in drug sensitivity must, in part, account for the relative lack of success with single agent chemotherapy for malignant glioma. The demonstration of differential chemosensitivity among clonal subpopulations of cell line P497 allows this aspect of human gliomas to be reproduced in an animal model. Acquired drug resistance in tumours may be caused by selective outgrowth of pre-existing resistant cells (15). Our in vitro chemosensitivity studies have demonstrated that clonal subpopulations exist within VMDk P497 which are considerably more resistant to VCR than is the parent cell line itself. We have been able to induce rapid chemoresistance to VCR in a cell line derived from an intracerebral P497 tumour treated in vivo with this agent. It is possible that this finding is due to the selective pressure of VCR therapy affecting only sensitive subpopulations of cells contained within P497 tumours. The derived cell line 497-V (2) may then contain a higher proportion of the VCR resistant clones. The VCR resistant cell line 497-V (2) exhibited cross-resistance to the related vinca alkaloid VDS and partial cross-resistance to ADM, a pattern of sensitivity previously observed in established VCR resistant cell lines (16, 17).

We believe that cell lines derived from the VM SMA offer a valuable model for the study of human glioma heterogeneity and acquired drug resistance.

SUMMARY

Six clones obtained from cell line VMDk P497, itself derived from the VM spontaneous murine astrocytoma (SMA), exhibit differential chemosensitivity in vitro particularly to the vinca alkaloids. The in vitro chemosensitivity of cell lines derived from in vivo drug treated P497 intracerebral tumours has been examined. Rapid acquisition of resistance to vincristine was observed in one of the derived cell lines, 497-V (2). This may be the result of overgrowth of vincristine resistant clones identified in the parent cell line.

KEY WORDS

Antineoplastic agents, Brain neoplasms, Drug resistance, Neoplasms experimental.

AKNOWLEDGEMENTS

RB is supported by a research training fellowship from the National Fund for Research into Crippling Disease. J.L.D. is supported by the Brain Research Trust and the Institute of Cancer Research.

REFERENCES

1. BARRANCO (S.C.), NOVAK (J.K.), HUMPHREY (R.M.): Studies on recovery from chemically-induced damage in mammalian cells. Cancer Res. **35**: 1194-1204 (1975).

2. BARRANCO (S.C.), DREWINKO (B.), ROMSDAHL (M.M.), HUMPHREY (R.M.): Differential sensitivities of human melanoma cells grown in vitro to arabinosylcytosine. Cancer Res. **32**: 2733-2738 (1972).

3. BARRANCO (S.C.), DREWINKO (B.), HUMPHREY (R.M.): Differential response by human melanoma cells to 1,3-bis-(2-chloroethyl)-1-nitrosourea and bleomycin. Mutat. Res. **19**: 277-280 (1973).

4. BARRANCO (S.C.), HAENELT (B.R.), GEE (L.): Differential sensitivities of five rat hepatoma cell lines to anticancer drugs. Cancer Res. **38**: 656-660 (1978).

5. HEPPNER (G.H.), DEXTER (D.L.), NUCCI (T. de), MILLER (F.R.), CALABRESI (P.): Heterogeneity in drug sensitivity among tumour cell subpopulations of a single mammary tumour. Cancer Res. **38**: 3758-3763 (1978).

6. SERANO (R.D.), PEGRAM (C.N.), BIGNER (D.D.): Tumourigenic cell culture lines from a spontaneous VM/DK murine astrocytoma (SMA). Acta Neuropath. **51**: 53-64 (1980).

7. PILKINGTON (G.J.), DARLING (J.L.), LANTOS (P.L.), THOMAS (D.G.T.): Cell lines (VMDk) derived from a spontaneous murine astrocytoma. Morphological and immunocytochemical characterization. J. Neurol. Sci. **62**: 115-139 (1983).

8. PILKINGTON (G.J.), DARLING (J.L.), LANTOS (P.L.), THOMAS (D.G.T.): Tumorigenicity of cell lines (VMDk) derived from a spontaneous murine astrocytoma. Histology, fine structure and immunocytochemistry of tumours. J. Neurol. Sci. **71**: 145-164 (1985).

9. THOMAS (D.G.T.), DARLING (J.L.), FRESHNEY (R.I.), MORGAN (D.): In vitro chemosensitivity assay of human glioma by scintillation autofluorography. In: Paoletti P., Walker M.D., Butti H., Knerich R., eds. Multidisciplinary Aspects of Brain Tumor Therapy. Amsterdam: Elsevier, 1979: 19-35.

10. MORGAN (D.), FRESHNEY (R.I.), DARLING (J.L.), THOMAS (D.G.T.), CELIK (F.): Assays of anticancer drugs in tissue culture: Cell cultures of biopsies from human astrocytoma. Br. J. Cancer **47**: 205-214 (1983).

11. BRADFORD (R.), DARLING (J.L.), THOMAS (D.G.T.): The in vitro chemosensitivity of three cell lines derived from the VM/Dk spontaneous murine astrocytoma. J. Neurol. Neurosurg. Psychiatry **49**: 1361-1366 (1986).

12. BIGNER (D.D.): Biology of gliomas: potential clinical implications of glioma cellular heterogeneity. Neurosurgery **9**: 320-326 (1981).

13. YUNG K-W (A.), SHAPIRO (J.R.), SHAPIRO (W.R.): Heterogeneous chemosensitivities of subpopulations of human glioma cells in culture. Cancer Res. **43**: 992-998 (1982).

14. KOBAYASHI (S.), HOSHINO (T.), DOUGHERTY (D.V.), ROSENBLUM (M.L.): Variable response to 1,3-bis (2-chloroethyl)-1-nitrosourea of human glioma cells sorted according to DNA content. J. Neuro-oncol. **2**: 5-11 (1984).

15. HARRUP (K.R.), JACKSON (R.C.): Biochemical mechanism of resistance to antimetabolites. In: Schabel F.M., ed. Fundamentals in Cancer Chemotherapy. Antibiotics and Chemotherapy, Vol. 23. Basel: Karger, 1978: 228-237.

16. WILKOFF (L.J.), DULMADGE (E.A.): Resistance and cross-resistance of cultured leukemia P388 cells to vincristine, adriamycin, adriamycin analogs and actinomycin-D. J. Natl. Cancer Inst. **61**: 1521-1524 (1978).

17. HILL (B.T.): Collateral sensitivity and cross-resistance. In: Fox B.W., Fox M. eds. Handbook of Experimental Pharmacology, Vol. 72. Berlin: Springer-Verlag, 1984: 673-697.

Assay of Anticancer Drugs in Tissue Culture: The Effect of Cell Kinetics and the Mode of Action of Drugs on the Chemosensitivity of Cultures Derived from Malignant Brain Tumours

J.L. DARLING and D.G.T. THOMAS (°).

INTRODUCTION

It is a common clinical observation that tumours of similar histology do not always respond identically to the same cytotoxic drugs. Although factors such as drug delivery and host-tumour interactions must play a role in this, other factors, in particular intrinsic drug sensitivity must also be important.

In this study, we have evaluated the response of a number of cultures derived from high grade, malignant gliomas, low grade gliomas and a small number of cerebral metastases and medulloblastomas to a panel of cytotoxic drugs with different modes of action.

MATERIALS AND METHODS

The experimental methodology for the preparation of cultures from human brain tumours and the performance of the in-vitro chemosensitivity assay has been published (1, 2). Briefly, exponentially dividing glioma cells at low passage levels (2 or 3) were treated in 96 well microtitration plates for 3 days with appropriate drug concentrations. Drugs were renewed daily. After drug removal, cells were washed and allowed a recovery period of between 1 and 3 cell generations (growth curves were performed in parallel, untreated, microtitration plates for each culture) and then treated with 2 μCi/ml ^{35}S-methionine for 4 hours. Cells were then washed, fixed in situ, treated with 10% w/v trichloroacetic acid to remove acid-soluble material and dried. Each well of the microtitration plate with the cells still in situ was filled with 0.02 ml of toluene-based scintillation fluid and a piece of blue-sensitive X ray film was placed against the base of each plate and held in place with polythene sponge. After exposure, in the dark, at -70°C for 24-48 hours, the film was detached and developed in high-contrast developer, fixed, washed and dried. The image was scanned with a scanning densitometer and dose-response curves generated by plotting peak height against drug concentration. The ID_{50} (dose of drug which inhibits protein synthesis by 50%) was determined from the dose-response curve.

RESULTS

Variation in chemosensitivity between cultures derived from tumours of the same histology

Cultures were treated as described in the methods section and the ID_{50} determined. It was clear that there was a considerable range of sensitivity between cultures derived from the same histological type of tumour. Drugs such as adriamycin (ADR), vincristine (VCR) and VP16-213 exhibited a wide range of sensitivity (ID_{50} range 3-10 logs) whilst the range of sensitivities to drugs like as CCNU, procarbazine (PCB) and AZQ tended to be smaller (ID_{50} range 1-3 logs). It was apparent that this range was widest for cell cycle-specific drugs (VCR, ADR and VP16-213). Ranges in drug sensitivity seemed to be smaller in cell-cycle non-specific alkylating agents (CCNU, PCB and AZQ).

(°) Gough-Cooper Department of Neurological Surgery, Institute of Neurology, National Hospital, Queen Square, London, WC1N 3BG, United Kingdom.

M. Chatel, F. Darcel and J. Pecker (eds.), Brain Oncology. ISBN-13: 978-94-010-8003-3

There appeared to be no convincing overall differences in chemosensitivity between different histological groups of tumour.

A panel of five cultures were screened for chemosensitivity to three drugs which have proved to be without appreciable clinical activity in human glioma: Bleomycin (BLM), 5-Fluorouracil (5-FU) and mithramycin (MITH). Two cultures were derived from grade IV astrocytomas, two from grade III oligodendrogliomas and one from a grade II astrocytoma. BLM produced a 19.3 fold range in ID_{50}, 5-FU produced a 3.1 fold range in ID_{50} and MITH only a 1.42 range in ID_{50}.

A sub-group of cultures were treated in duplicate plates with cytotoxic drugs as described in the methods section. One set of plates was processed for ID_{50} determination after a short recovery period of 4 hours (to allow equilibration of acid-soluble pools and efflux of unbound drug) and the second set of plates for each culture were allowed to recover for 1-3 cell generations before processing.

It was apparent that sensitivity to two alkylating agents, PCB and CCNU was rapidly lost, whilst sensitivity to a third agent, AZQ continued to accumulate during the recovery period. This pattern of accumulating damage was also seen in cultures treated with ADR and VP 16-213. The ID_{50}'s of cultures treated with VCR remained relatively stable during recovery.

Relationship between cell culture kinetics and drug sensitivity in vitro

It was apparent that culture doubling time, drug exposure time and length of recovery period did not influence chemosensitivity in vitro. The Spearman rank correlation coefficients (SRCC) for culture doubling times against chemosensitivity to PCB, CCNU and VCR were 0.529 ($p = 0.13$), -0.2297 ($p = 0.27$) and 0.787 ($p = 0.51$) respectively. The SRCCs for culture doubling times against chemosensitivity to ADR, AZQ or VP 16-213 were -0.03454 ($p = 0.85$), 0.1557 ($p = 0.403$) and 0.3146 ($p = 0.075$) respectively.

DISCUSSION AND CONCLUSIONS

For most drugs there was a wide range of chemosensitivity between cultures derived from different, but histologically similar, tumours. The widest ranges of sensitivity were found in cultures treated with cell cycle hyden specific agents. For some drugs like BLM, 5FU and MITH there was little difference in chemosensitivity between one culture and another.

Cell kinetic factors such as population doubling time and the length of drug treatment and recovery did not seem to influence in-vitro chemosensitivity. This would tend to indicate that for these drugs, at least, in-vitro sensitivity is unrelated to simple growth kinetic parameters and seems to be an independant cellular characteristic.

Human glioma cells appear to repair damage induced by CCNU and PCB rapidly although damage induced by another alkylating agent, AZQ, continues to accumulate after drug removal. It is possible that two separate mechanisms operate between these two classes of alkylating agents.

Cultures appear to continue to accumulate damage induced by both ADR and VP 16-213 following drug removal.

A knowledge of the in-vitro response of cultures of human brain tumours is crucial for the development of chemosensitivity assays to predict tumour response. In particular, the designation of a culture as sensitive or in-sensitive in relation to a panel of cultures derived from tumours of similar histology is important in determining relative in-situ chemosensitivity. The determination of the biochemical mechanisms of recovery from drug-induced cellular damage and how this is affected by factors such as the three dimensional structure of the tumour (perhaps using multicellular tumour spheroids as a model system) may well be important in the development of rational chemotherapy of malignant brain tumours.

KEY WORDS

Brain neoplasms, Drug testing, Antineoplastic agents.

ACKNOWLEDGEMENTS

This work was supported by grants from the Cancer Research Campaign and the Brain Research Trust.

REFERENCES

1. THOMAS (D.G.T.), DARLING (J.L.), FRESHNEY (R.I.), MORGAN (D.): In vitro chemosensitivity assay of human glioma by scintillation autofluorography. In: Paoletti P., Walker M.D., Butti G.H. and Knerich R. eds, Multidisciplinary Aspects of Brain Tumor Therapy. Amsterdam, Elsevier, 19-35, (1983).
2. MORGAN (D.), FRESHNEY (R.I.), DARLING (J.L.), THOMAS (D.G.T.), CELIK (F.): Assay of anticancer drugs in tissue culture: Cell cultures of biopsies from human astrocytoma. Br. J. Cancer **47**: 205-214 (1983).

Chemosensitivity Studies on Human Gliomas in Nude Mice Preliminary Results

V. BUDACH, M. BAMBERG, M. STUSCHKE, G. CZEGLARSKI, S. DUWE.

INTRODUCTION

Poor prognosis of patients suffering from malignant gliomas has not changed in the last decade. The 5-year survival rates are still disappointing (less than 5%). Chemotherapy is given either for adjuvant treatment or in case of relapse. The nitrosoureas play a leading role in chemotherapy of gliomas. They are of small molecular size, lipid soluble and are bound only minimally to protein, which enables them to cross the intact blood-brain-barrier ("bbb"). A similar penetration is known for Procarbazine (PCB). Other cytostatic agents e.g. Dacarbazine (DTIC), Ifosfamide (IFO) and Teniposide (VM-26) do not cross the "bbb". Various degrees of alterations in the "bbb" are known in patients suffering from brain tumours. This fact makes the prediction of the success following treatment with a given cytostatic drug difficult. Clinicians have looked for experimental models which enable valid preclinical screening of cytostatic drugs. One of the best models for this purpose is the athymic nude mouse. Subcutaneously implanted human gliomas can be directly observed for their response to different chemotherapies.

METHODS

More than 200 gliomas have been xenografted in nude mice during the last 6 years. The method of inoculation is readily done. Tumour slices of a freshly removed surgical specimen (about 5 mm diameter and 1 mm thickness) are subcutaneously inserted bilaterally to the flanks of nude mice in the milk-ridge levels. Metal clamps, which are removed 5 days later, serve to close the incisions. After tumour specific lag-phases in the range of some days to weeks the xenografts grow to nodules of about 1 cm diameter. The animals are then killed and the tumour transplanted to the next mouse passage. After 3 complete passages the grafts were subjected to the therapeutic trials. Each third passage the xenografts were compared to the original tumour with respect to growth behaviour, histomorphology, DNA-index and further properties if necessary. The studies were performed on groups of 8 to 10 animals (female nude mice) aged 8 to 10 weeks. The cytostatic drugs in the different experiments were given as single ip.-injections either dissolved in water (Lomustine (ACNU) 16,5 and 33,0 mg/kg, DTIC - 200 mg/kg, PCB - 300 mg/kg and Ifo - 150 and 300 mg/kg) or in alcohol (Carmustine (BCNU) and VM-26, 33 mg/kg each). The follow-up ranged from 3 to 4 weeks. We have chosen 3 astrocytomas and 1 oligodendroglioma (Kernohan's grading III/IV and III respectively) for the studies. The tumour growth was measured twice weekly by a slide caliper in two dimensions. The volume was calculated according to the formula: $V = \text{length} \times \text{width}^2 \times 0{,}5$. The growth delay was one analysed parameter and was defined as time to reach original or twice the original tumour volume. The mean tumour volumes at different dates of observation were plotted for growth curves of the treated and control animals.

RESULTS

Only 8 out of 100 human gliomas could be successfully established in nude mice (4%) for more than 3 subsequent passages. All gliomas showed significant growth delays following ACNU-, BCNU-, PCB-, DTIC- and Ifo-treatment. Only VM-26 was ineffective (fig. 2a). ACNU compared to BCNU revealed pronounced growth inhibition in 3 out of 4 gliomas (fig. 1a-b-c-d). For the "Li"-

(°) *Dep. of Radiooncology, West German Tumour Center. University of Essen, Hufelandstr. 55, D - 4300 Essen - 1.*

M. Chatel, F. Darcel and J. Pecker (eds.), Brain Oncology. ISBN-13: 978-94-010-8003-3

and "Re"-xenografts the significance was $p \leqslant 0{,}01$ and $p < 0{,}05$ for the oligodendroglioma. The results for the fourth glioma "Me" were statistically not significant ($p > 0{,}05$). For the "Me"- and "Li"-xenografts efficacy of PCB and DTIC could equally be demonstrated. The difference between the 2 drugs was not statistically evident because of the small number of animals tested in these groups (fig. 2a). In the "Me"-xenograft tumour growth could be inhibited more by 16,5 mg/kg ACNU than by 150 mg/kg Ifo ($p = 0{,}01$) (fig. 2b). A combination of both drugs in the same dosage was not significantly better than ACNU alone ($p = 0{,}05$) (fig. 3a). For the "Li"-xenograft the doses of both drugs were doubled (33 mg/kg ACNU and 300 mg/kg Ifo). This produced a higher growth delay for Ifo and ACNU compared to the "Me"-xenograft. The antiproliferative effect for ACNU was better than for Ifo ($p < 0{,}05$). The combination of both drugs in a dose of 16,5 mg/kg ACNU and 150 mg/kg Ifo was equally effective as ACNU alone ($p > 0{,}05$) in spite of reduced doses for the cytostatics (fig. 3b). Compared to earlier "Me"- and "Li"-grafts (passages 8 and 9) the tumour response to ACNU was clearly dose dependant.

DISCUSSION

A number of investigators have unsuccessfully tried to establish human brain tumours in various laboratory animals of immunocompetent origin. The anterior chamber of the guinea pig eye presented an exception to the above mentioned trials (8, 9). With the discovery of the athymic nude mice increasing success was achieved in xenotransplantation of human gliomas (5, 7). The "take - rates", which are reported for this type of tumours, differ in a wide range from 4% in our series up to 80% (2, 8). The reason may be either the different methodology or the definition of the term "take - rate". Therefore comparison of take - rates in different trials is difficult. A number of investigators have dealt with chemotherapy of gliomatous brain tumours in nude mice (6, 8, 9). Common drugs in these studies were the nitrosoureas and PCB, but no data are available for VM-26, Ifo and DTIC. Some authors could demonstrate definite cytostatic effects for ACNU and other nitrosoureas in nude mice and in monolayer cell cultures (3, 4, 6, 11). This is in agreement with our results, which showed a good response to both nitrosoureas (ACNU and BCNU) in 3 of 4 tested gliomas. PCB in our experiments was very effective in 2 tested gliomas. Schold reported on 5 human gliomas with good response to PCB, whereas Shapiro found one of 2 gliomas to be resistent to PCB (8, 10). Surprisingly good activity could be shown for DTIC in 2 of our gliomas, which is in agreement with preliminary results of Bradley and Bloom (1, 2). For VM-26 and Ifo corresponding data in nude mice are not available. Combined therapy using ACNU and Ifo had surprising results. When Ifo was added to ACNU in the "Me"-xenograft and additive effect was not seen. This contrasts to the results obtained from the "Li"-glioma, where in spite of reduced drug doses in the combined therapy by one half the effect was equivalent to 33 mg/kg of ACNU. For explanation, additive or synergistic mechanisms may be discussed. These results should be confirmed by further trials on a number of xenografted gliomas. The toxicity of the above mentioned combination seems to be in the same range as single drug therapy with 33 mg/kg ACNU or 300 mg/kg Ifo respectively. Our results underline the validity of this experimental model for preclinical testing of different drugs in human gliomas.

KEY WORDS

Gliomas, Chemotherapy, ACNU, BCNU, Procarbazine, Dacarbazine, Nude Mice.

REFERENCES

1. BLOOM (H.J.G.): Intracranial tumours: Response and resistance to therapeutic endeavours, 1970-1980. Int. J. Radiation Oncol. Biol. Phys. **8**: 1083-1113.

2. BRADLEY (N.J.), BLOOM (H.J.G.), DAVIES (A.J.S.) and SWIFT (S.M.): Growth of human gliomas in immune-deficient mice: A possible model for preclinical therapy studies. Br. J. Cancer **38**: 263-272.

3. HARADA (K.), KIYA (K.), OKAMOTO (H.), UOZUMI (T.): Comparative studies of the anti-tumor effect of nitrosoureas, ACNU and MCNU, on experimental brain tumors. In: Proceedings 13th International Cancer Congress, Sept. 8 - 15, 1982, Seattle, Washington USA, No. 3145.

4. HORI (M.), NAKAGAWA (H.), HASAGAWA (H.), MOGAMI (H.), HAYAKAWA (T.), NAKATA (T.): ACNU, a new nitrosourea compound, in the treatment of gliomas. Gann-t-Kagakuryoho, 1978, **5**: 773-778.

5. HORTEN (B.C.), BASLER (G.A.), SHAPIRO (W.R.): Xenograft of human malignant glial tumors into brain of nude mice. J. Neuropathol. Exp. Neurol., 1981, **40**: 493-511.

6. HOUCHENS (D.P.), OVEJERA (A.A.), RIBLET (S.M.), SLAGEL (D.E.): Human brain tumor xenografts in nude mice as a chemotherapy model. Eur. J. Cancer. Clin. Oncol., 1985, **19**: 799-805.

7. RANA (M.W.), PINKERTON (H.), THORNTON (H.), NAGY (D.): Heterotransplantation of human glioblastoma multiforme and meningioma to nude mice. Proc. Soc. Exp. Biol. and Med., 1977, **155**: 85-88.

8. SCHOLD (S.C.), jr., FRIEDMAN (H.S.): Human brain tumor xenografts. Prog. Exp. Tumor Res., 1984, **28**: 18-31.

9. SHAPIRO (W.R.), BASLER (G.A.), CHERNIK (N.L.), POSNER (J.B.): Human brain tumor transplantation into nude mice. J. Natl. Cancer Inst., 1979, **62**: 447-453.

10. SHAPIRO (W.R.), BASLER (G.A.): Chemotherapy of human brain tumors transplanted into nude mice, in Paoletti, Walker, Butti, Knerich, Multidisciplinary aspects of brain tumor therapy, pp. 309-316 (Elsevier, Amsterdam, 1979).

11. YAMASHITA (J.), HANDA (H.), TOKURIKI (Y.), HA (Y.S.), OTSUKA (S.I.): Intra-arterial ACNU therapy for malignant brain tumors. Experimental studies and preliminary clinical results. J. Neurosurg., 1983, **59**: 424-430.

1a

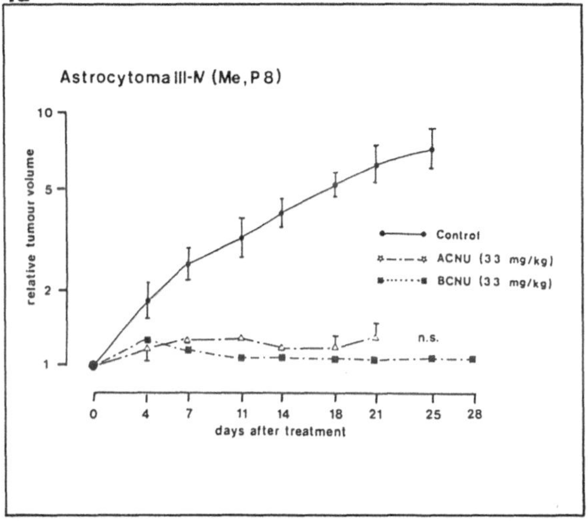

1b

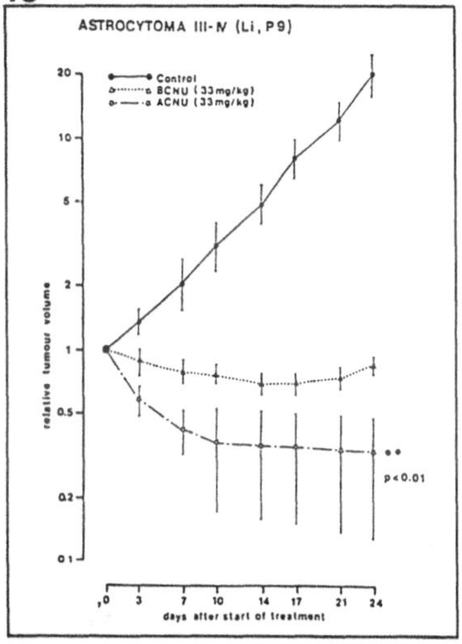

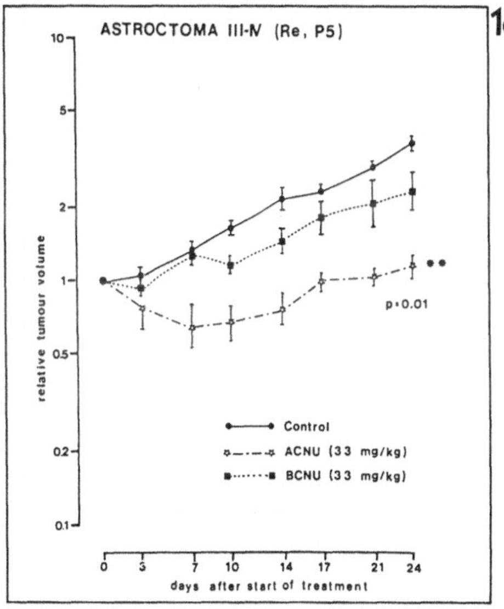

1c

1d

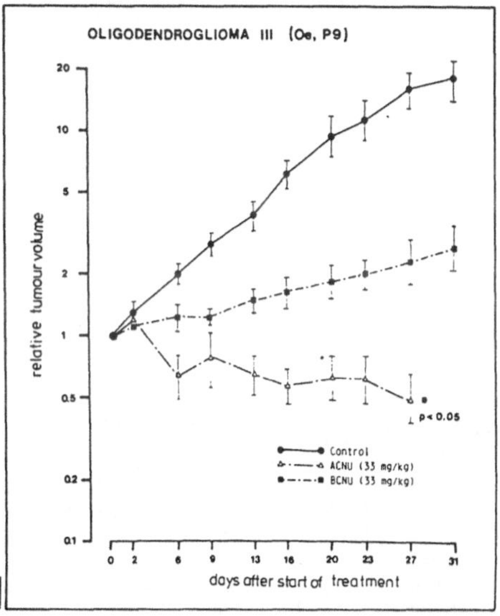

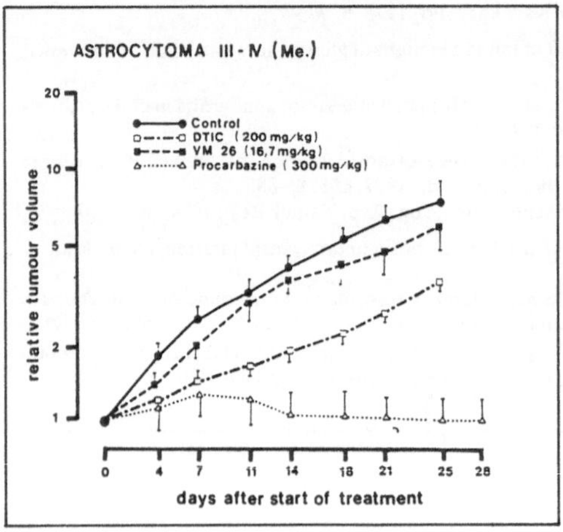

2a

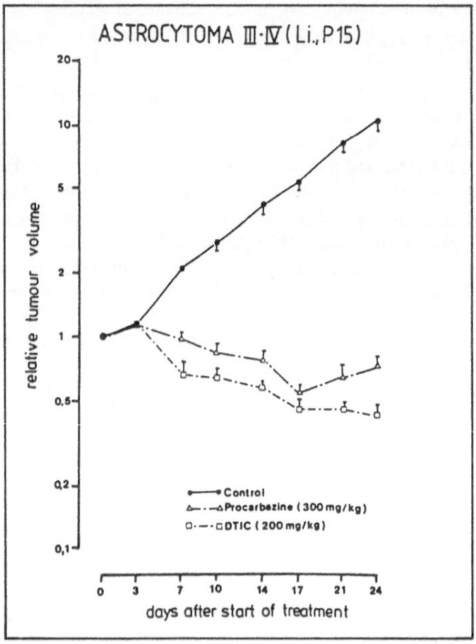

2b

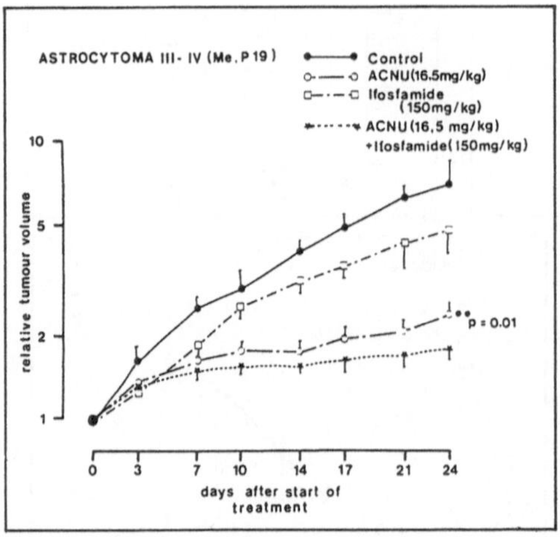

3a

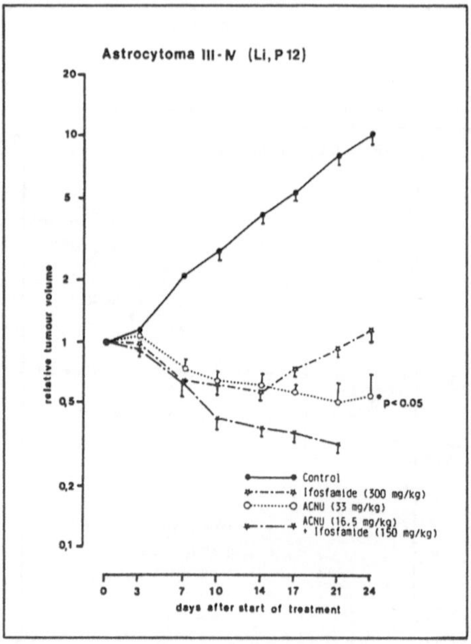

3b

FIGURE 1a-b-c-d:

Comparative studies with ACNU and BCNU on 4 different glioma xenografts ("Me", "Li", "Re", "Oe").

FIGURE 2a-b:

Chemotherapy with Procarbazine, Dacarbazine and VM-26 on 2 glioma xenografts ("Me" and "Li").

FIGURE 3a-b:

Combined chemotherapy with ACNU and Ifosfamide on 2 glioma xenografts ("Me" and "Li").

Rat Glioma Follow-Up by In-Vivo 31-Phosphorus Magnetic Resonance Spectroscopy: Activity of Two New Antineoplastic Agents

L. LE MOYEC (°), S. NARUSE, T. HIGUCHI, K. HIRAKAWA, H. WATARI (°°), B.P. ROQUES (°°°), J.D. de CERTAINES (°).

It has been previously shown that energy metabolism exploration by 31 phosphorus magnetic resonance spectroscopy (MRS) enables tumor evalution and therapy follow up using surface coils (1). This method begins to have clinical applications in spectrometers built to acquire successively an image and a spectrum from a particular region of interest. Another application of this technique could be to detect the effect of chemotherapies on animal tumor models in order to study pharmacologic characteristics of new antitumoral agents. This kind of experiment is carried out in an NMR probe using a surface coil. The anesthetized animal is set in the probe so that the tumor faces the coil in order to obtain acute localization. Two new antitumoral substances were tested by 31-P MRS on a brain tumor model subcutaneously implanted.

MATERIAL AND METHODS

Tumors were implanted by s.c. injection of 10^6 cells in the hind leg of male wistar rats. « In-vivo » spectra were acquired with a coil of 1 cm diameter, in a JEOL SCM 200 spectrometer operating at 80.75 MHz for phosphorus. Acquisition time is 20 min for 600 accumulations. « In-vitro » spectra were acquired on a Bruker AM 360 spectrometer operating at 146 MHz for phosphorus. Perchloric extracts were performed on tumoral tissue frozen in liquid nitrogen immediately after removal from the animal. The extract was lyophilised then dissolved in deuterated water at the moment of the NMR experiment and adjusted to pH 7.2-7.3. The first drug used was sarcosinamide *, a nitrosourea (fig. 1). It was i.p. injected at the single dose of 80 mg/kg (3). The second drug was Ditercalinium **, a DNA bis-intercalating agent (fig. 2) at the dose of 25 mg/kg i.p. injected (4).

RESULTS AND DISCUSSION

The rat glioma EA 285 can be qualified of slowly growing tumor because 5 to 6 weeks are required to have a 1 to 2 cm diameter tumor. At this phase, the typical phosphorus spectrum of this tumor is represented in fig. 3 showing as main resonances, phosphomonoesters (PME), high inorganic phosphates (Pi), low phosphocreatine (PCr), and successively, γ, α and β nucleoside triphosphates (NTP).

Control animals without any treatment have been followed by MRS during several days. Spectra from the same region within the tumor don't change during 6 to 9 days (fig. 4).

Treated animals received the drug after the acquisition of a first spectrum and were followed during 5 to 6 days.

A group of 11 rats was treated with sarcosinamide. Depletion of NTP peaks, 2 days after the injection, was found for 7 cases upon 11, while PME seemed to remain stable and Pi was increased (fig. 5). This type of effect has already been described on this model with other kind of therapy (2). Two animals not giving this type of response received a second injection one week later. Then, the proportion of NTP was decreased in the tumor.

This drug known to be active on some murine brain tumors, has never been tried on rat glioma. The dose of 80 mg/kg represents the highest optimal dose for other models. Size of tumors

* Gift from SANOFI, France. ** Gift from B.P. Roques, Dpt. Chimie Organique, Université Paris V, France.

Dept. of Neurosurgery, Kyoto prefectoral University of Medicine, Japan. (°) Laboratoire de RMN, Faculté de Médecine, Rennes, France, (°°) National Institute for Physiological Science, Okasaki, Japan, (°°°) Département de Chimie Organique, Université, Paris V, France.

M. Chatel, F. Darcel and J. Pecker (eds.), Brain Oncology. ISBN-13: 978-94-010-8003-3

and animal survival rate have been followed after the treatment but the wide individual variations, made impossible to get significant differences between control and treated groups.
Ditercalinium was injected to 9 rats. Only 3 cases showed the depletion of NTP peaks after 5 to 6 days (fig. 6). This result is more difficult to interprete because drug effect can interfere with the normal evolution of tumoral tissue after 5 days. But, this activity delay is in good agreement with data obtained « in-vitro » with cell cultures: several generations are needed to observe cytotoxic effect on colony formation (5).
On those « in-vivo » spectra, PME peak was not completely resolved. In order to determine the different components of this peak, we performed high resolution spectra on perchloric extracts. Spectrum at 146 MHz showed two main resonances in the region of PME (fig. 7): phosphoryl ethanolamine and phosphorylcholine. Glucose-6-phosphate has a higher chemical shift and AMP has also a resonance in this region. For the type of treatment used in this study, those substances, metabolites of phospholipids, do not seem to be involved. An increase of AMP due to depletion of NTP could also occur, but « in-vivo » resolution is not sufficient to detect AMP.

CONCLUSION

NTP peaks seem to be good markers of antitumoral activity on this model, and can provide informations about the activity delay because their variations are wide and don't present any quantification problem. PME peaks in relation with membrane structure are more difficult to interprete because of their heterogeneous composition. Those results show the importance of the chosen tumor model to study completely the activity of a substance. Thus in case of Sarcosinamide, lower or repeated doses could be tried on this model. On the opposite, the tumor is not adapted to study Ditercalinium because of its important activity delay giving interferences between the drug effect and the tumor evolution.

KEY WORDS

31 P-NMR, Chemotherapy, Energy Metabolism Nude Mice Xenografts.

REFERENCES

1. LE MOYEC (L.), BENOIST (L.), DE CERTAINES (J.): Perspectives d'application de la RMN du phosphore 31 à la surveillance des traitements anticancéreux. Bull. Cancer **72**: 506-515, (1985).
2. NARUSE (S.), HIRAKAWA (K.), HORIKAWA (Y.), TANAKA (C.), HIGUCHI (T.), VEDA (S.), NISHIKAWA (H.), WATARI (H.): Measurements of in vivo ^{31}p nuclear magnetic resonance spectra in neuroectodermal tumors for the evaluation of the effects of chemotherapy. Cancer Res., **45**, 2429-2433, (1985).
3. SUAMI (T.), KATO (T.), TAKINO (H.), HISAMATSU (T.): 2(chloroethyl) nitrosourea congeners of amino acid amides. J. Med. Chem., **25**, 829-832, (1982).
4. ROQUES (B.P.), PELAPRAT (D.), LE GUEN (J.), PORCHER (G.), GOSSE (C.), LE PECQ (J.B.): DNA bifunctional intercalators antileukemic activities of new pyridocarbazole dimers. Biochem. Pharmacol., **28**, 1811-1815, (1979).
5. ESNAULT (C.), ROQUES (B.P.), JACQUEMIN-SABLON (A.), LE PECQ (J.B.): Effects of New antitumor bifunctional intercalators derived from 7H-pyridocarbazole on sensitive and resistant 1210 cells. Cancer Res., **44**, 4355-4360, (1984).

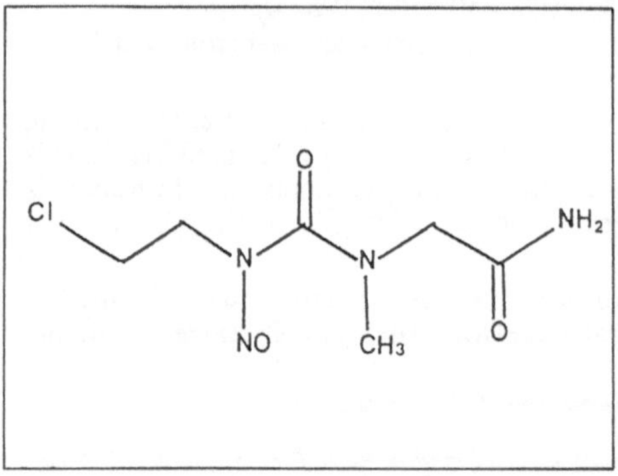

FIGURE 1. Sarcosinamide: 2-Chloroethyl Nitrosourea. Optimal Dose: 60 to 80 mg/kg (gift from Sanofi-France).

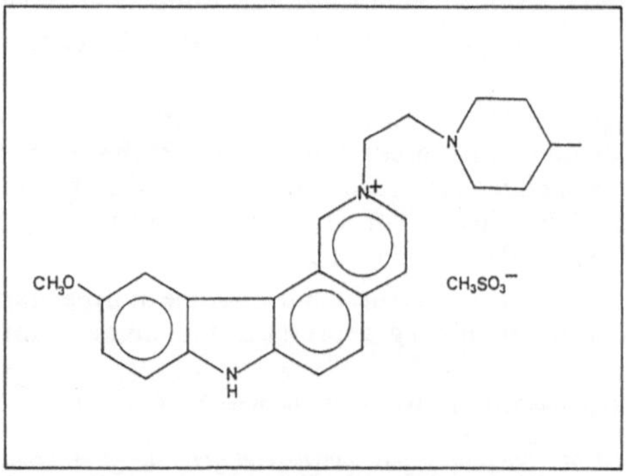

FIGURE 2. Ditercalinium: DNA Bis Intercalator. Usual dose for experimental studies: 25 mg/kg (gift from prof. B.P. roques, Dpt chimie organique, Paris V).

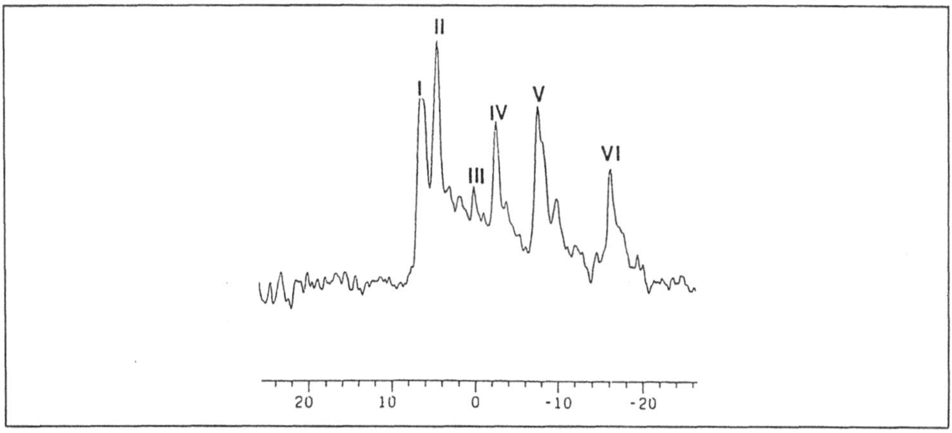

FIGURE 3. I: Phosphomonoesters (PME). II: Inorganic Phosphates (Pi). III: Phosphocreatine. IV: γ Nucleotide Triphosphates. V: α Nucleotide Triphosphates. VI: β Nucleotide Triphosphates.

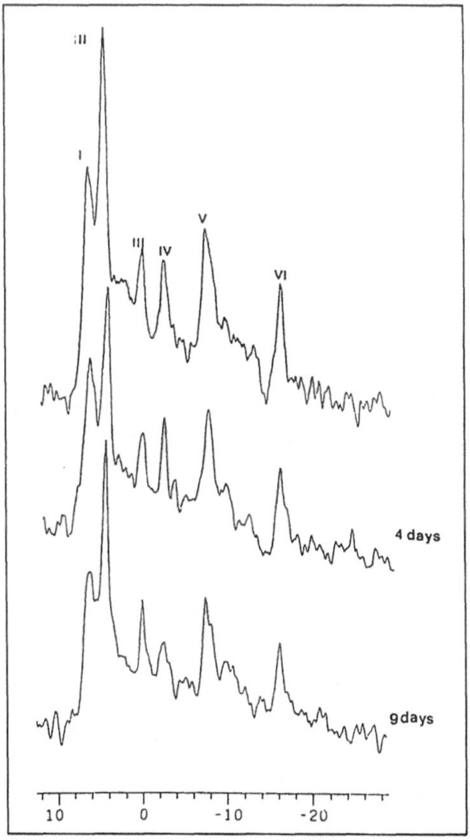

FIGURE 4. Rat Glioma: Control animal followed during 9 days.

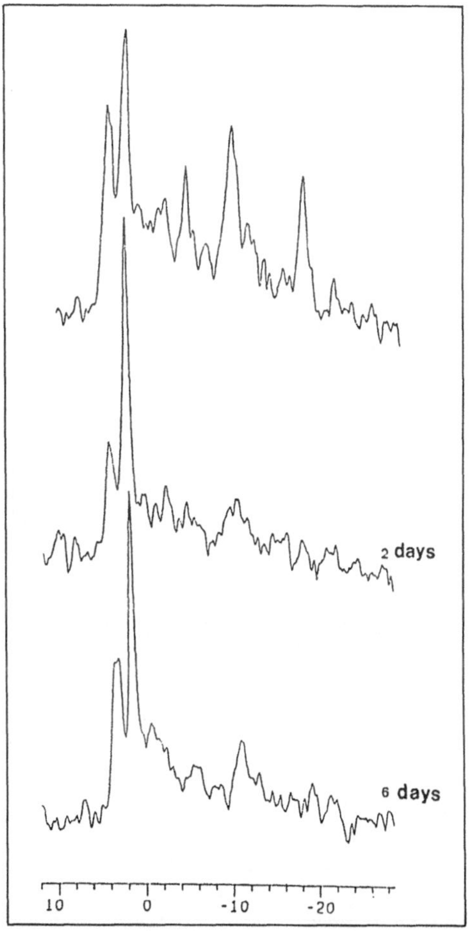

FIGURE 5. Rat Glioma: Treatment by sarcosinamide, 2 days and 6 days after injection.

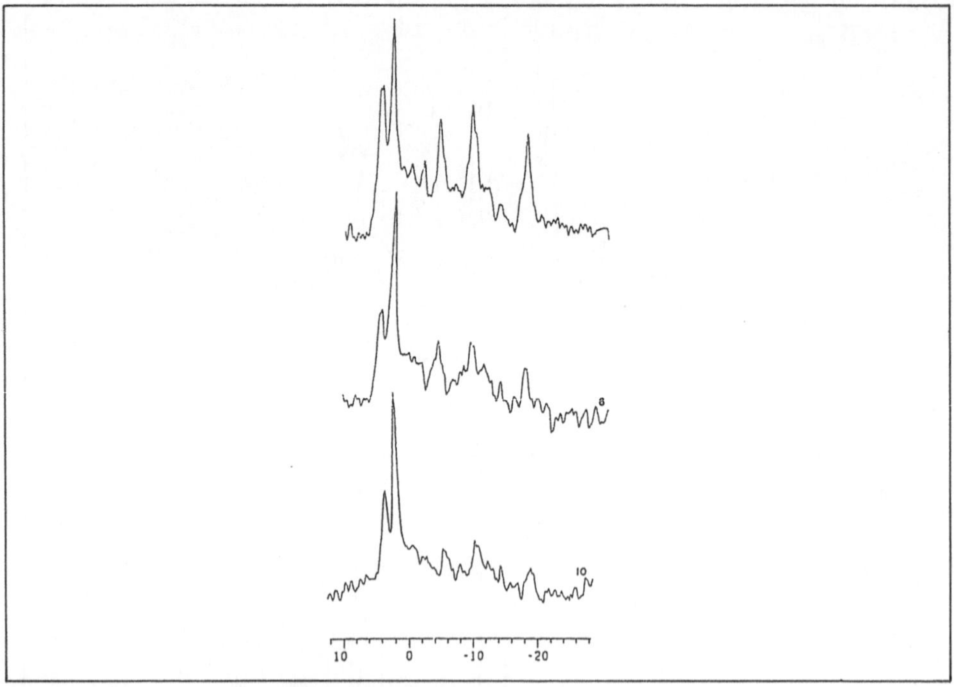

FIGURE 6. Rat Glioma: Treatment by ditercalinium, 6 and 10 days after injection.

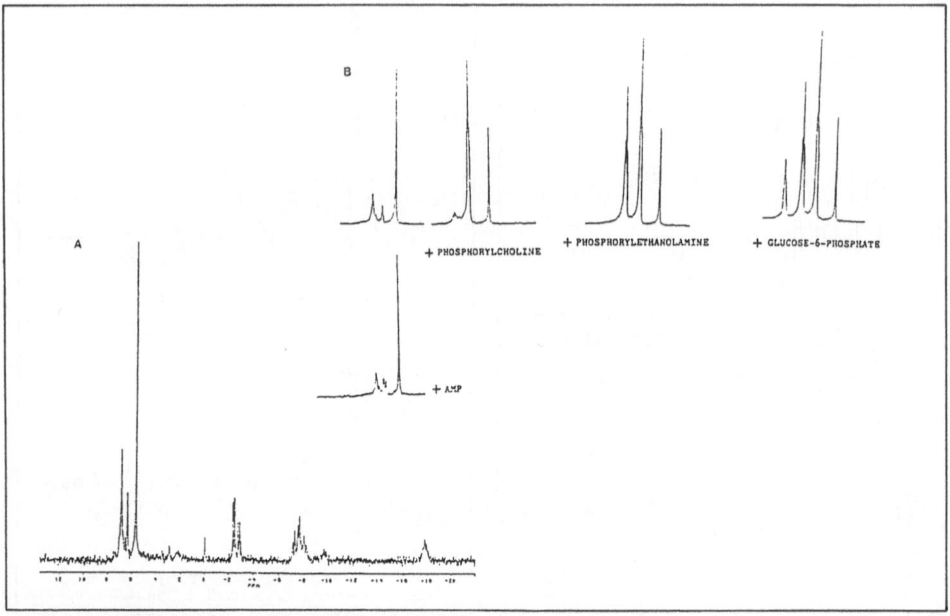

FIGURE 7. Perchloric extract of Rat Glioma. A: ^{31}P NMR Spectrum. B: PME region between 5 and 8 ppm.

31-P-NMR Spectroscopy in vivo of Human and Rat Brain Tumors Grafted on Nude Mice

C. REMY (°), J.P. ALBRAND (°°), S. LOTITO (°), M. JACROT (°°°),
A. FRANÇOIS (°), J. RIONDEL (°°°), M. DECORPS (°°), J.F. LE BAS (°), A.L. BENABID (°).

INTRODUCTION

NMR spectroscopy provides a unique way of measuring metabolite levels of tissues both in vivo (in living animals) and in vitro (in perchloric acid extracts). This opportunity was applied to the study of the energy metabolism changes by 31P-NMR induced in brain tumors by the neoplastic phenotype as compared to the normal brain metabolism observed in the normal rat brain. Previous studies (2, 5) described, in various kinds of extra-cerebral tumors, changes suggesting hypoxic phenomena and evolving with time along with the growth of the lesion. The present study was aimed at the description of in vivo metabolite patterns of brain tumors grafted on nude mice and at the identification of these metabolites by in vitro high resolution spectroscopy on perchloric acid (PCA) extracts.

MATERIAL AND METHODS

31P-NMR Spectroscopy:

All spectra were obtained at 4.7 Teslas in a CXP 200 or a WM 200 wide bore Bruker spectrometer. Three different spin echo sequences were used to obtain routine spectra as well as measurements of in vivo T1 and T2 relaxation times of the phosphorylated metabolites, with addition of selective refocusing Dante pulses to suppress the J modulation of ATP (7). Home-built probes were designed which could hold anesthetized nude mice or awake rats chronically implanted with surface coils (1, 7).

Animals:

Normal adult Sprague Dawley female rats (180-200 g) were chronically implanted with surface coils, as previously described (1), and used as controls for normal 31P-NMR spectra of the awake rat brain.

Nude mice were surgically grafted in the scapular region with tumor samples or cultured cell lines and examined for NMR spectroscopy at different times of the tumor evolution under Nembutal anaesthesia.

Tumors:

Several types of human brain tumors, including a gliosarcoma, were established as continuous models on nude mice and used in this study. A human ovarian cystadenocarcinoma served as comparison between human tumors.

The C6 cell line, derived from a chemically induced rat malignant glioma, was injected to nude mice (10^6 cells) and served as comparison between brain tumors in different species.

PCA extracts:

Tumors were freeze-clamped in vivo on the anaesthetized mice, ground in liquid nitrogen. PCA (0.6 M, 1/5-W/V) was added, the mixture was homogeneized with an Ultraturrax at 4°C. After centrifugation, K_2CO_3 5M was added to the supernatant until pH equals 7.4. After further

(°) LMCEC, Dept. of Biophysics, Grenoble University Medical School, 38700 La Tronche, France. (°°) RMBM, SPH/DRF, Centre d'Etudes Nucléaires, 85X, 38041 Grenoble Cedex, France. (°°°) Laboratoire d'Histologie, Grenoble University Medical School, 38700, La Tronche, France.

M. Chatel, F. Darcel and J. Pecker (eds.), Brain Oncology. ISBN-13: 978-94-010-8003-3

centrifugation, the supernatant was lyophilized, stored at -20°C until NMR processing and then added with 1 ml of TRIS 10 mM EDTA 50 mM pH 8.00.

RESULTS AND DISCUSSION

Characteristic features of the C6 rat glioma as compared to the normal rat brain:

There is no "tumor specific" peak. However, Uridine-di phospho glucose (UDPG) is observed on long accumulation time spectra of tumors but not of normal brain. The exact identification of this resonance remains to be precisely determined. There is no acidosis, the intracellular pH determined from the chemical shift of the inorganic phosphate (Pi) peak being equal to 7.2. As compared to the normal brain spectra, there is an elevation of the Pi peak and a decrease in Phosphocreatine (PCr). This is attributed to a hypoxic cell population within the tumor.

Characteristic features of the human tumors

— Compounds involved in the phosphoglycerides metabolism and in maturation:

Tumor tissues exhibit an increased amount of phosphomonoesters (PME), especially in the ovarian cystadenocarcinoma and a decrease in the phosphodiesters (PDE). The increase in PME is also observed in the immature brain of newborn infants or animals and could be related to maturation processes as it has been demonstrated (2, 3, 6) to be due to an increase in phosphorylethanolamine, a compound involved in membrane phospholipids metabolism. The decrease in PDE is apparent as compared to the normal human brain 31P spectrum where the PDE are much more elevated than in the rat brain: this could be due to the high amount of myelin in the human brain, which constitutes an accumulation of cell membranes.

— Compounds involved in glycogen synthesis:

Depending on the type of the tumor, there is a peak of variable amplitude corresponding to UDPG.

— Evolution of the spectra along with the growth of the tumors:

In our experience, the growth over one month of two tumors of different types (a gliosarcoma and an ovarian cystadenocarcinoma) dit not induce any significant change in the 31P-NMR pattern. This is different from previously reported data (2, 5) and could be related to the variable occurence of necrosis in the core of the tumor.

Characteristic features of the PCA extracts (fig. 1):

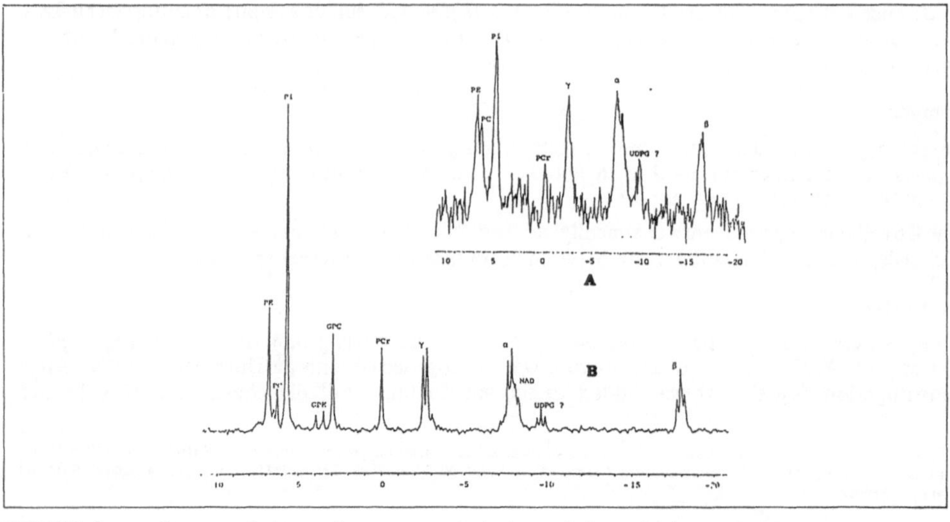

FIGURE 1. Comparative spectra of a human gliosarcoma: A - in vivo, grafted on nude mice. B - PCA extract.

— DPDE (Diphosphodiesters) region (-9.5 ppm):

Three peaks are observed in PCA extracts spectra of tumors (2) and not in mammalian normal brain (3, 6). They may correspond to UDPG, until further characterization.

— PDE region:

According to (2, 3, 6), the 3 ppm resonance corresponds to Glycerephosphorylcholine (GPC), the 3.5 ppm resonance to glycerophosphorylethanolamine (GPE), the 4 ppm peak remains unattributed.

— PME region:

The PME were first attributed to sugarphosphates (mainly ribose-5-phosphate). It was further demonstrated in tumors (2) and in mammalian brains (3, 6) that the resonances of this region correspond to Phosphorylcholine (PC) at 6.35 ppm and to Phosphorylethanolamine (PE) at 6.85 ppm. The precise assignment of these resonances remains to be done (using selective proton decoupling, titration curve of the chemical shift with respect to the pH, addition of the suspected compound) for each of our tumor models.

TABLE 1

Values of the ratio of relaxation times T1 and T2 of a C6 rat glioma to the corresponding T1 and T2 of the normal rat brain

Compound	T1 glioma/T1 normal	T2 glioma/T2 normal
PME	1.42	1.86
Pi	1.88	1.93
PCr	1.34	1.01
Gamma-ATP	1.5	1.32
Alpha-ATP	1.67	1.24
Beta-ATP	1.91	1.12

T1 and T2 relaxation times of phosphorylated compounds (Table 1):

T1 of all compounds, but mainly of Pi and ATP, are elevated in the C6 rat glioma grafted on nude mice, as compared to the values observed in the normal rat brain. The elevation of T2 is significant only for PME and Pi. At the present time, there is no available explanation of this original observation. We previously reported that, on stereotactic biopsies of human brain tumors, the proton relaxation times of these samples were increased by a ratio of about 2 and that this could be mainly related to an increased water content (4). Whether a similar cause could be involved in the increased values of the 31 P relaxation times should be demonstrated by further experiments.

CONCLUSION

31 P-NMR spectroscopy provides metabolic informations about brain tumors in vivo which can be correlated to precise identification of the observed compounds in vitro by high resolution NMR of PCA extracts. The detailed knowledge of these metabolic patterns could be useful in the prospect of future NMR spectroscopy and/or spectroscopic NMR imaging of brain tumors in human patients.

SUMMARY

Nude mice were grafted with human (gliosarcoma) and rat (C6 malignant glioma cell line) brain tumors and, for comparison, with extracerebral human tumors (ovarian cystadenocarcinoma). They were placed under pentobarbital anaesthesia in a laboratory built NMR probe, in a 4.7 Teslas 100 mm wide bore supraconducting magnet. 31P-NMR spectra were performed at 81MHz, using a Spin-Echo pulse sequence. Measurements of the T1 and T2 relaxation times of the high energy phosphates were made using a Spin-Echo sequence with a selective refocusing pulse. These values in the tumors grafted on nude mice were compared with those obtained on a normal rat brain equiped with a chronically implanted surface coil, as a control. In addition, perchloric acid extracts of the grafted tumors were used for high resolution NMR spectroscopy to identify the metabolite responsible for elevated amplitudes of some resonances. The 31P-NMR pattern of the grafted brain tumors, as compared to the normal rat brain, is made of a decreased peak of Phosphocreatine, an elevated peak of inorganic phosphate and a significant increase of the Phosphomonoester peak, which is even higher in the ovarian cystadenocarcinoma. The pH is not significantly decreased. Long term acquisition (2 hours) yields well resolved spectra where Uridine diphosphoglucose can be detected. Preliminary results of high resolution NMR spectroscopy of perchloric acid extracts of the gliosarcoma suggests that Ribose-5-phosphate and/or phosphorylethanolamine might be the major components of the increased phosphomonoester peak. The precise identification of these compounds in different types of tumors is in progress. T1 and T2 relaxation times are significantly elevated in rat brain tumors as compared to the normal rat brain. There is no available explanation of this original finding. Comparison may be made with what is known about the relationship between elevation of T1 and T2 in brain tumors and their elevated water content.

KEY WORDS

31-P NMR, Chemotherapy, Energy Metabolism, Nude Mice, Xenografts.

AKNOWLEDGEMENTS

This work has been supported in part by grants of MRT, MEN, MGEN, INSERM-CNAMTS, EPR Rhône-Alpes, LCC, ESPOIR and Grenoble University Scientific Council.

REFERENCES

1. DECORPS (M.), LEBAS (J.F.), LEVIEL (J.L.), CONFORT (C.), REMY (C.) and BENABID (A.L.): FEBS Lett., 168, 1-6 (1984).
2. EVANOCHKO (W.T.), SAKAI (T.T.), NG (T.C.), KRISHNA (N.R.), KIM (M.D.), ZEIDLER (R.B.), GHANTA (V.K.), BROCKMAN (R.W.), SHIFFER (L.M.), BRAUNSCHWEIGER (P.G.) and GLICKSON (J.D.): Biochim. Biophys. Acta, 805, 104-116 (1984).
3. GUYLAI (L.), BOLINGER (L.), LEIGH (J.S.), BARLOW (C.) and CHANCE (B.): FEBS Lett., 178, 137-142 (1984).
4. LE BAS (J.F.), LEVIEL (J.L.), DECORPS (M.) and BENABID (A.L.): Comput. Assist. Tomogr., 8, 1048-1057 (1984).
5. NG (T.C.), EVANOCHKO (W.T.), HIRAMOTO (R.N.), GHANTA (V.K.), LILLY (M.B.), LAWSON (A.J.), CORBETT (T.H.), DURANT (J.R.) and GLICKSON (J.D.): J. Magn. Res. 49, 271-286 (1982).
6. PETTEGREW (J.W.), KOPP (S.J.), DADOK (J.), MINSHEW (N.J.), FELIKSIK (J.M.), GLONEK (T.) and COHEN (M.M.): J. Magn. Res., 67, 443-450 (1986).
7. REMY (C.), ALBRAND (J.P.), BENABID (A.L.), DECORPS (M.), JACROT (M.), RIONDEL (J.) and FORAY (M.F.): Magn. Res. in Med., in press (1987).

Blood Brain Barrier Modification and Chemotherapy in Treatment of Malignant Gliomas

A. HORACZEK, G. BAUMGARTNER, P. GRUNERT, K. KITZ, E. KNOSP, P. VORKAPIC, K. HEIMBERGER, P. SAMEC.

INTRODUCTION

The results of chemotherapy of malignant gliomas were not satisfactory (1, 4). Blood-brain-barrier modification and intra-arterial application of MTX (2) prolonged the survival rate. Barrier modification with 76% angiografin and Thio-Tepa intra-arterial was reported to be successfull in treatment of malignant gliomas (3). Some groups argue, that blood-brain-barrier is not a factor of distribution of chemotherapy in brain tumors.

MATERIALS AND METHODS

17 patients were treated with polychemotherapy and hyaluronidase. 6 of them were treated before by barrier modification with 76% angiografin, Thio-Tepa was applicated intra-arterial.

In 1 patient blood-brain-barrier was disrupted with 25% mannitol, MTX applicated intra-arterial, cytoxan was infused i.v., 1 patient was treated with both methods.

3 patients were radiated as well.

All these patients had a malignant glioma and underwent surgery prior to chemotherapy.

Table I shows the histological data.

Polychemotherapy with hyaluronidase was performed i.v. for three days in cycles of every three weeks.

There was applicated: MTX, CCNU, ETOPOSID, CIS-PLATIN and 5 FLUOROURACIL. The patients recieved also every day 200.000 units of hyaluronidase i.v.

Blood-brain barrier modification was performed under general anesthesia either with 25% mannitol or with 76% angiografin.

Table II shows the pre-treatment.

TABLE I

HISTOLOGY	NR. of PAT
Glioblastoma multiforme	5
Glioblastoma IV	4
Anaplastic glioma	1
Anaplastic astrocytoma III - IV	1
Anaplastic astrocytoma III	4
Astro-oligodendroglioma III	1
Astrocytoma II - III	1

TABLE II

PRE-TREATMENT	N.
Radiation	3
Reversible blood-brain-barrier Modification with mannitol and I.A. application of MTX	1
Reversible blood-brain-barrier Modification with 76% angiografin and I.A. application of thio-tepa	6

RESULTS

All patients who were treated with blood-brain barrier modification experienced recurrency of the glioma and underwent surgery before treatment with polychemotherapy and hyaluronidase.

From these 17 patients neurological conditions improved in 7 patients, in 8 cases it was unchanged and deterioration was observed in 2 cases (Table III).

TABLE III

Neurological condition	
Improved	7
Unchanged	8
Deteriorated	2

M. Chatel, F. Darcel and J. Pecker (eds.), Brain Oncology. ISBN-13: 978-94-010-8003-3

Cat-Scan findings improved in 9 patients, while in 4 patients CAT-Scan remained unchanged (Table IV).

TABLE IV

CAT-Scan Findings	
Improved	9
Unchanged	4
Deterioriated	1
No Control CAT-Scan	3

In 1 patient progress of tumor growth was observed and in 1 case there was deterioration for the first time.

Two patients died because of pulmonary embolism during the therapy cycles, so now we applicate anticoagulant medication p.o.; one patient died because of toxic colitis and intracranial thrombopenic hemorrhage.

One patient deterioriated in his neurological condition as well as in his CAT-Scan findings. All other patients do well, no one of them has a recurrent tumor in CAT-Scan.

DISCUSSION

In our material using monochemotherapy with blood-brain-barrier modification we could not find the results as reported previously (3). Blood-brain-barrier disruption with mannitol and intra-arterial MTX and i.v. Cytoxan was reported to prolong survival rate (6).

Polychemotherapy with hyaluronidase seems to be an alternative method in treatment of recurrent gliomas, but the study is not finished yet.

SUMMARY

Reversible osmotic disruption of blood-brain-barrier by intra-arterial application of hyperosmolar substances makes chemotherapy more effective. We present two methods of barrier disruption, using neuroradiological technics. We report our results, and we present an other method of treatment of malignant gliomas, using polychemotherapy and hyaluronidase.

KEY WORDS

Blood-Brain-Barrier-Modification, Chemotherapy, Malignant Gliomas, Hyaluronidase.

REFERENCES

1. WALKER (M.D.) et al.: Randomized comparisons of radiotherapy and nitrosoureas for the treatment of malignant gliomas after surgery. N. Engl. J. Med. 1980, 303, 1323-1329.
2. NEUWELT (E.A.) et al.: Reversible osmotic BBBD in humans: implications for the chemotherapy of malignant brain tumors. Neurosurgery, 1980, 7, 47-52.
3. LEVIN (A.B.): Personal communication, Vienna, March 1986.
4. JELLINGER et al.: Ergebnisse der Kombinationsbehandlung maligner Gliome. Nervenarzt, 1981, 52, 41-50.
5. VICK (N.) et al.: Chemotherapy of brain tumors: The blood-brain-barrier is not a factor. Arch. Neurol., 1977, 34, 523-526.
6. HOWIESON (J.) et al.: Results of altered blood-brain-barrier chemotherapy of glioblastoma multiforme. Paper read at XIII. Symp. Neuroradiologicum, Stockholm, June 1986.

Human Central Nervous System Pharmacology of Antineoplastic Agents: Implications for the Treatment of Brain Tumors

D.J. STEWART (°).

INTRODUCTION

It has long been argued that the blood-brain barrier (BBB) may be a very important consideration in the chemotherapy of intracranial tumors. While it was initially felt that the BBB would prevent uptake of drug into intracerebral tumors, it was eventually recognized that the vasculature within brain tumors is highly abnormal (1) and that the BBB is at least partially disrupted to a variable degree within these neoplasms (1, 2).

It has also been argued that the area of the brain adjacent to tumor (BAT) is very important in brain tumor resistance to chemotherapy, since actively growing glioma cells may penetrate widely into this area, but the degree of BBB disruption is less in BAT than within tumor (2, 3, 4) and capillary permeability in BAT may even be less than that in normal brain (3, 4). Some authors feel that there would also be minimal diffusion of drug out from tumor to the BAT around large human brain tumors (3, 4). Thus, the tumor cells penetrating into the BAT would be relatively protected from the effect of agents that cannot cross the normal BBB (3, 4). The conclusion that the BBB is important in the treatment of brain tumors has also been supported by observations that: a) the most active drugs against brain tumors are lipid-soluble agents that readily cross the BBB (4, 5). b) Less methotrexate is taken up into intracerebral than subcutaneous animal tumors (6). c) Distribution of methotrexate in animal brain tumors is irregular, while being very uniform in extracerebral tumors (6). d) Capillary permeability is generally less in intracerebral than in subcutaneous rat tumors (7). e) Water-soluble drugs that are active against extracerebral tumors in animals are often less active against the same tumor if it is in the brain (8). f) Activity of different members of some classes of chemotherapeutic agents against rat brain tumors varies as a function of lipid solubility (9, 10). g) Patients with acute leukemia may develop meningeal relapse while other systemic disease is still in remission (11). h) In patients with solid tumors who are responding to chemotherapy, the brain may be the first site of tumor recurrence or progression (12).

However, despite the available evidence, it remains inconclusive whether or not a pharmacological sanctuary effect plays a major role in the chemotherapy of human brain tumors.

In an attempt to better understand the nature of the effect on the chemotherapy of brain tumors of drug central nervous system (CNS) pharmacology, we have undertaken studies of the uptake of a number of different antineoplastic agents into the human CSN, intracerebral tumors and extracerebral tumors.

METHOD

Non-toxic doses of chemotherapeutic agents were administered intravenously to consenting patients prior to surgical resection of intracerebral tumors (13-28). Tumor tissue that was not needed for histopathological examination was assayed for drug content. If any brain tissue was adherant to the resected tumor, it was also assayed for drug. If a lobectomy was required for surgical removal of a patient's tumor, drug concentration was determined in the resected brain samples as a function of distance from the grossly visible edge of the tumor. Blood samples were obtained from some patients by venipuncture or by insertion of a heparin lock.

(°) The Ontario Cancer Treatment and Research Foundation Ottawa Regional Cancer Centre and the University of Ottawa Faculty of Health Sciences.

M. Chatel, F. Darcel and J. Pecker (eds.), Brain Oncology. ISBN-13: 978-94-010-8003-3

Tissues samples were also collected from patients who had received chemotherapy drugs therapeutically and subsequently died and underwent autopsy (13-15, 22, 23, 29-33). Some patients receiving drugs therapeutically who had easily accessible extracerebral tumor also underwent biopsy of these intracerebral tumors to determine drug concentrations (14, 17, 21, 22, 24). Cerebrospinal fluid was also obtained from some patients receiving therapeutic doses of drugs (14, 17, 18, 20-23, 26). If the patient had an Ommaya reservoir in place, Ommaya reservoir puncture was used to obtain the cerebrospinal fluid samples. If there was no Ommaya reservoir in place, cerebrospinal fluid samples were obtained by lumbar puncture.

Different assay methods were used depending on which drug was being assayed. Flameless atomic absorption or x-ray dispersive fluorescence was used to assay samples for platinum after administration of cisplatin. A colorimetric assay was used for gallium nitrate. An enzyme inhibition assay was used for phosphonacetyl-L-aspartate (PALA). Radiochemical assays were used for vinblastine and Baker's antifol. High pressure liquid chromatographic (HPLC) assays were used for all other drugs.

RESULTS

Surgical tissue samples were obtained from the following numbers of patients: cisplatin - 8 patients, AZQ - 4, mitoxantrone - 10, AMSA - 4, 3-deazauridine - 4, IMPY - 1, methylglyoxyl bis (guanylhydrazone) (MGBG) - 6, PALA - 16, pentamethylmelamine - 10, vinblastine - 1, VM-26 - 29, VP-16 - 17, Baker's antifol - 6, tiazofurin - 16, gallium nitrate - 1. Autopsy tissue samples were obtained from the following numbers of patients: cisplatin - 31, AZQ - 1, mitoxantrone - 11, AMSA - 5, 3-deazauridine - 2, MGBG - 2, pentamethylmelamine - 1, vinblastine - 2. Cerebrospinal fluid samples were obtained from the following numbers of patients: cisplatin -8, AMSA - 4, 3-deazauridine - 3, MGBG - 3, PALA - 7, pentamethylmelamine - 5, vinblastine - 1, Baker's antifol - 7, tiazofurin - 2.

Potentially cytotoxic concentrations of each of these drugs were found in most intracerebral tumors from most patients. However, with some of the drugs, individual tumor samples had only very low concentrations of drug or no drug. The only patient in whom gallium nitrate was studied had only a low concentration of the drug in his tumor. With Baker's antifol, large quantities of radio-label were found in intracerebral tumors but it is probable that most of the label was attached to relatively inactive metabolites. For other drugs, concentration in intracerebral tumors was generally moderately high.

For the purposes of this manuscript, we converted results to a standard dose for each drug to facilitate comparisons of concentrations of the drug in different body compartments. The Student's t-test was used to test for statistical differences between drug concentrations in intracerebral tumors and in other compartments. Both intracerebral and extracerebral tumor samples were available for nine different drugs. For cisplatin and AMSA, the drug concentration in intracerebral tumor was significantly higher ($P < 0.05$) than in extracerebral tumor. For PALA the difference was of borderline significance ($P < 0.1$). Pentamethylmelamine and 3-deazauridine achieved slightly ($P < 0.1$) higher concentrations in intracerebral tumor than in extracerebral tumor. For mitoxantrone and VP-16, drug concentrations were significantly ($P < 0.05$) higher in extracerebral tumor than in intracerebral tumor. Only a single extracerebral tumor sample was obtained for MGBG. The concentration in this extracerebral tumor was somewhat higher than the mean concentration in intracerebral tumors, but it was within the range of the concentrations seen in intracerebral tumors. For vinblastine, 2 intracerebral tumor samples were obtained. An accurate assessment of the vinblastine concentration was possible for only one of these intracerebral tumors. This single evaluable intracerebral tumor specimen had a higher concentration of vinblastine than did any of the extracerebral tumor samples that were available for assay.

For all drugs that were studied, only low concentrations were noted in the cerebrospinal fluid. Statistical comparison between concentration in cerebrospinal fluid and in intracerebral tumor was possible for seven drugs. In each case, the concentration in cerebrospinal fluid was significantly ($P < 0.05$) less in cerebrospinal fluid than in intracerebral tumor. Either BAT or samples of brain distant from tumor were also available for all of the drugs except gallium nitrate. The concentration of drug in BAT was generally slightly lower than in the tumor itself, although it was actually higher than the concentration obtained in tumor for 3-deazauridine, IMPY and tiazofurin. There was significantly more drug in tumor than in BAT for pentamethylmelamine ($P < 0.05$), and for

PALA the difference approached statistical significance ($P < 0.1$). Apart from these two drugs, none of the differences between intracerebral tumor and BAT achieved significance, although significance levels could not be tested for four of the drugs (AZQ, IMPY, vinblastine and VP-16) since only single BAT samples were obtained. Brain distant from intracerebral tumor consistently had far lower drug concentrations than did the tumor itself. Statistical comparisons were possible for five of the drugs (cisplatin, mitoxantrone, AMSA, MGBG and 3-deazauridine) and the difference between distant brain and intracerebral tumor was statistically significant ($P < 0.05$) for the first three of these five drugs. No distant brain was available for analysis for IMPY, VM-26, Baker's antifol, tiazofurin and gallium nitrate. For seven drugs (cisplatin, AZQ, mitoxantrone, AMSA, 3-deazauridine, PALA, pentamethylmelamine, vinblastine and VP-16) both BAT and distant brain samples were available for assay. In each case, drug concentrations were lower in distant brain than they were in BAT.

Plasma samples drawn at times comparable to when tumor was sampled were available for all of the drugs except cisplatin and AMSA. Statistical comparison was possible for 11 of the drugs but was not possible for IMPY and gallium nitrate since plasma samples were only obtained from single patients for these two drugs. For IMPY the concentration of drug in this one plasma sample was comparable to the concentration of drug in intracerebral tumors and in brain adjacent to tumor, while with gallium nitrate, the concentration in plasma was far higher than the concentration in intracerebral tumor. The plasma concentration of drug was significantly higher than the intracerebral tumor drug concentration for AZQ, PALA, VP-16, and tiazofurin, whereas the plasma concentration of drug was significantly ($P < 0.05$) lower than the drug concentration in tumor for MGBG and Baker's antifol. The comparison for Baker's antifol was based on disintegrations per minute using radiochemical assay. As stated previously, a substantial amount of the radioactivity in tumor was actually in the form of metabolite rather than parent drug. The amount of radioactivity was significantly higher in intracerebral tumor than in plasma, but we could not determine what the relative concentrations of parent drug were. For other drugs, concentrations in plasma were comparable to those in intracerebral tumor, but minor differences generally existed. Drug concentration was somewhat higher in intracerebral tumor than in plasma for mitoxantrone, 3-deazauridine, pentamethylmelamine and vinblastine.

For cisplatin, tumor samples were available both after intravenous and intraarterial administration of drug. Tumor platinum concentration was significantly ($P < 0.025$) higher after intraarterial than after intravenous administration of cisplatinum.

Attempts were made to augment the uptake of VM-26 into human intracerebral tumors by a variety of manœuvres. Amphotericin-B results in increased uptake of antibiotics and antineoplastic agents into mammalian cells (34) and may also increase the penetration of some drugs across the BBB (35). We found no evidence that it increased the amount of VM-26 attainable in human intracerebral tumors, although the number of samples was small. Glycerol was also tested. Glycerol increases blood flow to areas around intracerebral mass lesions in baboons and humans (36). Increasing blood flow to a tumor could potentially increase the drug concentration attained in the tumor (37), although experimental data suggest that blood flow may be a relatively minor factor in determining the uptake of water-soluble drugs into brain tumors (38). Patients who had received glycerol prior to their I.V. VM-26 may have achieved a higher ($P < 0.1$) VM-26 concentration in their intracerebral tumors than did patients who did not receive glycerol. Twenty-four hour infusions of VM-26 were also tried on the assumption that a prolonged low-gradiant of drug might result in more drug entering deep tissue compartments than with a brief high gradiant (2). However the concentration of VM-26 attained in human intracerebral tumors after 24-hour infusion was substantially lower than the concentration attained with a one-hour infusion of the same dose of VM-26.

For some drugs such as MGBG, higher drug concentrations were attained in glioblastomas than in brain metastases, while the opposite was true for VM-26. For some drugs such as mitoxantrone, there was more drug in necrotic tumor than in viable tumor, while for others, such as MGBG and VP-16, there was more in viable tumor than in necrotic tumor. For some of the drugs, different pieces of a tumor were assayed. As a rule, drug concentration varied from one part of a tumor to another.

DISCUSSION

These pharmacology data indicate that potentially cytotoxic concentrations of many antineoplastic agents are attained in human intracerebral tumors. The concentration of a drug attained in CSF and normal brain tissue does not predict the concentration in human intracerebral tumors. Moreover, while the concentrations of drug in the BAT are frequently lower than the concentrations in the tumor itself, the concentrations in BAT are often still potientially cytotoxic and are higher than they are in more distant brain, contrary to the predictions from some animal studies (3, 4).

Comparisons of drug concentrations in human brain tumors to those in human extracerebral tumors also differed from that seen in animal models. Unlike the situation in animals (6, 7) penetration of many drugs into intracerebral tumor was no less than penetration into extracerebral tumors. The only exceptions to this were mitoxantrone and VP-16 (16, 24, 30). It is stressed however, that the comparisons we have made between intracerebral and extracerebral tumors in this study must be interpreted cautiously, since numbers of patients were small and since time from drug administration to sample acquisition varied from one patient to another. Dose also varied. We corrected the results for dose, but in doing so, we assumed that the uptake of drug into tumor was linear with dose. In any event, we can state that we have failed to demonstrate that substantially less drug penetrates into human intracerebral tumors than into extracerebral tumor for many antineoplastic agents. While our pharmacology data definitely do not prove that the BBB is of no consequence in the treatment of human brain tumors, they do indicate that it may possibly be of somewhat less importance than it is in small animal models.

In addition to our pharmacology data, there are also some other problems with accepting unquestionningly available evidence that the BBB is a major impediment to brain tumor chemotherapy:

a) Glioblastomas are actually a fairly responsive solid tumor rather than being a fairly resistant one: response rates of glioblastomas (5) are superior to those seen for many other solid tumors (39-43) and glioblastomas are one of only a handful of solid tumors where chemotherapy prolongs survival (44).

b) The importance of lipid solubility of a drug in treating brain tumors is somewhat of a self-fulfilling prophecy: since current biases dictate that drugs that cross the BBB are fare more likely than others to be evaluated against brain tumors, such drugs have a far higher chance of being shown to be active against brain tumors than do drugs which are not lipid soluble and hence not tested. A large number of water-soluble agents have never been tested properly against brain tumors.

c) BCNU, in addition to being lipid soluble, is also one of the more active drugs against glioblastoma tumor cells grown in tissue culture (45). Its superior activity against brain tumors may be due more to its cytotoxicity than to its pharmacology.

d) Many drugs that cross the normal BBB only very poorly are active against human and animal brain tumors (46-49).

e) In animal tumors, even lipid soluble drugs that should cross the BBB readily may be more active against extracerebral than against intracerebral tumors (50).

f) In different classes of antineoplastic agents, activity against intracerebral tumors is not directly proportional to degree of lipid solubility (9). Moreover, the optimal log P varies from one class of antineoplastic agents to another (9, 10) and from one type of intracerebral tumor to another (9).

g) Rather than measuring reduction in size of tumor or prolongation of survival from the development of tumor-related symptoms, as occurs in humans, animal studies comparing activity of antineoplastic agents against intracerebral vs extracerebral tumors generally measure survival from the time of tumor inoculation (8). Quite frequently the drug is administered on the same day the tumor is implanted or just a few days later (8). Intracerebral tumors will initially grow without inducing their own blood supply and the BBB becomes leaky only after induction of neovascularization by the tumor (51). Hence, it is very possible that the BBB could protect intracerebral tumors while they were very small, but this may bear little relationship to the effect of chemotherapy on a tumor that has developed its own blood supply.

h) In some studies, anaesthetic was used to implant the intracerebral tumors but not to implant extracerebral tumors (8). Such anaesthetics could potentially alter metabolism and activity of anticancer agents.

i) An extracerebral tumor has to be far larger than an intracerebral tumor to kill an animal because of the "closed box" effect of the skull, and intracerebral tumors kill animals by a different mechanism (impairment of blood flow to brain and infiltration of brain) than do extracerebral tumors.

j) Any drug that led to delayed rather than immediate cell killing could well be more advantageous against extracerebral tumors than against intracerebral tumors because the intracerebral tumor could prove lethal at a smaller size, before the onset of drug effect.

k) Animal tumors may not be good models for human tumors since human tumors are generally far larger than animal tumors are. Tumor blood flow, vascular permeability and presence of resistant tumor cell clones are markedly dependant on tumor size for many tumors (52-54).

l) While the meninges may be the first site of relapse of acute leukemia (11) and while central nervous system prophylaxis can prevent such relapses (55), effective CNS prophylaxis does not prolong the duration of marrow remission or survival in acute leukemia (56, 57) and the clinical factors that predict for meningeal relapse of leukemia are very similar to those that predict for early bone marrow relapse (58-61).

m) In a rat model of meningeal carcinomatosis, systemic drugs that do not ordinarily penetrate well into the CNS will be effective once the meningeal tumor deposits have had time to establish their own blood supply (62).

n) Patients with acute leukemia who have died of causes other than their leukemia have been found to have leukemia deposits in multiple other organs despite the bone marrow remaining in complete remission (63, 64). It is debateable whether one should claim that tumor deposits survive in the CNS because of a pharmacological sanctuary if one does not claim the same for residual leukemia deposits in these other organs such as the kidney, lymph node, testis, lung, bowel and liver.

o) Small cell lung cancer is held up as an example of a tumor where the CNS is frequently the first site of relapse or progression because of protection of the brain metastases by the blood-brain barrier (65); however, drugs which cross the BBB do not reduce the incidence of brain metastases (66), prophylactic cranial irradiation does not prolong median survival despite decreasing the rate of brain metastases (67), and sites other than brain are also frequently an isolated site of first progression (68).

p) There are many other types of malignancies which can be cured with systemic chemotherapy (69), but where isolated development of brain metastases is not a frequent occurrence.

q) Brain metastases are frequently highly responsive to front-line treatment with water-soluble IV chemotherapy (70-73).

It would be reasonable to speculate that meningeal and intraparenchymal brain metastases are protected from chemotherapy by an intact BBB until such time as the tumor induces its own blood supply. It is also reasonable to conclude that this may contribute to the establishment of brain metastases despite the response of tumor in other areas, but it does not prove that the BBB is of significance in the treatment of established brain metastases. In addition, the BAT phenomenon would be expected to have less impact on the treatment of brain metastases than on treatment of glioblastomas (if it actually has any major impact on the treatment of glioblastomas) since brain metastases tend to be far more sharply demarcated than glioblastomas, with less infiltration into surrounding brain.

A drug must gain at least some access to a tumor before it can kill it; however, even if very high concentrations of drug are achieved in tumor, the tumor will not be killed if the tumor cells are inherently resistant to the drug. In vitro sensitivity studies of glioblastoma cells have shown that cells from many tumors will remain viable even if exposed to high concentrations of various chemotherapeutic agents (23). Based on these in vitro sensitivity studies, and based on our pharmacology studies, it would be reasonable to assume that the major problem with the chemotherapy of glioblastomas at the present time is one of resistance of the tumor cells to drugs, rather than inadequate delivery of drug to tumor.

Therefore, we feel that studies against brain tumors should not be restricted to lipid soluble drugs and that both new and old water soluble drugs should also be tested. It is quite possible that if in vitro cytotoxicity were equal between 2 drugs, the more lipid soluble one would be more active in vivo than the more water soluble one, but even this remains to be proven in humans.

SUMMARY

We have studied the uptake of a number of different antineoplastic agents into human intracerebral tumors. Tumor drug concentrations were generally far higher than drug concentrations in normal brain and cerebrospinal fluid and slightly higher than in edematous brain adjacent to the tumor. They frequently approached and sometimes exceeded drug concentrations in plasma and extracerebral tumors. For some drugs, there were differences between gliomas and brain metastases, and between necrotic and viable tissue with respect to drug concentrations attained. Oral glycerol appeared to augment the penetration of VM-26 into human brain tumors. Based on our results we do not feel that drugs should be excluded from trials against brain tumors simply because they do not penetrate into the normal central nervous system. The role of the blood-brain barrier in resistance of human brain tumors to chemotherapy remains controversial. It is probable that with drugs that are currently available, tumor cell resistance to the drug is a far more important factor than is the drug's pharmacology.

KEY WORDS

Pharmacology, Antineoplastic Agents, Chemotherapy, Brain Tumours.

REFERENCES

1. HIRANO (A.), MATSUI (T.): Vascular structures in brain tumors. Hum. Pathol. **6**: 611-621 (1975).
2. BLASBERG (R.G.), GROOTHUIS (D.R.): Chemotherapy of brain tumors: physiological and pharmacokinetic considerations, Semin. Oncol. **13**: 70-82 (1986).
3. LEVIN (V.A.), FREEMAN-DOVE (M.), LANDAHL (H.D.): Permeability characterisation of brain adjacent to tumor in rats. Arch. Neurol. **32**: 785-791 (1975).
4. LEVIN (V.A.): A pharmacologic basis for brain tumor chemotherapy. Semin. Oncol. **2**: 57-61 (1975).
5. EDWARDS (M.S.), LEVIN (V.A.), WILSON (C.B.): Brain tumor chemotherapy: an evaluation of agents in current use for phase II and III trials. Cancer Treat Rep. **64**: 1179-1205 (1980).
6. TATOR (C.H.): Retention of tritiated methotrexate in a transplantable mouse glioma. Cancer Res. **36**: 3058-3066 (1976).
7. GROOTHUIS (D.R.), FISCHER (J.M.), VICK (N.A.), BIGNER (D.D.): Comparative permeability of different glioma models to horseradish peroxidase. Cancer Treat. Rep. **65** (suppl. 2): 13-18, 1981.
8. WODINSKY (I.), MERKER (P.C.), VENDITTI (J.M.): Responsiveness to chemotherapy of mice with L1210 lymphoid leukemia implanted in various anatomic sites. J. Natl. Cancer Inst. **59**: 405-408 (1977).
9. LEVIN (V.A.), KABRA (P.): Effectiveness of the nitrosoureas as a function of their lipid solubility in the chemotherapy of experimental rat brain tumors. Cancer Chemother. Rep. **58**: 787-792 (1974).
10. LEVIN (V.A.), CRAFTS (D.), WILSON (C.B.), KABRA (P.), HANSCH (C.), BOLDREY (E.), ENOT (J.), NEELY (M.): Imidazole Carboxamides: relationship of lipophilicity to activity against intracerebral murine glioma 26 and preliminary phase II trial of 5-[3,3-bis(2-chloroethyl)-1-triazeno]imidazole-4-carboxamide (NSC-82196) in primary and secondary brain tumors. Cancer Chemoth. Rep. **59**: 327-331 (1975).
11. AUR (R.J.A.), SIMONE (J.), HUSTU (H.), et al.: Central nervous system therapy and combination chemotherapy of childhood lymphocytic leukemia. Blood **37**: 272-281 (1971).
12. BENJAMIN (R.S.), WIERNICK (P.H.), BACHUR (N.R.). Adriamycin chemotherapy - efficacy, safety and pharmacologic basis of an intermittent single high dose schedule. Cancer **33**: 19-27 (1974).
13. STEWART (D.J.), MIKHAEL (N.), NANJI (A.), KACEW (S.), MAROUN (J.), HIRTE (W.): Human tissue cisplatin (CP) pharmacology: clinical implications. Proc. Am. Assoc. Cancer Res. **26**: 154 (1985).
14. STEWART (D.J.), LEAVENS (M.), MAOR (M.), FEUN (L.), LUNA (M.), BONURA (J.), CAPRIOLI (R.), LOO (T.L.), BENJAMIN (R.S.): Human central nervous system distribution of cis-diaminedichloroplatinum and use as a radiosensitizer in malignant brain tumors. Cancer Res. **42**: 2474-2479 (1982).
15. SAVARAJ (N.), LU (K.), FEUN (L.G.), LEAVENS (M.E.), STEWART (D.J.), BURGESS (M.A.), BENJAMIN (R.S.), LOO (T.L.): Intracerebral penetration and tissue distribution of 2,5-Diaziridinyl 3,6-bis(Carboethoxyamino) 1,4-Benzoquinone (AZQ NSC 182986). J. Neuro-Oncol. **1**: 15-20 (1983).
16. STEWART (D.J.), HUGENHOLTZ (H.), GREEN (R.), RICHARD (M.), BENOIT (B.), RUSSELL (N.), MAROUN (J.), THIBAULT (M.): Mitoxantrone hydrochloride: uptake into human brain tumors and phase II study in gliomas. J. Neuro-Oncol. **4**: 114 (1986).

17. ZHENGANG (B.), SAVARAJ (N.), FEUN (L.G.), LU (K.), STEWART (D.J.), LUNA (M.), BENJAMIN (R.S.), LOO (T.L.): Tumor penetration of AMSA in man. Cancer Invest. **1**: 475-478 (1983).

18. STEWART (D.J.), BENVENUTO (J.A.), LEAVENS (M.), HALL (S.W.), BENJAMIN (R.S.), PLUNKETT (W.), McCREDIE (K.D.), BURGESS (M.A.), LOO (T.L.). Penetration of 3-Deazauridine into human brain, intracerebral tumor and cerebrospinal fluid. Cancer Res. **39**: 4119-4122 (1979).

19. FONG (K.L.), HO (D.H.W.), YAP (B.S.), STEWART (D.J.), BROWN (N.S.), BENJAMIN (R.S.), FREIREICH (E.J.), BODEY (C.P.). Clinical Pharmacology of IMPY by radio-immunoassay. Cancer Treat. Rep. **64**: 1253-1260 (1980).

20. ROSENBLUM (M.), STEWART (D.J.), YAP (B.S.), LEAVENS (M.), BENJAMIN (R.S.), LOO (T.L.): Penetration of Methylglyoxal Bis (guanylhydrazone) into intracerebral tumors in humans. Cancer Res. **41**: 459-462 (1981).

21. STEWART (D.J.), LEAVENS (M.), FRIEDMAN (J.), BENJAMIN (R.S.), MOORE (E.C.), BODEY (G.P.), VALDIVIESO (M.), BURGESS (M.A.), WISEMAN (C.), LOO (T.L.): Penetration of N-(Phosphonacetyl)-L-aspartate into human central nervous system and intracerebral tumor. Cancer Res. **40**: 3163-3166 (1980).

22. STEWART (D.J.), BENVENUTO (J.), LEAVENS (M.), SMITH (R.), CABANILLAS (F.), BENJAMIN (R.S.), LOO (Ti Li): Human central nervous system pharmacology of Pentamethylmelamine and its metabolites. J. Neuro-Oncol. **1**: 357-364 (1983).

23. STEWART (D.J.), LU (K.), BENJAMIN (R.S.), LEAVENS (M.), LUNA (M.), YAP (H.Y.), LOO (T.L.): Concentrations of vinblastine in human intracerebral tumor and other tissues. J. Neuro-Oncol. **1**: 139-144 (1983).

24. STEWART (D.J.), RICHARD (M.), HUGENHOLTZ (H.), DENNERY (J.), BELANGER (R.), GERIN-LAJOIE (J.), MONTPETIT (V.), NUNDY (D.), PRIOR (J.), HOPKINS (H.): Penetration of VP-16 (Etoposide) into human intracerebral and extracerebral tumors. J. Neuro-Oncol. **2**: 133-139 (1984).

25. STEWART (D.J.), RICHARD (M.T.), HUGENHOLTZ (H.), DENNERY (J.), NUNDY (D.), PRIOR (J.), MONPETIT (V.), HOPKINS (H.S.): Penetration of teniposide (VM-26) into human intracerebral tumors: preliminary observations on the effect of tumor type, rate of drug infusion and prior treatment with amphotericin-B or oral glycerol. J. Neuro-Oncol. **2**: 315-324 (1984).

26. STEWART (D.J.), LEAVENS (M.), LU (K.), WANG (Y.M.), BENJAMIN (R.S.), HO (D.H.), YAP (H.Y.), LOO (T.L.): Central nervous system pharmacology of Baker's Antifolate (NSC 139 105) in man. J. Neuro-Oncol. **2**: 187-193 (1984).

27. STEWART (D.J.), GREEN (R.M.), HUGENHOLTZ (H.), RICHARD (M.T.), DENNERY (J.), MONTPETIT (V.), HOPKINS (H.S.), THIBAULT (M.): Human central nervous system pharmacology of Tiazofurin. In: Walker M., Thomas D. (eds): Biology of brain tumor. Martinus Nijhoff Publishers, Dordrecht, The Netherlands, 1986, pp. 425-429.

28. HALL (S.W.), YEUNG (K.), BENJAMIN (R.S.), STEWART (D.J.), VALDIVIESO (M.), BEDIKIAN (A.Y.), LOO (T.L.): Kinetics of gallium nitrate. A new anticancer agent. Clinc. Pharm. and Therap. **25**: 82-87 (1979).

29. STEWART (D.J.), BENJAMIN (R.S.), LUNA (M.), SEIFERT (W.E.), LOO (T.L.): Human tissue distribution of platinum after Cis-Diamminedichloroplatinum. Cancer Chemother. Pharm **10**: 51-54 (1982).

30. STEWART (D.J.), GREEN (R.M.), MIKHAEL (N.Z.), MONTPETIT (V.), THIBAULT (M.), MAROUN (J.A.): Human autopsy tissue concentrations of mitoxantrone. Cancer Treatment Rep. **10**: 1255-1261, 1986.

31. STEWART (D.J.), ZHENGANG (G.), LU (K.), SAVARAJ (N.), FEUN (L.G.), BENJAMIN (R.S.), KEATING (M.J.), LOO (T.L.): Human tissue distribution of 4'-(9-Acridinylamino)-Methanesulfon-m-Aniside (NSC 14159, AMSA). Cancer Chemother. Pharmacol. **12**: 116-119 (1984).

32. BENVENUTO (J.A.), HALL (S.W.), FARQUHAR (D.), STEWART (D.J.), BENJAMIN (R.S.), LOO (T.L.): Clinical pharmacology of 3-deazauridine. Cancer Res. **39**: 349-352 (1979).

33. STEWART (D.J.), ROSENBLUM (M.), LUNA (M.), LOO (T.L.): Disposition of Methylglyoxyl bis (Guanylhydrazone) (MGBG, NSC-32946) in Man. Cancer Chemother. Pharm. **7**: 31-35 (1981).

34. MEDOFF (J.), MEDOFF (G.), GOLDSTEIN (M.N.), SCHLESSINGER (D.), KOBAYASHI (G.S.): Amphotericin-B-induced sensitivity to actiomycin-D in drug-resistant HELA cells. Cancer Res. **35**: 2548-2552 (1975).

35. LEVIN (V.A.), LANDAHL (H.D.), FREEMAN-DOVE (M.A.): The application of brain capillary permeability coefficient measurements to pathological conditions and the selection of agents which cross the blood-brain barrier. J. Pharmacokin Biopharm **4**: 499-519 (1976).

36. MEYER (J.), FUKUUCHI (Y.), SHIMAZU (K.), MATHEW (N.), OHUCHI (T.): Effect on regional cerebral blood flow of compression by a mass lesion. Europ. Neurol. **8**: 83-81 (1972).

37. BISCHOFF (K.B.): Some fundamental considerations of the applications of pharmacokinetics to cancer chemotherapy. Cancer Chemother. Rep. **59**: 777-793 (1975).

38. BLASBERG (R.G.), GROOTHUIS (D.R.): Chemotherapy of brain tumors: physiological and pharmacokinetic considerations. Semin. Oncol. **13**: 70-82 (1986).

39. MOERTEL (C.G.), THYNNE (G.S.): Large bowel. In: Holland J.F., Frei E III, eds. Cancer Medicine, Philadelphia; Lea and Febiger (1982), p. 1848.

40. KLASTERSKY (J.), SCULIER (J.P.): Chemotherapy for non-small-cell lung cancer. Semin. Oncol. *4 (Suppl. 6)*: 38-48 (1985).

41. FALKSON (G.), MacINTYRE (J.M.), SCHUTT (A.J.), COETZER (B.), JOHNSON (L.A.), SIMSON (I.W.), DOUGLASS (H.O. Jr.): Neocarzinostatin versus M-AMSA or doxorubicin in hepatocellular carcinoma. J. Clin. Oncol. **2**: 581-584, 1984.

42. KERNION (J.B. de): Treatment of advanced renal cell carcinoma - traditional methods and innovative approaches. J. Urol. **130**: 2-7 (1983).

43. O'CONNELL (M.J.): Current status of chemotherapy for advanced pancreatic and gastric cancer. J. Clin. Oncol. **3**: 1032-1039 (1985).

44. SHAPIRO (W.R.): Therapy of adult malignant brain tumors: what have the clinical trials taught us? Semin. Oncol. **13**: 38-45 (1986).

45. BOGHDAN (U.): Chemosensitivity of malignant brain tumors: preliminary results. J. Neuro-Oncol. **1**: 149-166: (1983).

46. MAHALEY (M.), URSO (M.), WHALEY (R.), SILKER (R.), WILLIAMS (T.), GUASPARI (A.): Malignant glioma treatment with interferon. Proc. Am. Soc. Clin. Oncol. **3**: 65 (1984).

47. SKLANSKY (B.D.), MANN-KAPLAN (R.S.), REYNOLDS (A.F.), ROSENBLUM (M.L.), WALKER (M.D.): 4'-Demethyl-epidodophyllotoxin-β-D-thenylidene-glucoside (PTG) in the treatment of malignant intracranial neoplasms. Cancer **33**: 460-467 (1974).

48. STEWART (D.J.), O'BRYAN (M.), AL-SARRAF (M.), COSTANZI (J.J.), OISHI (N.): Phase II study of cisplatin in recurrent astrocytomas in adults. J. Neuro-Oncol. **1**: 145-147, 1983.

49. MELLET (L.B.): Physicochemical considerations and pharmacokinetic behaviour in delivery of drugs to the central nervous system. Cancer Treat. Rep. **61**: 527-531 (1977).

50. FREIDMAN (H.S.), SCHOLD (S.C. Jr.), BIGNER (D.D.): Chemotherapy of subcutaneous and intracranial human medulloblastoma xenografts in athymic nude mice. Cancer Res. **46**: 224-228 (1986).

51. YAMADA (K.), HAYAKAWA (T.), USHIO (Y.), ARITA (N.), KATO (A.), MAGAMI (H.): Regional blood flow and capillary permeability in the ethylnitrosourea-induced rat glioma. J. Neurosurg. **55**: 922-928 (1981).

52. VOGEL (A.W.): Intratumoral vascular changes with increased size of mammary adenocarcinomas: new method and results. J. Natl. Cancer Inst. **34**: 571-578 (1965).

53. BLASBERG (R.), KOBAYASHI (T.), PLATLAK (C.), SHINOHARA (M.), MIZOAKA (M.), RICE (J.), SHAPIRO (W.): Regional blood flow, capillary permeability and glucose utilization in two brain tumor models: preliminary observations and pharmacokinetic implications. Cancer Treat. Rep. *65 (Suppl. 2)*: 3-12 (1981).

54. GOLDIE (J.H.), COLDMAN (A.J.): The genetic origin of drug resistance in neoplasms: implications for systemic therapy. Cancer Res. **44**: 3643-3653 (1984).

55. HUSTU (H.), AUR (R.J.A.), VERZOSA (M.S.), SIMONE (J.V.), PINKEL (D.): Prevention of central nervous system leukemia by irradiation. Cancer **32**: 585-597 (1973).

56. MURIEL (F.S.), PAVLOVSKY (S.), PENALVER (J.A.) et al.: Evaluation of induction or remission, intensification, and central nervous system prophylactic treatment in acute lymphoblastic leukemia. Cancer **34**: 418-426 (1974).

57. Working Party on Leukemia in Childhood. Treatment of acute lymphoblastic leukemia: effect of "prophylactic" therapy against central nervous system leukemia. Br. Med. J. **2**: 381-384 (1973).

58. BAUMER (J.H.), MOTT (M.G.): Sex and prognosis in childhood acute lymphoblastic leukemia. Lancet **ii**: 128-129 (1978).

58a. WEST (R.J.), GRAHAM-POLE (J.), HARDISTY (R.M.), PIKE (M.D.): Factors in pathogenesis of central nervous system leukemia. Br. Med. J. **3**: 311-314 (1972).

59. GEORGE (S.L.), FERNBACH (D.J.), LU (E.T.): Early deaths in newly diagnosed cases of pediatric acute leukemia. A Southwest Oncology Group Study. Cancer **42**: 781-786 (1978).

60. STEWART (D.J.), KEATING (M.J.), McCREDIE (K.B.), SMITH (T.L.), MURPHY (S.G.), BODEY (G.P.), FREIREICH (E.J.): Natural history of central nervous system acute leukemia in adults. Cancer **47**: 184-196, 1981.

61. KEATING (M.J.), SMITH (B.S.), GEHAN (E.A.), MCCREDIE (K.B.), BODEY (G.P.), SPITZER (G.), HERSH (E.), GUTTERMAN (J.), FREIREICH (E.J.): Factors related to length of complete remission in adult acute leukemia. Cancer **42**: 2017-2029 (1980).

62. USHIO (Y.), POSNER (J.), SHAPIRO (W.): Chemotherapy of experimental meningeal carcinomatosis. Cancer Res. **37**: 1232-1237 (1977).

63. NIES (B.A.), BODEY (G.P.), THOMAS (L.B.), BRECHER (G.), FREIREICH (E.J.): The persistance of extramedullary leukemic infiltraten during bone marrow remission of acute leukemia. Blood **26**: 133-141 (1965).

64. SIMONE (J.V.), HOLLAND (E.), JOHNSON (W.): Fatalities during remission of childhood leukemia. Blood **39**: 759-770 (1972).

65. NUGENT (J.L.), BUNN (P.A.) Jr., MATTHEWS (M.J.), IHDE (D.C.), COHEN (M.H.), GAZDAR (A.), MINNA (J.D.): CNS metastases in small cell bronchogenic carcinoma. Increasing frequency and changing pattern with lengthening survival. Cancer **44**: 1885-1893 (1979).

66. ALEXANDER (M.), GLATSHEIN (E.J.), GORDON (D.J.), DANIELS (J.R.): Combined modality treatment for oat cell carcinoma of the lung: a randomized trial. Cancer Treat. Rep. **61**: 1-6 (1977).

67. SEYDEL (H.G.), CREECH (R.), PAGANO (M.), SALAZAR (O.), RUBIN (P.), CONCANNON (J.), CARBONE (P.), MOHUIDDIN (M.), PEREZ (C.), MATTHEWS (M.): Prophylactic versus no brain irradiation in regional small cell lung carcinoma. Am. J. Clin. Oncol. (CCT) **8**: 218-223 (1985).

68. LININGER (T.R.), FLEMING (T.R.), EAGEN (R.T.): Evaluation of alternating chemotherapy and sites and extent of disease in extensive small cell lung cancer. Cancer **48**: 2147-2153 (1981).

69. VITA (V.T. de) Jr.: Principles of chemotherapy. In: Cancer: Principles and Practice of Oncology. De Vita V.T. Jr., Hellman S., Rosenberg S.A. (eds). J. B. Lippincott Co, Philadelphia (1982), p. 115.

70. KOLARIC (K.), ROTH (A.), JELICIC (I.), MATKOVIC (A.): A preliminary report on antitumorigenic activity of cis-dichlorodiammineplatinum in metastatic brain tumors. Tumori**67**: 483-486 (1981).

71. ROSNER (D.), NEMOTO (T.), PICKREN (J.), LANE (W.): Management of brain metastases from breast cancer by combination chemotherapy. J. Neuro-Oncol. **1**: 131-137 (1983).

72. KANTARAJIAN (H.), FARHA (P.A.M.), SPITZER (C.), MURPHY (W.K.), VALDIVIESO (M.): Systemic combination chemotherapy as primary treatment of brain metastases from lung cancer. Southern Med. J. **77**: 426-430 (1984).

73. MAROUN (J.A.), STEWART (D.J.), YOUNG (V.), BELANGER (R.), CROOK (A.F.): Effectiveness of VM-26 in non-small cell carcinoma of the lung (NSCCL) with central nervous system (CNS) metastases. Preliminary Results. Proc. Am. Soc. Clin. Oncol. **1**: 140 (1982).

Intraarterial Chemotherapy for Brain Tumors: A Summary of the Ottawa Experience

D.J. STEWART (°).

INTRODUCTION

Intraarterial administration of chemotherapy results in augmentation of both local peak plasma concentration of the drug and local area under the concentration - times - time curve (AUC) during the drug infusion (1-4). It can be particularly advantageous to administer drugs with a rapid total body clearance intraarterially since if clearance is rapid, the usual AUC will be relatively small, and the local increase in AUC resulting from intraarterial administration will be proportionally quite large (3, 4). For some drugs, intraarterial administration would be expected to result in increased therapeutic efficacy, while for other drugs, there would be relatively little advantage (1-4). Augmentation of local tissue concentrations by intraarterial administration has been documented for some drugs (5-9), but not for others (10).

The first clinical trials of intracarotid administration of chemotherapy were reported more than 30 years ago, and since then, at least 23 different antineoplastic agents have been tested, and a few intracarotid drug combinations have also been tried (9, 11-20). In this manuscript, we present our experience to date in Ottawa with intracarotid chemotherapy.

METHOD

Five different intracarotid regimens have been tested in Ottawa over the past 4 years. Three have involved combinations of drugs and two have involved single agents only. The first study involved the intracarotid combination of BCNU, cisplatin, and VM-26 (teniposide) (21). This study was undertaken since each of the 3 drugs had previously been shown to be tolerable and effective when administered into the carotid arteries as single agents (22-25), since there was pharmacological evidence of an advantage for intraarterial administration for 2 of them (5-8) (VM-26 pharmacology after intraarterial administration has not been studied yet), and since preclinical studies had shown synergism between the 3 drugs (26-28). As this was a phase I study, the doses of the 3 drugs were gradually increased during the course of the study until toxicity became dose-limiting. For both this study and the other studies summarized here, a catheter was placed in the carotid artery using a transfemoral, fluoroscopically-guided approach. Each drug was given separately over 15-20 min in 100 ml 0.45 % saline. The line was flushed with saline between drugs and was removed immediately after the end of the infusion of the third drug. Dexamethasone 50 mg was given iv before and after each course of treatment in both this and the other intracarotid studies that were done. Parenteral narcotics were given as needed for ocular pain during BCNU. Mannitol 250 ml of a 20 % solution and 500 ml of dextrose 5 % in 0.45 % saline were given iv prior to the cisplatin to decrease nephrotoxicity. Treatments were repeated at 6-7 week intervals upon recovery from toxicity, providing tumor progression had not occurred. Hematological toxicity was monitored by doing blood counts once per week. Response status was monitored by repeating a CT scan of the brain prior to each course. Response was defined as unequivocal decrease in tumor size on CT scan.

The second study (29) used the same intracarotid regimen used in the first study, but additional drugs were added systemically between intracarotid courses, since each of these drugs had proven to be active against astrocytomas individually (30-34), and since there was synergism between some of them (35, 36). The intracarotid drug doses were BCNU 100 mg/m^2, cisplatin 60 mg/m^2, and VM-26 150 mg/m^2. The systemic drugs used were vincristine 2 mg iv on days 1, 8, 15, and 36 of each course, methotrexate 200 mg/m^2 iv on days 8 and 36 of each course (with citrovorum factor 20 mg im or po

(°) *The Ontario Cancer Treatment and Reseach Foundation Ottawa Regional Cancer Centre and the University of Ottawa Faculty of Health Sciences Ottawa, Canada.*

M. Chatel, F. Darcel and J. Pecker (eds.), Brain Oncology. ISBN-13: 978-94-010-8003-3

q6h for 8 doses beginning 24 hr after the methotrexate), bleomycin 30 units iv once weekly for the first 10 weeks on study, and procarbazine 100 mg/m^2 po on days 22 to 28 of each course. VM-26 was repeated iv on day 8 of each course because of its schedule-dependant activity. Oral glycerol 500 mg/kg q6h times 4 doses was given beginning 18 hr prior to the day 8 VM-26 because of pharmacological data suggesting that oral glycerol may possibly augment the uptake of VM-26 into human brain tumors (37), perhaps by increasing blood flow to the tumor. For this study and for studies 3,4 and 5, a 0.2 micron in-line filter was used during the intracarotid infusions because of the suggestion by Lehane et al (38) that this might reduce local toxicity. Monitoring of toxicity and response was the same as in the first study. Courses were repeated at 7 week intervals.

The third study (Stewart, unpublished data) used the same intracarotid doses of BCNU, cisplatin, and VM-26 on day 1 of each course as were used on day 1 of the second study. In addition, cytosine arabinoside 800-1,000 mg/m^2 was given iv over 30 min immediately after the intracarotid chemotherapy since this drug is synergistic with each of the 3 intracarotid drugs in some preclinical systems (39-42), since it is active against glioblastoma cells grown in vitro (43), and since the combination of cisplatin and cytosine arabinoside may be somewhat more effective against gliomas than is cisplatin alone (44, 45). For this regimen, intracarotid cisplatin and VM-26 ware repeated on day 22 of each 6 week cycle. Since local toxicity and not systemic toxicity was dose-limiting in the first study, we did not feel that we could add any additional intracarotid drug, but we felt that we might be able to give more of the same drugs systemically. Hence, cisplatin 20 mg/m^2 was given iv on days 2 and 23 of each course, and VM-26 25-50 mg/m^2 was given iv on days 2,3,23, and 24 of each course. Cytosine arabinoside 800-1,000 mg/m^2 was given iv after the other drugs on days 2, 22, and 23 in addition to day 1. Glycerol 500 mg/kg was given po 6 hr and immediately before the chemotherapy on each day and mannitol 250 ml of a 20 % solution was also given iv each day beginning 15 min before the chemotherapy and ending concurrently with it. The mannitol was given both to protect the kidneys from the cisplatin as well as to attempt to increase drug delivery to the tumor. Mannitol given iv increases blood flow to brain areas around mass lesions (46) and increases delivery to brain tumors of a least some drugs, including BCNU (47). The iv cisplatin and VM-26 were each given in 250 ml 0.45 % saline over 1 hr, while the cytosine arabinoside was given in 50 ml dextrose 5 % in water over 30 min. To help protect the kidneys from the effect of cisplatin, dextrose 5 % in 0.45 % saline was given with cisplatin (500 ml on days 1 and 22, and 250 ml on days 2 and 23 of each course). We have previously found that these fluid volumes adequately protect the kidney without causing excessive cerebral edema. Intracarotid drug delivery techniques and monitoring of toxicity and response were the same as in the first 2 studies.

The fourth study was a phase I-II study of the intraarterial administration of mitomycin-C (48, 49). The drug was mixed in 100 ml 0.45 % saline and given over 15 min. Treatments were repeated at 7 week intervals. This study was undertaken since intraarterial administration of mitomycin-C would be expected to be advantageous because of its rapid clearance (3, 4), since it has proven effective when administered into other arteries (50), and since some very preliminary data suggested that it would probably be well tolerated when given into the carotid (51).

The fifth study was a phase I study of the intracarotid infusion of the new nitrosourea, PCNU (16, 52). The drug was carefully reconstituted with dimethylacetamide and propylene glycol, then mixed in a volume of 0.45 % saline sufficiently large to give a final concentration of $\leqslant$ 0.5 mg/ml. Treatment courses were repeated at 7 week intervals. This study was conducted in the hope that intracarotid PCNU would cause less periorbital pain and retinal toxicity than does BCNU. When administered intravenously, PCNU appears to be comparable to BCNU in activity against gliomas (53, 54), and causes less gastrointestinal toxicity (53).

RESULTS

First Study : Intracarotid BCNU plus Cisplatin plus VM-26 :

A total of 38 patients were treated on this study, including 21 with primary brain tumors and 17 with brain metastases. Twenty-four had had prior cranial irradiation plus chemotherapy, 1 had had prior chemotherapy only, 1 had had radiotherapy only, and 5 very poor prognosis patients had had neither chemotherapy nor radiotherapy previously. In the 36 patients who were evaluable for response, the response rate was 64 %. Responses were seen in 70 % of patients with primary brain tumors, including 10 of 16 (63 %) with glioblastomas, 2 of 2 with ependymomas, and single patients with an oligodendroglioma and a primitive neuroectodermal tumor (PNET) respectively. Fifty-six percent of patients with brain metastases responded including 4 of 7 with lung adenocarcinomas, 1 of 3 with breast carcinoma, single patients with each of prostate carcinoma, large cell lung carcinoma, squamous cell lung carcinoma, and malignant melanoma. Single patients with colon carcinoma and testicular carcinoma did not respond.

The maximum tolerated doses of the 3 drugs when given in combination were BCNU 100 mg/m^2, cisplatin 60 mg/m^2, and VM-26 150 mg/m^2. When these or lower doses were used, the response rate was 57 % and the incidence of serious local toxicity was 9 %. At higher doses, the response rate was 100 % but the incidence of serious local side effects was unacceptably high at 56 %.

Vertebral artery infusion of BCNU resulted in marked cardiorespiratory depression if the BCNU was reconstituted with ethanol. This was not a problem if the drug was reconstituted in saline. Marked cardiorespiratory depression also occurred during VM-26 administration into the vertebral artery. This was diminished by slowing the rate of the infusion and by giving iv atropine. Vertebral artery doses were limited to BCNU 100 mg/m^2, cisplatin 40 mg/m^2 (to decrease the risk of ototoxicity), and VM-26 100 mg/m^2.

Second Study: Combined Intracarotid and Systemic Chemotherapy:

When multiple different systemic drugs were added to the intracarotid drugs, the response rate did not change appreciably. The response rate was 46 % if all patients were considered and was 63 % if only patients who were fully evaluable (i.e., who received the intracarotid chemotherapy and at least half the scheduled systemic chemotherapy of course 1) were considered. If only patients with gliomas were considered, the response rate was 50 % for all patients and 71 % for fully evaluable patients. The median survival was 17 wk from initiation of chemotherapy and 55 wk from diagnosis. Myelosuppression was noted in 56 % of courses, and was dose-limiting for the systemic chemotherapy. One patient (4 %) developed permanent ipsilateral blindness, and 3 (11 %) developed possible (1 patient) or probable (2 patients) permanent neurological toxicity. Since it offers no response or toxicity advantage over the 3 intracarotid drugs alone, we do recommend further studies of this particular regimen.

Third Study: Intracarotid plus Systemic Chemotherapy:

The study combining systemic cisplatin, VM-26, cytosine arabinoside, glycerol and mannitol with intracarotid BCNU, cisplatin, and VM-26 has only recently been initiated. Ten patients have been treated. It is too early to comment on the response rate. No retinal or neurological toxicity has been seen to date. Myelosuppression is profound, but rapidly reversible.

Fourth Study: Intracarotid Mitomycin-C:

Intraarterial mitomycin-C 7.5-18 mg/m^2 was given to 21 patients with intracerebral tumors. All of the patients had had prior cranial irradiation and most had had prior chemotherapy, 1 had a primitive neuroectodermal tumor, and 1 had a primary germ cell tumor of the brain. Six (46 %) of the patients with brain metastases and the single patient with the primary neuroectodermal tumor responded. None of the other patients responded. We concluded that this is a useful regimen in patients with recurrent brain metastases. The maximum tolerated dose of mitomycin-C was 15 mg/m^2. Neurological and ocular toxicity were comparable to that seen with other intraarterial chemotherapy, and were dose-limiting. Local skin toxicity was also seen in 3 patients. Vertebral artery infusion did not result in any cardiorespiratory depression, although one patient died of herniation due to increased edema following a vertebral artery infusion.

Fifth Study: Intracarotid PCNU:

Sixteen patients with recurrent gliomas or glioblastomas and 1 with recurrent brain metastases were treated with intracarotid PCNU. Seven (41 %) responded. Thrombocytopenia, neurological, and ocular toxicity were dose-limiting at a PCNU dose of 110 mg/m^2, although serious toxicity was also seen in one patient treated at the lowest dose studied (60 mg/m^2). Orbital pain was less than that seen with inracarotid BCNU, while transient neurological toxicity was more frequent than with BCNU. A single patient received a vertebral artery infusion of PCNU for a posterior fossa tumor. The infusion had to stopped after 25 mg/m^2 had been delivered since the patient developed a severe headache and marked restlessness.

While it is always hazardous to judge the worth of a treatment approach based on the results of a phase I trial, it was our feeling based on our preliminary observations that the apparent therapeutic index of intraarterial administration of PCNU was not sufficiently high to warrant further study.

DISCUSSION

Based on the studies we have undertaken to date, we feel that the 3 drug intracarotid combination of BCNU, cisplatin, and VM-26 is of value in the treatment of recurrent primary and metastatic brain tumors. While we have not proven that the 3 drug combination is superior to treatment with just 1 or 2 drugs, and while we have not proven that intraarterial administration is superior to iv administration, we feel that this treatment regimen is definitely active enough to warrant further investigation. We plan to continue to alter the schedule and to add different systemic medications to it in an attempt to further improve upon it. The systemic medications added in our second study did not appear to improve the efficacy of the 3 drug regimen, and it is still too early to judge the effect of the systemic medications added in our third study.

Intracarotid mitomycin-C definitely appears to be of value in recurrent brain metastases, but was not effective in a small number of patients with gliomas. We plan to initiate a study of intracarotid mitomycin-C combined with intracarotid cisplatin and VM-26 as treatment of recurrent brain metastases.

As stated previously, we do not feel that intracarotid administration of PCNU warrants further study. The response rate seen with iv administration of this drug (53, 54) is quite comparable to the response we obtained in this intracarotid study.

Intracarotid administration of chemotherapy is definitely more toxic than is iv administration. Serious local toxicity will occur in $\geqslant 10\ \%$ of patients. Despite this, many intracarotid regimens are active enough that there is a net gain in the therapeutic index and patient quality of life. At this point in time, we feel that intracarotid chemotherapy should still be regarded as being investigational, and should not be used routinely ; however, it is sufficiently promising that further studies are definitely warranted.

SUMMARY

Five different intracarotid regimens have been tested in Ottawa. The combination of BCNU, cisplatin, and VM-26 was effective against recurrent glioblastomas and brain metastases. Efficacy and toxicity were both dose-related. The addition of multiple systemic drugs to the 3 drug intracarotid regimen did not increase therapeutic efficacy. Studies have been initiated adding different systemic drugs. Intraar-rrial mitomycin-C was effective against recurrent brain metastases, but not against gliomas. Intraca-tid PCNU dit not appear to be any more effective than was iv PCNU. Overall, we feel that some ıtracarotid regimens are probably more effective against brain tumors than are iv regimens, but ıntracarotid chemotherapy can be quite toxic and should still be considered investigational.

KEY WORDS

Intra-arterial Chemotherapy, Brain Tumours.

REFERENCES

1. FENSTERMACHER (J.D.), COWLES (A.K.).Theoretic limitations of intracarotid infusions in brain tumor chemothe-1980).
2. CHEN (H-SG), GROSS (J.F.). Intra-arterial infusion of anticancer drugs: theoretic aspects of drug delivery and review of responses. Cancer Treat Rep **64**: 31-40 (1980).
3. COLLINS (J.) Pharmacologic rationale for regional drug delivery. J. Clin Oncol **2**: 498-504 (1984).
4. ENSMINGER (W.), GYVES (J.). Clinical pharmacology of hepatic arterial chemotherapy. Semin. Oncol. **10**: 176-182 (1983).
5. STEWART (D.J.), LEAVENS (M.), MAOR (M.), FEUN (L.), LUNA (M.), BONURA (J.), CAPRIOLI (R.), LOO (T.L.), BENJAMIN (R.S.): Human central nervous system distribution of Cis-Diaminedichloroplatinum and use as a radiosensitizer in malignant brain tumors. Cancer Research **42**: 2474-2479 (1982).
6. STEWART (D.J), MIKHAEL (N.), NANJI (A.), KACEW (S.), MAROUN (J.), HIRTE W: Human tissue cisplatin (CP) pharmacology: clinical implications. Proc Amer Assoc Cancer Res **26**: 154 (1985).
7. LEVIN (V.A.), KABRA (P.M.), FREEMAN-DOVE (M.A.). Pharmacokinetics of intracarotid artery 14C-BCNU in the squirrel monkey. Neurosurgery **48**: 587-593 (1978).
8. CARLSON (J.A. Jr.), LITTERST (C.L.), GREENBERG (R.A.), DAY (T.G. Jr.), MASTERSON (B.J.). Platinum tissue concentrations following intra-arterial and intravenous cis-diamine-dichloroplatinum II in New Zealand white rabbits. Am J Obstet Gynecol **148**: 313-317 (1984).

9. STEWART (D.J.), Novel modes of chemotherapy administration. In: ROSENBLUM (M.L.), WILSON (C.B.) (eds). Progress in experimental brain tumor research (S. Kargel Med & Scientific Publishers. Basel/Switzerland, 1984) **28**: 32-50.

10. MADAJEWICZ (S.), SPAULDING (M.), BHIMANI (S.), AVELLANOSA (A.), DE LOS SANTOS (R.), PERRY (A.), ZEIGLER (P.), KIRSHNER (J.). Phase I-II Diaziquone chemotherapy in brain tumors. Cancer Treat Rep **68**: 913-914 (1984).

11. BONSTELLE (C.T.), KORI (S.H.), REKATE (H.). Intracarotid chemotherapy of glioblastoma after induced blood-brain barrier disruption. AJNR **4** : 810-812 (1983).

12. FEUN (L.G.), LEE (Y.-Y.), YUNG (W.K.A.), CHARNSANGAVEJ (C.), SAVARAJ (N.), TANG (R.A.), WALLACE (S.). Phase II trial of intracarotid BCNU and cisplatin in primary malignant brain tumors. Cancer Drug Delivery **3**: 147-156 (1986).

13. YAMASHITA (J.), HANDA (H.), TOKURIKI (Y.), HA (Y.S.), OTSUKA (S.-I.), SUDA (K.), TAKI (W.). Intra-arterial ACNU therapy for malignant brain tumors : experimental studies and preliminary clinical results. J. Neurosurg **59**: 424-430 (1983).

14. BREMER (A.M.), KLERIGA (E.), NGUYEN (E.), BALSYS (R.), NORTHUP (H.M.), GONZALEZ (N.), DUARTE (P.), MILLER (R.I.). Complications associated with intra-arterial BCNU administered in combination with vincristine and procarbazine for the treatment of malignant brain tumors. J. Neuro-Oncol **2**: 129-132 (1984).

15. CALVO (F.A.), PASTOR (M.A.), DY (C.), ALGERIA (E.), APARICIO (L.M.A.), GIL (A.), HARGUINDEY (S.), ZUBIETA (J.L.), LAGE (M.M.). Intra-arterial and intravenous chemotherapy for the treatment of malignant glioma : preliminary results. Am J. Clin Oncol (CLT) **8**: 200-209 (1985).

16. STEWART (D.J.), GRAHOVAC (Z.), GUPTA (S.) GOUMNEROVA (L.), RICHARD (M.), HUGENHOLTZ (H.), MAROUN (J.): Phase I study of intracarotid PCNU. J Neuro-Oncol **4**: 114 (1986).

17. FEUN (L.G.). Intra-arterial chemotherapy for primary and metastatic brain cancer: Cancer Bulletin **36**: 57-61 (1984).

18. GREENBERG (H.S.), ENSMINGER (W.), LAYTON (P.), GEBARSKI (S.), MEYER (M.B.), BENDER (J.), GRILLO-LOPEZ (A.). A phase I-II evaluation of intra-arterial diaziquone (AZQ) for malignant tumors of the central nervous system. Proc Am Soc Clin Oncol 3: 256 (1984).

19. WEST (C.R.), AVELLANOSA (A.M.), BARUA (N.R.), PATEL (A.R.). Phase II study of intra-arterial (IA) BCNU plus VM-26 for malignant gliomas and for metastatic brain tumors. Proc Am Soc Clin Oncol **2**: 234 (1983).

20. MUGHAL (T.), GLODE (L.M.), BRAUN (T.J.), GEYER (M.), KINDT (G.). Phase I study of intra-arterial bis-chloroethyl nitrosourea and 2'-deoxy-5-fluoridine in malignant astrocytomas. Proc Am Assoc Cancer Res **25**: 198 (1984).

21. STEWART (D.J.), GRAHOVAC (Z.), BENOIT (B.), ADDISON (D.), RICHARD (M.T.), DENNERY (J.), HUGENHOLTZ (H.), RUSSELL (N.), PETERSON (E.), MAROUN (J.A.), VANDENBERG (T.), HOPKINS (H.S.). Intracarotid chemotherapy with a combination of 1, 3-Bis (2-chloroethyl)-1-nitrosourea (BCNU), cis-Diaminedichloroplatinum (Cisplatin) and 4'-O-Demethyl-1-0 (4,6-0-2-thenylidene-β-D-glucopyranosyl) epipodophyllotoxin (VM-26) in the treatment of primary and metastatic brain tumors. Neurosurg **15**: 828-833 (1984).

22. STEWART (D.J.), WALLACE (S.), FEUN (L.), LEAVENS (M.), YOUNG (S.E.), HANDEL (S.), MAVLIGIT (G.), BENJAMIN (R.S.). Intracarotid artery infusion of Cis-Diaminedichloroplatinum: phase I study in patients with recurrent malignant intracerebral tumors. Cancer Res **42**: 2059-2062 (1982).

23. FEUN (L.G.), WALLACE (S.), STEWART (D.J.), CHUANG (V.P.), YUNG (W-KA), LEAVENS (M.E.), BURGESS (M.A.), SAVARAJ (N.), BENJAMIN (R.S.), YOUNG (S.E.), TANG (R.A.), HANDEL (S.), MAVLIGIT (G.), FIELDS (W.S.). Intracarotid infusion of Cis-Diaminedichloroplatinum in the treatment of recurrent malignant tumors. Cancer **54**: 794-799 (1984).

24. MADAJEWICZ (S.), WEST (C.R.), PARK (H.C.), AVELLANOSA (A.M.), CARACANDAS (J.E.), TAKITA (H.), VINCENT (R.G.), JENNINGS (E.). Phase II study of intra-arterial 4'-0-demethyl-1-0-(4,6-0-2-thynylidene-β-D-glycopyranosyl) epipodophyllotoxin (VM-26) therapy of metastic bronchogenic adenocarcinoma to the brain. Proc Am Soc Clin Oncol **22**: 502 (1981).

25. MADAJEWICZ (S.), WEST (C.R.), PARK (H.C.), GHOORAH (J.), AVELLANOSA (A.M.), TAKITA (H.), KARAKOUSIS (C.), VINCENT (R.), CARACANDAS (J.), JENNINGS (E.). Phase II study - intraarterial BCNU therapy for metastatic brain tumors. Cancer **47**: 653-657 (1981).

26. DREWINKO (B.), GOTTLEIB (J.). Action of cis-dichlorodiamineplatinum (II) (NSC-119875) at the cellular level. Cancer Chemother Rep **59**: 665-673 (1975).

27. ISSELL (B.). The podophyllotoxin-derivatives VP-16-213 and VM-26. Cancer Chemother Pharmacol **7**: 73-80 (1982).

28. DEWAYNE (R.), PECK (C.), HILLIARD (S.), KARAS (J.). Response of L1210 leukemia to treatment with 1, 3-bis (2-chloroethyl)-1-nitrosourea plus 4'-demethylepipodophyllotoxin-9-(4,6-0-2-thenylidene-β-D-glucopyranoside). Cancer Res **41**: 3891-3895 (1981).

29. STEWART (D.J.), GRAHOVAC (Z.), HUGENHOLTZ (H.), BENOIT (B.), RICHARD (M.). RUSSELL (N.), MAROUN (J.), DENNERY (J.), PETERSON (E.), NABWANGU (J.). Intraarterial plus systemic chemotherapy in the treatment of intracerebral tumors. J. Neuro-Oncol **4**: 114 (1986).

30. DJERASSI (I.), SUN KIM (J.), SHULMAN (K.). High-dose methotrexate-citrovorum factor rescue in the management of brain tumors. Cancer Treat Rep **61**: 691-694 (1977).

31. ROSENSTOCK (J.G.), EVANS (E.), SCHUT (L.). Response to vincristine of recurrent brain tumors in children. J. Neurosurg **45**: 135-140 (1976).

32. TAKEUCHI (K.). A clinical trial of intravenous bleomycin in the treatment of brain tumors. Int J. Clin Pharmacol **12**: 419-426 (1975).

33. KUMAR (A.), RENAUDIN (J.), WILSON (C.), BOLDREY (E.), ENOT (K.), LEVIN (V.). Procarbazine hydrochloride in the treatment of brain tumors. J. Neurosurg **40**: 365-371 (1974).

34. SKLANSKY (B.), MANN-KAPLAN (R.), REYNOLDS (A.), ROSENBLUM (M.), WALKER (M.). 4'-Demethyl-epipodophyllotoxin-β-D-thenylidene-glucoside (PTG) in treatment of malignant intracranial neoplasms. Cancer **33**: 460-467 (1974).

35. BARRANEO (S.), KUE (J.), ROMSDAHL (M.), HUMPHREY (R.). Bleomycin as a possible synchronizing agent for human tumor cells in vivo. Cancer Res **33**: 882-887 (1973).

36. CHELLO (P.), SIROTVAK (F.), DORICK (D.), MOCCIO (D.). Schedule-dependent synergism of methotrexate and vincristine against murine L1210 leukemia. Cancer Treat Rep **63**: 1889-1894 (1974).

37. STEWART (D.J.), RICHARD (M.T.), HUGENHOLTZ (H.), DENNERY (J.), NUNDY (D.), PRIOR (J.), MONTPETIT (V.), HOPKINS (H.S.). Penetration of teniposide (VM-26) into human intracerebral tumors : preliminary observations on the effect of tumor type, rate of drug infusion and prior treatment with Amphotericin-B or oral glycerol. J. Neuro-Oncol **2**: 315-324 (1984).

38. LEHANE (D.E.), BRYAN (R.N.), HOROWITZ (B.), DE SANTOS (L.), EHNI (G.), ZUBLER (M.A.), MOIEL (R.), RUDOLPH (L.), ALDAMA-LEUBBERT (A.), MAHONEY (D.), HARPER (R.). Intraarterial cisplatinum chemotherapy for patients with primary and metastatic brain tumors. Cancer Drug Delivery **1**: 69-77 (1983).

39. BERGERAT (J.P.), DREWINKO (B.), CORRY (P.), BARLOGIE (B.), HO (D.H.). Synergistic lethal effect of cis-dichlorodiamineplatinum and 1-β-D-arabinofuranosylcytosine. Cancer Res **41** : 25-30 (1981).

40. KYRIAZIS (A.P.), KYRIAZIS (A.A.), MARTELO (A.J.). Response to single agent and combination chemotherapy of a human pancreatic carcinoma grown in nude mice. Proc Am Assoc Cancer Res **22**: 211 (1981).

41. SCHABEL (F.M.) Jr, LASTER (W.R.) Jr, TRADER (M.W.), CORBETT (T.H.), Griswold (D.P.) Jr. Combination chemotherapy with nitrosoureas plus other anticancer drugs against animal tumors. In : PRESTAYKO (A.W.), CROOKE (A.T.), BAKER (L.H.), CARTER (S.K.), SCHEIN (P.S.), (eds). Nitrosoureas: Current Status and New Developments. (Academic Press, New York, New York, 1981): 9-26.

42. OPFELL (R.), MUGGIA (F.). The role of VM-26 (teniposide: NSC 122819) in chemotherapy of cancer. Chemoterapia **1**: 98-101 (1982).

43. BOGHDAN (U.). Chemosensitivity of malignant brain tumors: preliminary results. J. Neuro-Oncol **1**: 149-166 (1983).

44. STEWART (D.J.), O'BRYAN (M.), AL-SARRAF (M.), COSTANZI (J.J.), OISHI (N.). Phase II study of cisplatin in recurrent astrocytomas in adults. J. Neuro-Oncol **1**: 145-147 (1983).

45. STEWART (D.J.), RICHARD (M.), HUGENHOLTZ (H.N.), BENOIT (B.), RUSSEL (N.), DENNERY (J.), PETERSON (E.), MAROUN (J.A.). Cisplatin plus cytosine arabinoside in adults with malignant gliomas. J. Neuro-Oncol **2**: 29-34 (1984).

46. MEYER (J.), FUKUUCHI (Y.), SHIMAZU (K), MATHEW (N.), OHUCHI (T.). Effect on regional cerebral blood flow of compression by a mass lesion. Europ Neurol **8** : 83-91 (1972).

47. VILLEMURE (J.G.), personal communication.

48. STEWART (D.J.), GRAHOVAC (Z.), RICHARD (M.T.), BENOIT (B.), MAROUN (J.A.), HUGENHOLTZ (H.), RUSSEL (N.), DENNERY (J.), PETERSON (E.), LUKE (B.), VENTUREYA (E.G.), GIRARD (A.), HOPKINS (H.S.). Phase I study of intraarterial mitomycin-C for recurrent intracerebral tumors. In: WALKER (M.), THOMAS (D.) (eds) *Biology of Brain Tumor* (Martinus Nijhoff Publishers, Dordrecht, The Netherlands) (1986): pp. 469-474.

49. STEWART (D.J.), GRAHOVAC (Z.), MAROUN (J.), HUGENHOLTZ (H.), BENOIT (B.), RICHARD (M.), RUSSEL (N.), DENNERY (J.), PETERSON (E.), LUKE (B.), HOPKINS (H.). Intraarterial (IA) chemotherapy (CT) for brain tumors (BT). Proc Amer Soc Clin Oncol **4**: 132 (1985).

50. MISRA (N.C.), JAISWAL (M.), SINGH (R.), DAS (B.). Intrahepatic arterial infusion of combination of mitomycin-C and 5-fluorouracil in the treatment of primary and metastatic liver carcinoma. Cancer **39**: 1425-1429 (1977).

51. TAKAKURA (K.). Chemotherapy of metastatic brain tumors with particular reference to continuous intracranial infusion of mitomycin-C and a radiosensitizing agent BUDR. Jpn J. Cancer Clin **17**: 263-268 (1971).

52. STEWART (D.J), GRAHOVAC (Z.), RIDING (M.), GUPTA (S.), HUGENHOLTZ (H.), DA SILVA (V.), RICHARD (M.), BENOIT (B.), RUSSEL (N.), MAROUN (J.), VERMA (S.). Intracarotid (IC) PCNU: an NCI Canada study. Proc Am Soc Clin Oncol **5**: 136 (1986).

53. STEWART (D.J.), BENJAMIN (R.S.), LEAVENS (M.), VALDIVIESO (M.), BURGESS (M.A.), BODEY (G.P.). Phase I study of intravenous 1-(2-Chloroethyl)-3-(2,6-Dioxo-3-Piperidyl)-1-Nitrosourea (PCNU, NSC 95466) in adults with solid tumors. Cancer Res **40**: 3750-3754 (1980).

54. FEUN (L.G.), STEWART (D.J.), LEAVENS (M.E.), BURGESS (M.A.), SAVARAJ (N.), BENJAMIN (R.S.), BODEY (G.P). A phase II trial of 1-(2-Chloroethyl)-3-(2,6-Dioxo-3-Piperidyl)-1-Nitrosourea (PCNU, NSC 95466) in recurrent malignant brain tumors. J. Neuro-Oncol **1**:45-48 (1983).

Intra-Arterial Chemotherapy Using Extra-Intracranial by-Pass for the Treatment of Malignant Gliomas

Technical Note

Y. GUEGAN (°), M. BEN HASSEL (°°), P. BOURGUET (°°), J. PECKER (°).

Intra-carotid administration of antineoplastic agents (ACNU, BCNU and CISPLATIN) is being explored as an alternative route of drug administration for the treatment of malignant gliomas, in several centres [3, 4, 14-19].

In most of these studies, the infusions are made by catheterization of the internal carotid artery (Seldinger's method or direct approach to the carotid artery in the neck).

Although these techniques have been improved, a number of important problems are still to be solved:

1) the true approach to the tumor site leads to a greater selectivity in catheterization [7, 8]; other procedures have been described in which the cerebral blood-flow is modified [5].
2) the high incidence of complications due to the toxicity of the drugs; the most frequently reported local toxicity is retinal damage following infusion of an antineoplastic agent into the infra-ophtalmic segment of the internal carotid artery; focal sites of cerebral toxicity and haemorrhagic infarction have been observed in animal studies and clinical trials [2, 4, 6, 9, 11]. Blacklock has recently shown that patients who had received intracarotid BCNU developed late focal brain damage outside the tumor site [1]. Intravascular drug streaming resulting in non-uniform drug delivery is a possible cause of focal toxicity and the author studied the distribution of drug delivery after internal carotid artery infusion in Rhesus monkeys.
3) drug delivery (number of injections, rate, dosage, concentration); repeated catheterization and the presence of a catheter in the arterial blood flow for several hours increase the risk of complications. A totally implantable system for the continuous and bolus delivery of intra-arterial chemotherapeutic agents to obviate these problems has been described [12].

In the light of these problems, we have evolved a new technical approach using:

— A subcutaneous injection chamber * positioned in the subclavian region, allowing all types of drug delivery.
— An extra-intracranial anastomosis, performed as near as possible to the tumor site and on the main tumor artery.
— The chamber is connected to the anastomosis by a sub-cutaneous catheter ** inserted through the superficial temporal artery (STA).

It must be stressed that this report is restricted to the description of a technique used for research purposes in the difficult problem of treating malignant gliomas of the central nervous system (the research programme has been approved by the Ethics Committee of the Société de Neurochirurgie de Langue Française).

ANATOMICAL BASIS

The superficial temporal artery divides into posterior and anterior branches above and beyond the tragus.

— One of these branches is used for the extra-intracranial anastomosis. The exact position of the anastomosis is determined by the arteriographical findings and stereotactic localization (a biopsy is performed in cases of unresectable gliomas during the latter), or by CT scan-guided exploratory surgery.

* Port-A-Cath System. PHARMACIA AB. S-75882. UPPSALA. SWEDEN. ** Dimensions: ID = 0.50 mm, OD = 0.86 mm.

(°) Clinique Neurochirurgicale, C.H.U. 35000 Rennes, France, (°°) Centre Régional de Lutte contre le Cancer, 35000 Rennes, France.

M. Chatel, F. Darcel and J. Pecker (eds.), Brain Oncology. ISBN-13: 978-94-010-8003-3

— The other branch receives the catheter which is carefully attached to it (Fig. 1).

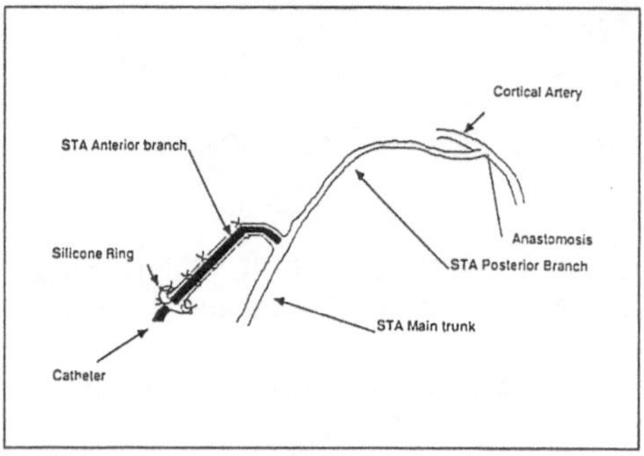

FIGURE 1

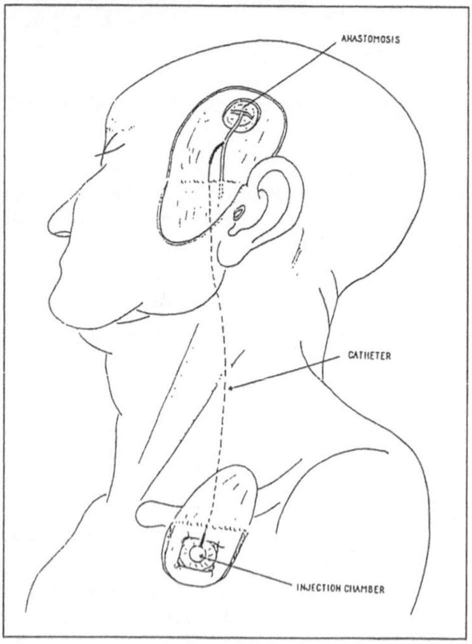

FIGURE 2

TECHNICAL PROCEDURE

The patient is positioned so that the intracranial tumor site and the sub-clavian region can be approached simultaneously (Fig. 2).

Step 1 — the brain/skull:
The two branches of the STA are dissected as far as the commun trunk. Craniectomy faces the tumor site. The dura mater is opened and the receiving cortical artery selected according to the arteriographical data or local operative conditions. One of the STA branches (usually the posterior) is then used for the anastomosis, which must be both perfectly watertight and permeable.

Step 2 - sub-clavian:
The injection chamber is put into place and attached to the pectoral fascia.

Step 3 - catheterization:
The catheter is fixed to the chamber and then pushed subcutaneously to the tumor site. The catheter-chamber complex is then filled with a solution of heparin (5 ml of heparin at 1000 u/ml in 125 ml of isotonic saline water solution).

Step 4 - introduction and fixation of catheter:
The STA branch to be used is dissected at approximately 4 cm from its base. A suitable length is dissected and the catheter inserted until its distal extremity reaches the lumen of the part of the STA that has been selected for the extra-intracranial anastomosis.
A silicone ring is fixed on to the catheter (9/0) and sutured to the artery wall. A number of ligatures are also done around the intra-arterial catheter (Fig. 1).
The heparin solution is then slowly injected to check that the complex is permeable and functions correctly.

Post-operative care:
A heparinized solution must be injected into the chamber to avoid the risk of thrombosis. This is done daily for the first three days then once a week.

RESULTS

Technetium-99 (99-Tcm) was infused into the chamber to check that the complex worked well and to assess cerebral distribution. These results were compared with those obtained by intravenous infusion of 99-Tcm.

Six patients were fitted with the complex. All had histologically confirmed glioblastoma and the tumor was recurrent in three cases.

Thrombosis caused by the complex led to failure in the first **two patients.** The most probable explanation is that the catheter was badly positioned. In both of these cases, the catheter had been inserted into the anterior STA, but its distal extremity did not reach the lumen of the branch used for the anastomosis.

The complex was perfectly **permeable** in the last **four patients** (Photo 1). The scintigrams of the tumor following intravenous infusion of 99-Tcm and injection via the catheter chamber complex concorded perfectly. The radio-isotope delivered via the injection chamber demonstrated uniform distribution in the tumor. The comparison of tumor concentration of 99-Tcm and normal brain tissue concentration gave a value of 2 for intravenous administration and 6 by extra-intracranial anastomosis (Photo 2).

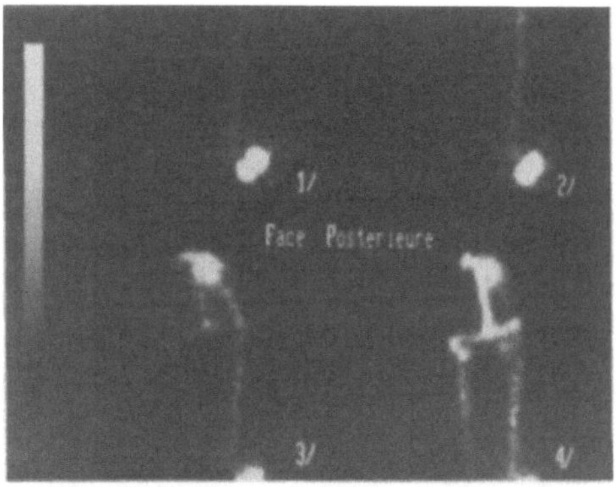

PHOTO 1: Dynamic study after injection of Technetium 99 into the injection chamber.

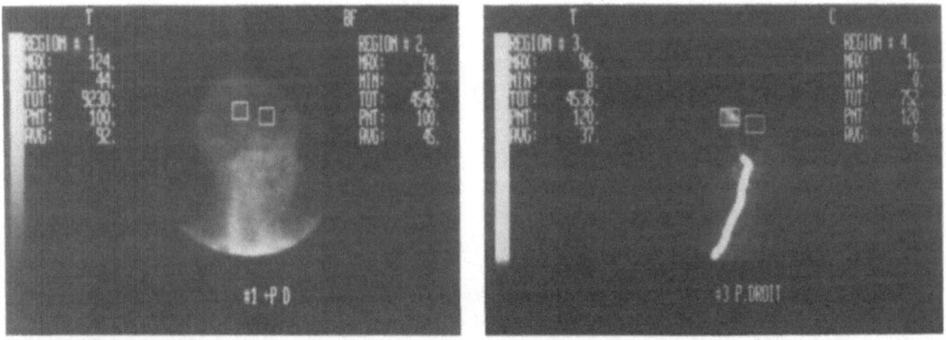

PHOTO 2: Comparison of tumor concentration of 99-Tcm and normal brain tissue:
A: Intravenous administration. Value of 2 (92/45)
B: Intraarterial administration. Value of 6 (37/6).

DISCUSSION

This technique presents considerable difficulties, and, in particular, insertion of the catheter into the STA which is often less than 1 millimetre in diameter. The catheter must be attached with precision, otherwise it can move out of the artery during the postoperative period. A sound knowledge of microsurgery and especially of extra-intracranial anastomosis is therefore necessary.

The main problem, in our opinion, is linked to the thrombosis of the complex at short or medium term and therefore its reliability. This demands rigourous monitoring and a weekly wash-out with an heparin solution.

The materials for implantation at our disposal was well tolerated and none of our patients developed infections. Conditions during surgery were meticulously aseptic.

When the complex has been shown to work perfectly, the administration of cytotoxic drugs can be considered. The method of delivery is simple: the chamber is punctured through the skin. Any combination of rate, dosage, dilution and type of injection (a single bolus, rapid or slow, slow perfusion using an electronic syringe with a constant flow-rate) can therefore be used.

Because an extra-intracranial anastomosis has to be performed, this technique is limited in application to these tumours with a readily accessible vascular system and hence these connected to the superficial sylvian network.

CONCLUSION

Our preliminary results are encouraging. Neither the implantation of the complex nor the administration of the drugs caused any morbidity or any mortality.
The number of patients studied is too small and the period considered too short to speculate on the success of the technique.
It must, however, be emphasized that, as yet, no effective treatment for malignant gliomas of the central nervous system has been found.
Chemotherapy is a promising field of research.
Intra-arterial drug administration has been the subject of a number of interesting articles. Besides an experienced medical team, it requires repeated catheterization, which represents an additional burden for patients who have often undergone surgery and radiation therapy. The quality of survival of such patients must be very carefully weighed up.
The present study only describes a new technique, but we feel it is a promising line of research in the treatment of patients with malignant glioma.

SUMMARY

The authors are reporting a new technical procedure for intra-arterial administration of antineoplastic agents, using:
- *a subcutaneous injection chamber positioned in the subclavian area,*
- *an extra-intracranial anastomosis performed as near as possible to the tumor site and on the main tumor artery,*
- *the chamber is connected to the anastomosis by a sub-cutaneous catheter inserted through the superficial temporal artery.*

After surgery, Technetium-99 was infused into the chamber to check that the complex worked well and to assess cerebral distribution. These results were compared with those obtained by intravenous infusion of 99-Tcm.
6 patients were fitted with the complex. Thrombosis led to failure in the first two patients. The complex was perfectly permeable in the last 4 patients.

It must be stressed that this report is only a description of a technique used for research purposes; but our preliminary results are encouraging and we feel that it is a line of research which may be worth considering in the difficult problem of treating malignant gliomas of the central nervous system.

KEY WORDS

Chemotherapy - Intra-arterial drug delivery - Malignant Glioma - EICA by-pass.

REFERENCES

1. BLACKLOCK (J.B.), WRIGHT (D.C.), DEDRICK (R.L.), BLASBERG (R.G.), LUTZ (R.J.), DOPPMAN (J.L.), and OLDFIELD (E.H.): Drug streaming during intra-arterial chemotherapy, J. Neurosurg., **64**: 284-291, (1986).
2. BREMER (A.M.), KLERIGA (E.), NGUYEN (T.Q.), BALSYS (R.), NORTHUP (H.M.), GONZALES (N.), DUARTE (P.), MILLER (R.I.): Complications associated with intra-arterial BCNU administered in combination with vincristine and procarbazine for the treatment of malignant brain tumors, J. Neuro-Oncol., **2**: 129-132, (1984).
3. FAUCHON (F.), CHIRAS (J.), ROSE (M.), DORMONTNSMINGER (W.D.), CHANDLER (W.F.): Intaarterial BCNU chemotherapy for treatment of malignant gliomas of the central nervous system, J. Neurosurg., **61**: 423-429, (1984).
4. GREENBERG (H.S.), ENSMINGER (W.D.), CHANDLER (W.F.): Intraarterial BCNU chemotherapy for treatment of malignant gliomas of the central nervous system. J. Neurosurg., **61**: 423-429, (1984).
5. KAPP (J.P.): Vascular Diversion in Chemotherapy of Brain Tumors, Surg. Neurol., **25**: 33-38, (1986).
6. KAPP (J.P.), VANCE (R.B.), PARKER (J.L.), SMITH (R.R.): Limitations of high dose intraarterial BCNU chemotherapy for malignant gliomas, Neurosurgery, **10**: 715-9, (1982).
7. KAPP (J.L.), PARKER (J.L.), TUCKER (E.M.): Supraophthalmic carotid infusion for brain chemotherapy. Experience with a new single-lumen catheter and maneuverable tip, J. Neurosurg., **62**: 823-825, (1985).

8. KAPP (J.P.), ROSS (R.L.), TUCKER (E.M.): Supraophthalmic carotid infusion for brain-tumor chemotherapy. Technical note, J. Neurosurg., **58**: 616-618, (1983).

9. LAYTON (P.B.), GREENBERG (H.S.), STETSON (P.L.): BCNU solubility and toxicity in the treatment of malignant astrocytomas, J. Neurosurg., **60**: 1134-1137, (1984).

10. LEVIN (V.A.), KABRA (P.M.), FREEMAN-DOVE (M.A.): Pharmacokinetics of intracarotid artery C-BCNU in the squirrel monkey, J. Neurosurg., **48**: 587-593, (1978).

11. OMOJOLA (M.F.), FOX (A.J.), AUER (R.N.): Hemorrhagic encephalitis produced by selective non-occlusive intracarotid BCNU injection in dogs, J. Neurosurg., **57**: 791-796, (1982).

12. PHILLIPS (T.W.), CHANDLER (W.F.), KINDT (G.W.), ENSMINGER (W.D.), GREENBERG (H.S.), SEEGER (J.F.), DOAN (K.M.), GYVES (J.W.): New implantable continuous administration and bolus dose intracarotid drug delivery system for the treatment of malignant gliomas, Neurosurgery, **11**: 213-218, (1982).

13. ROSS (R.L.), KAPP (J.P.), HOCHBERG (F.): Solvent systems for intracarotid 1,3-bis (2-chloroethyl)-1-nitrosourea (BCNU) infusion, Neurosurgery, **12**: 512-514, (1983).

14. SAFDARI (H.), MOMPEON (B.), DUBOIS (J.B.), GROS (C.): Intraarterial 1,3-Bis (2-Chloroethyl)-1-Nitrosourea chemotherapy for the treatment of malignant gliomas of the brain: A preliminary report, Surg. Neurol., **24**: 490-497, (1985).

15. STEWART (D.J.), GRAHOVAC (Z.), BENOIT (B.), ADDISON (D.), RICHARD (M.T.), DENNERY (J.), HUGENHOLTZ (H.), RUSSELL (N.), PETERSON (E.), MAROUN (J.A.), VANDERBERG (T.), HOPKINS (H.S.): Intracarotid chemotherapy with a combination of 1,3-bis (2-chloroethyl)-1-nitrosourea (BCNU), cis-diaminodichloroplatinum (Cisplatin), and 4'-0-demethyl-1-0-(4,6-0-2)-thenylidene--D-glucopyranosyl) epipodophyllotoxin (VM 26) in the treatment of primary and metastatic brain tumors, Neurosurgery, **15**: 828-33, (1984).

16. VILLEMURE (J.G.), THERON (J.), TYLER (J.), WORTHINGTON (C.), DROP (D.): Infusion artérielle supersélective de BCNU dans les gliomes malins cérébraux: résultats préliminaires et corrélation avec la tomographie d'émission de positron, Neurochirurgie, **2**: 179, (1986).

17. WEST (C.R.), AVELLANOSA (A.M.), BARUA (N.R.): Intraarterial 1,3-bis (2-chloroethyl)-1-nitrosourea (BCNU) and systemic chemotherapy for malignant gliomas: a follow-up study, Neurosurgery, **13**: 420-426, (1983).

18. YAMASHITA (J.), HANDA (H.), TOKURIKI (Y.): Intra-arterial ACNU therapy for malignant brain tumors. Experimental studies and preliminary clinical results, J. Neurosurg., **59**: 424-430, (1983).

19. YUMITORI (K.), HANDA (H.), TERAUBA (T.): Treatment of malignant brain tumors with ACNU and phenobarbital: continuous infusion of ACNU into internal carotid artery and systemic administration of phenobarbital, ACTA Neurochir., **70**: 155-168, (1984).

Intra-Arterial Chemotherapy With BCNU. Correlations between Tumour Growth and Red Blood Cell Polyamine Levels.

J. THERON (°), J.Ph. MOULINOUX (°°), A. CASASCO (°), V. QUEMENER (°°), P. COURTHEOUX (°), F. ALACHKAR (°), J.M. DERLON (°°°).

Intraarterial chemotherapy of high grade gliomas has been undertaken for 13 months in our institution. This was the continuation of the work performed by one of us (9) (10) at the Montreal Neurological Hospital. However, the protocol was modified on a major point: knowing the efficacy of the BCNU on the gliomas (4) but also its toxicity on the normal brain (5), our goal was to treat, if possible with lower doses, the tumour before the post surgical recurrence can be recognized on the clinical signs and on the CT findings.

Determination of polyamine blood levels (7) seems to provide interesting informations for the therapeutic strategy and specially, as recently reported (8), when the correlations between the Spermine and Spermidine levels are studied: the findings permit to determine the proliferative or non proliferative state of the tumour.

In this series, the intraarterial chemotherapy technique consisted in a catheterization of the intracranial internal carotid with positionning of a silastic (2,5 F) catheter above the ophthalmic artery (2) associated or not, depending on the tumoral location, to the catheterization of the controlateral internal carotid (fig. 1) and to the catheterization of the basilar artery.

The dose of chemotherapy was 50 to 150 mg infused on 3 hours. The radiotherapy was given between the first and the second session of chemotherapy.

The positionning of the catheter above the ophthalmic artery has totally ruled out the orbital complications (3) and was prefered to a more distal catheterization of cortical branches wich does not permit the infusion of the whole tumoral vascular territory (9). It seemed also very important to treat the controlateral hemisphere and the posterior cerebral artery when the tumor involved their territory to decrease the risk of controlateral (frontal tumour) or posterior (temporal tumour) recurrence wich may happen when only a portion of the tumour is treated.

The treatment was infused on 3 hours to increase the chances of treating the tumour during the phase of reproduction of the ADN (6).

A first series of 22 patients has been treated with 4 sessions of chemotherapy. There were 6 weeks between two sessions of chemotherapy. The polyamine blood levels have been determinated before and after each session showing in some cases an important decrease but also in other cases a transitory increase wich could correspond to a release of the intratumoral polyamines due to the necrosis of the tumour (fig. 2A, fig. 2B).

The diagram of correlations between Spermine and Spermidine levels, that we used at the end of this first series of patients, has showed three points that seem to us retrospectively quite interesting.

1) A few patients, although their polyamine levels fluctuated, had a point of correlation between Spermine and Spermidine remaining in the proliferative tumoral area of the diagram, even when their CT and their clinical neurological status dit not show any modification (fig. 3B). Such post chemotherapy no-response seems to us quite important to help in the decision of changing the type of chemotherapy and testing other drugs before new clinical or radiological signs have appeared.

2) For a few patients, the diagram showed that the chemotherapy was given when the point of correlation between Spermine and Spermidine was not in the proliferative tumoral area (fig. 2B). Knowing the risks of cerebral toxicity, it seems that, in the future, it could be better not to treat these patients and to wait for a new proliferation phase demonstrated on the follow up polyamine levels. It is

(°) Neuroradiology Department, C.H.U. Côte-de-Nacre, Caen, France, (°°) Histology and Cytology Department, C.H.U. Pontchaillou, Rennes, France, (°°°) Neurosurgery Department, C.H.U. Côte-de-Nacre, Caen, France.

M. Chatel, F. Darcel and J. Pecker (eds.), Brain Oncology. ISBN-13: 978-94-010-8003-3

also possible that the toxicity of the drug on the normal brain is increased when the tumour is not in a proliferative phase.

3) It is not sure that high doses of chemotherapy are necessary to get a therapeutic response. The work performed in Montreal (10) using labelled BCNU studied on PET has showed that the intratumoral concentration of the drug was at least 50 times higher when the drug was given by intraarterial intracerebral catheterization as compared to the systemic administration. In our series, the polyamine levels were modified and the point of correlation between Spermine and Spermidine was displaced out of the proliferative area with doses sometimes markedly lower than the doses usually given. It also appears that, as demonstrated on the Montreal study, the uptake of the drug is quite variable from one tumour to another and that the use of a biological marker is particulary interesting to study the responsiveness of each tumour to a given chemotherapy and adapt the dose at each type of tumour.

CONCLUSION

It is too early to give final conclusions from this study but a few points should be emphasized:

1) From a technical point of view, the infusion of the whole vascular tumoral territory is necessary and the positionning of the catheter above the ophthalmic artery rules out the orbital complications.

2) The question on how long time the infusion should be given remains pending but, in our opinion, it seems that, even if the laminar flow (1) makes the concentrations of drug less homogenous, the chances of reaching the tumor cells during the phase of reproduction of the ADN are higher with slow infusion than with a bolus.

3) The study of the polyamine blood levels and the diagram of correlation between Spermine and Spermidine seem particulary interesting as a marker of the tumoral proliferation and permits to « personalize » the treatment of a brain tumour whose various metabolic types cannot be distinguished on the usual investigations. They will permit to: 1. - appreciate the evolutivity of the tumour in the postsurgical follow-up, 2. - treat the tumour when it proliferates and not to treat it when it does not proliferate as to decrease the toxic risks of the chemotherapy, 3. - adapt the type of chemotherapy and its dose depending on the tumoral response.

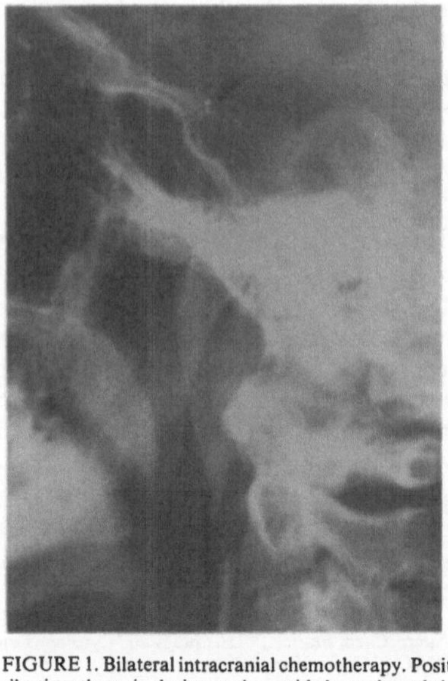

FIGURE 1. Bilateral intracranial chemotherapy. Positionning of a silastic catheter in the internal carotid above the ophthalmic artery on each side.

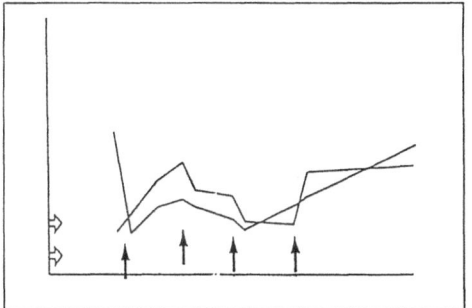

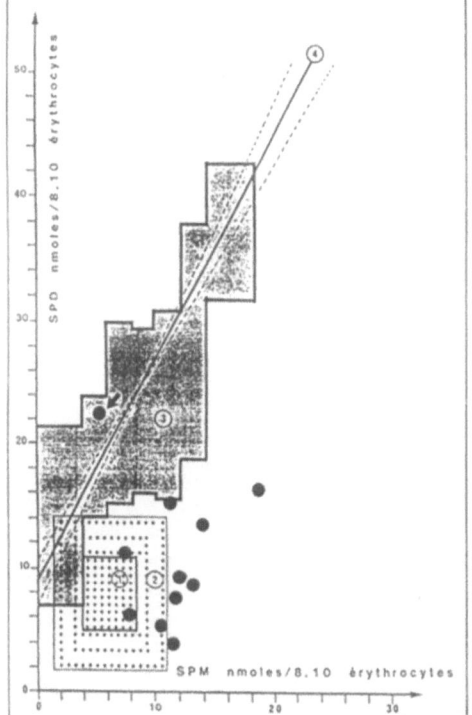

FIGURE 2 (A and B). Astrocytoma grade IV, presently well controlled with the chemotherapy.

A - Blood levels of Spermine and Spermidine. There is a crossing of the two lines wich would be characteristic of a tumoral necrosis. One notes the fluctuations of the levels after chemotherapy (closed arrows). The two open arrows represent the normal levels of Spermine and Spermidine.

B - Diagram correlating the blood levels of Spermine (SPM) and Spermidine (SPD). Are represented: the couples of numbers of a normal population at 1 SD (1) and at 2 SD (3), the graphic representation of the theoric linear regression of a malignant glial proliferation (4). On this patient, one notes only one couple of numbers (arrow) in the glial malignant proliferative area corresponding to the state before chemotherapy. All the other numbers are out of this area.

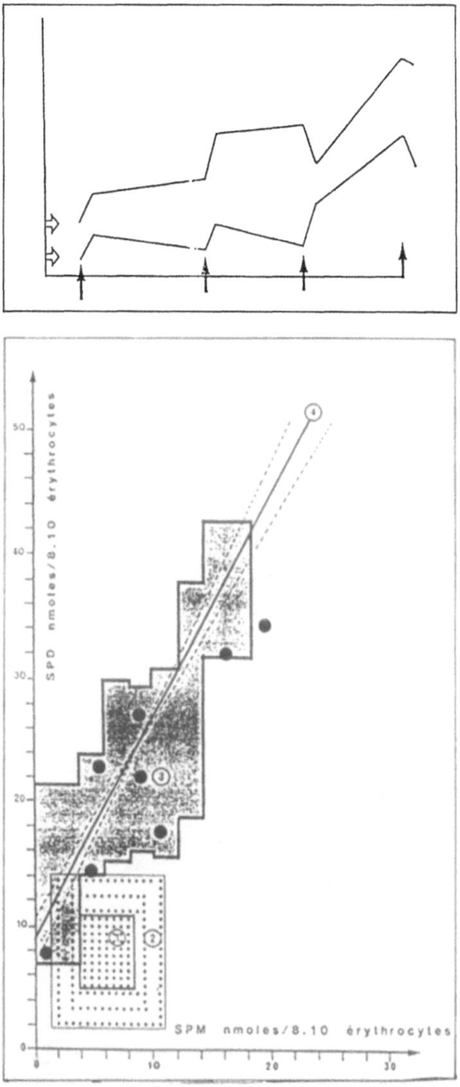

FIGURE 3 (A and B). Astrocytoma grade IV. Patient who has presented for a few months after surgery a good clinical status with minor modifications on the CT until the onset of severe neurological signs and who rapidly died.

A - Fluctuations of the SPD and SPM blood levels with progressive increase of the levels although the patient was treated by chemotherapy.

B - Diagram correlating the SPD and SPM blood levels. The patient has remained in the « poliferative malignant glial area » because the chemotherapy was inefficient although the clinical status and the CT findings remained apparently stabilized for a few months.

KEY WORDS

Gliomas, Chemotherapy, Intra-Arterial Chemotherapy, Polyamines.

REFERENCES

1. BLACKLOCK (J.B.), WRIGHT (D.C.), DEDRICK (P.D.) et al.: Drug streaming during intraarterial chemotherapy. J. Neurosurg., **64**: 284-291, 1986.
2. DEBRUN (G.M.), DAVIS (K.R.), HOCHBERG (F.H.): Superselective injection of BCNU through a latex calibrated-leak balloon. AJNR, **4**: 399-400, 1983.
3. GEBARSKI (S.S.), GREENBERG (H.S.), GABRIELSEN (T.O.), VINE (A.K.): Orbital angiographic changes after intracarotid BCNU chemotherapy. AJNR, **5**: 55-58, 1984.
4. GREENBERG (H.S.), ENSMINEGER (W.D.), CHANDLER (W.F.) et al.: Intraarterial BCNU chemotherapy for the treatment of malignant gliomas of the central nervous system. J. Neurosurg. **61**: 423-429, 1984.
5. KAPP (J.), VANCE (R.), PARKER (J.L.), SMITH (P.R.): Limitations of high dose intraarterial 1, 3bis (2-Chloroethyl) -1-Nitrosourea (BCNU) chemotherapy for malignant gliomas. J. Neurosurg. **10**: 715-719, 1982.
6. LEHNINGER (A.L.): Biochimie, Bases moléculaires de la structure et des fonctions cellulaires, 3e édition, traduction P. Cartier & P. Kamoun, Flammarion Médecine - Sciences, p. 982.
7. MOULINOUX (J.Ph.), QUEMENER (V.), LE CALVE (M.), CHATEL (M.), DARCEL (F.): Polyamines in human brain tumors. J. of Neuro Oncology, **2**: 153-158, 1984.
8. MOULINOUX (J.Ph.), QUEMENER (V.), HERCOUET (H.), DARCEL (F.), CHATEL (M.): Red blood cell polyamines in malignant glioma patients, Spermine and Spermidine blood levels and tumour evolution. To be published in the J. of Neuro Oncology.
9. THERON (J.), VILLEMURE (J.G.), WORTHINGTON (C.), TYLER (J.): Superselective intracerebral chemotherapy of malignant tumours with BCNU. Neuroradiology **28**: 118-125, 1986.
10. TYLER (J.), YAMAMOTO (Y.L.), DIKSIC (M.), THERON (J.), VILLEMURE (J.G.), WORTHINGTON (C.), EVANS (A.), FEINDEL (W.): The pharmacokinetics of superselective intraarterial and intravenous 11C-BCNU evaluated by PET. J. Nucl. Med. **27**: 775-780, 1986.

Effects of Intra-Arterially Administered 1,3-bis[2-chloroethyl]-1-nitrosurea (BCNU) on the Electroretinogram of the Rabbit
A Study on the Retinal Toxicity of BCNU

N. ROOSEN (°), S. SCHREINER (°) (°°), M. SCHIRMER (°), and U. WEBER (°°).

INTRODUCTION

Malignant gliomas of the brain have a poor prognosis despite surgery and radiotherapy and/or systemic chemotherapy (10, 11). Therefore, alternative ways of administering chemotherapeutic agents have been developed, as for instance the intra-arterial (ia) route, which has been used for BCNU, ACNU, cisplatin, and other drugs (3, 6, 13). Although local complications have been reported with various chemotherapeutic agents, the retinotoxicity of these ia administered cytostatics has received relatively minor attention in the clinical literature (5, 7, 9), and experimental investigations on this subject have been performed rarely (2).

We designed a study to evaluate the effects of ia BCNU on the retina of the rabbit. In this investigation neurophysiologic long term effects of intra-carotid BCNU infusion were monitored using electroretinography (ERG), a reliable and standardized method to evaluate retinal function (14). Morphologic studies of the infused retinae, and morphologic-neurophysiologic correlations are still in progress and will be presented in future communications.

STUDY DESIGN AND METHODS

Rabbits. Eleven adult, or , Bastard Chinchilla rabbits, each weighting between 3.0 and 3.5 kg, were studied. For ERG recording the animals were anesthetized with intramuscular injection of Ketanest®* and Rompun®*. The operative procedure was performed during anesthesia with Hypnorm®* and Valium®*.

Electroretinography. The ERG was elicited by short (10μs) white Xenon flashes with a frequency of 30 flashes/min. Flash intensity was varied from I to V on the scale of the KNOTT-Lightstimulator LT 1001. A central field of 35° was illuminated during the flashes. HENKES' corneal electrodes were used. ERG was recorded under light (room lights, approx. 450 cd/m^2) and dark adaptation (recordings were made after 3, 10 and 15 minutes of dark adaptation). Three ERG's were obtained before infusion: mean values and standard deviations of the mean of the various ERG components were determined for standardization. Thereafter sequential ERG recordings were performed on postoperative days 1, 2, 7, 18, 28, and 60. The ERG parameters we analyzed for this report, were the standard amplitude at the lowest flash intensity I [SA], the maximal amplitude of the a- and b-waves [$A(a_{max})$ and $A(b_{max})$]. Several other parameters such as a- and b- wave latencies, and oscillating potentials, have not been analyzed yet.

(*) 15 mg/kg Ketanest® [Ketamine]; 6 mg/kg Rompun® [Xylazine];
0.5 ml/kg Hypnorm® [100 mg Fluanisone & 2 mg Fentanyl/10 ml];
1.5 mg/kg Valium® [Diazepam].

(°) Neurosurgical Clinic and (°°) Ophtalmological Clinic, Hospital of the University of Düsseldorf, 4000 Düsseldorf, 1, Federal Republic of Germany.

M. Chatel, F. Darcel and J. Pecker (eds.), Brain Oncology. ISBN-13: 978-94-010-8003-3

Surgery and ia infusion. The left carotid artery was microsurgically exposed. After applying two temporary vascular microclamps a small arteriotomy was performed. An infusion catheter was introduced into the carotid artery and advanced 0.5 cm into the external carotid artery. The retinal arterial supply in rabbits mainly derived from the external carotid artery by way of the external ophthalmic artery (Fig. 1): The internal ophthalmic artery-internal carotid artery does not contribute significantly to the vascularization of the retina. During 20 minutes 10 ml of a solution (either 5% glucose in H_2O [≡(5% GLUC)], 0.3% ethanol in 5% glucose in H_2O [≡(0.3% ALC)], and 100 or 200 mg BCNU in 0.3% ethanol in 5% glucose in H_2O [≡(100 mg BCNU) or (200 mg BCNU)]) were ia infused. After finishing the infusion, the catheter was withdrawn and the arteriotomy was sutured carefuly without obliterating the blood vessel. Finally, the wound was closed.

RESULTS (Table)

The largest effects of the different infusions were noted on $A(a_{max})$, whereas SA and $A(b_{max})$ were influenced less.

$A(a_{max})$ (Fig. 2). After infusion of (5% GLUC) we recorded hypernormal a-waves. (0.3% ALC) caused only a slight and transient increase of $A(a_{max})$, which was present at days 2, 7, 18 and 28. After (100 mg BCNU) we saw the most prominent effect on $A(a_{max})$. An increase of the a-wave amplitude up to 800-900% was seen. These amplitudes were diminishing again toward the end of follow-up (days 28 and 60), approaching normal values. A less pronounced $A(a_{max})$ increase was noted after infusion of (200 mg BCNU); however, the amplitude reduction, recorded during the last follow-up examinations, was more marked than after (100 mg BCNU) and levels below 1 standard deviation under the mean values were seen.

SA. (100 mg BCNU) and (200 mg BCNU) resulted in a decrease of SA, both under photopic and scotopic conditions.

$A(b_{max})$. Slight hypernormal amplitudes were seen after (100 mg BCNU) infusion. At the higher BCNU concentration [(200 mg BCNU)] the amplitudes tended towards subnormality.

DISCUSSION

We found several effects of ia infusion of (5% GLUC), (O.3% ALC), (100 mg BCNU) and (200 mg BCNU) upon the ERG of the rabbit, which was followed-up during two months. The most marked effect of the different infusions was seen on the photoreceptors, as demonstrated by the changes of $A(a_{max})$. (5% GLUC) had an amplitude increasing influence, that was inhibited by addition of ethanol [(0.3% ALC)]. BCNU seemed to facilitate and shorten this amplitude increasing glucose effect at the medium dosis of 100 mg [(100 mg BCNU)], whereas a high dose BCNU infusion [(200 mg BCNU)] did not result in the same extreme and transient $A(a_{max})$ increase, and even resulted in an amplitude reduction after 60 days. These results may allow a "quantification" of the BCNU effects on the retinal photoreceptors. Furthermore, hypernormal often occur prior to subnormal amplitudes, as for example in canthaxantine (12) and glycol intoxication (8) of the retina. Therefore the photoreceptors seem to react in a nonspecific way, irrespective of the single toxic agent used: an amplitude reduction follows transient hypernormal amplitudes in case of a large enough lesion.

Several ERG parameters can be altered in chorioretinitis, and changes in $A(b_{max})$ are known to occur in ischemic retinopathy (1). We do not know the exact nature of the retinal changes causing the ERG abnormalities, that we saw, yet. This awaits further pathologic examination of the infused retinae. It seems, however, that BCNU, at least in the doses used in these experiments, is more retinotoxic than (0.3% ALC). But the ERG changes after ia infusion of (0.3% ALC) suggest, that an alcohol solution may be also harmful to the retina if infused intra-arterially.

CONCLUSIONS

On the basis of our preliminary findings, we conclude, that in clinical practice the alcohol content of the solvent used in ia chemotherapy of brain tumors with the lipophilic and alcohol soluble drug BCNU, should be as low as possible, and that further efforts should be undertaken to reduce the chemotherapeutic burden to the ipsilateral retina in intra-carotid chemotherapy of malignant cerebral gliomas with BCNU.

TABLE

ERG results [SA, $A(a_{max})$ & $A(b_{max})$] as related to the duration of dark adaptation [photopic & scotopic ERG] and the different infused solutions

ERG Wave	S A				$A(a_{max})$				$A(b_{max})$			
Duration of Dark Adaptation (Minutes)	0	3	10	15	0	3	10	15	0	3	10	15
Infused Solutions												
{5% GLUC}	~	~	~	~	↑↑↑	↑↑↑	↑↑↑	↑↑↑	~↑	~	~	~
{0.3% ALC}	~↓	~↓	~	~	↑|↓	↑|↓	↑|~	↑|~	~	~	~	~
{100 mg BCNU}	↓↓	↓↓	↓	~	↑↑↑|~	↑↑↑|~	↑↑↑|~	↑↑↑|~	~↑	~↑	~↑	~↑
{200 mg. BCNU}	↓	↓	↓	↓	↑↑|↓	↑↑|↓	↑↑|↓	↑↑|↓	~↓	~↓	~↓	~↓

~ : unchanged
~↑ : slight increase
~↓ : slight decrease
↓ : 1 standard deviation decrease
↓↓ : 2 standard deviations decrease
↓↓↓ : 3 standard deviations decrease
↑ : 1 standard deviation increase
↑↑ : 2 standard deviations increase
↑↑↑ : 3 standard deviations increase
↑|↓ : transient increase, then decrease
↑↑|↓ : transient increase, then decrease
↑|~ : transient increase, than unchanged
↑↑↑|~ : first increase, then unchanged
{5% GLUC} : see text
{0.3% ALC} : see text
{100 mg BCNU} : see text
{200 mg BCNU} : see text
Increase, decrèase and unchanged refer to the mean value (100 %, see Fig. 2)

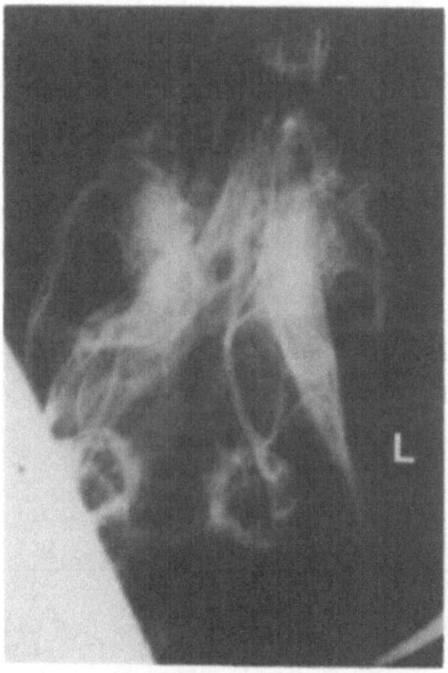

FIGURE 1. Selective angiography of the left external carotid artery demonstrates a capillary blush, which clearly outlines the retina in the left orbit.

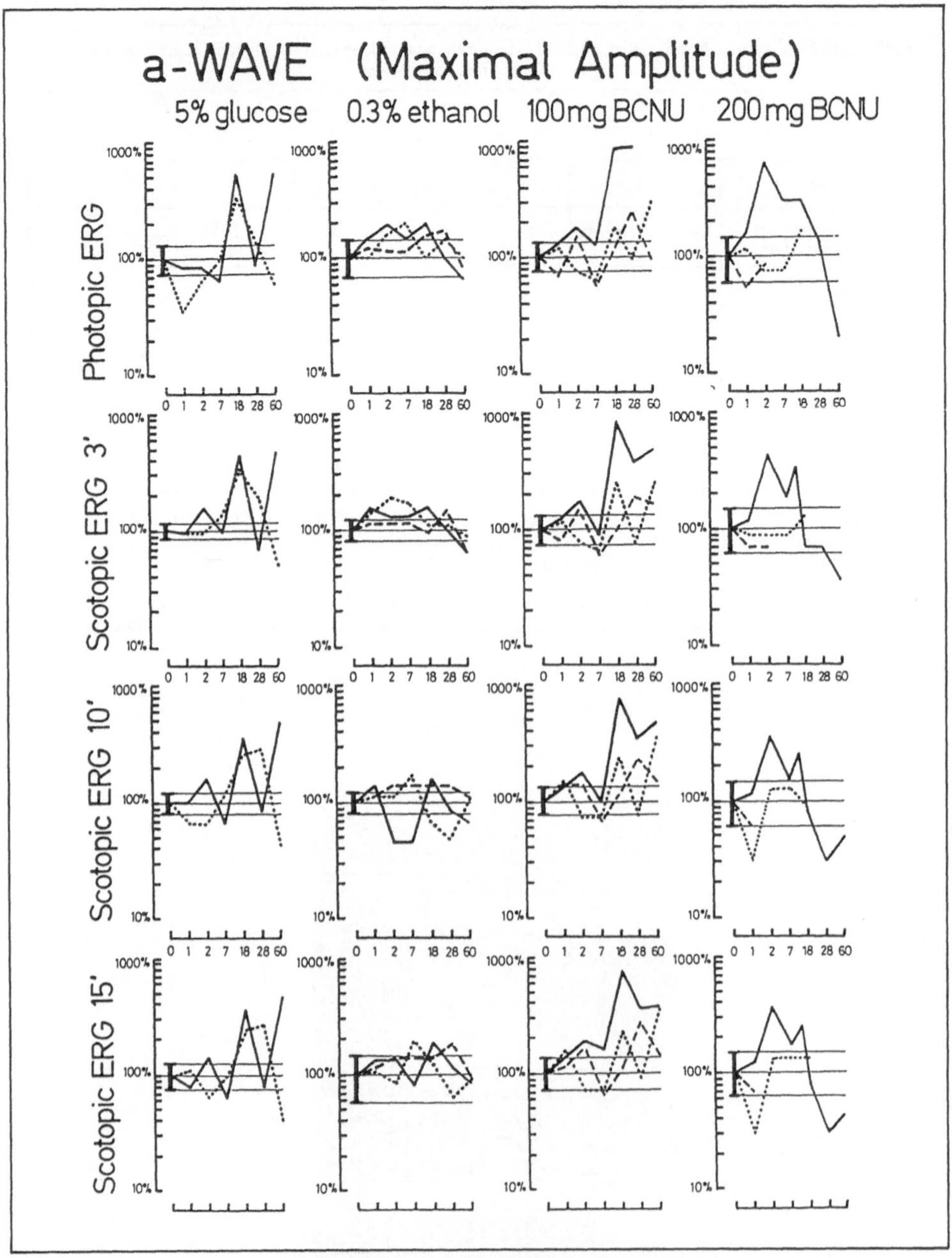

FIGURE 2. Effects of ia infusion of 5% glucose [Ξ(5% GLUC)], 0.3% ethanol [Ξ(0.3% ALC)], 100 mg BCNU [Ξ(100 mg BCNU)], and 200 mg BCNU [Ξ(200 mg BCNU)] on the maximal a-wave amplitude of the photopic and scotopic ERG, after 3, 10 and 15 minutes dark adaptation, as recorded preoperatively (day 0) and postoperatively (day 1, 2, 7, 18, 28 and 60). Note that the y-axis has a logarithmic scale.

KEY WORDS

Intraarterial Chemotherapy, Toxicity, Eye Toxicity, Brain Tumours.

REFERENCES

1. BABEL (J.), STANGOS (N.), KOROL (S.), SPIRITUS (M.): Ocular electrophysiology - a clinical and experimental study of electroretinogram, electrooculogram, visual evoked response. Georg Thieme Publishers, Stuttgart, 1977.
2. DE WYS (W.D.), FOWLER (E.H.): Reports of vasculitis and blindness after intracarotid injection of 1,3-bis(2-chloroethyl)-1-nitrosurea (BCNU; NSC-409962) in dogs. Cancer Treat Rep 1973; 57: 33-40.
3. FEUN (L.G.), WALLACE (S.), YUNG (W.K.A.), LEE (Y.Y.), LEAVENS (M.E.), MOSER (R.), SAVARAJ (N.), BURGESS (M.A.), PLAGER (C.), BENJAMIN (R.S.), TANG (R.A.), MAVLIGIT (G.M.), FIELDS (W.S.): Phase-I trial of intracarotid BCNU and cisplatin in patients with malignant intracerebral tumors. Cancer Drug Delivery 1984; 1: 239-245.
4. FISHMAN (C.A.): Basic principles of electroretinography. Retina 1985; 5: 123-126.
5. GEBARSKI (S.S.), GREENBERG (H.S.), GABRIELSEN (T.O.), VINE (A.K.): Orbital angiographic changes after intracarotid BCNU chemotherapy. AJNR 1984; 5: 55-58.
6. KAPP (J.P.), VANCE (R.B.): Supraophthalmic carotid infusion for recurrent glioma: rationale, technique, and preliminary results for cisplatin and BCNU. J. Neuro-Oncol. 1985; 3: 5-11.
7. MILLER (D.F.), BAY (J.W.), LEDERMAN (R.J.), PURVIS (J.D.), ROGERS (L.R.), TOMSAK (R.L.): Ocular orbital toxicity following intracarotid injection of BCNU (carmustine) and cisplatinum for malignant gliomas. Ophthalmology 1985; 92: 402-406.
8. ROSSA (V.), WEBER (U.), KERN (W.): Experimental glycol poisoning of the rabbit retina. A morphological and electroretinographic study (in prep.).
9. SHINGLETON (B.J.), BIENFANG (D.C.), ALBERT (D.M.), ENSMINGER (W.D.), CHANDLER (W.F.), GREENBERG (H.S.): Ocular toxicity associated with high-dose carmustine. Arch. Ophthalmol. 1982; 100: 1766-1772.
10. TAKAKURA (K.), ABE (H.), TANAKA (R.), KITAMURA (K.), MIWA (T.), TAKEUCHI (K.), YAMAMOTO (S.), KAGEYAMA (N.), HANDA (H.), MOGAMI (H.), NISHIMOTO (A.), UOZUMI (T.), MATSUTANI (M.), NOMURA (D.): Effects of ACNU and radiotherapy on malignant glioma. J. Neurosurg. 1986; 64: 53-57.
11. WALKER (M.D.), ALEXANDER (E. jr), HUNT (W.E.), MacCARTY (C.S.), MAHALEY (M.S. jr), MEALEY (J. jr), NORRELL (H.A.), OWENS (G.), RANSOHOFF (J.), WILSON (C.B.), GEHAN (E.H.), STRIKE (T.A.): Evaluation of BCNU and/or radiotherapy in the treatment of anaplastic gliomas. A cooperative clinical trial. J. Neurosurg. 1978; 49: 333-349.
12. WEBER (U.), KERN (W.), NOVOTNY (G.E.K.), GOERZ (G.), HANAPPEL (S.): Experimental carotenoid retinopathy. I. Functional and morphological alterations of the rabbit retina after 11 months dietary carotenoid application (in prep.).
13. YUMITORI (K.), HANDA (H.), TERAUA (T.), YAMASHITA (J.): Treatment of malignant brain tumours with ACNU and phenobarbital: continous infusion of ACNU into internal carotid artery and systemic administration of phenobarbital. Acta Neurochir. 1984; 70: 155-168.

Cerebral Toxicity Following Supraophthalmic Intracarotid Infusion of BCNU: Study of 4 Malignant Gliomas

F. MIKOL (°), J. MORET (°°), J. MIKOL (°°°),
A. BOUCHAREINE (°), M.L. AUBIN (°°), C. FISCH (°°).

Intra-arterial infusion of BCNU provides a substantial advantage over intravenous administration for treatment of malignant gliomas (4, 6). The ocular complications, which reduce this modality of therapy (5), are avoided by selective supraophthalmic carotid artery infusion (2, 8).

We report serious cerebral complications in four patients treated with this technique and emphasize the peculiarity of CT scan features and neuropathologic findings.

METHODS

The four patients have been previously treated — IV chemotherapy or surgical procedure — (table 1). IA perfusion of BCNU was performed as clinical impairment, CT scan, angiography demonstrated recurrent malignant gliomas.

A calibrated-leak balloon microcatheter was introduced and positioned distal to the ophthalmic artery origin (cases 2, 3 and 4) or proximal to the middle cerebral artery (case 1). BCNU was infused at a total dose of 300 mg (except for case 4) every 2 months; each 100 mg of BCNU was dissolved in 3 ml of alcohol, further diluted with 27 ml of 5% glucose in water and infused each hour. Dexamethasone (24 mg IV) was given on the day of infusion and two days after.

TABLE 1: Summary of clinical data in 4 patients

	Age	Sex	Site of tumour	Histological diagnosis *	Prior treatment	Delay before 1st IA infusion	BCNU doses (mg)
1	52	M	Lt parietal	astrocytoma II **	IV chemotherapy (Teniposide; Lomustine)	18 months	300,300,300
2	73	F	Rt parietal	astrocytoma III	surgical removal	6 months	300,300
3	56	F	Lt frontal	astrocytoma III	surgical removal	3 months	300,300
4	60	F	Lt frontal	glioblastoma	surgical removal	4 months	300,150,150

* grading according to WHO's system. ** biopsy.

CLINICAL RESULTS

The four patients showed marked tumour regression and clinical stabilisation during the procedure of therapy. In the 4 cases, fast gradual clinical impairment arose after the 2nd ou 3rd IA infusion (table 2). CT scan showed extensive hypodensity (fig. 1B, fig. 2) and new enhancing lesions (fig. 1B, fig. 3).

Two patients died (cases 1 and 2).

PATHOLOGIC STUDIES

Macroscopic findings included an extensive hemispheric edema predominant in the corona radiata (case 2); a softened necrotic frontal white matter, an incisural herniation of lingula and the fusiform gyrus associated to necrosis of the anterior limb of the internal capsule and softened appearance of the dorsal part of midbrain and pons (case 1).

(°) Service de Neurologie, Fondation Rothschild, Paris, (°°) Service de radiologie, Fondation Rothschild, Paris, (°°°) Service d'Anatomo-pathologie, Hôpital Lariboisière, Paris.

M. Chatel, F. Darcel and J. Pecker (eds.), Brain Oncology. ISBN-13: 978-94-010-8003-3

TABLE 2: Deterioration after supraophtalmic BCNU infusion in 4 patients

	Delay after the last IA infusion	Clinical features	CT findings without contrast	CT findings with contrast	Fate
1	1 month	seizures hemiplegia coma	increased initial hypodensity	annular enhancement in ant. limb int. caps. (remote from originate tumour site)	death
2	5 weeks	seizures hemiplegia coma	severe hypodensity in ipsilateral white matter		death
3	3 weeks	hemiplegia aphasia	diffuse ipsilateral white matter hypodensity	wide-spread festoon annular enhancement	chronic state
4	4 days	hemiplegia aphasia	ipsilateral white matter hypodensity	festoon annular enhancement in temporal lobe (remote from originate tumour site)	chronic state

At histological examination, few tumour cells were present. Polymorph vascular abnormalities were predominant in case 2: they consisted of haemorrhagic distension of the Virchow-Robin spaces, cellular intramural arteriolar infiltration, hyalinosis of the capillaries and an ischaemic infarct in the right lenticulo-striate territory. These abnormalities were distant from the residual tumour.

COMMENTS

Cerebral complications after intracarotid BCNU administration were known in animal studies (3, 11) and in human chemotherapy (6, 7); our neuropathological findings were in agreement with previous report (7).

This toxic cerebral necrosis seems to be related to cumulative and/or repeated infusion of BCNU (7); immediat nearness of irradiation therapy (6); age and high blood flow pressure (our case 2); concentration of the ethanol diluent (5, 9, 12); low infusion rates (1, 10) or, on the other hand, bolus injection (12).

Further studies to determine this therapy and to define accurate indications are needed.

SUMMARY

In four patients with malignant supratentorial gliomas, treated with supraophthalmic intracarotid infusion of chemotherapeutic agents (300 mg of BCNU dissolved in 9 ml of alcohol), serious cerebral complications arose after the 2nd or 3rd infusion; two patients died one month after the last injection.

CT scan showed white matter large hypodensity and/or annular enhancement outside the originate tumour site. Necropsy of two cases revealed severe white matter edema and numerous vascular abnormalities: these findings were distinct from residual tumour.

KEY WORDS

Intra-arterial chemotherapy, BCNU, glioma, cerebral toxicity.

REFERENCES

1. BLACKLOCK (J.B.), WRIGHT (D.C.), DERRICK (R.L.), BLASBERG (R.G.), LUTZ (R.J.), DOPPMAN (J.L.) and OLDFIELD (E.H.): Drug streaming during intra-arterial chemotherapy. J. Neurosurg. **64**: 284-291 (1986).
2. DEBRUN (G.M.), DAVIS (K.R.) and HOCHBERG (F.H.). Superselective injection of BCNU through a latex calibrated-leak balloon. AJNR, **4**: 399-400 (1983).
3. DE WYS (W.D.) and FOWLER (E.H.): Report of vasculitis and blindness after intracarotid injection of 1,3-Bis (2-chloroethyl)- 1-nitrosourea (BCNU; NSC-409962) in dogs. Cancer Chemother. Rep **57**: 33-40 (1973).

4. GREENBERG (H.S.), ENSMINGER (W.D.), SEEGER (J.F.), KINDT (G.W.), CHANDLER (W.F.), DOAN (K.) and DAKHIL (S.R.): Intra-arterial chemotherapy for the treatment of malignant gliomas of the central nervous system: a preliminary report. Cancer Treat. Rep., **65**: 803-810 (1981).

5. GREENBERG (H.S.), ENSMINGER (W.D.), CHANDLER (W.F.), LAYTON (P.B.), JUNCK (L.), KNAKE (J.) and VINE (A.K.): Intra-arterial BCNU chemotherapy for treatment of malignant gliomas of the central nervous system. J. Neurosurg., **61**: 423-429 (1984).

6. HOCHBERG (H.S.), PRUITT (A.A.), BECK (D.O.), DEBRUN (G.) and DAVIS (K.): The rationale and methodology for intra-arterial chemotherapy with BCNU as treatment for glioblastoma. J. Neurosurg., **63**: 876-880 (1985).

7. KAPP (J.P.), VANCE (R.), PARKER (J.L.) and SMITH (R.R.): Limitations of high dose intra-arterial, 1,3-Bis (2-Chlorethyl)- 1-nitrosourea (BCNU) chemotherapy for malignant gliomas. J. Neurosurg., **10**: 715-719 (1982).

8. KAPP (J.P.), ROSS (R.L.) and TUCKER (E.M.): Supraophthalmic carotid infusion for brain-tumor chemotherapy. J. Neurosurg., **58**: 616-618 (1983).

9. LAYTON (P.B.), GREENBERG (H.S.), STETSON (P.L.), ENSMINGER (W.D.) and GYVES (J.W.). BCNU solubility and toxicity in the treatment of malignant astrocytomas. J. Neurosurg., **60**: 1134-1137 (1984).

10. LUTZ (R.J.), DEDRICK (R.L.), BORETOS (J.W.), OLDFIELD (E.H.), BLACKLOCK (J.B.) and DOPPMAN (J.L.). Mixing studies during intracarotid artery infusions in an *in vitro* model. J. Neurosurg., **64**: 277-283 (1986).

11. OMOJOLA (M.F.), FOX (A.J.), AUER (R.N.) and VINUELA (F.V.). Hemorrhagic encephalitis produced by selective non-occlusive intracarotid BCNU injection in dogs. J. Neurosurg., **57**: 791-796 (1982).

12. THERON (J.), VILLEMURE (J.G.), WORTHINGTON (C.) and TYLER (J.L.): Superselective intracerebral chemotherapy of malignant tumours with BCNU. Neuroradiol., **28**: 118-125 (1986).

COMPUTED TOMOGRAPHIES

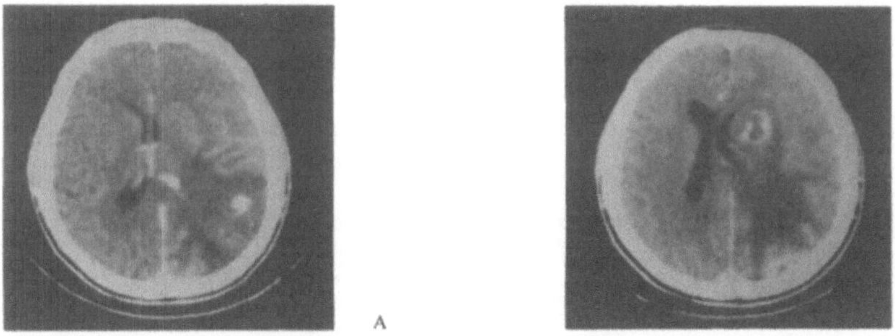

A B

FIGURE 1. Case 1 - LEFT PARIETAL GLIOMA.
A) Contrast-enhanced CT-scan shows Lt parietal hyperdensity (tumour) and surrounding edema.
B) Four months after intracarotid infusion of BCNU, disappearance of Lt parietal enhancement; annular enhancement in anterior limb of internal capsule is present.

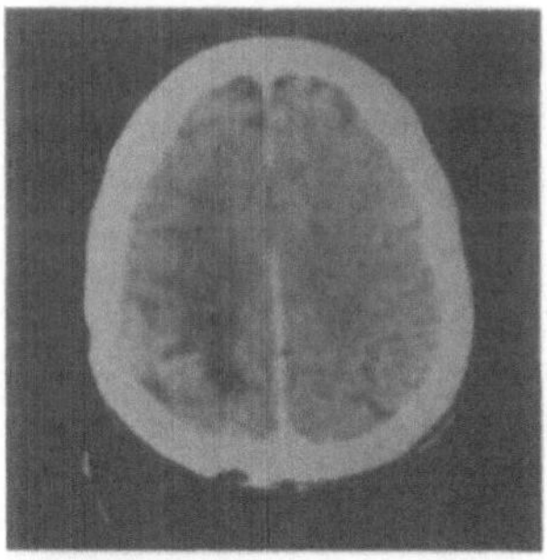

FIGURE 2. CASE 2 - RIGHT PARIETAL GLIOMA. Partial removal.
Two months after second infusion of BCNU, the size of tumour is reduced but ipsilateral white matter hypodensity is largely extended.

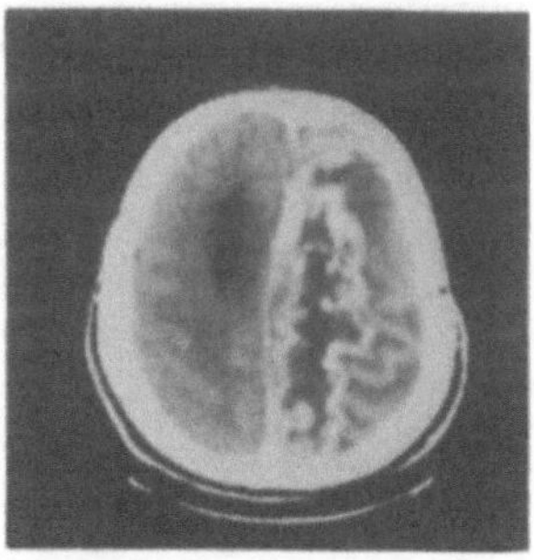

FIGURE 3. CASE 3 - LEFT ANTERIOR FRONTAL GLIOMA. Complete removal.
Five months after second infusion of BCNU, a wide-spread festoon annular enhancement is present.

Preliminary Experience With Menogaril in the Treatment of Recurrent Glioblastomas

D.J. STEWART (°).

INTRODUCTION

While chemotherapy can definitely prolong survival of patients with glioblastomas, this tumor remains incurable (1). It has generally been assumed that drugs that do not readily cross the normal blood-brain barrier would be unlikely to be effective against glioblastomas. While the blood-brain barrier is frequently disrupted in brain tumors, animal studies suggest that the disruption may be variable from one part of a tumor to another (2). In addition, actively growing tumor cells may penetrate into the area of the brain surrounding the tumor where the blood-brain barrier may be less disrupted than it is within the tumor itself (3). However, a number of pharmacological studies have indicated that potentially cytotoxic concentrations of different antineoplastic agents are frequently achieved within human intracerebral tumors even if the antineoplastic agent does not penetrate well into the normal central nervous system, and drug concentrations attainable in human brain tumors appear to generally be quite comparable to those achieved in extracerebral tumors (4-18). In addition, it is frequent to find moderatively high concentrations of drug in brain for at least several millimetres beyond the grossly visible border of the tumor (5-7, 9-11, 14-17). Hence, while it might be necessary to use drugs that penetrate well into the normal central nervous system to **cure** glioblastomas, palliation should be possible with drugs that do not cross the normal blood-brain barrier, provided the drug is cytotoxic to glioblastoma cells. Thus, it would be reasonable to conduct studies of any new antineoplastic agent in patients with glioblastomas whether or not the drug does cross the intact blood-brain barrier.

Menogaril is a new antineoplastic agent related to doxorubicin (Adriamycin) and other anthracycline antibiotics (19). While little is known about the central nervous system pharmacology of menogaril, related anthracyclines do not generally cross the blood-brain barrier very well. We are currently conducting a Phase I study of menogaril administered intravenously once per week. This schedule of administration was chosen because of evidence that anthracyclines cause less cardiac toxicity when administered once per week than when administered in higher doses once every three weeks (20). In animal studies, menogaril caused less cardiac toxicity than did the anthracyclines (19). Patients with glioblastomas have been included in our Phase I study.

MATERIALS AND METHODS

To be eligible for this study, patients had to have a histologically proven malignancy that was incurable by standard means. They had to have a Zubrod performance status of 0 (completely asymptomatic) to 3 (bedridden more than 50% of the day because of tumor-related symptoms but not completely bedridden). Renal and hepatic function had to be normal or near normal. The patient could not have any major heart disease and could not have received any more than 250 mg/m^2 of adriamycin previously. Patients had to give informed consent.

The drug was administered intravenously in $\geqslant$250 ml of dextrose 5% in water over 1-2 hours. It was imperative to avoid any chloride in the solution, as contact of the drug with chloride would cause precipitation of the drug. Treatments were repeated once weekly if the patient had adequately recovered from toxicity of prior treatments. When possible, a Hickman catheter or Port-a-cath (permanent central venous catheter) was used, since the drug frequently caused severe arm vein phlebitis.

(°) The Ontario Cancer Treatment and Research Foundation Ottawa Regional Cancer Centre and the University of Ottawa Faculty of Health Sciences, Ottawa, Ontario.

M. Chatel, F. Darcel and J. Pecker (eds.), Brain Oncology. ISBN-13: 978-94-010-8003-3

The first dose used (5 mg/m^2 per week) was equivalent to 10% of the LD_{10} in mice. The dose was doubled in subsequent groups of 3 patients per group until minimal toxicity was noted. Fifty per cent dose escalations were then used in subsequent groups of 3 patients each. Once true toxicity was noted, 25% dose escalations were used to define dose-limiting toxicity and the maximum tolerated dose. Dose escalations were allowed in individual patients if no toxicity was noted in the first eight courses at their initial dose. Blood counts were monitored twice weekly. Serum chemistry, clotting factors, urinalysis and physical examination were monitored once weekly. An electrocardiogram was done before and after each treatment. Blood pressure and pulse were checked at regular intervals for 48 jours after each treatment.

For glioblastomas, response was defined as unequivocal reduction in the enhancing area on CAT scan without neurological deterioration.

Thirty-four patients have been entered on the study to date, including 8 patients with glioblastomas and 26 patients with extracerebral tumors. Among the glioblastoma patients, the median age was 47 years with a range of 29-55 years. The Zubrod performance status among glioblastoma patients was 1 for three patients, 2 for two patients and 3 for three patients. All eight glioblastoma patients had received both prior radiotherapy and chemotherapy.

RESULTS

The first group of three patients was treated at a dose of 5 mg/m^2 per week. Doses were subsequently escalated in groups of three patients each to 10, 20, 40, 60, 75, 90, and 115 mg/m^2. A total of six patients were treated at 75 and 90 mg/m^2 and we plan to treat at least six patients at a dose of 115 mg/m^2. Patients who had received prior mytomycin-C developed granulocytopenia at menogaril doses as low as 40 mg/m^2 per week. However, granulocytopenia was inconsistant: only one third to one half of patients with prior mitomycin-C exposure developed granulocytopenia at higher doses. A decision was made not to attempt dose escalation above 90 mg/m^2 in this patient population. For patients who had not received prior mitomycin-C, granulocytopenia was very uncommon. In patients without prior mytomycin-C, two out of eight treated at a dose of 75 mg/m^2 developed granulocytopenia (including one patient with extensive prior irradiation), whereas none of six patients treated at 90 mg/m^2 and no patient treated at a dose of below 75 mg/m^2 developed granulocytopenia. Three patients have been treated at a dose of 115 mg/m^2, but it is too early to assess whether or not myelosuppression will be dose-limiting at this dose. No patient developed thrombocytopenia. Mild anemia was seen in a few patients, but was not dose-limiting.

Arm vein phlebitis was the major non-hematological toxicity seen. There was no clear-cut evidence that it was dose-related. In some patients, it was quite severe, causing marked inflammation of the arm. It was frequently acute in onset, with blockage of the vein during the actual drug infusion, such that in some patients it was not possible to complete their infusion. This complication was completely circumvented by administering the drug through a central vein using a permanent central venous catheter such as a Hickman catheter or Port-a-cath.

The second most common non-hematological complication was fatigue. This was seen at all dose levels and was noted in 28% of patients overall. Gastrointestinal toxicity was generally quite mild with only two patients developing vomiting. Other toxicity that was seen occasionally included anorexia, diarrhea, abdominal bloating, constipation, pruritic rash, stomatitis, drug fever, dyspnoea with cough, mild alopecia, headache, and arthralgias. Extravasation of the drug occurred in five patients. None of these patients developed tissue ulceration or other severe local reaction after the extravasation. Moderate increases and decreases in blood pressure were noted frequently following drug administration. It was uncertain whether these blood pressure alterations were in any way related to the drug. They were not severe or life-threatening. Premature ventricular and atrial contractions were also seen occasionally. They were of no major clinical significance, and again it is unclear whether they were related to the drug. Two patients developed acute myocardial infarctions while on the treatment. In one of these two patients, the acute myocardial infarct was felt to be due to fluid overload. He was an elderly patient with hypercalcemia secondary to a renal cell carcinoma, who was being treated with large volumes of intravenous saline. It is unclear whether the menogaril contributed to the development of the acute myocardial infarct in either patient. Another patient died suddenly at home shortly after receiving a dose of menogaril of 20 mg/m^2. It was felt that her death was due to tumor rather than due do the drug, but this could not be proven unequivocally. One patient who had previously received high doses of metronidazole developed a peripheral neuropathy while receiving menogaril. The peripheral neuropathy cleared despite the continuation of the menogaril. It was felt that the neuropathy was due to the previous metronidazole rather than being due to the menogaril. Several of the patients were found to have traces of albumin in their urine. This was not clinically significant in any patient. A number of patients also had minor rises in serum levels of lactic dehydrogenase, alkaline phosphatase, and transaminases. It was unclear whether or not these were due to the menogaril. They were not clinically significant in any patient and did not require discontinuation of the drug or reduction in its dose.

Of the eight glioblastoma patients treated, two are still too early to evaluate for response as they only began treatment in the past two weeks. On the six evaluable patients, three (50%) have responded with reduction in size of the tumor on CAT scan and with neurological improvement. The other three glioblastoma patients have failed, with progression of tumor. Among other tumor types, seven of nine patients with renal cell carcinoma are evaluable for response and one (14%) of the evaluable patients has responded. An additional four (57%) of the renal cell carcinoma patients are stable, including two who have had objective responses but less than 50%. Among the 17 patients with other extracerebral tumors (7 with colon carcinoma, 4 with non-small cell lung carcinoma, 2 with sarcomas, and 1 each with malignant melanoma, prostatic carcinoma, head and neck carcinoma and squamous cell carcinoma of unknown origin) 15 are evaluable and none have responded. Six of these patients with other extracerebral tumors (40%) are stable.

DISCUSSION

Based on the preliminary observations in this Phase I study, we feel that menogaril administered intravenously once per week may possibly be active against previously treated glioblastomas. It is stressed that it is hazardous to draw conclusions about response rates based on only small numbers of patients, and a Phase II study including a far larger number of patients will be needed to more accurately define the response rate and to confirm that the drug is active. Overall the drug appears to be very well tolerated, with arm vein phlebitis, fatigue, and granulocytopenia being the main toxicities seen to date. We have not yet defined the maximum tolerated dose of the drug when it is administered on a once per week schedule, but our experience to date indicates that it will be at least 90 mg/m^2 per week for those patients who have not received previous mitomycin-C. When the drug is given intravenously on a q 3-4 week schedule, the maximum tolerated dose is 200 mg/m^2 administered once every four weeks (21); hence, the dose-intensity that is tolerated on a weekly schedule appears to be substantially higher than that which is possible on other schedules tested to date. The reason for this is not clear. We are currently conducting pharmacology studies in an attempt to determine whether the pharmacology of the drug on a weekly schedule is different than is the pharmacology of a higher dose administered on a different schedule.

SUMMARY

Thirty-four patients, including 8 with glioblastomas, have been treated on a Phase I study of weekly IV menogaril. Three of six glioblastoma patients evaluable for response have responded. All glioblastoma patients had previously received both radiotherapy and chemotherapy. The maximum tolerated dose of menogaril has not yet been determined. A dose of 115 mg/m^2 per week is currently being evaluated. Granulocytopenia has been noted occasionally. The major non-hematological toxicity has been arm vein phlebitis requiring administration of the drug through a central line. Other toxicity has been minimal. We plan to conduct a full Phase II study of IV weekly menogaril in glioblastoma patients. The dose intensity achievable with weekly administration of menogaril appears to be considerably higher than that achievable with other schedules.

KEY WORDS

Menogaril, Chemotherapy, Gliomas.

REFERENCES

1. SHAPIRO (W.R.): Therapy of malignant brain tumors; what have the clinical trials taught us? Semin. Oncol. **13**: 38-45 (1986).
2. GROOTHUIS (D.R.), FISCHER (J.M.), VICK (N.A.), BIGNER (D.D.): Comparative permeability of different glioma models to horseradish peroxidase. Cancer Treat. Rep. **65 (suppl. 2)**: 13-18 (1981).
3. LEVIN (V.A.), FREEMAN-DOVE (M.), LANDAHL (H.D.): Permeability characteristics of brain adjacent to tumor in rats. Arch. Neurol. **32**: 785-791 (1975).
4. HALL (S.W.), YEUNG (K.), BENJAMIN (R.S.), STEWART (D.J.), VALDIVIESO (M.), BEDIKIAN (A.Y.), LOO (T.L.): Kinetics of gallium nitrate: a new anticancer agent. Clin. Pharmacol. Therap. **25**: 82-87 (1979).
5. STEWART (D.J.), BENVENUTO (J.A.), LEAVENS (M.), HALL (S.W.), BENJAMIN (R.S.), PLUNKETT (W.), McCREDIE (K.D.), BURGESS (M.A.), LOO (T.L.): Penetration of 3-Deazauridine into human brain, intracerebral tumor and cerebrospinal fluid. Cancer Res. **39**: 4119-4122 (1979).
6. STEWART (D.J.), LEAVENS (M.), FRIEDMAN (J.), BENJAMIN (R.S.), MOORE (E.C.), BODEY (G.P.), VALDIVIESO (M.), BURGESS (M.A.), WISEMAN (C.), LOO (T.L.): Penetration of N-(Phosphonacetyl)-L-aspartate into human central nervous system and intracerebral tumor. Cancer Res. **40**: 3163-3166 (1980).
7. FONG (K.L.), HO (D.H.W.), YAP (B.S.), STEWART (D.J.), BROWN (N.S.), BENJAMIN (R.S.), FREIREICH (E.J.), BODEY (G.P.): Clinical pharmacology of IMPY by radio-immunoassay. Cancer Treat. Rep. **64**: 1253-1260 (1980).
8. ROSENBLUM (M.), STEWART (D.J.), YAP (B.S.), LEAVENS (M.), BENJAMIN (R.S.), LOO (T.L.): Penetration of methylglyoxal bis (guanylhydrazone) into intracerebral tumors in humans. Cancer Res. **41**: 459-462 (1981).
9. STEWART (D.J.), LEAVENS (M.), MAOR (M.), FEUN (L.), LUNA (M.), BONURA (J.), CAPRIOLI (R.), LOO (T.L.), BENJAMIN (R.S.): Human central nervous system distribution of cis-diaminedichloroplatinum and use as a radiosensitizer in malignant brain tumors. Cancer Res. **42**: 2474-2479 (1982).
10. SAVARAJ (N.), LU (K.), FEUN (L.G.), LEAVENS (M.E.), STEWART (D.J.), BURGESS (M.A.), BENJAMIN (R.S.), LOO (T.L.): Intracerebral penetration and tissue distribution of 2,5-Diaziridinyl 3,6bis(Carboethoxyamino) 1,4-Benzoquinone, (AZQ NSC 182986). J. Neuro-Oncol. **1**: 15-20 (1983).
11. STEWART (D.J.), LU (K.), BENJAMIN (R.S.), LEAVENS (M.), LUNA (M.), YAP (H.Y.), LOO (T.L.): Concentrations of vinblastine in human intracerebral tumor and other tissues. J. Neuro-Oncol. **1**: 139-144 (1983).
12. ZHENGANG (G.), SAVARAJ (N.), FEUN (L.G.), LU (K.), STEWART (D.J.), LUNA (M.), BENJAMIN (R.S.), LOO (T.L.): Tumor penetration of AMSA in man. Cancer Investig. **1**: 475-478 (1983).
13. STEWART (D.J.), BENVENUTO (J.), LEAVENS (M.), SMITH (R.), CABANILLAS (F.), BENJAMIN (R.S.), LOO (T.L.): Human central nervous system pharmacology of Pentamethylmelamine and its metabolites. J. Neuro-Oncol. **1**: 357-364 (1983).
14. STEWART (D.J.), RICHARD (M.), HUGENHOLTZ (H.), DENNERY (J.), BELANGER (R.), GERIN-LAJOIE (J.), MONTPETIT (V.), NUNDY (D.), PRIOR (J.), HOPKINS (H.): Penetration of VP-16 (Etoposide) into human intracerebral and extracerebral tumors. J. Neuro-Oncol. **2**: 133-139 (1984).
15. STEWART (D.J.), LEAVENS (M.), LU (K.), WANG (Y.M.), BENJAMIN (R.S.), HO (D.H.), YAP (H.Y.), LOO (T.L.): Central nervous system pharmacology of Baker's Antifolate (NSC 139 105) in man. J. Neuro-Oncol. **2**: 187-193 (1984).
16. STEWART (D.J.), RICHARD (M.T.), HUGENHOLTZ (H.), DENNERY (J.), NUNDY (D.), PRIOR (J.), MONTPETIT (V.), HOPKINS (H.S.): Penetration of teniposide (VM-26) into human intracerebral tumors: preliminary observations on the effect of tumor type, rate of drug infusion and prior treatment with Amphotericin-B or oral glycerol. J. Neuro-Oncol. **2**: 315-324 (1984).
17. STEWART (D.J.), GREEN (R.M.), HUGENHOLTZ (H.), RICHARD (M.T.), DENNERY (J.), MONTPETIT (V.), HOPKINS (H.S.), THIBAULT (M.): Human central nervous system pharmacology of Tiazofurin. In: Walker M., Thomas D. (eds). *Biology of Brain Tumor* (Martinus Nijhoff Publishers, Dordrecht, The Netherldands), 1986, pp. 425-429.
18. STEWART (D.J.), HUGENHOLTZ (H.), GREEN (R.), RICHARD (M.), BENOIT (B.), RUSSEL (N.), MAROUN (J.), THIBAULT (M.): Mitoxantrone Hydrochloride: uptake into human brain tumors and phase II study in gliomas. J. Neuro-Oncol. **4**: 114 (1986).
19. McGOVERN (J.P.), NEIL (G.L.), DENLINGER (R.H.), HALL (T.L.), CRAMPTON (S.L.), SWENBERG (J.A.): Chronic cardiotoxicity studies in rabbits with 7-con-O-methylnogarol, a new anthracycline antitumor agent. Cancer Res. **39**: 4849-4855 (1979).
20. WEISS (A.J.), MANTHEL (R.W.): Experience with use of Adriamycin in combination with other anticancer agents using a weekly schedule with particular reference to the lack of cardiac toxicity. Cancer **40**: 2046-2052 (1977).
21. DODION (P.), SESSA (C.), JOSS (R.), CRESPEIGNE (N.), WILLEMS (Y.), KITT (M.), ABRAMS (J.), FINET (C.), BREWER (J.E.), ADAMS (W.J.), EARHART (R.H.), ROZENCWEIG (M.), KENIS (Y.), CAVALLI (F.): Phase I study of intravenous menogaril administered intermittently. J. Clin. Oncol. **4**: 767-774 (1986).

Chemotherapy in the Management of Pineal Region Germinomas

D. GEDOUIN (°), M. BEN-HASSEL (°), H. GALLOUX (°),
R. GADAN (°°), J.J. MOREAU (°°°), G. de CHAMBENOIT (°°°), R. RAVON (°°°).

The authors report the treatment by chemotherapy of three cases of pineal region germinoma and attempt to define its role in the management of such tumours.

Case 1:

PL presented in April 1981 with raised intra-cranial pressure and Parinaud's syndrome. He was 16 at the time. The CT scan demonstrated uptake in a mass in the pineal region and dilatation of the ventricles. A ventriculo-peritoneal shunt was inserted. No neoplastic cells were found in the cerebral spinal fluid and there was no increase in tumour marker serum levels. Sub-total resection of a highly necrosed pineal tumour was performed by the sub-occipital and supra-tentorial approach. The tumour corresponded to a typical germinoma. Post-operative radiotherapy was delivered to the pineal region at 55 Gy over a 5-week period. Disease course was favourable. Ten months later, the patient complained of drowsiness. This was caused by the shunt functioning badly. Ascites was also found. A laparoscopy for biopsy was carried out and the existence of multiple metastases from the pineal germinoma confirmed. Chemotherapy, bases on the protocol for tumours of the testicle (adriamycin -vinblastine - bleomycin - actinomycin D - cyclophosphamide) dried the ascites as of the first cycle and disease course appeared favourable throughout chemotherapy (14 months). Two months after chemotherapy has finished, Parinaud's syndrome appeared. The CT brain scan showed an enhanced area which extended from the fourth ventricle to the ependyma outside the radiation field. Six months later, a single metastasis was found at the level of the cauda equina. Removal was partial and the metastasis was found to be identical to the primary tumour. Local radiotherapy was rapidly effective, but the patient died from pneumonia (Klebsiella) 32 months after the diagnosis had been made.

Case 2:

JYF presented in March 1984 at the age of 12 with raised intra-cranial pressure and precocious puberty syndrome. The CT scan showed an enhanced lesion in the pineal region. Surgical removal was only partial due to haemorrhage.

Histological examination confirmed an embryonic carcinoma. Post-operative tumour marker serum levels were elevated for β-HCG (8000 μml) and for α-fetoprotein (6400 μml). Parinaud's syndrome and diabetes insipidus were also found. Chemotherapy with VP 16 (100 mg/m^2 D1, D2, D3), bleomycin (30 mg D1, D2, D3, continuous perfusion) and cisplatinum (100 mg/m^2 on D3) was started on month after surgery and the patient completed 4 cycles (1 every 3 weeks). He improved rapidly (tumour markers and CT scan returned to normal).

Radiotherapy was administered to the whole brain (40 Gy in 4 weeks) with a 10 Gy boost to the tumour site. Twenty-eight months after diagnosis, the patient is still in complete remission, with negative tumour markers, normal CT scan and a left lateral homonymous hemianopsia consequent to the surgery.

Case 3:

AR, aged 28, presented with raised intra-cranial pressure, Parinaud's syndrome and a bilateral pyramidal syndrome in May 1984. The CT scan demonstrated a homogeneous enhanced mass in the pineal region, well-delineated, and dilated ventricles. A shunt was put into place as an emergency.

(°) Centre Régional de Lutte Contre le Cancer, Rennes. (°°) Service de Neurochirurgie, Pontchaillou, Rennes. (°°°) Service de Neurochirurgie, Neurotraumatologie, CHU, Limoges.

M. Chatel, F. Darcel and J. Pecker (eds.), Brain Oncology. ISBN-13: 978-94-010-8003-3

A biopsy was performed in stereotactic conditions and the diagnosis of germinoma made. Radiotherapy to the tumour site was quickly started, but had to be interrupted after 6 sessions as the tumour markers showed α-feto-protein at 400 μg/ml and β-HCG at 18 mU/ml. The patient had two cycles of chemotherapy at an interval of 3 weeks: VP 16 (100 mg/m^2, D1, D2, D3), bleomycin (30 mg, D1, D2, D3 by continuous perfusion) and cisplatinum (100 mg/m^2 on D3), and his clinical condition improved. Tumour marker levels returned to normal. The side-effects of the chemotherapy, however, led to medical treatment being stopped and radiotherapy was used again, with a total of 60 Gy being delivered to the tumour site. Clinical, biological and CT scan findings confirm that the patient is still in complete remission 26 months after diagnosis.

DISCUSSION

These three cases correspond to standard descriptions given in the literature:

— clinical features: Parinaud's syndrome, precocious puberty, diabetes insipidus and raised intracranial pressure;

— surgery by the sub-occipital route leading to partial or complete tumour removal and histological diagnosis;

— radiotherapy is effective in cases of recurrence and metastatic spread (case 1);

— chemotherapy is effective in the event of peritoneal metastases linked to the ventriculo-peritoneal shunt (case 1);

— tumour markers are important, especially pre-operatively, when a tumour is suspected in the pineal region.

Furthermore:

— intravenous chemotherapy is effective on the primary tumour site, thus confirming the absence of blood brain barrier in the pineal region;

— chemotherapy was only administered intravenously. The intra-thecal route was never used;

— the chemotherapy protocols were those used for testicular germ cell tumours with metastases to the brain and viscera.

CONCLUSION

In the light of these three case reports, the management of pineal region tumours may be redefined and the importance of chemotherapy specified.

A tumour in the pineal region with increased β-HCG and/or α-feto-protein levels means a non-seminomatous germ cell tumour. Surgery is no longer advisable to confirm diagnosis.

Radiotherapy remains the treatment of choice for pure germinomas. A rise in tumour markers corresponds to choriocarcinoma or embryonic carcinoma and therefore the risk of local recurrence is high. Chemotherapy should then be the first treatment, followed by radiotherapy to the tumour site, but the role of radiation therapy has yet to be defined.

Extensive surgery may lead to serious sequelae. When extemporaneous histological diagnosis is made, tumour removal should be avoided. Cytoreductive chemotherapy followed by radiotherapy should again be preferred.

KEY WORDS

Germinoma, Tumour Markers, Chemotherapy.

The Effectiveness of Chemotherapy in a Case of Childhood Esthesioneuroblastoma

E. LE GALL (°), M. ROUSSEY (°°), I. CASADEVALL (°), H. JOUAN (°°°),
M. BEN-HASSEL (°°°°), G. LE CLECH (°°°°°), M. CARSIN (°°°°°°), C. LE FRANÇOIS (°°).

Esthesioneuroblastoma or olfactory neuroblastoma is a rare tumour of neuronal origin (14) arising in the olfactory epithelium of the nasal vault. It is more frequently encountered in adults. Conventional treatment, consisting of surgical resection and/or radiation therapy, does not prevent local recurrence. The prognosis in cases of extensive disease is worse than in those of limited disease (5, 10). Good results in childhood neuroblastomas have been obtained with chemotherapy (7, 8). Various trials have therefore been proposed for certain olfactory neuroblastomas. The promising results encouraged us to use chemotherapy as the treatment of choice in a child of 4 suffering from an advanced form of the disease, given the consequences of surgery of radiotherapy at that age.

Case Report:

B. was admitted to hospital in June 1985 at the age of 4 for unilateral rhinorrhea which had persisted for a month. A right, intra-nasal tumour associated with moderate homolateral exophthalmia was found. Clinical examination was otherwise normal. Plain radiography and CT brain scans demonstrated involvement of the ethmoid, the nasal fossae, the maxillary sinuses and the posterior part of the internal wall of the orbits. On the post contrast CT scan, a mid-line intracranial budding was seen in the region of the sphenoid and ethmoid. Histological examination of a biopsy specimen showed a malignant tumour with islets of cells dispersed in a well vascularized pseudo-mixoid stroma. The cells were larger than lymphocytes with more or less dense chromatin. These findings favoured a diagnosis of esthesioneuroblastoma with emboli in the lymphatics. Urinary excretion of catecholamine was normal. There was no meningeal spread. The bone marrow was normal on the myelogram and on bone biopsy. No primary tumour was found. There was no uptake of 121-iodine-labelled meta-iodobenzylguanidine in the tumour.

The diagnosis of non-secretory and non-metastasized olfactory neuroblastoma with extension to the sphenoid and ethmoid was therefore made. The child first received 6 cycles of chemotherapy: 300 mg/m^2 cyclophosphamide D1 et D5, 1.5 mg/m^2 vincristine D1-D5 and 60 mg/m^2 doxorubicin on D5, at 3 week intervals. The exophthalmia disappeared after the first cycle. On completion of the third cycle, B. was in complete remission (confirmed histologically and by CT scan). At the end of the 6 cycles, B. was very well and presented no signs of recurrence: clinical examination, CT brain scan and CSF were all normal. Chemotherapy was maintained with 1.5 mg/m^2 vincristine on D1 and 150 mg/m^2 cyclophosphamide D1-D5 every 3 weeks.

After 10 months of favourable course, a cerebellar syndrome appeared, with dysarthria, hand tremor, a broader base for walking, then difficulty in swallowing and ataxia. The CSF contained 40 malignant cells/mm^3 and 11.50 g/l of protein. A CT brain scan and NMR imaging refuted a diagnosis of local recurrence. It was concluded that the localization was meningeal and treatment by methotrexate at 6 g/m^2 by intravenous perfusion over 24 hours was begun. At the end of the perfusion, blood and CSF methotrexate were 56.3 gamma/ml and 46.8 gamma/ml respectively. There was a moderate improvement. After a week, the child convulsed and went into a coma which regressed favourably in 4 days. The treatment was completed by radiation therapy of 20 Gy delivered to the brain with a weekly intrathecal injection of 15 mg/m^2 methotrexate. Given the marked improvement in B.'s condition (only moderate hand tremor remained), it was decided to

(°) Unité Oncologie Pédiatrique, Hôpital Sud, Rennes (Pr C. Jézéquel). (°°) Service de Pédiatrie B, Hôpital Pontchaillou, Rennes (Pr Sénécal). (°°°) Laboratoire d'Anatomie Pathologie, Hôpital Pontchaillou, Rennes (Pr. B. Ferrand). (°°°°) Service de Radiothérapie, Centre Eugène-Marquis, Pontchaillou, Rennes. (°°°°°) Service ORL, Hôpital Pontchaillou, Rennes (Pr J. Bourdinière). (°°°°°°) Service de Radiologie, Hôpital Pontchaillou, Rennes (Pr Simon).

M. Chatel, F. Darcel and J. Pecker (eds.), Brain Oncology. ISBN-13: 978-94-010-8003-3

perform a lipiodol myelography to look for a blockage. An almost total blocakge was found at D_1 level and the lipiodol at the level of the lumbar spine was inhomogeneously distributed. Before the 30 Gy irradiation of the spinal cord could be administered, signs of medullary compression with paraplegia and compression of the cauda equina appeared, but all regressed favourably after the radiotherapy.

DISCUSSION

Esthesioneuroblastoma usually occurs between the ages of 11 and 20 and between 51 and 60 (5). It is uncommon in the under-fives and only 6 case reports have been documented so far (3, 13). Diagnosis is based on histological examination. Three forms have become standards: neuroepithelioma (1), neuroblastoma (12) and neurocytoma (2). A more recent study has distinguished between neuroblastomas with or without olfactory differentiation and neuroendocrine carcinomas (13). It is sometimes difficult to differentiate between an esthesioneuroblastoma where maturation towards a ganglioneuroblastoma is possible (13) and a neuroblastoma. It is for this reason that the diagnosis of metastatic sympathoblastoma, which usually secretes catecholamine, should be ruled out before confirming the diagnosis of olfactory neuroblastoma, when the patient is a child.

The prognosis depends on disease extension at the time of diagnosis (10). In a series of 79 patients, mainly made up of adults treated by surgery and/or radiotherapy, survival at 5 years was 75% for localized forms and 41% for extended forms. Local recurrence that can be checked occurs in one third of cases, lymph node involvement in 10% and distant metastases in 8%. Metastases sometimes appear several years after the onset of the disease.

According to Kadish's classification (10), the present cases was an extensive Grade C with spread to the orbits and the lymphatics. Complete surgical resection would have been impossible and too mutilating. Radiotherapy would have resulted in a facial dysmorphy which the parents found unacceptable. We therefore proposed chemotherapy as the first treatment, using a combination of vincristine, cyclophosphamide and doxorubicin. Complete remission resulted. We found in the literature 15 patients treated by chemotherapy who could be evaluated (3, 6, 15). Chemotherapy is rarely the treatment of choice and the protocols differ. Of the 15 patients, complete remission was obtained in 6 and partial remission in 4. Apart from the drugs used in the present case, the following would also seem efficient: nitrogen mustard, thiotepa and dimethyltriazenoimidazole-carboxamide. A dose effect may well exist as one patient did not response to cyclophosphamide at the conventional dosage, whereas high-dose cyclophosphamide followed by autologous bone marrow transplantation proved effective (11). The drugs used, however, do not prevent extension to the CSF. Our patient was under cyclo-phosphamide when the meningeal involvement appeared with no sign of local recurrence. A 24-hour perfusion of 6 g/m^2 of methotrexate by intravenous route gave a high level of methotrexate in the CSF. Clinical improvement was immediate and rapid but compression of the spinal cord became evident two weeks later. We therefore recommend prophylactic treatment of the central nervous system as soon as complete remission is obtained in cases of esthesioneuroblastoma.

SUMMARY

The authors report a case of esthesioneuroblastoma with local extension to the sphenoid and ethmoid in a 4-year old child. Chemotherapy cycles using cyclophosphamide, vincristine and doxorubicin administered at intervals of 21 days resulted in complete remission. The treatment, however, did not prevent spinal meningeal involvement with blockage of the cerebral spinal fluid but with no signs of local recurrence. We therefore recommend prophylactic treatment of the central nervous system in the event of complete response to chemotherapy.

KEY WORDS

Esthesioneuroblastoma, Childhood, Chemotherapy.

REFERENCES

1. BERGER (L.), LUC (R.): L'esthesioneuroepitheliome olfactif. Bull. Cancer, 13, 410-421 (1924).
2. BERGER (L.), COUTARD (H.): L'esthesioneurocytome olfactif. Bull. Cancer, 15, 404-414 (1926).
3. CHAMPS (C. de), DEMEOCQ (F.), MERLE (P.), PALCOUX (J.B.), MORH (M.), HARTMANN (O.): Neuroblastome olfactif révélé par une cécité chez une fillette de 9 mois. Arch. Fr. Ped., 42, 119-121 (1985).
4. DEUTSH (M.), MERCADO (R.), PARSONS (J.A.): Cancer of the naso-pharynx in children. Cancer, 41, 1128-1133 (1978).
5. ELKON (D.), HIGHTOWER (S.I.), LIM (M.L.), CANTRELL (R.W.), CONSTABLE (W.C.): Esthesioneuroblastoma. Cancer, 44, 1087-1094 (1979).
6. FERTILO (A.), MICHEAU (C.): Infantile olfactory neuroblastoma. A clinicopathological study with a review of the literature. ORL, 41, 40.45 (1979).
7. FERNBACK (D.J.), WILLIAMS (T.E.), DONALDSON (M.H.): Neuroblastoma. In Sutow W.W., Vietti T.J., Fernback D.J.. Clinical Pediatric Oncology (St Louis: CV Mosby, 506-537, 1977).
8. GREEN (A.A.), HAYES (F.A.), HUSTU (H.O.): Sequential cyclophosphamide and doxorubicin for induction of complete remission in children with disseminated neuroblastoma. Cancer, 48, 2310-2317 (1981).
9. HAMILTON (A.E.), RUBINSTEIN (L.J.), POOLE (C.J.): Primary intracranial esthesioneuroblastoma (olfactory neuroblastoma). J. Neurosurg., 38, 548-556 (1973).
10. KADISH (S.), GOODMAN (M.), WINE (C.C.): Olfactory neuroblastoma: a clinical analysis of 17 cases, Cancer, 37, 1571-1576 (1976).
11. O'CONNOR (G.T.), DRAKE (C.R.), JOHNS (M.E.), CAIL (W.S.), WINN (H.R.), NISKANEN (E.): Treatment of advanced esthesioneuroblastoma with high-dose chemotherapy and autolagous bone marrow transplantation. Cancer, 55, 347-347 (1985).
12. PORTMANN (N.M.), BONNARD (E.T.), MOREAU (J.J.): Sur un cas de tumeur nerveuse des fosses nasales (esthesioneuroblastome). Acta Otolaryngol. 13, 52-57 (1928).
13. SILVA (E.G.), BUTLER (J.J.), MACKAY (B.), GOEPFERT (H.): neuroblastomas and neuroendocrine carcinomas of the nasal cavity. A proposed new classification. Cancer (50, 2388-2405 (1982).
14. TROJANOWSKY (J.Q.), LEE (V.), PILLSBURY (N.), LEE (S.): Neuronal origin of human esthesioneuroblastoma demonstrated with anti-neurofilament monoclonal antibodies. N. Engl. J. Med. 307, 159-161 (1982).
15. WADE (P.M.), SMITH (R.E.), JOHNS (M.E.): Response of esthesioneuroblastoma of chemotherapy. Report of five cases and review of the literature. Cancer, 53, 1036-1041 (1984).

Renaissance of Intratumoural Chemotherapy

B. RAMA, J. JANSEN, H.D. MENNEL, E. DINGELDEIN (°).

INTRODUCTION

The use of chemotherapeutic drugs in the therapy of brain tumours is obviously hindered by the blood brain barrier (bbb). The application of a chemotherapeutic drug directly into the brain tumour is often practised, but without the expected success.

Experimentally the advantages of intraneoplastic (i.n.) administration of chemotherapeutic drugs could be shown. The concentration of a drug applied i.n. was higher and remained at a higher level for a longer period of time than by i.v. application.

In order to avoid repeated injections and to cope with the problem of the concentration decay, carriers were used from which the drug is able to diffuse.

Our own experiment was based on the premise that Polymethylmethacrylate (PMMA) might be capable of carrying MTX as well as Gentamycin.

By implanting the MTX-PMMA-pellets stereotactically into the brain tumour, we can avoid the negative effect of the "bbb" on the MTX-concentration within the tumour.

MATERIAL AND METHODS

The brain tumour used in our model is induced transplacentally by intraperitoneal (i.p.) injection of 40 mg Ethylnitrosourea (ENU)/kg body weight on 15th day after conception. One descendant of this rat developed a tumour located in the spinal cord and died after 253 days. This tumour — named G XIII — was transplanted intracerebrally on other BD-IX-rats.

The tumour is regarded histologically as a mixed glioma with oligodendroglia- and astrocyte- like cells.

A cell-suspension containing 20,000 tumour cells/10 μl was transplanted into the brain stereotactically.

The PMMA pellets (diameter 1 mm, length 5 mm) contain 1.4 mg MTX, corresponding to 7.1 mg MTX/kg body weight.

For stereotactic implantation the pellets were fixed to a micromanipulator and implanted 5 mm below the skull. The coordinates of the pellet implantation are the same as for the tumour suspension injection.

The tumour volume was calculated by integration utilizing the tumour's measurements with the help of a "videoplan computer" on every 15 μm tumour bearing slice.

The assignment of an animal to a given group was performed randomly.

The animals surviving 60 days after transplantation were killed.

1. Groups of treated animals

1.1. MTX-PMMA given i.n. on day 14 post tumour injection (p.t.i.), perfusion 24th day p.t.i., measurement of tumour volume (n = 9).

1.2. MTX-PMMA given i.n. on day 14 p.t.i., observing of survival time (n = 8).

(°) *Klinik und Poliklinik fur Neurochirurgie, Universitat, Göttingen.*

M. Chatel, F. Darcel and J. Pecker (eds.), Brain Oncology. ISBN-13: 978-94-010-8003-3

2. Control groups

2.1. Perfusion 14th day p.t.i., measurement of tumour volume (n = 9).

2.2. Perfusion 24th day p.t.i., measurement of tumour volume (n = 10).

2.3. No therapy, observing of survival time (n = 18).

2.4. PMMA-pellet (placebo) given i.n. on day 14 p.t.i., observing of survival time (n = 11).

RESULTS

1. The median survival time — post tumour transplantation — of animals treated with MTX as opposed to untreated animals was increased by 69%. Those animals treated only with PMMA (placebo) exhibited a survival time shortened by 12% (Gehan-test: $p < 0.001$):

	(n)	Range (days)	Median (days)	%
MTX treatment	(8)	28 - 59	44	169
No treatment	(18)	17 - 42	26	100
Placebo	(11)	18 - 59	23	88

2. The median tumour volume 14 days after the tumour injection was 1.5 μl (range 0.45 - 15 μl). 10 days later the median tumour volume increased 25 fold: 38.5 μl (range 8.3 - 291 μl).

Therapy of 10 day duration with MTX-PMMA pellets reduced the tumour volume 16 fold to 0.09 μl (range 0.02 - 1.7 μl).

CONCLUSION

As a result of our experiments we can state the efficiency of MTX applied i.n. We may suggest to develop procedures enabling the MTX to diffuse more constantly, or repeated implantation of pellets and the combination of i.n. MTX treatment with systemic application of chemotherapeutics in order to increase the effectiveness of MTX treatment.

KEY WORDS

Brain Tumours, Intratumoural Chemotherapy.

Chemotherapy of Malignant Supratentorial Gliomas: Achievements and Prospectives

J. HILDEBRAND (°).

Several recent reviews have been devoted to this subject (1, 2, 3). The aim of this presentation is not to be exhaustive, but instead, to stress the main achievements of a great effort made, during the last two decades, to improve the outcome of patients with malignant gliomas by means of chemotherapy. Our subject will be restricted to the most common primary brain neoplasia of the adult: the malignant supratentorial gliomas.

METHODOLOGICAL ACHIEVEMENTS

Evaluation criterias

The effectiveness of a given drug or drug combination may be related to the criteria chosen for its evaluation.

In phase-III type studies aiming to assess the role of adjuvant chemotherapy three parameters may be measured. The mean or median survival, and the free interval (or time to recurrence) vary in parallel (4, 5, 6), but the percentage of long term survivors, the third parameter, may be modified undependently of the two others.

In phase-II type studies the most meaningfull evaluation criteria is the rate and length of objective remissions. Objective remission is usely defined as a clearcut improvement of the neurological status. It may be produced either by the administration of corticosteroids, which act primarily on the peritumoral oedema, or by cytotoxic agents, which reduce the tumor volume. Because in patients with signs of tumor recurrence, the two therapies are frequently initiated concomitantly, their effects are difficult to differentiate even with the help of X-ray or MR-scans.

This difficulty largely accounts for the discrepancies found in the litterature reporting phase-II type trials.

Prognostic factors

Retrospective and prospective analyses of phase-III type studies have revealed several prognostic factors. The strongest and those found most consistently are **age, performance status** (P.S., Karnowsky index) and **pathology.**

Younger patients and those with higher PS survive significantly longer, whereas patients with glioma multiforme have a shorter life expectancy than those with anaplastic astrocytomas, ependymoblastomas or oligodendrogliomas. These prognostic factors are so important that they should be regarded as minimal subsets to be reported in any publication. The prognostic value of other patient characteristics such as tumor location or the extend of surgical removal appear less crucial, but survival is definitely shorter when operation is limited to a biopsy (7).

Effects of corticosteroids in phase-III type studies

As mentioned previously the administration of corticosteroids appears today as the most effective therapy to relieve temporarely symptoms and signs due to brain neoplasms. On the contrary, despite the possibility that corticosteroids may act as cytotoxic agents in malignant gliomas (8) it has been shown that intermittent monthly administration of high dose of methyl-prednisolone 400 mg/m^2 day X 5 has no effet on the median survival nor on the percentage of long term survivors (9).

(°) Service de Neurologie, Hôpital Erasme, Université Libre de Bruxelles.

M. Chatel, F. Darcel and J. Pecker (eds.), Brain Oncology. ISBN-13: 978-94-010-8003-3

Therefore the administration of corticosteroids does not interfere with the evaluation of chemotherapeutic agents in phase-III type studies.

RESULTS OF PHASE-II TYPE STUDIES

Single agent chemotherapy

Objective remissions have been obtained in malignant gliomas with several agents but the list of inactive drugs far exceeds the actives (2).

Nitrosoureas (BCNU, CCNU and methyl-CCNU) have emerged as first choise chemotherapy in the experience of various authors. The rate of objective remissions varies from about 15 to 50 percent (10, 11), the difference being due primarily to the operational definition. The median duration of objective remission ranges from 6 to 9 months.

The activity of procarbazine appeared similar to that of nitrosourea derivatives in some studies (10). However, we were unable to improve the neurological status with this drug in patients who failed to respond to CCNU or VM26 plus CCNU.

Other agents such as AZQ, DDMP, or cisplatinium are less active yelding a rate of objective remissions equal of even inferior to 10 percent (12, 13).

Anaplastic astrocytoma are more sensitive to chemotherapy than glioblastoma multiforme and it is likely that less malignant tumors (grade II astrocytoma for instance) are even more sensitive, at least to nitrosoureas. Regardless to pathology malignant supratentorial gliomas of younger patients respond better to chemotherapy.

Combination therapy

The heterogeneity of human brain tumors and rapid drug resistance are the main reasons to use drug combinations. Several "clever" combinations have been tried.

Yet despite occasionally observed benefits, therapy still revolves around single agents, mainly nitrousourea derivatives (2).

RESULTS OF PHASE-III TYPE STUDIES

Mainly nitrosoureas; BCNU and CCNU have been tested as adjuvant chemotherapy in phase-III type studies. Neither of them prolonges significantly the mean on median survival time nor the time to recurrence. In the trials conducted by the NCI Brain Tumor Group the percentage of survivors at 18 and/or 24 months was significantly increased (14, 25). Similar results were also reported by Chang et al. (16), at least for a selected group of patients aged 40 to 60 years.

Such a benefit, however, was not observed with CCNU nor the combination of VM26 plus CCNU in trials performed by the EORTC Brain Tumor Group (4, 5). More recently Afra et al. (17) have confirmed their previous results showing that the combination of dibromodulcitol given during irradiations and of CCNU significantly improves both the median survival and the percentage of long term survivors.

CONCLUSION AND PROSPECTIVES

At present time the optimal treatment of supratentorial malignant gliomas combines:

a) as large resection as possible of the tumor;

b) followed by irradiation with 6000 rads, lower doses are less effective and higher doses do not improve the therapeutic results;

c) BCNU is used at adjuvant chemotherapy by those who feel that a modest increase of the percentage of long-term survivors is a meaningfull benefit. In this respect predictive tests concerning chemosensitivity of individual tumors are desperatly needed;

d) At recurrence any single nitrosourea combined with corticosteroids will improve the clinical condition of about 50% of patients during a median period of approximatively 6 months.

All these treatments are characterised by a very low therapeutic index. Increasing of this index is a major prospective for a better therapy.

One such approach is the administration of drugs via internal carotid. Compared to systemic administration this route increases substantially the concentrations of certain drugs in the tumor, but also in the surrounding normal brain. The advantage of intra-carotid administration is only present during the first passage. Therefore the drug chosen must be rapidely extracted and retained by tumor cells, and should have a sizeable increase in log cell-kill for the increase of concentration achieved by the procedure. Besides theoretical advantages, intracarotid administration has an increased toxicity for the eye and the brain and cannot be repeated easily.

Finally its therapeutic superiority over systemic routes of administration has not been clearly established.

Another prospective is the synthesis of new drugs. Important discoveries in the field of molecular biology of malignant gliomas such as:

— the production by these tumor through oncogenes of several factors essential for their growth 18),
— or the production by rapidely growing tumor such as medulloblastomas of polyamines, which play regulatory functions in cellular growth (19),

may lead the development of more specific and hopefully more active tools against malignant brain tumors.

SUMMARY

Effects of chemotherapy in adults with supratentorial malignant gliomas in phase-II or phase-III type studies are reviewed separately.

Phase-II type trials measuring the rate and length of objective remissions are performed in patients with signs of recurrence. The number of active agents is limited; nitrosoureas and possibly procarbazine are the most active. No combination chemotherapy has been shown to be definitely superior to single-agent therapy.

Cooperative phase-III type studies have revealed several prognostic factors; the most important are: age, performance status and pathology. In these studies adjuvant chemotherapy does not prolong the duration of the median survival nor the time to recurrence. However BCNU, but not CCNU, increases moderately yet significantly the percentage of survivors at 18 and/or 24 months.

KEY WORDS

Gliomas, Chemotherapy.

REFERENCES

1. WALKER (M.D.) and STRIKE (T.A.): The treatment of malignant glioma in controlled studies. In Paoletti P., Walker G., Butti R. et al. (eds): Multidisciplinary Aspects of Brain Tumor Therapy. Amsterdam, Elsevier-North Holland, 267-274, (1979).
2. LEVIN (A.): Chemotherapy of primary brain tumors. Neurologic Clinics 3: 855-866, 1985.
3. HILDEBRAND (J.) and DELECLUSE (F.): Malignant glioma in randomized trials in cancer. Editors Slevin M.L. and Staquet M.J. Raven Press, 15: 583-604, 1986.
4. EORTC Brain Tumor Group: Effect of CCNU on survival rate of objective remission and duration of free interval in patients with malignant brain glioma: First evaluation. Eur. J. Cancer, 12: 41-45, 1976.
5. EORTC Brain Tumor Group: Evaluation of CCNU, VM-26 plus CCNU and procarbazine in supratentorial brain gliomas. J. Neurosurg. 55: 27-31, 1981.
6. EORTC Brain Tumor Group: Misonidazole in radiotherapy of supratentorial malignant gliomas in adult patients: A randomized double-bind study. Eur. J. Cancer. Clin. Oncol. 19: 39-42 (1983).
7. BYAR (D.P.), GREEN (S.B.) and STRIKE (T.A.): Prognostic factors for malignant glioma. Oncology of Nervous System (Nijhooff in press).
8. CHEN and MEAKEY (J.Jr.): Effects of corticosteroids on protein and nuclei acid synthesis in human glial tumor cells. Cancer Res. 33: 1721-1723, 1973.
9. GREEN (S.B.), BYAR (D.P.), WALKER (M.D.) et al.: Comparisons of carmustine, procarbazine and high dose methylprednisolone as additions to surgery and radiotherapy for the treatment of malignant glioma. Cancer Treat. Rep. 67: 121-132, 1983.

10. WILSON (C.B.), GUTIN (P.H.), BOLDREY (E.B.) et al.: Single-agent chemotherapy of brain tumors: A 5-year review. Arch. Neurol. 33: 739-744, 1976.

11. HILDEBRAND (J.): Current status of chemotherapy of brain tumours. Prog. Exp. Tumor Res., F.C. Rose and W.S. Fields editors, 219: 152-166, 1985.

12. EORTC Brain Tumour Group: Effect of DDMP (2,4-Diamino-5-3',-4'dichlorophenyl-6-methylpyrimidine) on brain gliomas. A phase II study. Eur. J. Cancer 12: 41-45, 1980.

13. EORTC Brain Tumour Group: Effect of AZQ (1,4-cyclohexadiene-1,4-diacarbonic acid, 2,5-bis (1-aziridinyl-3,6-dioxo-dyethylester) in recurring supratentorial malignant brain gliomas. A phase II study. Eur. J. Cancer clin. Oncol. 21: 143-146, 1985.

14. WALKER (M.D.), ALEXANDER (E.Jr)., HUNT (W.E.) et al.: Evaluation of BCNU and/or radiotherapy in the treatment of anaplastic gliomas: A cooperative clinical trial. J. Neurosurg. 49: 333-343, 1978.

15. WALKER (M.D.), GREEN (S.B.), BYAR (D.P.) et al.: Randomized comparisons of radiotherapy and nitrosoureas for the treatment of malignant glioma after surgery. N. Engl. J. Med. 303: 1323-1329, 1980.

16. CHANG (C.H.), HORTON (J.), SCHOENFELD (D.) et al.: Comparison of post-operative radiotherapy and combined postoperative radiotherapy and chemotherapy in the multidisciplinary management of malignant gliomas. Cancer 52: 997-1007, 1983.

17. AFRA (D.), KOCSIS (B.), KERPEL-FRONIUS (S.) and ECKHARDT (S.): Dibromodulcitol based combined postoperative chemotherapy of malignant astrocytomas and gliomas. J. Neuro-Oncology 4: 65-70, 1986.

18. WESTERMARK (B.), NISTER (M.) and HELDIN (C.H.): Growth factors and oncogenes in human malignant glioma. Neurologic Clinics 3: 785-800, 1985.

19. MOULINOUX (J.Ph.), QUEMENER (V.), LE CALVE (M.), CHATEL (M.), DARCEL (F.): Polyamines in human brain tumors. A correlative study between tumor, cerebrospinal fluid, and red blood cell. Free polyamine levels. J. Neuro-Oncology 2: 153-158, 1984.

Early Phase II Study of the Adoptive Immunotherapy of Human Brain Tumors with Lymphokine-Activated Killer (LAK) Cells and Recombinant Interleukin-2 (rIL-2)

K. SHIMIZU (°), Y. OKAMOTO (°), Y. MIYAO (°), S. NAKATANI (°), M. YAMADA (°), and H. MOGAMI (°).

INTRODUCTION

Various attempts have been made to carry out adoptive immunotherapy with cytotoxic T lymphocytes (CTL), which have the capacity to lyse autologous tumor cells specifically (1, 11). One of serious problems encountered in these attempts, however, was how to obtain tumor-specific CTL in large quantities. Previously, our laboratory demonstrated that culture of peripheral blood lymphocytes (PBL) with human recombinant interleukin-2 (rIL-2) resulted in the generation of lymphokine-activated killer (LAK) cells, which were capable of lysing fresh autologous glioblastoma cells (9). Now, adoptive transfer of autologous or homologous LAK cells was performed in 5 patients with meningeal dissemination derived from some brain tumors.

MATERIALS AND METHODS

Interleukin-2 (IL-2): Human rIL-2 was kindly supplied by Takeda Chemical Industries, Ltd., Osaka, Japan and was used for the induction of LAK cells.

Production of LAK Cells: The lymphocyte fractions were obtained from patients through multiple leukaphereses (using CS-3000 Blood Cell Separator, Fenwal Laboratories, Deerfield, IL, USA), and the PBL were collected with lymphocyte separation medium (LSM, obtained from Litton Bionetics, Kensington, Maryland, USA). The PBL were activated to generate LAK cells by **in vitro** incubation for 3 to 4 days in complete medium consisting of RPMI 1640*, containing 2% heat-inactivated human AB serum (MA Bioproducts, MD, USA), 2 mM of L-glutamine*, 0.01 mM of sodium pyruvate*, 1 ml of 100x non-essential amino acids*/dl (* Flow Laboratories, Virginia, USA), 5×10^{-5}M 2-Mercaptoethanol (2-ME), and 5 mg of gentamicin/dl. (3, 8). Then rIL-2 was added at a final concentration of 500 units/dl.

Adoptive Transfer of LAK Cells: Two to 3×10^8 PBL were immediately cultured in complete medium with rIL-2 for an initial adoptive transfer, and the rest of the PBL were cryopreserved after leukapheresis. When subsequent adoptive transfer was scheduled, the same count of PBL was thawed and cultured as described above. One to 2×10^8 of LAK cells were administered intrathecally through an Ommaya reservoir or a valve of ventriculoperitoneal (VP) shunt twice or three time a week. For first two cases, 500 units of rIL-2 were diluted in 50 ml of normal saline and infused intravenously over 15 minutes during the period of LAK cells administration. But for last three cases, 25 to 50 units of rIL-2 were administered intrathecally with LAK cells during this treatment.

RESULTS

Case 1:

This 29-year-old man presented in June, 1984, with a 4-month history of progressive neurological deterioration (double vision and clumsiness of the right limbs), which began with occasional nausea and vomiting. A computerized tomography (CT) scan showed a slightly high density area (about

(°) Department of Neurosurgery, Osaka University Medical School, 1-1-50, Fukushima, Fukushima-ku, Osaka 553, Japan (TEL: 06-451-0051).

M. Chatel, F. Darcel and J. Pecker (eds.), Brain Oncology. ISBN-13: 978-94-010-8003-3

2 cm in diameter) in the middle cerebellum, adjacent to the roof of the fourth ventricle. This area was markedly enhanced with contrast medium. He had undergone suboccipital craniectomy with subtotal removal of a cerebellar tumor (anaplastic astrocytoma) on November 6, 1984. The radiotherapy with a total dose of 60 Grays was delivered to the whole brain, postoperatively. Then, he was fully recovered. Five months later, he developed severe headache, and gait disturbance with bilateral ankle clonus. A CT scan revealed areas of slightly high density at the bilateral anterior horn of the lateral ventricle, which were remarkably enhanced with contrast medium. Numerous malignant glioma cells were found by cytological examination of the cerebrospinal fluid (CSF), and this patient was diagnosed as having meningeal gliomatosis. 1.5×10^9 LAK cells in total were intrathecally administered to the patient through the valve of the VP shunt over one month. The patient improved steadily and led a normal life (Karnofsky scale 80%) with left ankle clonus. The malignant cells were no longer detected in his CSF. Seven months later, he was suddenly suffocated to death at home after general convulsion.

Case 2:

This 56-year-old man presented in January, 1985, with a 2-week history of persistent headache, a slight fever and double vision. He was alert, and had bilateral sixth nerve palsies and bilateral swollen cervical lymph nodes. The biopsy of cervical lymph nodes led to a diagnosis of metastasis of unknown origin (squamous cell carcinoma). A brain CT scan showed no abnormal findings. Many malignant cells were detected by cytological examination of the CSF. and this patient was diagnosed as having meningeal carcinomatosis. Two $\times 10^9$ LAK cells in total were transfered intrathecally through Ommaya reservoir over one month. After this treatment, malignant cells were no longer detected in his CSF. The patient improved steadily and has been leading a normal life (Karnofsky scale 90%) with slight double vision for up to 14 months.

Case 3:

A 6-year-old boy presented in March, 1985, with one-week history of headache, vomiting and gait disturbance. On April 2, he had undergone suboccipital craniectomy with partial removal of a cerebellar tumor (medulloblastoma) at another hospital. Postoperative radiation and chemotherapy were performed from May to December, 1985. Numerous malignant cells were detected by careful cytological examination of the CSF, and he entered to our hospital in January, 1986. On admission, he had severe bone marrow suppression. A CT scan showed the remaining tumor mass in the middle of the cerebellum. This mass was remarkably enhanced with contrast medium. Two weeks after his admission, he had undergone subtotal removal of the remaining tumor. Adoptive transfer of homologous (one-haplotype identical matching) LAK cells from his mother was scheduled postoperatively. The tissue typing tests of this patient and his mother were (A11, 24, B7, w62, Cw4, w7, DR1, 4.2, w53, DQw1, w3), and (A11, 24, B54, w62, Cw1, w4, DR4.2, w9, w53, DQw3), respectively. Seven $\times 10^9$ LAK cells in total were transferred intrathecally through Ommaya reservoir, and the malignant cells were eradicated from his CSF. This patient has been leading a normal life (Karnofsky Scale 100%) without complaints for 3 months.

The profile of 5 patients with meningeal dissemination from brain tumors was showed in the Table 1. Complete tumor regression occurred in one patient with meningeal carcinomatosis. Partial responses occurred in one patient with anaplastic astrocytoma and one with medulloblastoma. Fever, hydrocephalus and increased protein in the CSF were the main side effects of this therapy, although all side effects resolved upon termination of IL-2 therapy.

DISCUSSION

It is difficult to treat the patients with malignant gliomas, despite the combined use of surgery, radiation and any kinds of anticancer agents. Diffuse or multifocal invasion of the leptomeninges by malignant glioma (meningeal gliomatosis) is rare, but their neurological signs and symptoms of meningeal gliomatosis (MG) are sometime serious and its treatment by chemotherapy is not so effective. In the cases reported here, we tried an alternative therapeutic approach utilizing adoptive transfer of the tumoricidal effector cells, which were generated from autologous and homologous PBL by rIL-2 (9, 10).

TABLE 1

Profile of 5 patients with meningeal dissemination from brain tumors

Case N°	Age (yrs) Sex	Diagnosis	Previous Therapy	Phase II Treatement: rIL-2 Units	Phase II Treatement: LAK cells	Cytospin of CSF	Follow-Up Period
1	29, M	anaplastic astrocytoma	1: craniectomy for tumor removal (subtotal) 2: whole-brain radiation (60 Grays)	5×10^2/day (iv)	1.5×10^9 (it)	(+) ↓ (—)	dead (7 mos)
2	56, M	meningeal	none	5×10^2/day (iv)	2×10^9 (it)	(+) ↓ (—)	14 mos
3	6, M	medulloblastoma	1: craniectomy for tumor removal (subtotal) 2: whole-brain & spine radiation (60 Grays & 40 Grays) 3: VCR	25/2-3 days (it)	7×10^9* (it)	(+) ↓ (—)	3 mos
4	5, M	medulloblastoma	1: craniectomy for tumor removal 2: whole-brain & spine radiation (60 Grays & 30 Grays) 3: MTX. VCR	50/day (it)	3×10^9* (it)	(+) ↓ (+)	dead (2 mos)
5	30, M	germinoma	1: whole-brain & spine radiation (50 Grays & 30 Grays)	50/day (it)	6×10^9 (it)		2 mos

Tumor-specific immunotherapy by monoclonal antibodies or cytotoxic T lymphocytes (CTL) has been documented in the last few years (1, 5, 7). However, their clinical application may be limited because of some difficulties in preparing individual agents for each patient. Rencently, Rosenberg et al. reported the adoptive immunotherapy by LAK cells and rIL-2 in patients with advanced cancers, and they observed a distinct clinical response in 11 patients within 25 cases (8).

We have previously demonstrated that the incubation of murine spleen cells or human PBL with rIL-2 generated lymphoid effector cells, which were able to lyse NK-resistant tumor cells but not normal cells. However, several workers have reported that cytotoxic cells exhibiting potent cytotoxicity **in vitro** are not very effective for **in vivo** adoptive immunotherapy (2, 6). One of possible reasons is that sufficient amount of effector cells cannot reach the target organs of the patients after the intravenous administration. Lotze et al. reported that the activated killer cells, which were injected into patients intravenously, appeared in the lung at first and were subsequently re-distributed to the liver and spleen (4). Therefore, we transferred a total of $1.5 - 7 \times 10^9$ LAK cells with rIL-2 intrathecally. 24 hours after adoptive transfer of III_{I_n} oxine labeled LAK cells, most of the LAK cells were detected in the whole cerebrospinal space (unpublished data). After this treatment, the neurological findings of these three improved in five patients with meningeal dissemination derived from some brain tumors, and malignant cells were no longer detected in the CSF.

This therapy is an attractive approach for the treatment of malignant tumors that have poor immunogenicity or are insensitive to several anticancer agents, and for patients with severe immunosuppressive conditions which are induced by repeated radiation therapy or chemotherapy.

SUMMARY

A total of two to 10×10^9 autologous or homologous LAK cells, with 25 to 50 units of rIL-2 through Ommaya reservoirs, were intrathecally transfered into 5 patients with meningeal dissemination derived from some brain tumors (two with medulloblastomas, one with germinoma, cerebellar astrocytoma, and metastatic tumor). Complete tumor regression occured in one patient with meningeal dissemination of epipharyngeal cancer and has been sustained for 14 months after therapy, and partial responses occurred in two patients with medulloblastoma and cerebellar astrocytoma. Thus, this therapy is an attractive approach for the treatment of malignant tumors that are insensitive to several anticancer agents.

KEY WORDS

Adoptive immunotherapy, Interleukin-2, Lymphokine-activated killer (LAK) cells, Meningeal gliomatosis, Meningeal carcinomatosis.

REFERENCES

1. CHEEVER (M.A.), GREENBERG (P.D.), FEFER(A.) and GILLIS (S.): Augmentation of the antitumor therapeutic efficacy of long-term cultured T lymphocytes by **in vivo** administration of purified interleukin-2. J. Exp. Med. **155**: 968-980 (1982).

2. DAILY (M.O.), FATHMAN (C.G.), BUTCHER (E.C.), PILLEMER (E.) and WEISSMAN (I.): Abnormal migration of T lymphocyte clones. J. Immunol. **128**: 2134-2136 (1982).

3. JACOBS (S.K.), WILSON (D.J.), KORNBLITH (P.L.), GRIMM (E.A.): In vitro killing of human glioma by interleukin-2 activated autologous lymphocytes. J. Neurosurg. **64**: 114-117 (1986).

4. LOTZE (M.T.), LINE (B.R.), MATHISEN (D.J.), ROSENBERG (S.A.): The in vivo distribution of autologous human and murine lymphoid cells grown in T cell growth factor (TCGF); Implications for the adoptive immunotherapy of tumors. J. Immunol. **125**: 1487-1493 (1980).

5. MILLER (R.A.), MALONEY (D.G.), McKILLOP (J.) and LEVY (R.): In vivo effects of murine hybridoma monoclonal antibody in a patient with T-cell leukemia. Blood **58**: 78-86 (1981).

6. MILLS (G.B.), CARLSON (G.) and PAETKAU (V.): Generation of cytolytic lymphocytes to syngeneic tumor by using co-stimulator (Interleukin-2). J. Immunol. **125**: 1904-1909 (1980).

7. RITZ (J.), PESANDO (J.M.), SALLAN (S.E.), CLAVELL (L.A.), NOTIS-MCCONARTY (J.), ROSENTHAL (P.) and SCHLOSSMAN (S.F.): Serotherapy of acute lymphoblastic leukemia with monoclonal antibody. Blood **58**: 141-152 (1981).

8. ROSENGERG (S.A.), LOTZE (M.T.), MUUL (L.M.), LEITMAN (S.), CHANG (A.E.), ETTINGHAUSEN (S.E.), MATORY (Y.L.), SKIBBER (J.M.), SHILONI (E.), VETTO (J.T.), SEIPP (C.A.), SIMPSON (C.) and REICHERT (C.M.): Observations on the systemic administration of autologous lymphokine-activated killer cells and recombinant interleukin-2 to patients with metastatic cancer. NEJM **313**: 1485-1492 (1986).

9. SHIMIZU (K.), OKAMOTO (Y.), MIYAO (Y.), WAKAYAMA (A.), NAKATANI (S.) and MOGAMI (H.): Lysis of malignant gliomas by syngenic murine splenocytes or autologous human peripheral blood lymphocytes activated **in vitro** with recombinant interleukin-2. J. Neurol. (Berlin) **232 (Suppl.)**: 179 (1985).

10. SHIMIZU (K.), MIYAO (Y.), OKAMOTO (Y.), MATSUI (Y.), USHIO (Y.), TSUDA (N.), HAYAKAWA (T.), ISHIDA (N.): The antitumor efficacy of lymphokine-activated killer (LAK) cells induced **in vitro** from peripheral blood lymphocytes of patients with malignant gliomas. Brain and Nerve (Tokyo) **38**: 265-271 (1986).

11. SLANKARD-CHAHINIAN (M.), HOLLAND (J.F.), GORDON (R.E.), BECKER (J.) and OHNUMA (T.): Adoptive autoimmunotherapy cytotoxic effect of an autologous long-term T-cell line on malignant melanoma. Cancer **53**: 1066-1072 (1984).

Immunotherapy in Recurrent Malignant Brain Tumors

K. FUJISAWA, T. KANNO, K. YOKOI, N. SUZUKI, F. MITSUYAMA, V.K. JAIN.

INTRODUCTION

Malignant brain tumors have a bad prognosis (1). Most often we cannot remove them completely by surgery. Radiation is not fully effective. Therefore various types of chemotherapies and immunotherapies have been tried (2, 3, 4). Though the patients may become symptom free after first surgery, they soon come back with recurrence of their tumors. This study was conducted to see the therapeutic effects of immuno-agent interferon-γ (IFN-γ) alone and it was compared with the three other chemotherapies i.e. Intersleukin-2 (IL-2), IFN-β + IL-2, and IFN-β + ACNU + Radiation.

MATERIAL AND METHOD

This study consists of a total of 35 cases of recurrent malignant brain tumors (Table 1). IL-2, 1000 IU/day $\times$ 2 months was used in 6 cases. IFN-γ, 9×10^6 IU/day $\times$ 1-2 months was used for 14 cases. The combined therapy of irradiation, ACNU (100 mg/sqm. on second day) and IFN-β (1×10^6 IU/day $\times$ 1 week, third day onwards) was used in 9 cases. IL-2 + IFN-β, combined therapy was used in six cases.

TABLE 1

Cases (Malignant astrocytoma, Glioblastoma, Metastatic tumor)	
1. Interferon - γ alone	14
2. Interleukin - 2 alone	6
3. Combined therapy (I) (Interferon - β, ACNU, Radiation)	9
4. Combied therapy (II) (Interferon - β, Interleukin - 2)	6
TOTAL	35

Change of tumor mass on CT scan was used for response criteria as follow: Complete remission (CR) - the disappearance of all known disease, Partial remission (PR) - decrease in size by at least 50%, No change (NC) - decrease in size by less than 50% or increase of less than 25%, and Progressive disease (PD) - increase over 25% or appearance of a new lesion. Clinical grades used to compare clinical status before and after the therapy were as follow: Gr. 0 = full activities of daily life, Gr. 1 = minimum disturbance of activities of daily life, Gr. 2 = moderate disturbance of activities of daily life, Gr. 3 = severe disturbance of activities of daily life, Gr. 4 = activities of daily life not possible.

RESULTS

IFN-γ therapy -- Fourteen cases were treated with IFN-γ (Table 2). Basic schedule of total dose was 9×10^6 units, per day. This daily dose was continued for 4 weeks at least. If we consider CT criteria, 6 patients showed progressive disease, 5 cases showed no change, and only two patients had partial remission. However none of the patients showed a good clinical response.

Il-2 therapy -- Six patients were treated with IL-2. The treatment was given for 4 weeks except in 2 cases who died early. 4 patients showed progressive disease, and one showed no change. None of the patients showed partial resission or complete remission.

M. Chatel, F. Darcel and J. Pecker (eds.), Brain Oncology. ISBN-13: 978-94-010-8003-3

TABLE 2

INF-γ therapy on malignant brain tumor

Case	Age	Sex	Diagnosis	Total Dose	Response	
					CT	PS
1. S.O.	12	M	Medulloblastoma	4.5×10^6 U $\times$ 10 days 3×10^6 U $\times$ 23 days	—	4 ▸ Dead
2. T.T.	24	M	Astrocytoma Gr IV	9×10^6 U $\times$ 56 days	PR (-62%)	2 ▸ 2
3. H.S.	50	M	Astrocytoma Gr IV	9×10^6 U $\times$ 47 days	PD	4 ▸ 4
4. H.O.	75	F	Astrocytoma Gr IV	9×10^6 U $\times$ 38 days	NC	4 ▸ 4
5. M.S.	42	M	Astrocytoma Gr III	9×10^6 U $\times$ 56 days	PD	4 ▸ 4
6. C.T.	12	F	Astrocytoma Gr III	9×10^6 U $\times$ 42 days	PD	2 ▸ 2
7. S.S.	3	F	Astrocytoma GR III	4.5×10^6 U $\times$ 3 days 3×10^6 U $\times$ 53 days	PR (-61%)	3 ▸ 3
8. M.I.	38	M	Metastatic Tumor	9×10^6 U $\times$ 35 days	NC	3 ▸ 4
9. S.H.	54	F	Astrocytoma Gr III	9×10^6 U $\times$ 22 days	PD	4 ▸ 4
10. O.K.	38	M	Oligodendroblastoma	9×10^6 U $\times$ 52 days	PD	3 ▸ 3
11. M.O.	48	M	Astrocytoma Gr III	9×10^6 U $\times$ 44 days	NC	2 ▸ 2
12. T.O.	64	M	Astrocytoma Gr IV	9×10^6 U $\times$ 40 days	PD	3 ▸ 3
13. S.E.	35	M	Metastatic Tumor	9×10^6 U $\times$ 50 days	ST	4 ▸ 4
14. T.K.	36	F	Astrocytoma Gr III	9×10^6 U $\times$ 17 days	ST	2 ▸ 2

Combined therapy (IFN- β + ACNU + Radiation) -- Nine patients were treated with this combined therapy (Table 3). None of the patients showed progressive disease. The size of tumor remained unchanged in 6 cases. 3 patients showed improvement. Their tumor decreased in size. One of them showed clinical improvement also.

TABLE 3

Combined therapy (IFN-β, ACNU, Radiation on malignant tumor)

Case	Age	Sex	Diagnosis	Total Dose* (Number of Cycle)	Response	
					CT	PS
1. K.O.	42	F	Astrocytoma Gr IV	1	NC	3 ▸ 3
2. H.H.	53	F	Astrocytoma Gr IV	2	PR	2 ▸ 2
3. M.D.	52	F	Astrocytoma Gr IV	2	NC	3 ▸ 3
4. E.S.	40	M	Astrocytoma Gr IV	1	PR	3 ▸ 2
5. U.O.	48	M	Astrocytoma Gr III	2	PR	2 ▸ 2
6. T.N.	65	M	Astrocytoma Gr III	1	NC	3 ▸ 3
7. Y.F.	43	F	Astrocytoma Gr III	1	NC	3 ▸ 3
8. Y.H.	14	F	Astrocytoma Gr III	1	NC	1 ▸ 1
9. S.I.	37	M	Astrocytoma Gr III	1	NC	3 ▸ 3

* Cycle : ACNU 100 mg, IFN-β 3×10^6 U $\times$ 7 days
Radiation 40 Gy (total dose)

Combined therapy (IL-2 + IFN-β) -- Six patients were treated with combined therapy of IL-2 and IFN-β (Table 4). Two patients showed complete remission, one patient showed no change, and 3 patients showed progressive disease.

TABLE 4

Combined therapy (IL-2, IFN-β)

Case	Age	Sex	Diagnosis	Total Dose*	Response	
					CT	PS
1. A.N.	57	M	—	4 W	CR	2 ➧ 1
2. I.K.	38	F	Astrocytoma IV	4 W	CR	2 ➧ 1
3. H.H.	43	F	Astrocytoma IV	4 W (+ACNU)	PD	3 ➧ 3
4. K.N.	60	M	Metastatic tumor	4 W (+Rad)	CR	2 ➧ 2
5. U.I.	55	M	Metastatic tumor	4 W (+Rad)	PD	2 ➧ 2
6. S.S.	54	F	Astrocytoma III	4 W	PD	4 ➧ 4

* Dose : IL-2 1000 u/day
IFN-β 1 (3) × 10^6 U/day

DISCUSSION

Application of only IFN-γ has little effect on recurrent malignant brain tumors. 17% cases had partial remission. This therapy was found better than IL-2 alone, where there was no case with partial remission, and progressive disease was seen in 67% of the patients. IFN-γ or IL-2 alone is not very useful for recurrent brain tumors, but have very little side effects. IFN-γ may be used as an adjuvant therapy, because it was found to be effective in 17% of the cases in this study. Therefore it may be more effective if used with other agents. IL-2 which is one of the biological response modifier + IFN-γ (or -β) may be useful if combined with ACNU or Radiation. By combination therapy of IFN-β, ACNU and Radiation, no case had progression of the disease and 30% had partial remission. However all cases of this group had side effects of myelosuppression. Therapy of only ACNU and radiation was found to be effective in 15 to 20% of the cases. This combined therapy was more effective. Another immuno-combined therapy of IL-2 and IFN-β showed complete remission in 33% and Progression of the disease in 50% of the cases (Table 5).

TABLE 5

Results

Therapy	RESPONSE ON CT				Side Effects
	CR	PR	NC	PD	
IFN-γ	—	2 (15%)	5 (39%)	6 (46%)	Transient fever
IL-2	—	—	1 (17%)	4 (67%)	Transient fever
IFN-β ACNU Radiation	—	3 (33%)	6 (67%)	—	Myelosuppression (WBC, Plat)
IFN-β IL-2	(2) (33%)	—	1 (17%)	3 (50%)	Transient fever

This study suggests combined therapy of IFN-γ (or -β) with IL-2 is one of the effective therapeutic method for recurrent malignant brain tumors. However, we must continue to search the best combination, ideal dose, and the schedule of therapy.

SUMMARY

The immunotherapy, Interferon-γ, was used in recurrent malignant brain tumors as the only treatment and the results were compared with other therapies (Interferon-β + ACNU + Radiation, Interleukin-2 + Interferon-β, and Interleukin-2). Interferon-γ was effective in two patients in reducing the size of tumor. Six patients treated with Interleukin-2 did not show any benefit. Combination therapy (Interferon-β + ACNU + Radiation) was effective in reducing the size of the tumor in three patients and in arresting the further growth in four patients. But this therapy caused bone-marrow suppression. Interferon-β + Interleukin-2 therapy resulted in complete remission in 2 of the 6 cases. Combining Interferon-γ or Interferon-β with other adjuvants may be more useful for the treatment of recurrent malignant brain tumors.

KEY WORDS

Recurrent malignant brain tumor, Interferon-γ, Interleukin-2, Brain Tumors.

ACKNOWLEDGEMENTS

We are deeply indebted to Assistant Professor Koji Ezaki, Department of Hematology, for his generous support.

REFERENCES

1. WILSON (C.B.), GUTIN (E.), BOLDREY (B.): Single agent chemotherapy of brain tumors, A five-year review. Arch. Neurol. 33: 739-744, 1976.

2. NAGAI (M.), ARAI (T.), KOHNO (S.), and KOHASE (M.): Interferon therapy for malignant brain tumors, in: The Clinical Potential of Interferons, ed. by R. Kono, and J. Vilcek, Univ. Tokyo Press, pp. 257-272, 1982.

3. SALFORD (L.G.), BORGSTROM (S.), BISMAR (J.), BRUN (A.), CRONQUIST (S.) et al.: Intratumoral and systemic interferon treatment of astrocytomas grade III - IV, U.S. - Japanese Conference on Brain Tumor Therapy, Oct., Nikko, pp. 14-16, 1981.

4. JACOBS (S.), WILSON (D.J.), KORNBLITH (P.L.) and GRIMM (E.A.): Interleukin-2 or Autologous Lymphokine-activated Killer Cell Treatment of Malignant Glioma: Phase I Trial, Cancer Research 46, 2101-2104, April 1986.

INDEX OF KEY WORDS (°)

(°) Only the commonly used data bank keywords are listed.

AUTHORS